JEFFREY M. ROBBINS, DPM, DABPPH, DABPOPPM

Professor of Podiatric Medicine
Director, Podiatric Primary Care Residency
Ohio College of Podiatric Medicine
Cleveland, Ohio

PRIMARY PODIATRIC MEDICINE

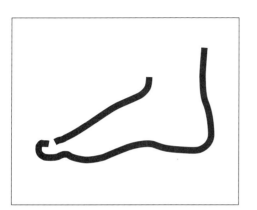

W.B. SAUNDERS COMPANY

A Division of Harcourt Brace & Company

Philadelphia
London Toronto Montreal Sydney Tokyo

W.B. SAUNDERS COMPANY
A Division of
Harcourt Brace & Company

The Curtis Center
Independence Square West
Philadelphia, Pennsylvania 19106

Library of Congress Cataloging-in-Publication Data

Primary podiatric medicine / edited by Jeffrey M. Robbins.

    p.   cm.

ISBN 0–7216–4363–9

1. Podiatry.   I. Robbins, Jeffrey M.
    [DNLM: 1. Podiatry.   WE 890 P952 1994]

RD563.P73 1994

617.5′85—dc20

DNLM/DLC   93-17926

Primary Podiatric Medicine   ISBN 0–7216–4363–9

Printed in the United States of America.

Last digit is the print number: 9   8   7   6   5   4   3   2   1

This book is dedicated to
my wife Barbara,
daughter Carly,
and son Jay,
for their
inspiration, dedication, support, and devotion,
and most importantly,
their love

CONTRIBUTORS

Georgia J. Anetzberger, PhD
Adjunct Assistant Professor, School of
Medicine, Case Western Reserve
University, University Heights, Ohio;
Associate Director for Community
Services, The Benjamin Rose
Institute, Cleveland, Ohio
Psychosocial and Behavioral Components

Corliss L. Austin, DPM
Private practice, Atlanta, Georgia
Podiatric Peripheral Vascular Diseases

**Myron A. Bodman, DPM,
DABPOPPM**
Associate Professor of Podiatric
Medicine, Department of Podiatric
Medicine and Department of General
Medicine, Ohio College of Podiatric
Medicine, Cleveland, Ohio
Pedal Nail and Skin Problems

Marvin Boren, DPM
Private practice, Canton, Ohio
Communication

Myron Boxer, DPM
Clinical Professor, College of
Podiatric Medicine and Surgery,
University of Osteopathic Medicine
and Health Sciences, Des Moines,
Iowa; Director, Department of
Podiatry, Gouverneur Hospital, New
York, New York; Director,
Department of Podiatry, Peninsula
Hospital Center, Queens, New York;
Director Emeritus, Division of
Medical Sciences, New York College
of Podiatric Medicine, New York, New
York
Quality Assurance and Utilization Review

James L. Canterbury, DPM
Assistant Professor, Ohio College of
Podiatric Medicine, Cleveland, Ohio
Pedal Manifestations of Systemic Disease

Mark Caselli, DPM
Chairman, Department of
Orthopedics, New York College of
Podiatric Medicine, New York, New
York
Quality Assurance and Utilization Review

Howard Darvin, MD
Vascular Surgeon, Mt. Sinai Medical
Center, Cleveland, Ohio
Podiatric Peripheral Vascular Diseases

Steven L. Friedman, DPM
Associate Professor, Department of
Podiatric Medicine, Ohio College of
Podiatric Medicine; Staff Member,
Division of Podiatric Medicine, Mt.
Sinai Medical Center, Cleveland,
Ohio
Palliative Care

**Christiane H. Gardner, DPM,
DABPOPPM**
Formerly, Assistant Professor,
Department of Orthopedics, Ohio
College of Podiatric Medicine,
Cleveland, Ohio; Private Practice,
Rockport Maine
Interpretation of Laboratory Values

Eugene P. Goldman, DPM
Surgery Staff, Podiatry Section,
Community Hospital Medical Center,
John C. Lincoln Hospital and Medical
Center, Phoenix Baptist Hospital and
Medical Center, Phoenix, Arizona
Podiatric Rheumatology

Arthur E. Helfand, DPM, DABPPH, DABPOPPM
Professor and Chairman, Department of Community Health and Aging, Pennsylvania College of Podiatric Medicine; Adjunct Professor, Department of Orthopedic Surgery, Jefferson Medical College of Thomas Jefferson University, Philadelphia, Pennsylvania
Introduction
Ambulatory Care

Warren Joseph, DPM
Associate Professor of Medicine, Chief, Infectious Diseases, Pennsylvania College of Podiatric Medicine, Philadelphia, Pennsylvania
Foot Infections

Steven M. Krych, DPM, DABPOPPM
Clinical Faculty, University of Texas Health Sciences Center, Clinical Faculty, Audie L. Murphy Memorial Veterans Hospital, San Antonio, Texas; Podiatrist, Austin Diagnostic Clinic, Austin, Texas
Podiatric Surgery

Todd Laughner, DPM
Medical Director, Diabetic Foot Care Centers, Philadelphia, Pennsylvania
The Diabetic Foot

Leonard A. Levy, DPM, MPH, DABPPH
Dean and Professor of Podiatric Medicine, College of Podiatric Medicine and Surgery, University of Osteopathic Medicine and Health Sciences, Des Moines, Iowa
Podiatric Prevention
Community Health

James E. Lichniak, DPM
Assistant Professor, Ohio College of Podiatric Medicine, Cleveland, Ohio
Sports Medicine

Jeffrey Lynn, DPM
Mt. Sinai Medical Center, Cleveland, Ohio
Podiatric Peripheral Vascular Diseases

Robert Marcus, DPM, DABPOPPM
Associate Professor, Division of Orthopedic Sciences, New York College of Podiatric Medicine, New York, New York; Former Director, Podiatric Orthopedic Residency Program, Department of Veterans Affairs, Montrose, New York; Director, Foot and Ankle Center of Teaneck, Teaneck, NJ; Attending, Gouverneur Hospital, New York, New York
Quality Assurance and Utilization Review

Franklin J. Medio, PhD
Formerly, Director of Educational Resources, School of Osteopathic Medicine, University of Medicine and Dentistry of New Jersey, Newark, New Jersey; Currently, Private Consulting Practice, Chicago, Illinois
Self-Directed Learning

Stephen J. Morewitz, PhD
Lecturer, Department of Sociology, DePaul University; Lecturer, Consultation Liaison Psychiatry, Department of Psychiatry, Humana/Michael Reese Hospital and Medical Center, Chicago, Illinois
Self-Directed Learning

Robert M. Palmer, MD, MPH
Associate Professor of Medicine, Case Western Reserve University, University Heights, Ohio; Head, Section of Geriatric Medicine, Cleveland Clinic Foundation, Cleveland, Ohio
Geriatric Assessment

Rock G. Positano, DPM, MSC, MPH
Professor, Applied Biomedical Engineering, Cooper Union for the Advancement of Science and Art, New York, New York; Assistant Professor, New York Medical College, Valhalla, New York; Assistant Professor, Cornell University Medical College, New York, New York; Co-Director, Foot and Ankle Orthopedic Institute, The Hospital for Special Surgery, New York, New York
Development of a Foot Health Program in an Occupational Setting

Jeffrey M. Robbins, DPM, DABPPH, DABPOPPM
Professor of Podiatric Medicine, Director, Podiatric Primary Care Residency, Ohio College of Podiatric Medicine, Cleveland, Ohio
Communication
Pedal Manifestations of Systemic Disease
Podiatric Peripheral Vascular Diseases

Brad G. Samojla, DPM
Formerly, Assistant Professor of Anatomy and Clinician, Ohio College of Podiatric Medicine, Cleveland, Ohio; Kern Hospital, Warren, Michigan
The Diabetic Foot
Interpretation of Laboratory Values

Jacquelyn Slomka, PhD
Assistant Staff, Department of Bioethics, Cleveland Clinic Foundation, Cleveland, Ohio
Ethical Considerations

Martin L. Smith, STD
Associate Staff, Department of Bioethics, Cleveland Clinic Foundation, Cleveland, Ohio
Ethical Considerations

Allan M. Spencer, DPM, LHD (Hon)
Professor, Ohio College of Podiatric Medicine; Department of Veterans Affairs Medical Center, Cleveland, Ohio
Podiatric Biomechanics and Orthopedics

Patricia M. Sullivan, DPM
Private practice, Worcester, Massachusetts
Interpretation of Laboratory Values

William F. Todd, DPM
Director of The Diabetic Foot Center and Director of Clinics, Kern Hospital, Warren, Michigan
The Diabetic Foot

Rodney Tomczak, DPM, EdM
Professor, University of Osteopathic Medicine and Health Sciences, College of Podiatric Medicine and Surgery, Des Moines, Iowa
Teaching and Learning Clinical Problem Solving

Marvin H. Waldman, DPM, MPH
Chief, Podiatry Section, Surgical Service, Department of Veterans Affairs Medical Center, Allen Park, Michigan
The Medical Literature: Epidemiology and Biostatistics

PREFACE

The definition of primary care is fairly abstract. It subsumes characteristics rather than definitive lines of domain. Primary care includes serving as the entry point to the health care system, managing commonly occurring conditions, caring for patients on a long-term basis, and coordinating additional referrals as needed. Primary care emphasizes the total care of the patient and the families in time of crisis. One major area of primary care, which has traditionally received less attention, is the psychosocial domain. This book will present psychosocial aspects of patient care as well as the medical aspects of patient care.

The scope and domain of the primary care practitioner is much more difficult to define. With the current national emphasis on primary care, student education, resident training, and continuing medical education will be driven by the developing domain of primary care podiatric medicine. The new board in primary podiatric medicine has defined a body of knowledge that it considers the scope of practice. This process of definition will continue as the specialty itself becomes better defined. The initial response by the profession to this new board has been enthusiastic.

The purpose of this book is to continue the process of defining primary podiatric medicine as a specialty of medicine. It will serve as a reference for students, residents, and practitioners who seek to explore, examine, and study the concepts and precepts of primary podiatric medicine. It is a given that the health care system is dynamic. Hence, this book seeks to serve as an initial effort in establishing the body of knowledge that is primary podiatric medicine.

JEFFREY M. ROBBINS
CLEVELAND, OHIO

CONTENTS

PART TWO

Practice of Podiatric Primary Care

PART ONE

Components of Podiatric Primary Care

CHAPTER 1

INTRODUCTION

Arthur E. Helfand

In 1989 the House of Delegates of the American Podiatric Medical Association defined the area of primary podiatric medicine in the context of a primary medical physician as "One who provides comprehensive podiatric medical care, predominantly in an ambulatory setting, who has demonstrated advance education and expertise in the provision of that service, and, in addition, has demonstrated advanced education and skills in cognitive areas such as, but not limited to: General Medicine, Geriatrics and Gerontology, Behavioral Sciences and Preventive Podiatric Medicine."

THE NATURE OF PRIMARY PODIATRIC MEDICAL CARE

From a clinical perspective, much of the care provided by practitioners of podiatric medicine has as its basis primary care services that focus on the immediate patient care needs and symptoms that are generally related to pain. The nature of primary podiatric medical care can be characterized as an array of services that are accessible and acceptable to the patient, comprehensive, and coordinated and continuous over time. The practitioner is accountable for the quality and potential effects of these services, reflected as the outcome of intervention. In a sense, the primary podiatric medical practitioner is engaged in the general or family practice of podiatric medicine, utilizing other special clinical services in the profession (e.g., podiatric surgery, podiatric orthopedics, and podiatric public health) and special services in other professions as referral and supporting sources. Primary care includes such elements as podiatric radiology, podiatric dermatology, and general podiatric medicine as components of the concept of primary care.

Primary podiatric medical care is distinguished by being "front line" or "first contact" care, person centered (rather than disease, organ system, or procedure centered), and comprehensive, rather than focused on foot and related illness episodes or on the procedure and/or service process involved. Primary podiatric medical care is distinguished from other levels of care by the scope, character, and integration of services provided. The service forms the basis of the distinction between primary and other levels of care. These other special areas of care include podiatric surgery and podiatric orthopedics as well as the administrative aspects of podiatric public health, thus providing a separate and distinct but coordinated area of public need.

Primary podiatric practitioners interact with ambulatory patients as the initial contact between the patient and the health care system. Patients present with a variety of foot and related illnesses and concerns that represent the early stages of disease, deformity, impairment, dysfunction, and disability and may not easily be classified by diagnostic label or system. Often patients have multiple problems, and a rational approach to one problem may complicate another. Primary podiatric medical care thus provides an integrating function, balancing the multiple requirements of the patient's problem, using information developed from many sources, and developing a strategy for optimal resolution of the patient's condition.

Perhaps the best three examples of need are diabetic foot care, arthritis, and the care of the aging patient who presents with foot problems. The *Standards of Care* published by the American Diabetes Association clearly consider primary foot care services as preventive, given the potential to reduce amputations by 50% to 75% with continuing and preventive foot care. In addition, foot problems in the diabetic have been identified as one of the five major complications of diabetes mellitus. The projections by the US Public Health Service call for the reduction of amputations as a national goal, which cannot be achieved without the continuing delivery of primary foot care services, best provided by doctors of podiatric medicine.

The degree of disability and dysfunction in the arthritic patient again illustrates the need for improved services. For the most part, these services are not initiated as surgical or as orthotic. They represent a podiatric medical approach to the relief of pain and maintenance of function. If the arthritic disease progresses, then the components of orthotics and surgery can be integrated with primary podiatric medical services.

The potential number of older patients in the United States in the next 30 to 40 years is projected as approaching 50 million. Clearly recognized is the fact that 90% to 95% of these patients will require some form of foot care, which will be primary and essential for these persons to remain ambulatory, functional, and independent. The care settings will include ambulatory, consulting hospital, and long-term care, with some components of geriopsychiatric units. The management of onychial and keratotic lesions in the older patient may be the primary need. Given the changes in the *Standards for Long Term Care* issued by the Joint Commission on Accreditation of Healthcare Organizations, the Department of Veterans Affairs, and the Health Care Finance Administration, which now includes foot care and podiatric services as a quality assurance issue, the podiatric profession must provide access to practitioners who can demonstrate additional skills and education in a manner equal and compatible with other health care and professional services.

THE PRACTITIONER

At the core of primary podiatric medical care are the practitioner, the patient, the problem, and the clinical process of care by which the patient and practitioner deal with the problem. The process usually involves multiple encounters, with the practitioner and other health care professionals as needed. The reason for the visit for care or a problem, at any given time or visit, may be pain, an illness, a social problem, or a health concern, but clearly the focus must be on what concerns the patient. In addition, there are other primary environments that relate to the patient and practitioner as well as their interaction. These include the social structure, which is often the family, the community, the practice or program, and the health care system, since it provides for reimbursement and establishes issues of need and quality.

Primary care practitioner considerations also include location and practice styles, the use of protocols and practice guidelines, and communication with patients and consultants. In addition to technical skills, practitioners must possess an interpersonal style that promotes trust and confidence in the patient. Many times the initial diagnosis is an impression and not a final definition of the problem. The ability to explain and to reassure the patient and to provide initial relief of pain and discomfort is essential.

Primary care practitioners must assimilate large volumes of information, and the practitioner must remain current on the advances in knowledge and procedures. The ability to determine which management protocols are effective and which are ineffective or outmoded is most important. The ability to balance costs, financial incentives, and patient preferences as well as medicolegal considerations is important as practice patterns change over the years.

There is a need for practitioners to process a wide variety of physiologic and social data on each patient to integrate care to meet the individual needs of each patient. Because patients often seek care for pain, the podiatric practitioner may be the first portal of entry for the patient into the health care system, or it may be the podiatric practitioner who first diagnoses a new medical problem that requires care by other medical disciplines. The responsibility to coordinate care and referral mandates significant communication skills, to assure follow-up care and to assure confidentiality for the patient.

THE PATIENT

Patient considerations focus on the individual patient and the special needs of groups of patients. Some patient concerns in the primary care process include medical decision making, adherence to practitioner advice, health-related behaviors, values associated with health states, satisfaction with the process of health care, and the strategies associated with changes in the care provided to individual patients and the delivery system in general.

Components often not considered in the delivery process include race, ethnicity, and age, as well as patient health beliefs and behaviors. The value of primary and preventive services is also related to the patient's impressions of continuity, coordination, and comprehensive nature of the care provided. Social and cultural factors also blend into the patient's concerns, desire to seek care, and focus on appreciation of the services provided.

We know that a person's health behavior is a major determinant of health. Several of the leading causes of death could be reduced by modifying smoking, dietary, and exercise behaviors. We can recognize that most infants are born with normal feet. But between birth and the age of 65, the 95% of normal becomes the 95% of abnormal in relation to foot problems, related to aging, misuse, disuse, deformity, disease, and dysfunction.

Future concerns in health care will also focus on the outcome of treatment and management. What is important to recognize is that, by definition, many of the conditions that involve the human foot are chronic particularly in the adult and elderly. This means that management rather than cure emerges as the direction for care. It also emphasizes the secondary prevention of chronic disease. Loss of function, discomfort, distress, and pain are usually the prime factors that cause a patient to seek care for foot problems. Associated with beliefs about outcomes are the perceptions of the condition, the types and levels of care, the frequency of visits, and the duration of symptoms. Also recognized is the fact that the same condition produces a different response in patients, mandating customizing care, which may vary from established protocols. Patient satisfaction with care and the practitioner is another factor that relates to all levels of care, but particularly ambulatory care, since the patient can easily seek alternatives.

As the health care system changes, costs, accessibility, and availability become critical factors in what services are included as reimbursable. Patient–practitioner relationships may be less of a critical issue under managed care plans. Because of costs, patients accept limitations in their younger years, which then need to be managed by other reimbursement programs in aging. Is that a cost-effective means of health care delivery? In relation to foot care, "routine foot care" is usually an exclusion. But what is "routine foot care"? There may be coverage definitions, but there is no valid medical definition, no more than there is for routine medical or dental care.

Health problems are strongly influenced by

a person's social environment. Changes in society that have modified the traditional family structure and community networks have given rise to special population risk categories. Many of these special patient populations have a direct relationship to demographics and health needs. Often podiatric care is not included in special program areas that magnify the potential for complications and have the potential to create wards of society. Because of financial, logistical, physical, mental, cultural, and personal reasons, foot care many not be perceived as needed until institutionalization is required for proper management. The projections that relate to the management of the diabetic patient and foot care are perhaps the best examples of this point. Other examples, although not related to podiatric care, are high-risk pregnant women and their infants, alcohol and drug dependence, human immunodeficiency virus infection, and the increase in venereal diseases.

Persons with disabilities do not always have access to proper foot care. It is estimated that there are about 3 million disabled persons in the United States younger than 65 years of age. Availability and financing are compounded by logistics, access, transportation, escorts, and interpreters. The Americans With Disabilities Act of 1990 may solve some of the problems in the future but does not focus on need, reimbursement, and preventive services. Foot care affects the mental and physical well-being of the disabled. Even when walking is not possible, multiple types of foot problems occur and require appropriate podiatric care. The ability to prevent impairments and additional disability is a concern for all age groups. The environmental concern for proper footwear for the disabled is a form of preventive care, as is proper patient education.

A clear podiatric need may be evident in 95% of elderly patients. Availability, costs, and long-term care are major policy issues. But how foot care and podiatric services are to be provided must form a basis for decisions. In addition, today, about one fourth, or 7 million, of the elderly are disabled. The advances in medicine and health care have given rise to the old, old patient. More patients with Alzheimer's disease and related dementias add to the continuing need for foot evaluation and

care. Low-income elderly, minority elderly, caregiver demands, rural and urban changes, housing needs, and health and social demands all contribute to the social segregation of the older population.

The potential modifications required for the organization and delivery of primary care services to an increasing older population are significant. Services in general have been diversified into multiple models for the delivery of noninstitutional services. The evolution of the managed care model as well as of individual provider concerns has placed greater restrictions on primary foot care services than in the past. Access is often limited until a complication develops, which reduces the art of prevention. Meeting care needs for the older person living alone provides an additional concern. Many are on low incomes, live in rural areas, and are considered poor, not only in an economic sense but also in their ability to understand their own health problems. Without a concerned caregiver, foot health and care is often neglected until hospitalization is required.

Podiatric practitioners must be concerned with the total patient and his or her needs. The concern for the quality and appropriateness of care received by the elderly is critical because as many as 95% of the older population will develop some form of foot discomfort and/or care need during their later years. Treatment needs to focus on functional capacities and on preventing complications associated with chronic diseases.

Although foot problems may not be the primary concern of the person with human immunodeficiency virus infection or the acquired immunodeficiency syndrome (AIDS), they do tend to surface in relation to comfort and the management of onychial and fungal conditions. Podiatric care is one of the special needs and support services that may be required for patients with AIDS and other diseases and infirmities as the health care system is stressed in future years.

The podiatric practitioner who provides primary care must respond to a wide variety of patient problems that may be focal or may manifest as complications of chronic diseases, such as diabetes mellitus, multiple forms of arthritis, arterial insufficiencies, and neuropathies. These problems relate to symptoms, chronic illnesses, environmental issues (e.g., footwear, flooring), medication, and behavioral and other risk factors. In addition, the practitioner must deal with a variety of administrative concerns in primary care that include third-party carriers, disability, and lifestyle. How patients seek podiatric care is an issue that must be considered as the patients learn what to expect in relation to foot care and that feet need not hurt.

Often patients present with clustered symptoms as opposed to a clearly defined diagnosis. Practitioners must delineate among self-limiting conditions, those that require definitive care, and those that require continuing management. The practitioner must also provide some degree of prognosis and develop a plan to deal with the problem presented. Adding to this is the need to be cost effective and not overuse diagnostic tests. Clearly, at times, defensive health care becomes a part of the consideration in management. Primary care needs to be directed toward the care of a person rather than toward the treatment of a disease or a condition.

THE CLINICAL PROCESS OF PRIMARY PODIATRIC CARE

Primary podiatric care presents a challenge with a broad range of management concerns. There is a need to communicate as a therapeutic adjunct so that information processing, management, referrals, and outcomes maintain continuity, are comprehensive, are coordinated and accessible, and are acceptable. Primary podiatric care is at the front line of the health care system, striking a balance between self and specialty care. The initial step is the recognition of illness. Given the fact that most patients do not present with a clearly defined diagnosis, the primary podiatric practitioner must respond to the patient's problem and relieve initial pain and discomfort. He or she must plan a course of treatment or management that may involve diagnostic studies and specialty consultation.

The practitioner must then sort the myriad signs and symptoms presented and provide an explanation of the problem presented to the patient. Part of that focus is a management plan and a prognosis. Also needing recognition is that prevention is a fundamental objective of primary care and that health education is the first step toward meeting that goal. For example, how can the practitioner motivate, inform, and assist a patient in making changes in his or her foot health or care direction to eliminate potential complications in the future? Perhaps the best example of this is in relation to diabetes mellitus and the need to reduce the number of amputations. In this example, different disciplines, working together, might potentiate their impact on patient risk factors.

In most cases, problems presented at the primary level have multiple causes. For the older patient, anxiety may be an important factor in management. For the diabetic, the fear of the loss of a limb might be a primary concern. The need to determine the cause and provide remediation are key components to primary podiatric care. Treatment effectiveness is measured by the patient, the practitioner, and the health care system. Health care effectiveness emphasizes the patient preferences for outcomes in terms of improvement in health status, functional capacity, and the quality of life, rather than on clinical measures. The success of a procedure in an anatomical sense that does not make the patient function at a better level might not be considered as a good outcome. How services are provided, how referrals are developed and made, and how determinants are manifested are all related aspects of primary care.

Medical decision making in the deliver of primary podiatric care services is also an area that needs to be emphasized. Patient ambiguity and limited patient response are issues that relate to developing a diagnosis. These factors are especially important in the care of the older patient. Decisions that consider risk and benefits in relation to treatment again are important factors, especially in the very young and older patient. The quality of care is yet another focus of primary care. The evaluation made not only by the patient and practitioner but also by the insurance carrier becomes an equal concern. Factors include the scope of the primary service as well as the recognition of need and the effects of therapy.

The practitioner–patient relationship is the

foundation of the clinical process of primary care. The practitioner must go beyond the diagnosis and understand the implications of illness. There needs to be a consideration of those elements of primary care that contribute to the continuity of care and increase patient responsibility and participation in decision making. The primary care podiatric practitioner often becomes the confidante of the patient, and this trend accelerates as the patient ages. Two of the key factors that have always been related to podiatric medicine and care are touch and the ability to provide almost immediate relief of pain.

Primary care practitioners in podiatric medicine must also consider the social environment of the patient as it relates to the care process. Families and social structure exert a strong influence on health-related behaviors, as well as the nature and course of health problems. Families are de facto members of the primary care team since they may reinforce or undermine the provider's efforts to care for patients. Other members of the family may also become future patients since they may seek care for conditions that have been left untreated.

SUMMARY

Most primary podiatric care is delivered by solo practitioners or single specialty groups. The influence of the care setting is a component of service. The setting may be urban community based, institutionally related, or rural or have a focus on underserved populations. Given the projections for an older population, the patient mix may change in the future to include more older patients, those with significant chronic disease complications, and patients at greater risk. Regardless of the setting, several factors emerge that will provide a focus for future care:

■ Health status measurement
■ Special considerations for the care provided to the homeless
■ Health promotion
■ Disease prevention
■ Increased health knowledge for low-income groups

■ Reduction in nonfinancial barriers to care
■ Assessment of quality of care

The implications of the delivery of podiatric care as a part of a managed health care system are also a future focus. Under current provisions, for the most part, care is limited and services are unmet. Many patients must go outside their system to obtain podiatric primary care or must develop serious complications before care can be obtained. The best example is not providing periodic primary services for a patient with a diabetic foot and thus permitting the patient to develop an ulceration, possibly resulting in hospitalization and the potential for limb loss. It has been estimated that the cost of one hospital admission and one lost diabetic limb could provide preventive care for multiple patients for a lifetime and maintain the quality of life for these at-risk patients.

Medical liability issues will also continue to influence primary care, the range of services provided, and perhaps even the choice of career for a potential student. Despite the emphasis on risk management, little data exist to demonstrate the effectiveness, or a lessening, of the number of liability suits. Thus practice guidelines, utilization review, and peer review may or may not have made a change in the care levels of patients.

Some of the factors that relate to future demographics in primary care include our aging population, the baby boom generation, a declining younger population, racial and ethnic diversity, and changes in the family unit. The disparity between rich and poor and limited public budgets may determine who might be eligible for primary foot care services, regardless of the degree of the provider. Aging, lifestyle, technology, AIDS, and the environment also will have a focus on the delivery of foot and podiatric care in the future. Access and limitations will also provide a key focus in our future health care system. Additional factors that relate to health care delivery include organizational complexity and diversity, corporate health care benefits, the shift from professional values to managerial values, the shift from inpatient to outpatient care, the changing nature of long-term care, mental health programs, and health care personnel activities. As a final factor, one needs to consider professional education, its financing, and its future curriculum.

Primary podiatric care is a vital link in the total comprehensive care system. The changes in the age of podiatric patients and the potential for increases in chronic disease in this older population will place a greater strain on the delivery and services provided by the podiatric profession. Rising costs, shrinking resources, potential rationing, and the reimbursement system may well determine what constitutes a needed health service. What is important to recognize is that foot health and care represents a needed service to maintain an ambulatory and productive society.

BIBLIOGRAPHY

American Diabetes Association: Therapy for Diabetes and Related Disorders. Alexandria, VA, American Diabetes Association, 1991.

American Podiatric Medical Association: Proceedings of the 1989 House of Delegates, American Podiatric Medical Association, Bethesda, MD, 1989.

Baran R, Dawber RPR: Diseases of the Nails and Their Management. Oxford, England, Blackwell Scientific Publications, 1984.

Beaven DW, Brooks SE: Color Atlas of the Nail in Clinical Diagnosis. Chicago, Year Book Medical Publishers, 1984.

Bild DE, et al: Lower-extremity amputation in people with diabetes: Epidemiology and prevention. Diabetes Care 12:23–31, 1989.

Calkins E, Davis PJ, Ford AB (eds): The Practice of Geriatrics. Philadelphia, WB Saunders, 1986.

Davidson JK: Clinical Diabetes Mellitus. New York, Thieme Medical Publishers, 1986.

Eisdorfer C (ed): Annual Review of Gerontology and Geriatrics, vol 4. New York, Springer Publishing Co, 1984.

Eng W: Geriatric Podiatry. Geriatric Curriculum Resource Guides for Health Professionals. Richmond, VA, Virginia Commonwealth University, Geriatric Education Center, 1986–1987.

Helfand AE (ed): Clinical Podogeriatrics. Baltimore, Williams & Wilkins, 1981.

Helfand AE (ed): Public Health and Podiatric Medicine. Baltimore, Williams & Wilkins, 1987.

Helfand AE: Feet First. Harrisburg, Pennsylvania Diabetes Academy, 1992.

Helfand AE, Bruno J (eds): Rehabilitation of the Foot. Clin Podiatr 1(2), 1984.

Jahss MH (ed): Diseases of the Foot. Philadelphia, WB Saunders, 1991.

Jessett DF, Helfand AE: Foot problems in the elderly. In Pathy MSJ (ed): Principles and Practice of Geriatric Medicine, ed 2. Edinburgh, John Wiley & Sons, 1991.

Kozak GP, Hoar CS Jr, Rowbotham JL, et al: Management of the Diabetic Foot. Philadelphia, WB Saunders, 1984.

Levin ME, O'Neal LW (eds): The Diabetic Foot, ed 4. St. Louis, CV Mosby, 1988.

Libow LB, Sherman FT (eds): The Core of Geriatric Medicine. St. Louis, CV Mosby, 1981.

McCarthy DJ (ed): Podiatric Dermatology. Baltimore, Williams & Wilkins, 1986.

Neale D, Adams I (eds): Common Foot Disorders, Diagnosis and Management, ed 2. Edinburgh, Churchill Livingstone, 1985.

Reichel W (ed): Clinical Aspects of Aging, ed 2. Baltimore, Williams & Wilkins, 1983.

Samitz MH: Cutaneous Disorders of the Lower Extremities, ed 2. Philadelphia, JB Lippincott, 1981.

Samman PD, Fenton DA: The Nails in Disease, ed 4. London, William Heinemann Medical Books, 1986.

Scardinia RJ: Diabetic foot problems: Assessment and prevention. Clin Diabetes 1983, March/April, pp 1–7.

Steinberg FU: Care of the Geriatric Patient, ed 6. St. Louis, CV Mosby, 1983.

US Department of Health and Human Services, Public Health Service, National Institutes of Health: Feet First. Publication No. 0-388-126. Washington, DC, US Government Printing Office, 1970.

US Department of Health and Human Services: A Research Agenda for Primary Care. Washington, DC, Public Health Service, 1991.

US Department of Health and Human Services: A Report on the Pew Health Professions Commission, Health America, Practitioners for 2005, An Agenda for Action for US Health Professional Schools, Pew Commission, Washington, DC, 1991.

Williams TF (ed): Rehabilitation in the Aging. New York, Raven Press, 1984.

Wilson LB, Simon SP, Baxter CR (eds): Handbook of Geriatric Emergency Care. Gaithersburg, MD, Aspen Systems Corporation, 1984.

Witkowski JA (ed): Diseases of the Lower Extremities. Clin Dermatol 1(1), 1983.

Yale I, Yale JF: The Arthritic Foot and Related Connective Tissue Disorders. Baltimore, Williams & Wilkins, 1984.

Yale JF: Yale's Podiatric Medicine, ed 3. Baltimore, Williams & Wilkins, 1987.

CHAPTER 2

PODIATRIC PREVENTION

Leonard A. Levy

A major component of primary care is prevention and health promotion. Today the concept of prevention has broadened considerably to include far more than efforts to avoid acquiring a disease or disorder. Prevention, whether in podiatric medicine or any other health care specialty, is concerned with the interruption of the natural history of any disease as early as possible.

LEVELS OF PREVENTION

Obviously, the ultimate goal is for prevention to occur before any disease is acquired. However, if such early action does not take place and a disease or disorder develops, prevention is still possible by focusing on the early detection of the condition and intervening to either stop or delay its progress or, in some instances, to eradicate or cure it completely. Often, early detection does not occur and the natural history of a disease advances to the point at which the process causes considerable damage to the human host. In such situations the next level of prevention is rehabilitation, which is efforts designed to maximize remaining function and avoid further disability or death.

Each of these aspects of prevention, referred to as primary, secondary, and tertiary prevention, are summarized in Table 2–1. Primary prevention includes activities that take place before the time when a person has any disease. This is referred to as the period of prepathogenesis. One type of primary prevention is referred to as health promotion, which is not disease specific. Health promotion activities are designed to improve the state of wellness using such measures as good eating habits; health education; avoidance of smoking; elimination or reduction of alcohol consumption; using seat belts and having a motor vehicle equipped with air bags, good brakes, and well-maintained tires; provision of adequate housing; proper hygiene and sanitation; and establishment of a regular physical fitness program.

The second type of primary prevention in-

TABLE 2-1. **Levels of Prevention and Goals**

Level of Prevention	Goals
Primary	
Health promotion	Positive improvement of state of health
Disease prevention	Prevention of specific diseases or disorders
Secondary	Early diagnosis and prompt treatment of diseases or disorders
Tertiary	Rehabilitation: maximize or improve remaining capacities

cludes measures to prevent specific diseases and disorders. These measures may include immunizations; use of specific nutrients; protection from occupational hazards (e.g., steel-toed shoes, use of masks, protective clothing); elimination of carcinogens from the home and the workplace; safe, well-maintained highways; and the avoidance of allergens.

Secondary prevention also has two categories, one of which is early diagnosis with the objective of identifying and arresting a health problem before it causes signs and symptoms. This includes case finding through the use of effective screening surveys and selective examinations. Examples include blood glucose and cholesterol examinations, blood pressure or hypertension screening, regularly scheduled mammograms and Papanicolaou smears, foot screening for diabetes, and glaucoma testing.

Another type of secondary prevention is called disability limitation. It includes adequate treatment as early as possible in the natural history of a disease to either arrest or slow down its course so that complications and other sequelae can be avoided or reduced in frequency or intensity. This type of secondary prevention requires proper podiatric medical facilities to provide such care, such as well-staffed and equipped community resources including trained health care professionals in community practices, clinics, and hospitals.

Rehabilitation, the third level of prevention, includes the provision of hospitals and community resources for retraining and educating victims of disease by preparing them to maximally use their remaining capacities. It also includes increasing the awareness of the public and industry to employ disabled persons to the maximum degree possible.

To best depict prevention it is appropriate to show it as part of a continuum rather than as a static concept. This can be done diagrammatically by placing it as part of a timeline representing the course or natural history of any disease or disorder (Fig. 2-1).

The period of prepathogenesis is that component of the natural history when the person is considered to be well. When the person begins to develop changes even at the cellular level as a result of a disease process, even if not detectable by the most sophisticated technology and through employing outstanding

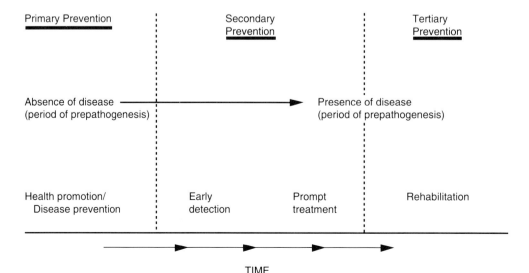

FIGURE 2-1. Prevention as a continuum.

physical diagnostic skills, the period of pathogenesis has been reached.

AGENT, HOST, AND ENVIRONMENTAL FACTORS

The optimum goal of health care is to interrupt the natural history of any disease or disorder before a person becomes a victim of that condition. It is during that period that a person is considered to be in the state of wellness or good health. Therefore, health is defined in a much broader context, not simply the absence of disease but also the presence of physical, mental, and social well-being. This involves the establishment of an equilibrium in the environment with the numerous agents associated with disease and disorders and those factors intrinsic to the human host (Fig. 2–2). As long as the equilibrium is maintained, the person will be free of any disease. If such factors as a poorly functioning immune system, inadequate nutrition, obesity, genetic deficiencies, hormonal dysfunction, and poor dietary habits overwhelm the host or increase susceptibility, the probability of various physical, biological, clinical, or mechanical agents upsetting the equilibrium between health and disease is increased. Such a person would then

no longer be considered well but instead be someone who is diseased.

In recent years there has been greater awareness of the importance of environmental conditions as one of the factors responsible for, or contributing to, disease and disorders. Environmental conditions including chemicals, pollution, noise, climate, stress, and socioeconomics may affect the equilibrium. This may result in the host's becoming affected by disease, defect, or disability or may even cause death.

Therefore, the concept that all diseases and disorders are multifactorially caused is appropriate. That is, every disease, illness, or injury is a result of the contribution of agent, host, and environmental factors (Table 2–2), and a combination of all of these interacting factors is what can lead to the disease state. Simplistically, for example, one may say that a virus is the cause of plantar warts. Actually, this is only part of the response to the question "What is the cause of plantar warts?" A more appropriate answer would also include host and environmental factors. In the case of the wart, it could include conditions of the immune system in the human host, environmental conditions that inoculated the person (e.g., nail in a shoe or other minor, often overlooked,

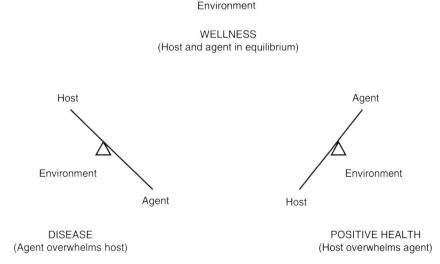

WELLNESS
(Host and agent in equilibrium)

DISEASE
(Agent overwhelms host)

POSITIVE HEALTH
(Host overwhelms agent)

FIGURE 2–2. The concept of equilibrium in health and disease.

trauma), and the viral agent. Indeed all three factors need to interact to produce the warts. Most of us are in environments in which there is a high concentration of the virus that causes warts yet because our immune system does not allow us to host the disease and perhaps also because the organism does not become inoculated into our body, we do not present with this clinical condition.

SAMPLE CASE: FOOT ULCERS IN DIABETES MELLITUS

A specific example of prevention and its relationship to foot ulcers associated with diabetes mellitus is provided in the perspective of a map of the natural history of a diabetic with an ulceration affecting the foot (Fig. 2–3). The map divides the period of prepathogenesis when no diabetic ulcer is present from the period of pathogenesis when the podiatric complications of diabetes begin to occur. The period of prepathogenesis provides opportunities for both the patient, family, and practitioner to interrupt the natural history of the process so that no ulcer occurs and a normal state remains. During the period of prepathogenesis, proactive measures include both health promotion and specific protection. These range from maintaining good general health to the elimination of various situations that could stimulate the human host to produce a foot ulcer (e.g., burn, biomechanical defect, tight shoe). Should these measures of primary prevention not be employed, and the natural history of the process be allowed to move forward, changes begin in the tissues that are not clinically detectable during the early period of pathogenesis. This is the time when even the most sophisticated clinical and laboratory studies employed by a clinician would not detect an abnormality. It is depicted on the chart as being below the clinical horizon, somewhat analogous to the iceberg that cannot be seen below the water line. If the disease process is permitted to progress, signs and symptoms appear that are detectable by examination either by the patient or by the practitioner. These are depicted on the chart as being above the clinical horizon, perhaps beginning with a small area of erythema, a vesicle, or other skin defect. Through secon-

TABLE 2–2. Factors Associated in the Natural History of Diabetic-Associated Ulcers

Agent Factors
Loose- or tight-fitting shoes
Improperly fitting hose
Height of heel of shoe
Foreign body projecting from part of shoe
Pointed shoes
Excessive heat/cold
Smoking
Trauma: minor/major
Hyperhidrosis

Host Factors
Age, sex, ethnic group
Occupation
Congenital/genetic
Osteoarthritis or other arthritides
Varus rotation of toe
Shape and length of toe bone
Exostosis
Fusion of phalanges
Subtalar varus—forefoot valgus and varus
Personal habits and customs
Circulatory abnormalities
Neurologic deficits
Other dermatologic abnormalities
Variation of skin responses to intermittent trauma
Muscular imbalance
Hyperhidrosis
Dry skin/xerosis
Ingrowing and/or dystrophic nails
Fissures
Dermatophytosis
Arteriosclerosis obliterans
Neuropathy, including anesthetic foot

Environmental Factors
Social and economic factors
  Custom and shoe styles
  Low income (e.g., cost of podiatric and other health
    care, cost of shoes, socks)
  Available podiatric facilities
  Nutrition
  Awareness of importance of foot care
Cultural barriers
Physical factors
  Climate
  Flooring materials and covering

dary prevention measures, the process most frequently can be interrupted with early diagnosis, prompt treatment, and activities designed to limit or avoid disability.

Unfortunately, in some patients the natural history of the disease process continues to progress, leading to foot ulcers complicated by infection, necrosis, and sometimes precipitation of major or minor lower-extremity amputations. Here, too, we try to intervene with tertiary preventive measures designed to reduce the extent of the amputation if it cannot be

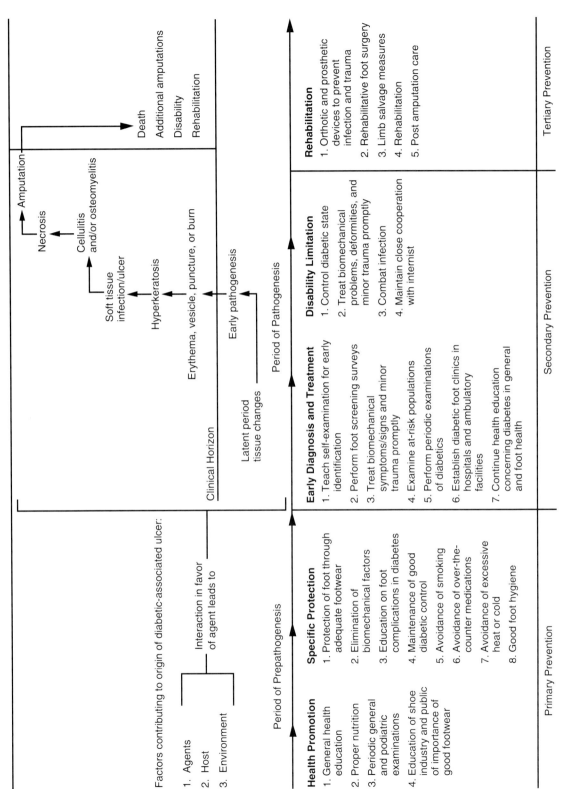

FIGURE 2–3. Natural history of a diabetic patient with ulceration of the foot.

prevented. Another component of tertiary prevention is the rehabilitation of the patient after an amputation so that further amputation of the same extremity is not necessary, the other limb can be salvaged, or rehabilitation with orthoses or prostheses can be accomplished. In addition, death, which too frequently occurs after amputation, can be prevented.

SUMMARY

Prevention of disease is a far broader concept than simply avoidance of disease. It is a multilevel activity that includes promotion of health, prevention of disease (primary prevention), early detection and prompt treatment of disease, limitation of disability (secondary prevention), and rehabilitation (tertiary prevention). The health care community should try to interrupt the natural history of a disease through primary prevention. Should that not be possible, secondary and even tertiary preventive measures should be employed. Considering prevention throughout the natural history of a disease is an effective but often overlooked part of the health care provided to communities and individuals.

BIBLIOGRAPHY

Levy LA: Epidemiology and prevention of diabetic foot disease. In Frykberg RG (ed): The High Risk Foot in Diabetes Mellitus, pp 25–31. New York, Churchill Livingstone, 1991.

Levy LA: Epidemiology of podiatric medical diseases and disorders. In Helfand AE (ed): Public Health and Podiatric Medicine, p 91. Baltimore, Williams & Wilkins, 1987.

Levy LA: The natural history of podiatric disorders—establishing priorities for our profession and its teaching institutions. J Am Podiatr Assoc 63(9), 1973.

Roht LH, et al: Principles of Epidemiology: a Self-Teaching Guide, pp 26–28. New York, Academic Press, 1982.

CHAPTER 3

AMBULATORY CARE

Arthur E. Helfand

As the health care delivery system changes, new models for the delivery of care continue to evolve. In addition to the services provided by practitioners in their offices, some programs that have surfaced provide care in community facilities. These include ambulatory care centers in hospitals, outpatient clinics, union health centers, health maintenance organization facilities, community health centers, and other similar facilities. In these instances, patients come to a particular facility as opposed to a practitioner's office for their primary care and ambulatory care needs. The inclusion of podiatrists in the professional component of these facilities and programs permits comprehensive services to be provided. Examples of such programs can also be found in the military and in the Department of Veterans Affairs ambulatory care programs.

In these types of programs and facilities the primary purpose of the podiatric service is to provide a comprehensive foot care service to patients, who may be eligible to receive ambulatory care as part of the particular program or health plan. In these cases, all aspects of podiatric care should be included to permit appropriate diagnostic considerations, therapeutic approaches, and elements of prevention, including health education, within the program definitions and the delineation of privileges for individual practitioners. In general, the best program provides a primary entry of the patient for podiatric care and includes a referral mechanism for care provided as part of a comprehensive approach to total patient management. The ability to serve as the primary portal of entry when the complaint or pain is in the foot is cost effective, since services can be provided at the initial visit and can include appropriate referrals, studies, and care to meet the symptoms of each individual patient.

WHAT IS AMBULATORY CARE?

The United States National Ambulatory Care Medical Survey, which was initiated in 1973, defined the ambulatory patient as "an individual presenting himself/herself for personal services, who is neither bedridden nor currently admitted to any health care institution." The ambulatory patient may also include the homebound patient and a person who has most of the responsibility for his or her own care. These patients generally administer most or all of their own treatments, monitor their own symptoms and functional status, adapt their activities to their degree of illness, and then decide how to deal with new problems when they arise. In a sense, because we in podiatric medicine deal so much with ambulation, the vast majority of podiatric services are in that classification. Much of the care provided can also be termed *primary podiatric medicine.* In addition, with the increase in the older population, many current as well as future patients will fall into the category of the aging or aged.

Most visits include some form of diagnostic service, which includes a limited history and physical examination as well as some form of treatment or therapy. In addition, a portion of the visit may be devoted to counseling or health education. In many cases, ambulatory care involves conditions that the practitioner is familiar with and includes patients whom he or she has seen before.

Telephone encounters and home visits are also elements of ambulatory care for noninstitutionalized persons. In most cases, these same elements translate to office visits on an ambulatory basis in the future.

Before making visits to any practitioner, the patient usually attempts to diagnose and treat his or her own symptoms, for example, with nonprescribed medications. Self-care of the feet may result in a complication, since the patient usually attempts some procedure with untoward results. When self-care fails, the patient seeks advice and treatment. For the practitioner, what is seen are usually the failures of self-management. In a sense, self-care before professional care is the way that the patient makes the decision about ambulatory care and who provides the service.

Once the patient is seen by the practitioner, there are several dimensions to care. Some include the significance of the recent symptoms, the advisability and need for referral, how well the patient will adhere to recommended care,

what is the impact of treatment on the patient's health, and what impact the condition and treatment will have on the patient's activities of life. Another focus must also deal with reimbursement, which may have multiple restrictions in relation to the care of the foot and its related problems. To some degree, although much of ambulatory care is related to preventive services, we as a society have yet to recognize the need for prevention. In real terms, if one computes the cost of hospitalization, subsequent amputation, and life care needs for an older diabetic as compared with preventive and primary foot care services, the focus of need becomes apparent.

GOALS OF AMBULATORY CARE

The goals for the patient are determined by the fact that the patient resides at home and not in an institution and that his or her activities can modify the outcome depending on compliance with therapy. Clearly the patient expects to maintain his or her lifestyle, activities, and occupation during the course of treatment. The patient also expects to be able to take care of his or her own personal needs, such as nutrition, clothing, hygiene, and travel. The patient expects to be free of pain as well as of physical and emotional symptoms that might modify lifestyle and activities. The patient will deal with the expectations of life at home rather than being in the hospital, where there is concern about discharge and the period of perhaps extended recovery.

For the practitioner, there must be a decision about how the patient is responding to the treatment as well as the patient's own expectations. There needs to be an assessment of wellness and a means to plan for additional care and monitoring. There is also a need to determine what care needs to be modified and when active treatment needs to end.

The practitioner must also have a working knowledge of epidemiology to identify the course of disease and be able to project usual outcomes. Making a working diagnosis, understanding the natural history of the condition, and planning and monitoring treatment are all components of this basic knowledge. The primary components used in making the diagnosis include a single diagnostic test, a quantitative deviation in physiologic function, and the presence of information that includes the symptoms, signs, and duration of the condition.

Communication and patient education are also important components of ambulatory care. Measurable or attainable goals are important for the patient and to step-manage the patient. Perhaps the terms *doctor–patient relationship* and *bedside manner* best describe what needs to be identified.

The clinical records must reflect the patient's social profile and should elicit a problem list from the patient. A preventive care profile is another area for future consideration, since the reduction of risk, particularly in those patients who are older or may have multiple chronic diseases, can prevent serious future complications. Subjective findings, assessment, objective findings, and a plan or progress report are components of the clinical record of ambulatory care.

Care must also be coordinated with need and referral. All of the special areas of podiatric practice should be employed in care and include, as examples, podiatric medicine, podiatric radiology, podiatric dermatology, podiatric orthopedics, podiatric surgery, and podiatric public health, all of which enhance the preventive component of patient management.

Cost containment and policy guidelines for reimbursement are additional components of ambulatory care, because without reimbursement a patient may defer care until complications arise. Payment is often made for technical and procedural activities, and consideration is not provided for inquiry, counseling, primary care, and preventive services.

AMBULATORY PODIATRIC MEDICAL CARE

As a general statement of intent, the following elements are suggested as initial considerations for the delivery of podiatric care in an office, ambulatory, or outpatient setting:

1. The facility should be adequate to deliver a quality podiatric service. This refers to the physical structure as well as to the equipment in each podiatric operatory.

2. The staff should be qualified and competent to deliver an appropriate podiatric service and should be properly appointed. Delineation should be consistent with state laws and the professional, moral, and ethical standings of individual practitioners.

3. The standards of care should be consistent with established norms and criteria as documented in acceptable elements of the medical literature. The quality of care should consider the major elements of history, examination, and records; diagnostic management; and treatment and follow-up.

4. Comprehensive, intermediate, limited, brief, and minimal visits and services should be utilized, when appropriate, with all records included on the appropriate and approved form, compatible with and supportive to other clinical services and programs.

5. Care provided to patients should be consistent with the appropriate state practice act and the delineation for each individual practitioner. The training, education, judgment, and ability of each practitioner is reflected in the reviews that determine individual delineations for clinical privileges and relate directly to patient care services.

6. Podiatric examination should include appropriate procedures and tests, including history, physical examination, radiographs, laboratory studies, and other special diagnostic tests, such as those in biomechanics and vascular analysis.

7. Primary podiatric care should deal with primary complaints and foot discomfort. The term *primary* in a sense refers to two distinct areas: the initial visit and the types of services provided.

8. Pain should be explored to its fullest extent with the use of all appropriate diagnostic modalities.

9. Appropriate specialized medical consultation should be employed when indicated, when the diagnosis is in doubt, and when systemic disease is present and contributing as a complicating factor. Clinical care should be multidisciplinary and based on total patient need.

10. Neurologic, vascular, and other related conditions should be managed in a primary sense.

11. Appropriate laboratory and other dermatologic tests should be available and employed when indicated.

12. Primary care for hyperkeratotic lesions and their sequelae should be provided with acceptable means of initial and continuing management. Debridement, pathomechanical, foot orthopedic, biomechanical, radiographic, orthotic, and dermatologic procedures should be employed as elements of total patient management.

13. Appropriate topical, systemic, and controlled drugs should be prescribed based on the diagnosis and therapeutic indications and should be consistent with local legal requirements under the provisions of the Drug Enforcement Administration.

14. Verrucae and related conditions should be managed in the appropriate manner, suited to each individual patient. Conservative as well as surgical management may be performed in the operatory or, if appropriate, in the ambulatory operating room, a short procedure unit, or another hospital operating room facility.

15. Mycotic conditions, infections, and conditions involving the sweat glands should be managed by appropriate methods.

16. Dermatologic lesions and ulcerations should be managed in the proper manner with adequate consultation and combined management, when indicated, such as with diabetic ulcers, to ensure appropriate medical and podiatric care for the patient.

17. Onychial care should be provided in a proper manner, depending on the diagnosis and patient outcome projections. Onychial surgical approaches may be managed in the primary setting and in an ambulatory operating unit, a short procedure unit, or an institutional operating room, depending on the diagnosis, surgical procedure, and risk for the patient. Mechanical debridement and dermabrasive techniques should be used as appropriate and as part of total patient care. Therapeutic agents should be used when indicated according to the diagnosis and desired patient outcome. At-risk patients with concomitant systemic disease, such as diabetes, should receive patient instruction and education as part of special patient education programs.

18. Primary inflammatory conditions of the foot should be appropriately managed. Therapeutic agents should be employed as indicated. Appropriate physical modalities and procedures should be available as part of patient management and to complement mechanical and orthotic procedures.

19. Congenital and acquired deformities of the foot should be managed by appropriate biomechanical and foot orthopedic measures in the clinical setting with radiographic analysis and orthotics employed when required.

20. Health education should be provided freely for individual patients, in group educational settings, and as part of a total interdisciplinary approach to preventive care.

21. All podiatric surgical care should conform to individual podiatric delineations and should be completed in the appropriate setting, be that the ambulatory clinical facility, outpatient operating room, short procedure unit, or hospital operating room, with appropriate podiatric admitting privileges to all such facilities.

22. Emergencies should be managed in the prescribed manner and may include cardiopulmonary resuscitation, supportive measures, transfer to an emergency facility, or admission to a hospital floor or other intensive care unit.

23. Continuing education should be a constant element of the facilities program to permit interdisciplinary improvement in the total approach to patient care and to permit the development of special programs pertaining to individual diseases and/or age groups.

These guidelines provide a total approach to ambulatory podiatric care in those programs that are institutionally based or are part of a system of care to selected populations or groups.

CARE SERVICES FOR THE MENTALLY ILL AND RETARDED

Although care programs that relate to the mentally ill and retarded are often classed as long-term care, it should be noted that most governmental agencies and programs separate this aspect of care and modify programs from those with traditional long-term care elements that primarily deal with the elderly and chronically ill. In addition, with the changes in philosophy regarding these two groups, much of this care is now community based and thus ambulatory.

From a conceptual point, one could project the following components for such a program:

1. The program must provide or make arrangements for comprehensive diagnostic and treatment services for each client from qualified personnel including licensed podiatrists, either through organized podiatric services in house or through arrangement.
2. Podiatric practitioners must participate, as appropriate, in the development, review, and updating of patient care policies as a part of the interdisciplinary process of care.

Diagnostic services should include the following:

1. A complete podiatric examination, using all diagnostic aids necessary to properly evaluate the client's foot health
2. Periodic examination and diagnosis performed at least annually, including radiographs when indicated and detection of manifestations of systemic disease
3. A review of the results of the examination and entry of the results in the client's podiatric and/or medical record

Podiatric treatment should include the following:

1. Provision of emergency (acute) podiatric treatment on a continuing basis by a licensed podiatrist
2. Podiatric care, including medical, biomechanical, and surgical care, needed and appropriate for the relief of pain
3. Comprehensive diagnostic services, including a complete initial examination, periodic follow-up examinations, and entry of the results in the client's podiatric records
4. Comprehensive podiatric treatment as required

PRACTITIONER ASSESSMENT FACTORS

In general, the following guidelines are examples of assessment factors for podiatric practitioners:

1. Current license to practice podiatric medicine
2. Adequate delineation of clinical privileges, which are specific to procedures and not diagnostic classifications and are based on moral, ethical, and professional competence, ability, and judgment
3. Demonstrated quality and appropriateness of care based on adequate and fair review in relation to the accepted practice of podiatric medicine
4. Appropriate review procedures that permit continuing revisions to delineations, based on demonstrated documentation for change as well as clinical ability, judgment, moral and ethical character, and proper health status.
5. General guidelines to be utilized for assessment, recognizing that all need not or should not be applied in all cases:
   a. Licensure
   b. Approved residency training, fellowships, and/or preceptorships
   c. Years of administrative and/or clinical experience supported by appropriate profiles and documentation
   d. Board certification, eligibility, and/or equivalent activity in special areas of podiatric practice
   e. Special society fellowship, associateship, or membership, both professional and interprofessional or interdisciplinary
   f. Continuing education as evidenced by licensure requirements or by the American Podiatric Medical Association's Podiatrist's Recognition Award and other specialized training and education
   g. Additional clinical, administrative, institutional, or educational experience

h. Institutional or agency affiliations

i. Recommendations as deemed as appropriate and verification of all education, licensure, training, memberships, and affiliations.

6. Ongoing review procedures equal to other professional components

7. Ongoing review of factors such as utilization, quality assurance, and medical necessity as appropriate

8. Current focused evaluations and reviews as appropriate

9. Compliance as applied to other professional categories and disciplines to provide process and procedures that are compatible with and supportive of the needs and objectives of the program.

SUMMARY

We have seen a change in the delivery of health care that as a result of an attempt to control costs has expanded the concept of ambulatory care to replace much of institutional care. As we move to the next century, these trends will continue.

What is important to recognize is that without the ability to walk, much of what is projected as ambulatory care is impossible. Thus, podiatric medicine is a key catalyst to our future health care system.

BIBLIOGRAPHY

American Diabetes Association: Therapy for Diabetes and Related Disorders. Alexandria, VA, American Diabetes Association, 1991.

Barker LR, Burton JR, Zieve PD: Principles of Ambulatory Medicine, ed 2. Baltimore, Williams & Wilkins, 1986.

Calkins E, Davis PJ, Ford AB (eds): The Practice of Geriatrics. Philadelphia, WB Saunders, 1986.

Davidson JK: Clinical Diabetes Mellitus. New York, Thieme Medical Publishers, 1986.

Eisdorfer C (ed): Annual Review of Gerontology and Geriatrics, vol 4. New York, Springer Publishing Co, 1984.

Eng W: Geriatric Podiatry, Geriatric Curriculum Resource Guides for Health Professionals. Richmond, VA, Virginia Commonwealth University, Geriatric Education Center, 1986–1987.

Helfand AE (ed): Clinical Podogeriatrics. Baltimore, Williams & Wilkins, 1981.

Helfand AE (ed): Public Health and Podiatric Medicine. Baltimore, Williams & Wilkins, 1987.

Helfand AE, Bruno J (eds): Rehabilitation of the foot. Clin Podiatr 1(2), 1984.

Jessett DF, Helfand AE: Foot problems in the elderly. In Pathy MSJ (ed): Principles and Practice of Geriatric Medicine, ed 2. Edinburgh, John Wiley & Sons, 1991.

Kozak GP, Hoar CS Jr, Rowbotham JL, et al: Management of the Diabetic Foot. Philadelphia, WB Saunders, 1984.

Levin ME, O'Neal LW (eds): The Diabetic Foot, ed 4. St. Louis, CV Mosby, 1988.

Levy LA, Hetherington VJ: Principles and Practice of Podiatric Medicine. New York, Churchill Livingstone, 1990.

Libow LB, Sherman FT (eds): The Core of Geriatric Medicine. St. Louis, CV Mosby, 1981.

McCarthy DJ (ed): Podiatric Dermatology. Baltimore, Williams & Wilkins, 1986.

Neale D, Adams I (eds): Common Foot Disorders: Diagnosis and Management, ed 2. Edinburgh, Churchill Livingstone, 1985.

Rakel RE: Textbook of Family Practice, ed 4. Philadelphia, WB Saunders, 1990.

Reichel W (ed): Clinical Aspects of Aging, ed 2. Baltimore, Williams & Wilkins, 1983.

Steinberg FU: Care of the Geriatric Patient, ed 6. St. Louis, CV Mosby, 1983.

US Department of Health and Human Services, Public Health Service, National Institutes of Health: Feet First. Publication No. 0-388-126. Washington, DC, US Government Printing Office, 1970.

Williams TF (ed): Rehabilitation in the Aging. New York, Raven Press, 1984.

Wilson LB, Simon SP, Baxter CR (eds): Handbook of Geriatric Emergency Care. Gaithersburg, MD, Aspen Systems Corporation, 1984.

Yale I, Yale JF: The Arthritic Foot and Related Connective Tissue Disorders. Baltimore, Williams & Wilkins, 1984.

Yale JF: Yale's Podiatric Medicine, ed 3. Baltimore, Williams & Wilkins, 1987.

CHAPTER 4

COMMUNICATION

Jeffrey M. Robbins
Marvin Boren

Communication is the transfer of information, ideas, understanding, or feelings between persons. Effective communication is essential for the well-being of any medical practice.

Communication occurs when the sender obtains his or her intended results from the receiver. The sender has a message to communicate to another person, the receiver (Fig. 4–1). The sender must first encode the message in such a way that the receiver will understand the message. The channel or medium of transmission can be in verbal or nonverbal form, such as speaking, writing, drawing, or body language. After transmission of the message the receiver must then decode the message to his or her own frame of reference, thereby understanding the message. The receiver then responds to the message in the form of feedback and allows the sender to know that the message was accurately received. Feedback is essentially the same transmission process except now the receiver becomes the sender and vice versa.

Although the communication process is simple enough, there are many barriers or obstacles along the path to effective communication. These barriers are present at each step of the process. The sender may not convey the message clearly. Often there are multiple competing or conflicting messages. As an example, suppose a practitioner has an office policy that pediatric patients are not to be left unattended. Yet in need of assistance, the practitioner hurriedly summons a nurse to another treatment room. Obviously, the nurse must choose between two conflicting messages.

Unintended messages are another source barrier. These are often in nonverbal form. For example, reassuring forgiveness verbally accompanied by a look of disgust sends a conflicting message.

Barriers in transmission are particularly ominous when the message must follow a chain of command. A practitioner informs the office manager that a specific patient should take her medication *only when she needs it*. The office manager tells the patient to take the medication *whenever she needs it.* The office manager has misinterpreted the practitioner's instruction and passed the wrong message to the patient. The greater the number of channels through which the message must pass, the more likely that the message will be altered.

The receiver's behavior can also present as a barrier. For example, if a practitioner is speaking to an internist about a mutual patient's progress, the internist may be prejudgmental because of his or her attitude toward podiatry. Other barriers in the receiver may include lack of interest, misinterpretation, and thinking about a response rather than listening.

Barriers in feedback are essentially the same as in transmission since now the receiver becomes the sender.

In practice, the podiatrist communicates with three general populations. He or she communicates with patients, office staff, and other health care professionals. Both patient communication and office staff communication are typically related to directing and controlling performance and therefore considered downward communication. The key to success with both of these audiences is to make sure that this downward communication does not lead the receiver into thinking that he or she is being talked down to.

Communication between colleagues and other health care professionals is considered lateral communication and generally involves the transfer of information.

PHYSICIAN–PATIENT COMMUNICATION

One of the greatest challenges for the new practitioner is learning to communicate effectively with patients. A great deal has been said about doctors' poor bedside manner or their inability to communicate effectively with patients. Some doctors have a natural ability to communicate with patients, while others are ill at ease and seem to struggle through the process. Nonetheless, practice can help even the most awkward practitioner.

The presumed goal of the practitioner is to accurately diagnose a patient's condition so that an effective management strategy can be developed. Patients will occasionally present with a dichotomy of thought. They will want to supply enough information needed to diagnose their problem, and, at the some time, they may select what information they reveal for fear of a life-threatening diagnosis or a painful test or procedure. Other patients may be poor historians for a variety of other reasons, including age and mental capacity. Using effective communication techniques, the effective practitioner is able to obtain all the data necessary to manage patients' problems.

The patient information transfer process

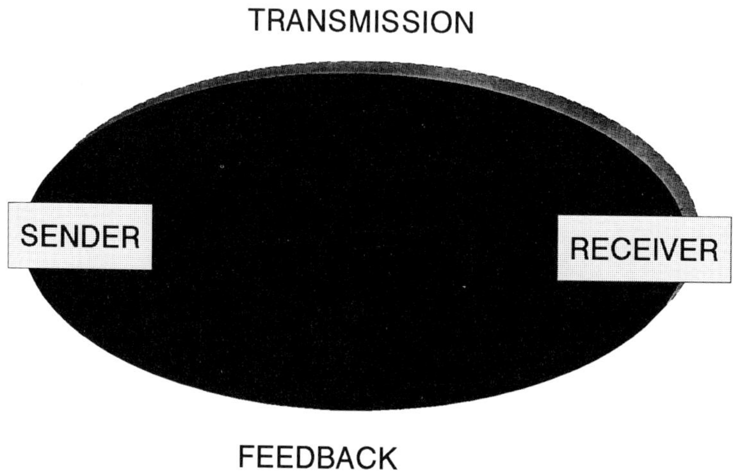

TRANSMISSION

SENDER

RECEIVER

FEEDBACK

FIGURE 4–1. Fundamental factors in communication.

can be broken down into three communication dimensions: facilitation, transition, and action.

Facilitation

The facilitation dimension begins the communication process by establishing rapport with the patient. This will set the tone for the rest of the practitioner–patient interaction. Failure to establish an effective rapport with the patient may jeopardize the entire process.

The first meeting of any two persons is anxiety producing; add the potential for "pain," and it becomes frightening for some patients. Thus, it is important for the practitioner to project warmth and empathy during the first encounter with the patient to elicit the respect and confidence from the patient that the practitioner needs to be effective. Projecting empathy seems to be one of the most important parts of facilitation. We have all had experiences with health care practitioners whom we thought were the "best in town" because they seemed to understand our problems. There are few persons who can "fake" empathy, and most patients can tell if they are being patronized.

Negative judgment of the patient is a common pitfall in establishing a rapport. It is human nature to make first-impression judgments, both good and bad; however, the practitioner must not allow a negative first impression to interfere with establishing the trust and respect that patients must have in their health care providers.

Respect must be obtained in the facilitation process. This works both ways. As a physician, the practitioner must show respect for the patient by treating him or her with respect. The patient must respect the practitioner as the physician through his or her conduct during the initial visit and subsequent treatment visits. When a patient is referred by another physician or patient, that patient brings with him or her a certain amount of respect. The rest is up to the practitioner. Respect is earned, not demanded.

Verbal Communication. The practitioner should communicate with patients on their level. Using long, complicated terms does not impress but, rather, confuses and sometimes irritates patients. Patients like to feel that their physician really understands their needs. The most common complaint by patients is that the physician does not listen or allow them to ask questions. By taking time with the patient and showing compassion, the practitioner is likely to see rapport develop more quickly.

Nonverbal Communication. Nonverbal communication from the patient can be very helpful to the practitioner. Body language is often a subconscious display of one's feelings or emotions. The practitioner should observe these clues. For instance, a patient with his or her legs and arms crossed will probably be a little less trusting and may require more explaining than the patient who seems more open. Observe the patient's facial expression and posture.

The best initial method of projecting warmth and caring is through nonverbal means. A practitioner's pleasant, caring smile will make a patient more comfortable than a stern serious expression. It is also important not to invade a patient's "private space." A person's "private space" represents 8 to 10 inches from his or her body. Violating "private space" will make the patient uncomfortable and defensive. This is considered personal territory, and breaking this boundary is threatening to patients.

The human touch is one of the most effective methods of projecting a warm, caring attitude. Each time a practitioner touches a patient he or she will project a message based on touch. In addition a practitioner can "read" how a patient is feeling by touch. A patient who is anxious may react by pulling away slightly when first touched. Gently holding a foot while taking a pulse can project warmth and show the patient gentle caring. Of course one must be sure the circumstances are appropriate, since some patients might receive the wrong message. Male physicians must be cautious with female patients and vice versa. In this situation we recommend having an office assistant present for examinations or leaving the room door open during an examination.

THE FIRST ENCOUNTER

The approach to the patient on the first encounter should seem unhurried. A firm handshake, a smile, and immediate eye contact tells the patient that he or she is the most important person in the room and the focus of attention. The practitioner should introduce himself or herself and any other personnel in the room at this time. This should be conducted in a formal but cordial manner. The next few minutes are spent in light social conversation until a more easy-going atmosphere is established. At this point the practitioner can elicit the reason the patient has sought out advice and counsel concerning a foot problem.

THE INITIAL INTERVIEW: INQUIRY STRATEGY

The initial interview seeks to establish the purpose of the patient's visit as well as to articulate the practitioner's role. The chief complaint as stated by the patient is the most logical place to start. This initial query should use an open-ended type of question, such as "What brings you to the office today?" The practitioner must also determine the competency level of the patient as a historian. This determination will direct which type of inquiry strategy to use.

The doctor must control the interview if efficient information transfer is to occur. Some patients will ramble aimlessly if allowed and must be kept focused and controlled until a diagnostic conclusion is reached. Tangential conversation confuses both the patient and the interviewer and may obscure important clinical clues. Controlling questions and answers involves interview strategy, which employs two question types, direct and indirect, and four question subtypes, open ended, closed ended, leading, and loaded.

During the initial data-gathering exchange it is recommended that a combination of direct and indirect questions be used. The use of statements designed to express concern and empathy for the patient's problem will help put the patient at ease and facilitate information gathering. The physician might say, "I understand your concern, tell me more about how this happened."

Direct Questions. Direct questions can be open or closed and are true questions in that they require specific information from the patient. Simple, direct questions are short, to the point, and require a "yes" or "no" answer. An example is "Does your foot hurt at night?"

These types of questions are challenging to the patient because they are direct and should be used only when necessary so patients do not become defensive.

Indirect Questions. Indirect questions are less threatening because they can be posed as statements requiring differentiation or affirmation. An example might be, "I imagine this pain makes walking very difficult." This type of question is not confrontational and will facilitate the interview. The patient is invited to respond with a short affirmation or expand on how the pain limits activities. If a patient volunteers too much information with this type of question, a more focused type of inquiry strategy may be necessary.

Open-Ended Questions. The short, open-ended question is generally used to obtain the chief complaint. For example, the practitioner might ask, "What brings you to the office?" This type of question solicits information and encourages the patient to answer in his or her own fashion. It will offer an insight into the patient's emotional reaction to the illness, as well as the patient's competence as a historian. The open-ended question gives the practitioner a significant amount of information and will direct the rest of the interview strategy.

Closed-Ended Questions. Closed-ended questions focus on specific details of the chief complaint. They will clarify, quantify, and qualify the clinician's suspicions and test differential diagnostic hypotheses. These question should not be biased or lead the patient into a particular answer but rather should be neutral and unbiased so that the information elicited is accurate. Examples include "When did the pain start?", "How much does it hurt?", and "What type of pain is it?"

Leading Questions. A leading question is used to test the reliability of information gathered. It will suggest to a patient one answer over another and is therefore biased. For example, after obtaining a history that seems to lead to the conclusion of intermittent claudication, the following leading question may sum up the clinician's suspicions: "Would you say that the calf pain always occurs after walking one block and is relieved by standing still?"

Loaded Questions. Loaded questions are also biased and are used to study the reaction of the patient. They tend to be confrontational, and thus significant rapport and trust are needed before using this type of question. "Do you really want to lose your foot?" might be asked of a noncompliant diabetic who has not followed home care for an infected ulcer, and "Do you want to develop a nonunion of this fracture?" might be asked of an athlete who insists on participating on a fractured metatarsal.

Transition

The second dimension is the transition dimension. Now that the practitioner has laid the basis of trust, respect, and caring, he or she must begin to get more specific and somewhat more threatening to the patient. If good rapport has been established, this dimension will be easier.

Now the practitioner should expect the patient to become more concrete or specific. To accomplish this, the practitioner must be more concrete or specific in his or her questioning of the patient. Genuineness and self-disclosure are two strategies that will facilitate information gathering.

Genuineness refers to the physician's ability to be real or honest. The level of honesty must be timed so as not to "turn off" the patient by being too brutal. This genuineness will help build trust and confidence in the physician–patient relationship.

The following case illustrates the importance of persevering with honest disclosure during the transition stage:

Case Study

A patient who was hemiplegic due to a recent stroke presented to our office. She had progressive contracture of the digits on her left side and walked with the assistance of a walker. She was a worrier and cried about her inability to control her left side, expressing her frustration and determination to recover full function. Significant time was devoted to listening to the patient's problem and expressing understanding and concern for her problems. She was not a surgical candidate and was assured that we would do everything conservatively to make her as comfortable as possible and return as much function as was possible. Her ability as a receiver of information was selective; she heard what she wanted to and blocked out the rest. As a selective listener, she heard that everything would be done and that she would be back to "normal."

On the second visit, the patient asked when she could expect her foot to return to normal. Since significant time had been devoted to establishing a rapport with the patient, on this visit she was told more specifically that the stroke had damaged her left foot and that it would not improve, but that she was fortunate that she was able to walk and get around as well as she did. This was communicated in a sincere and gentle manner expressing the genuineness and honesty required. The patient was upset about the permanence of her condition and required some time to accept her condition.

The empathetic tone of the explanation by the clinician facilitated the transfer of information and avoided a confrontation. The patient left the office with a much more positive attitude, recognizing her problem for what it was and grateful she had as much function as she had.

The timing of this confrontation (which is part of the next dimension) was important in this case. Sometimes a practitioner has to give bad news to a patient. If he or she can do it in a positive manner, it makes it easier for the patient. One analogy that might be used is to describe a glass filled halfway with water. The glass may be viewed as being half full or half empty. The practitioner's glass should always be half full.

Another strategy that facilitates information transfer is self-disclosure. Self-disclosure refers to the physician's calming the patient's fears by sharing of his or her experience or another patient's experience with the same condition the patient has. This has to be used with caution so as not to risk "stealing the spotlight" from the patient.

Action

The third and final dimension is action. This is the most threatening and confrontational dimension.

Confrontation refers to the inevitable point of assisting patients to face the reality of their situation. This is more easily accomplished when rapport is well established and the progression of information gathering and information delivery is developed properly.

A common patient attitude is "I do not care what you do, just fix my foot problem." This attitude places all responsibility for the patient's problem on the podiatrist. It is up to the podiatrist to explain that the condition is the patient's and that only through the combined efforts of podiatrist and patient can it be effectively managed.

The action dimension involves the essential information transfer from practitioner to patient. Here the provisional diagnosis is explained to the patient and the management strategy is discussed. Once presented with all of the treatment options, the practitioner makes his or her recommendation to the patient. It is important to remember that the treatment option is the patient's choice.

MANAGEMENT PRINCIPLES

The diagnosis and treatment of a patient's problem are explained clearly in words the patient is likely to understand. A diagram board (nonverbal communication) can be used to illustrate procedures and diagnosis and to facilitate understanding. An informed patient will have greater confidence in the doctor and in the patient's own ability to make a decision. The use of unpleasant words such as "pain" or "shot" should be avoided. Instead, words such as "discomfort" or phrases such as "we are going to put some medicine in there" can be used. This delivers the message in a less-threatening manner. Certain words, such as "always," "never," "permanent," and "I'm sure," should rarely be used. Instead, one can use "usually," "rarely," "it shouldn't recur," and "I'm confident" in their place. Many persons take what the physician says literally. For example, after being told an ingrown nail will be permanently corrected, the patient may be very upset if it recurs. It is important to inform patients of all the common complications of treatment. Informed consent is a patient's right.

PATIENT EDUCATION

The success of treatment will depend on how well the patient follows instructions for treatment, such as taking medications as prescribed, changing dressings properly, and using the correct soaking solutions. Patients must be properly educated to ensure the success of treatment plans. They must be educated to recognize signs and symptoms of developing problems as well as understand basic treatment skills. The best way to educate patients is through a combination of verbal and written instructions.

Some therapies are confusing and complicated, as illustrated on the following example:

Case Study

A 78-year-old man presents with chronic tinea pedis. The following strategy is recommended: "Soak your feet three times daily in a quart of warm, not hot, water and 1 tablespoon of Epsom salts. Soak for 15 to 20 minutes each time. After you soak make sure that you dry your feet well by patting and not by rubbing, making sure to dry between each toe. I have given you a prescription for an antifungal cream that I want you to apply twice daily after your soak. Preferably this should be after your first soak and your last soak. Your condition is a chronic one and will require treatment for at least 4 to 6 weeks and then additional prophylactic hygiene care thereafter. This will include continued care in drying your foot after bathing, daily use of antifungal foot powder, and spraying of a disinfectant to your shoes once weekly."

Even the most attentive patients would probably have trouble remembering everything in this plan. A 78-year-old person may have additional cognitive problems that may serve as an additional barrier to information transfer and compliance. Written instructions are one of the best facilitators for lengthy and complicated management strategies. They provide patients with a reference and help them follow instructions precisely, improving the chances for success. Written instructions will also enable the patient to participate to the degree the health care provider expects and will lessen patient frustration. Figure 4–2 is an example of the written instructions for this case.

COMMUNICATION WITH OTHER HEALTH CARE PROFESSIONALS

The next level of communication to be explored is between the doctor and other health care professionals. This is considered lateral communication since persons involved are of similar status.

In this category, the medical record is perhaps the single most important communication tool in medical practice. It allows for information organization and recall for the practitioner and communicates the relevant facts about the patient to other health care personnel.

In addition to the medical record, *referrals* and *consultations* involve communication with other health care professionals.

Problem-Oriented Medical Records

The problem-oriented system of medical records, originally developed by Weed in 1969,

establishes a logical system for patient care and the documentation of facts pertaining to the patient's care. It organizes the clinical reasoning process and allows clinicians to address multiple clinical problems. The basic components of the problem-oriented record are listed below:

1. The database. This list includes the chief complaint, present illness, patient profile, review of systems, physical examination, and laboratory results.
2. The complete problem list. This is usually a single sheet in the front of the chart that lists the patient's current and past problems.
3. Initial plans. Each problem on the problem list has a plan for diagnostic workup, a management strategy, and patient education goals.
4. Progress note. The progress note consists of the *s*ubjective or symptomatic, the *o*bjective, the *a*ssessment, and the *p*lan (SOAP):

∎ The *subjective* section is a description of how the patient interprets the problem. This is a statement made by the patient and is usually placed in quotation marks. If the patient is unable to communicate,

John Doe, DPM
123 Main Street
Anytown, USA 11111
(999) 555-1212

Patient _____ Date _____

You have a chronic fungal infection of your feet. The following home treatment guide is provided for your convenience. Please call our office if you have any questions or concerns.

SOAKS
1. Fill a container large enough for both feet with 1 gallon of warm water and 4 tablespoons of Epsom salts.
2. Soak your feet three times daily.

PROPER DRYING
3. Dry foot by patting, not rubbing dry; make sure to dry between each toe.

TOPICAL ANTIFUNGAL AGENT
4. Apply the prescribed cream to entire foot and between toes *once daily, twice daily*, or (other) _____

DISINFECTANT
5. Spray Lysol into shoes once weekly to disinfect shoes.
6. Use an antifungal foot powder daily.

PREVENTIVE CARE
7. Because this is a chronic condition, steps 3, 5, and 6 should be performed regularly.
    Dry foot by patting, not rubbing dry; make sure to dry between each toe.
    Spray Lysol into shoes once weekly to disinfect shoes.
    Use an antifungal foot powder daily.

FIGURE 4–2. An example of written instructions for a patient with chronic tinea pedis.

then an indication of who is doing the communicating is necessary in the subjective.

■ The *objective* should include all facts that are independently observed and are unbiased. This section should be arranged by each practitioner in a specific sequence for consistency, such as blood pressure, pulses, description of lesions or observable findings, laboratory results, and so on.

■ The *assessment* includes the diagnosis as well as how data are analyzed (probable diagnosis) and/or how the current or past treatment is supported by the observable data in the objective.

■ The *plan* includes all of the diagnostic and therapeutic modalities used in the management process. It should list the medications used, examination and laboratory procedures, diagnostic tests, patient education, and instructions for follow up. The plan acts as the practitioner's memory for the next visit so that continuity is maintained.

Referrals

Referral letters are sent when the podiatrist thinks that the patient's condition would be

best treated by another podiatrist or health care specialist. These circumstances will differ from practitioner to practitioner based on levels of training and competencies. A letter of referral should be brief and include the following information:

1. Introduction
   ■ Request examination and treatment
   ■ Identify the patient
   ■ Briefly explain the patient's problem

2. Patient data
   ■ History
   ■ Physical examinations
   ■ Special examinations
   ■ Laboratory examinations

3. Interpretation of data
   ■ Hypothesis
   ■ Differential diagnosis

4. Closing

See Figure 4–3 for a sample referral letter.

Consultations

A consultation letter or report of findings is sent in response to a letter of referral that the podiatrist has received from the patient's pri-

---

John Doe, DPM
123 Main Street
Anytown, USA 11111
(999) 555-1212

Dear Dr. _____ :

I am referring Mrs. Jane Doe to your office for evaluation and treatment of her severe calf pain, which I believe is due to occlusive arterial disease. Jane Doe is a 58-year-old woman who has been complaining of severe calf pain for the past 3 months.

Pertinent history and physical examination revealed the following results:

Calf pain when walking one block that is relieved with standing
Smoking history of 40 pack-years
Nonpalpable dorsalis pedis and tibialis posterior pulses in both feet
Ankle–arm index 0.54 left and 0.6 right

Based on my clinical examination, I believe this patient has some type of occlusive arterial problem. I am referring Mrs. Doe for evaluation and treatment of her vascular condition. I will continue to provide podiatric care for her.

Please contact me with your findings at your earliest convenience.

Sincerely,

John Doe, DPM

FIGURE 4–3. A sample referral letter.

John Doe, DPM
123 Main Street
Anytown, USA 11111
(919) 555-1212

Dear Dr. _____ :

Thank you for referring _____ to our office. We greatly appreciate the confidence you
have shown in us. As you know, _____ presented with a chief complaint of
_____ .

Examination revealed:

Diagnosis:

Treatment:

Plan:

Once again, thank you for allowing me to see your patient.

Sincerely,

John Doe, DPM

FIGURE 4–4. A sample letter of consultation.

mary physician, or whenever the podiatrist believes that a consultation is indicated. The format is basically the same as that of the referral letter, except that the podiatrist is reporting his or her findings as opposed to requesting an examination. In this letter the podiatrist is responding to the referring physician's request for examination or treatment (Fig. 4–4).

Immediate consultations are performed over the telephone and usually involve patients currently being treated. When a question arises about a patient care issue, it is often necessary to contact another treating physician for information or guidance.

Consideration for the patient's time as well as for the consulting physician's schedule mandates an efficient process for this communication. The chart and all pertinent data should be readily available when the podiatrist is ready to speak to the consultant.

Yet another form of communication with other physicians is to send a letter of progress concerning a new mutual patient (Fig. 4–5). The letter should be brief and include diagnosis, treatment plan, and prognosis as well as an invitation to call if there are any questions. This letter serves several purposes. First, it informs the physician of what the podiatrist treats. Second, it informs the physician that the podiatrist is also seeing the patient. If the

physician receives favorable feedback from his or her patient, referrals are likely to follow. Thank you letters for referrals serve the same purpose.

COMMUNICATION WITH STAFF

Effective interoffice communication is essential to a successful, efficient, and cost-effective primary care office. When communicating with staff, it is critical that mutual respect exists. Rather than command respect, the practitioner must earn it by showing genuine concern and compassion for support staff. Furthermore, the staff will have greater respect when the podiatrist exhibits confidence and self-assurance.

It is often difficult for the student or resident to make the transition into a position of "being the boss." The new practitioner may feel uneasy around older subordinates. In addition, it is not unusual to be uncomfortable with the new title of "doctor." However, as a matter of respect, the practitioner should have office staff address him or her by his or her title rather than by his or her first name.

The opposite of the unassuming new practitioner is the egotistical new practitioner. Now in a position of power and authority, this practitioner feels a need to remind others of his or her position and thus is often overbearing. It is easy to see how the overnight acquisition of such power and authority can go to one's head. Although managing with an "iron fist" may produce a desired result, subordinates act out of fear rather than respect. This typically leads to frustration or burnout, which ultimately causes turnover in staff. A cardinal rule in any business is that turnover is counterproductive. It is therefore of utmost importance that communication with staff be on a level of mutual respect.

A considerable barrier in communication with staff is that the practitioner and staff have different levels of education. This must be recognized so that a common plane of reference can be achieved. Another barrier is that the practitioner often does not realize the needs of subordinates for information that would help them perform their tasks. The practitioner withholds information from subordinates that he or she believes may cloud the tasks at hand. Too much filtering may diminish subordinates' ability to work independently since they are not as well informed.

For example, a common shortcoming in many podiatry offices is that the podiatrist is not explicit enough in scheduling patients for their next appointment. Thus the practitioner loses valuable time from his or her schedule while the staff adjusts to the unexpected. A key to any successful practice is a well-informed staff who are able to anticipate what will be expected of them throughout their daily routine.

A key to establishing effective communication in the podiatric office is to establish a good communication network. If the practitioner must deal with his or her staff when every little question or problem arises, it will divert a great deal of time and energy away from seeing patients. Therefore the practitioner must set up a chain of command or hierarchy within the office. With a small staff there may be no office manager or clearly defined leader. In such a case, responsibilities may be divided with perhaps a clinical leader and a business leader or front office and back office leaders. The goal is to funnel information up and down the hierarchy so that the practitioner is primarily dealing with major decision making. This is not a perfect arrangement, and therefore as a "safety valve" the practitioner should have an "open door policy" allowing staff to bypass the normal chain of command in some instances.

By scheduling regular staff meetings, most

John Doe, DPM
123 Main Street
Anytown, USA 11111
(999) 555-1212

Dear Dr. _____ :

The following progress report concerns a mutual patient of ours, _____ . If you should have any questions regarding his (her) care, please feel free to contact me.

Chief Complaint:

Diagnosis:

Treatment:

Plan:

Sincerely,

John Doe, DPM

FIGURE 4–5. A sample letter of progress.

of these confrontations can be defused, since the entire staff will have the opportunity to air their feelings, opinions, and observations. The podiatrist should encourage staff members to open up and contribute at such meetings. Since much of the staff works independently from the practitioner, the meeting is an excellent opportunity for informing the podiatrist of what is going on in the office. For instance, the podiatrist may have no idea that the patients are complaining about having to wait too long to get an appointment. Or perhaps a particular office policy is outdated and in need of change. It is likewise important for the practitioner to meet with the office manager regularly to keep informed.

One of the greatest measures of job satisfaction among subordinates is feeling appreciated. Therefore the aloof or inattentive practitioner, or one who shows a lack of trust on subordinates, risks low morale and, consequently, less than optimum job performance.

In many offices, individual staff members have no idea how the practitioner perceives their job performance. It is important that the podiatrist has annual employee performance reviews with appropriate salary increases. Such a review should include evaluation of individual job duties and personal characteristics. At the conclusion of the review, goals should be established for the employee to work toward in the coming year. The doctor should praise the staff both collectively and individually when appropriate. When a patient praises the staff for being helpful or kind, the compliment should be passed on to the staff. The staff can also be rewarded collectively when the office performs well.

SUMMARY

The communication process is rife with barriers and obstacles. Understanding this process and having an awareness of the barriers provide the practitioner with the appropriate tools for effective communication. For many it will require time and practice to become proficient. Since medicine is a service industry it is imperative that the practitioner possess good communication skills to be successful. Given adequate clinical results, patients have no idea how good the podiatrist really is. Such judgment is typically based on the image that the podiatrist projects and how well he or she communicates with patients. This perception of quality of care may be independent of true clinical expertise; yet in the eyes of the patient, perception is reality.

Bibliography

Bates B: A Guide to Physical Examination, ed 3. Philadelphia, JB Lippincott, 1983.

Bernstein A: The Practice Builder. CA 5(9), 1987 and 7(6), 1989.

Blondis MN, Jackson BE: Nonverbal Communication with Patients: Back to the Human Touch. New York, Wiley Medical, 1977.

Burnside JW, McGlynn TJ: Physical Diagnosis, ed 17. Baltimore, Williams & Wilkins, 1987.

Eisenberg JM: The Physician's Practice. New York, Wiley Medical, 1980.

Hampton DR: Management. New York, McGraw-Hill Book Company, 1986.

Hurst JH, Walker HK: The Problem Oriented System, pp 23–50. New York, Medcom Press, 1972.

Judge RD, Zuidema GD: Physical Diagnosis: The Physiologic Approach to the Clinical Examination, ed 2. Boston, Little, Brown & Co, 1968.

Judge RD, Zuidema GD, Fitzgerald FT: Clinical Diagnosis, ed 5. Boston, Little, Brown & Co, 1989.

Marcinko DE (ed): Medical and Surgical Therapeutics of the Foot and Ankle, Baltimore, Williams & Wilkins, 1992.

Reschke EM: The Medical Office: Organization and Management. Hagerstown, MD, Harper & Row, 1980.

Sachs L: Do it Yourself Marketing for the Professional Practice. Englewood Cliffs, NJ, Prentice-Hall, 1986.

Seidel HM, Ball JW, Dains JE, et al: Mosby's Guide to Physical Examination. St. Louis, Mosby–Year Book, 1991.

Young CR: Making Your Practice Grow: A Useful Guide for the Medical Care Professional. Detroit, Bracey, 1984.

CHAPTER 5

PSYCHOSOCIAL AND BEHAVIORAL COMPONENTS

Georgia J. Anetzberger

Comprehensive podiatric care requires a holistic perspective. This means that foot disorders can best be understood within a larger context of interrelationships that consider physical well-being as affecting and being affected by personality and culture. Seen in this light, podiatrists must familiarize themselves with the various psychosocial and behavioral problems that patients may present and develop strategies for effectively assessing and dealing with them. Limiting primary care to foot disease and disorder alone may have limited impact when problem dynamics include individual, family, ethnic, and other psychosocial dimensions.

Selected psychosocial and behavioral components of podiatric primary care are examined in this chapter. Particular attention is given to the following:

- Impact of self-concept and self-esteem on health status
- Importance of a wellness perspective for preventing illness
- Effect of ethnicity and minority status on health care
- Sources of community support for patients with identified needs
- Methods for assessing and treating substance abuse and family violence

These certainly are not the only topics that could be included within the context of psychosocial and behavioral components of care. The topics selected, however, do reflect major considerations in the field and provide an opportunity to showcase the diversity of approaches for addressing psychosocial and behavioral problems podiatrists may encounter among their patients.

SELF-CONCEPT AND SELF-ESTEEM

Self-concept and self-esteem may affect individual reaction to disease and impairment. As patients, how we see ourselves (self-concept) and how we feel about ourselves (self-esteem) can impact our ability to resist disease, our willingness to seek help, and our feeling of worth with disability or disfiguring conditions. For instance, a child with a clubfoot may become isolated rather than deal with the rejection of peers. An elderly man may resign himself to the pain of gout in misperception that such health problems are an inevitable part of the aging process.

Likewise, self-concept and self-esteem can influence our capacity to function as health care professionals. Podiatrists with poor self-concept and low self-esteem may have difficulty interacting with patients and their families, responding to patient needs, or recognizing their ability to affect change. Understanding self-concept and self-esteem, therefore, is central to the podiatrist–patient relationship.

Components of Self-Concept

Self-concept represents everything that we identify as characteristic of ourselves. It has four components: (1) body image, (2) role performance, (3) personal identity, and (4) self-esteem.[1]

Body image reflects our concept of physical being and personal space. Although body awareness begins early in life, the concept of physical self changes over time, influenced by social stimuli and physical alteration. Certain experiences tend to disrupt how one's body is perceived. These include loss of body parts, decreased body functioning, and disfigurement. For example, patients with foot amputations may feel "less than whole" or "imperfect." They may refuse to look at or discuss the missing part. They may not recognize their remaining strengths and abilities. Some may even withdraw from social interaction, because they see themselves as "grotesque."

Role performance relates to how well persons fulfill behavioral expectations associated with the positions in society that they occupy. Role performance tends to be compromised under circumstances of role strain, role conflict, and role ambiguity. For instance, a man who sees himself as the family breadwinner may negatively evaluate his performance of that role if an accident and resulting bone fractures keep him out of work for an extended period. Also,

conflict can arise if his wife finds it necessary to return to the work force instead of remaining at home to care for their children.

Personal identity is our sense of individuality. It is what we regard as unique about ourselves and different from others. Personal identity includes our appearance, abilities, goals, talents, values, and personality. It also consists of such memberships and situational characteristics as race, ethnic group, marital status, and schooling. Impairment can disturb personal identity. For an athlete, the onset of arthritis can be devastating. It can be seen as altering personal goals, relationships with team members, and sources for achievement and self-satisfaction.

Self-esteem is perceived as self-worth. It represents our feelings about ourselves. Self-esteem can be positive or negative, depending on the variance between perceived self (how we are seen by ourselves and others) and ideal self (how we would like to be seen). Where the variance is large, low self-esteem can result.

Low self-esteem is illustrated in behaviors that suggest distorted thinking. For example, a woman who cannot accept needing a wheelchair for movement may feel that other persons are staring at her and evaluating all that she does on the basis of her impairment of mobility. She may think, "If diabetes can affect my feet, it can affect other parts of my body as well. What will I lose next?" If she is promoted in her job, she may believe that it has nothing to do with her competencies, but only with an attitude of pity on the part of her employer or her employer's interpretation of disabled rights laws.

Development of Self-Esteem

Four factors relate to the development of self-esteem: (1) significant others, (2) role expectations, (3) crises of psychosocial development, and (4) coping styles.[2]

Significant others are persons who are important during a particular life stage. They can include parents, teachers, friends, and employers. Interaction with these persons provides us with perceptions about ourselves. Their judgments of us tend to become our judgment of ourselves, thereby contributing to our self-esteem.[3]

Every social position has associated with it certain expected behaviors. Persons occupying these positions are evaluated in their successful performance of the expected behaviors. Successful performance typically results in praise, which can foster positive self-esteem. Failure usually results in criticism or blame, which often leads to low self-esteem.

Persons are also expected to master certain developmental tasks throughout their lives. If these tasks are not mastered, problems of self-esteem may result. Eric Erikson has offered eight stages of psychosocial development.[4] They are listed in Table 5–1, along with associated tasks and behaviors suggesting unsatisfactory achievement of these tasks that podiatrists may see exhibited in their patients.

Finally, how persons cope with difficult situations will affect their self-esteem. When they appropriately assert themselves and show effective problem-solving ability, self-esteem is enhanced. On the other hand, when persons fail to claim their just due or pursue unsuccessful courses of action, self-esteem is diminished. Ineffective coping can cause depression, with such symptoms as fatigue, loss of interest in life, difficulty in making decisions, irritability, and social isolation.

Intervention Strategies for Podiatrists

Podiatrists will encounter patients with altered self-concept and self-esteem as a result of illness, disability, or other life experiences. When this occurs, they should consider intervention strategies designed to deal with these problems. Such strategies may include the following:

■ Providing clear and accurate information about the illness or disability
■ Allowing patients to express feelings and concerns
■ Showing support and understanding
■ Emphasizing remaining strengths and abilities
■ Encouraging the receipt of help from significant others
■ Promoting interaction with persons having similar illness or disability

■ Emphasizing independence and self-care, whenever appropriate
■ Referring patients to other professionals and services, when indicated

Although some of these strategies will be discussed in greater detail later in the chapter, two warrant special attention at this time: (1) social support and (2) mutual aid.

SOCIAL SUPPORT

Studies have shown that perception of social support from significant others is more important than the amount of assistance or number of support sources. Factors influencing that perception include the history of the relationship between the helper and recipient as well as the appropriateness of help given.[5, 6]

Help offered by significant others can be informational, emotional, or tangible. It is usually important, however, for the recipient to view the extension of this help as reciprocal. Persons benefit from perceiving that they, too, have something to give in the relationship, that help is not a one-sided phenomenon. Podiatrists can facilitate this perception by pointing out mutual gains from assistance. For instance, the husband who needs help and is unable to work temporarily because of fractures may also be more available to assist his wife with child care.

MUTUAL AID

Likewise, mutual aid can promote positive self-esteem. Contact with others who have the same illness or disability can promote problem solving, a sense of belonging, and empowerment.

Mutual aid can happen during informal interaction or through formal associations, usually designated as self-help groups. The number of self-help groups has grown considerably during the past decade. Many are disease specific, such as those for persons with cancer, multiple sclerosis, or spinal cord injury. Others are age based, like the Older Women's League or the Gray Panthers. The functions of self-help groups include resource sharing, skill training, role modeling, peer support, and advocacy. Self-help groups ordinarily involve small numbers of persons who meet on a reg-

TABLE 5–1. **Examples of Patient Behaviors Suggesting Unsatisfactory Achievement of Erikson's Stages of Psychosocial Development**

Stage	Task	Patient Behavior Suggesting Unsatisfactory Task Achievement
Infancy	Trust vs. mistrust	Unable to request or accept treatment or care
Toddlerhood	Autonomy vs. shame and doubt	Cannot challenge questionable health practices
Early childhood	Initiative vs. guilt	Expresses fear about each new treatment regimen
Early school years	Industry vs. inferiority	Does not follow through with care plans
Adolescence	Identity vs. role confusion	Accepts what professionals say without question
Early adulthood	Intimacy vs. isolation	Avoids close contact with other persons, including those who might offer assistance
Middle age	Generativity vs. stagnation	Always talks about own health problems; does not show concern for others
Old age	Integrity vs. despair	Demands unnecessary care and attention

ular basis. Meetings focus on discussions of member concerns, although occasionally professionals may be invited to address the group.

Certain cautions must be raised in the use of self-help groups to increase self-esteem. Group interaction is not for everyone. Persons who are loners or introspective may be uncomfortable with group activity or self-disclosure. Moreover, a certain amount of monitoring is needed for most group experiences to ensure that individual members positively contribute to group interaction and neither inhibit nor destroy the benefits of exchange.

WELLNESS AND ILLNESS

The Wellness Perspective

Wellness is a lifestyle choice that focuses on preventing illness and avoiding injury. It requires attending to the whole person and makes health maintenance and disease prevention a personal responsibility. Those who adopt a wellness perspective set goals that promote a positive outlook, good nutrition and physical fitness, healthy habits in response to change, balanced stimulation and stability, and nurturing and supportive relationships.

The wellness perspective recognizes the im-

portance of education, skill development, and advocacy in this process. It expects continuous self-evaluation to determine changing health status and needs. Wellness also encourages persons to seek and cooperate with health care professionals for early detection and treatment of disorders.

In recent years, wellness and health promotion have become national pastimes.[7, 8] There probably are several reasons for this:

■ Publication of various research findings that suggest correlations between diseases, such as cancer and stroke, and life choices, such as smoking and diet

■ Recognition that it may be more cost effective to prevent illness and injury than to deal with their consequences

■ Concern of aging "baby boomers" with their changing physical ability, personal appearance, and health

■ Desire to reduce health disparities among Americans

Individual adoption of a wellness perspective can contribute to positive self-concept. For example, body image is enhanced with the weight loss, better muscle tone, and increased physical ability that comes from controlled diet and more exercise. Similarly, self-esteem benefits from goal achievement and increased competencies in areas of health promotion as well as from praise received from significant others who acknowledge the improved attitude and appearance of someone adopting the wellness perspective.

The wellness perspective is framed on the recognition of human needs and the advancement of behaviors that address these needs. Major human needs are security and dependency, growth and independence, and personal uniqueness.[9] In the wellness model, seeking nurturing and supportive relationships recognizes the human need for security and dependency. Promoting balanced stimulation and stability relates to the need for growth and independence. Finally, the emphasis on personal responsibility and action in the wellness perspective acknowledges the human need for personal identity, uniqueness, and development.

When a person adopts a wellness perspective, the relationship between patient and health care professional changes. Because the wellness model is energizing and empowering, those who employ it tend to assume responsibility for their role in health promotion, establish partnerships with health care professionals in the prevention and treatment of disorders, and seek information about their illnesses or injuries and explore the benefits and risks of recommended treatment strategies.

Reactions to Illness

Underlying the wellness perspective is an understanding of illness and the behavioral responses to it. Each of the four attributes of illness can affect the person experiencing it and significant others: identity, causes, duration, and consequences.[10]

The identification of illness, including its symptoms and diagnosis, can be frightening and confusing. Those involved wonder what is happening and who can help. The causes of illness may lead to judgments regarding lifestyle or heredity. For example, those who suffer leg pain from a work accident may receive more sympathy and support from significant others than those incurring such pain from obesity caused by overeating. Furthermore, although acute illness may be temporarily disruptive, chronic illness can significantly disrupt lives for many years. Finally, the consequences of illness can be financial, social, or personal, draining resources at every level.

It is little wonder then that the reactions to illness are many and varied. Among the most common are anxiety, hostility, dependence, and rejection. The podiatrist needs to be aware of these possible reactions and have strategies to blunt their potential negative effect.

Anxiety is probably the most common reaction to illness. Anxiety connotes uneasiness and dread. For instance, the person with newly diagnosed diabetes asks, "What does this mean for me? How will my life change?"

Anxious persons may perspire, pace, or speak in a shaking voice. They may appear breathless or have difficulty concentrating. The podiatrist should be alert to these signs and recognize when the anxiety state increases to the point that individual perception is impaired.

Mild anxiety can enhance primary care. The patient's awareness of and interest in therapeutic procedures is heightened at this time. Therefore, learning the details of care and treatment is greater. On the other hand, severe anxiety interferes with primary care, because the patient may panic and distort what is happening. For mild anxiety, patient care should reinforce behaviors and provide feedback to individual activity. For severe anxiety, podiatrists should keep their communication with patients brief and simple. Complicated instructions or discussions of the illness would be missed during this state.

Hostility is one of the most difficult illness reactions to confront. At best it leaves its object uncomfortable, at worst defensive and afraid. Patient hostility is illustrated in argumentative, critical, demanding, or uncooperative behavior at one extreme and threatening, abusive, or destructive behavior at the other.

It is essential to appropriately assess hostility in a patient. Sometimes uncooperativeness, for example, has nothing to do with hostility but rather reflects patient concern about a given procedure. Likewise, patients who demand information to better understand their health status are not being hostile.

Genuine hostility on the part of patients requires measured response. The podiatrist should acknowledge that the patient is distressed and permit expression of these feelings. Limits have to be set when destructive behaviors are exhibited. Patients cannot be allowed to break things or hit anyone under any circumstances. Alternative means of expression or "time out" should be encouraged. When the episode subsides, the podiatrist can resume discussion around the patient's feelings of hostility, seeking causes and resolutions using appropriate problem-solving techniques.

Dependence is another frequent response to illness, with patients sometimes regressing to earlier developmental stages characterized by helplessness, self-absorption, and lack of responsibility. A certain amount of dependence is often necessary to achieve wellness. For instance, the elderly man with gout in his foot may need help with housekeeping when the condition is acute. Dependence is inappropriate, however, when the assistance demanded is unnecessary. This would be the case if the elderly man also demanded help with eating and grooming.

Finally, *rejection* can be a response to illness, especially when the illness is long term or stigmatized. Persons with chronic impairments may feel cut off from significant others and lonely. They may believe that no one cares. Those with stigmatized disorders, including athelete's foot, may sense a rejection or avoidance from others at certain times.

Podiatrists should validate feelings of rejection when they are expressed by patients, commenting that these are within the range of human emotions that all of us experience occasionally. Podiatrists should also demonstrate acceptance of patients and their illness, as they explore with them past measures found successful in alleviating feelings of rejection that may be helpful now as well.

ETHNIC ISSUES ON HEALTH CARE

The United States has always been characterized by ethnic diversity. From our beginnings, various cultures, races, and religions were found in most geographic areas. What has changed, however, is our recognition of ethnic diversity and belief that it should be nurtured.

In our early history, Americans emphasized assimilation for immigrant groups. It was expected that new arrivals to this country would conform to prevailing norms and customs. Later, amalgamation was popularized in the metaphor of America as a "melting pot," where persons from all over the world would come together and fuse, producing a new and better amalgam that combined the best of each of the ethnic groups represented. More recently, accommodation has been valued. Here the emphasis is on cultural pluralism, with immigrants becoming Americanized at the same time that they retain some of their distinct cultural heritages.[11]

Despite its popular appeal, it is unlikely that the melting pot theory ever completely applied to the United States, where some immigrant groups were forced to maintain ethnic ties almost in self-defense and others did so in steadfast belief in the superiority of their culture over others. The Japanese and Amish illustrate these respective patterns.

The discrediting of the melting pot theory began with the civil rights movement of the 1960s and 1970s. For the first time, various ethnic groups wanted acknowledgment on the basis of their distinctiveness and demanded the same opportunities as anyone else without having to camouflage this distinctiveness. In addition, the attitude toward immigrant groups has changed in recent years. As our country has become more settled and jobs and land scarcer, Americans have been less welcoming to new arrivals, even those coming here as a result of oppression, civil unrest, or economic disaster in their homelands. This lack of welcoming attitude may have resulted in a prolonged maintenance of ethnic ties. Finally, myths and stereotypes about genetic or cultural inferiority increasingly have been called into question as various ethnic groups have achieved material success in the United States after arriving here destitute. The Jews and Vietnamese illustrate this pattern.

Current emphasis on ethnicity may reflect other phenomena as well. Some of the newer ethnic groups have been so large in certain locales that they have dominated politics and culture there. This is true of Cubans in Miami, Florida, and Mexicans in San Antonio, Texas. Moreover, Glazer and Moynihan[12] suggest that ethnic identity may have replaced occupational identity as important among working-class Americans, since the occupational identities among this class have lost much of their glamor. Although these researchers made their observation in the late 1960s, this tendency may have more significance today, with further decline of labor unions, rise in education, increase in white collar jobs, and growing participation of women in the labor force.

Definitions of ethnicity focus on the characteristics of persons that distinguish them from others. These characteristics reflect cultural heritages that are passed on from generation to generation. All ethnic groups have some ethnocentrism or belief in their own heritage as superior to all others. Sometimes, however, ethnocentrism results in attitudes and behavior that subordinate other groups. A minority group is one that is set apart or subordinated from another group. It is usually smaller in size, but not always. On the other hand, it always has unequal access to power.

In the United States, ethnicity and minority status sometimes go hand-in-hand. African Americans and Hispanics are both ethnic and minority groups. Women, however, although not an ethnic group, are a minority group, and German Americans, although possibly an ethnic group, do not represent a minority one.

The 1990 US census presents the following breakdown of Americans by major racial or ethnic grouping: 80.3% white, 12.1% black, 9% Hispanic, 2.9% Asian, 0.8% Native American, and 3.9% others. Metropolitan areas have the greatest racial and ethnic diversity, with Los Angeles, California, the most diverse, and Dubuque, Iowa, the least. Among the states, New Mexico, with its large percentages of Native Americans and Hispanics, is the most racially and ethnically diverse, and Vermont, the least.[13]

It is important for podiatrists and other health care professionals to be aware of ethnicity and minority status and their effect on health care. Part of this awareness relates to the podiatrist's own culture and status, so they are not imposed on patients without knowledge of the consequences. Part, too, relates to the culture and status patients bring to health care that serve to guide their health practices and decisions.

The influence of culture on health has long been recognized.[14, 15] Certain illnesses have been identified as culture bound rather than resulting from biological or psychological malfunctioning.[16, 17] Likewise, treatment strategies have been found beneficial that stress the principles of cultural care.[18] Assessment tools, for example, have been developed that are based on the premise that patients have a right to their cultural beliefs and practices, and these factors should be recognized and respected.[19, 20]

Various domains listed in culturological assessments suggest the ways in which ethnic groups differ and the influence this can have on health practices. For instance, gender roles may be important for determining who makes decisions relative to health care. In Mexican American families, it is typically the father; among Jews, it is the mother. Ethnic differences in respect for age can have a similar effect. The Native American regard for advanced age means that the opinion of elderly family members may be more highly valued than that of younger members.

Language and communication patterns can impact understanding of health issues. If podiatrists and patients speak different languages, the description of symptoms may not be clear, leading to inaccurate diagnoses. Even body language can influence professional–patient relationships and ultimately health care. Podiatrists should recognize that each culture attaches its own meaning to eye contact and personal space. Although Anglo-Americans may like eye contact, Asians may find it disrespectful. Immigrants from southern European countries prefer closer distance when talking than do those from northern European countries. Time is also viewed differently across ethnic groups. Middle-class Americans are more future oriented and willing to schedule medical appointments well in advance. Present-oriented Hispanics would rather attend to health care on an as-needed or even crisis basis.

Ethnic food preferences can influence compliance with care plans. Some patients may reject a special diet, if it includes unfamiliar foods or violates religious doctrine. Similarly, ethnic attitude about the role of family may affect health decisions. In cultures that emphasize the extended family, as many Native American ones do, the needs of the family as a whole may be prioritized over those of any individual member. Finally, pain, suffering, or grief may be differently expressed by culture. African Americans tend to be more open in grieving the loss of a loved one than are Japanese Americans.

Just as ethnicity can influence health beliefs and practices, so, too, can minority status. The major effect here, however, is the creation of access barriers to health care. Discrimination and social inequities can deny persons access to quality health care. Lack of financial resources, including health insurance as a result of unemployment or employment in the secondary labor market, may reduce the use of health care or delay treatment until very advanced stages. Different definitions of what constitutes health, framed in expectations resulting from differential socialization, may result in a failure to appreciate health promotion strategies and a continuance of risky behaviors.

Folk Medicine

The importance of folk medicine cannot be overstated in dealing with ethnic groups. For many, folk remedies may be the first and preferred treatment, with traditional Western medicine considered only when folk remedies have failed. As a result, it is useful for podiatrists to determine what folk remedies have been employed and benefits derived before recommending further treatment. At times it may be desirable to encourage patients to continue these remedies, provided there are no ill effects and they promote the patient's well-being.

Folk remedies are many and varied and include herbs, roots, charms, and voodoo. They are preferred by many groups over traditional Western medicine as being more humanistic, familiar, practical, holistic, and inexpensive. Also, since traditional Western medicine encourages much treatment in hospitals or other institutions by professionals, rather than at home by family and friends, it is regarded as more frightening and alien than folk medicine.

Each of the four major racial or ethnic groups in the United States has a long history

in the use of folk medicine and home remedies. For example, among rural, southern blacks the "old lady" or "granny" is the local consultant for common ailments and is well versed in the use of herbs, roots, and home remedies.[21] Among Native Americans are several types of healers, including those who only heal; those who only identify the causes of illness; those who also can cause illness; those who offer specialized treatment, such as herbologists; those who heal the soul; and those who cure by singing.[22]

Guidelines for the Practitioner

Working with patients representing various ethnic and minority groups requires podiatrists to be knowledgeable, sensitive, and encouraging. More specifically, it is important to

- Understand that ethnic and minority groups are not monolithic
- Learn the beliefs, values, and practices of those groups found in the geographic area served
- Convey respect for individual and group beliefs, values, and practices
- Begin with the patient's definition of the illness, and appreciate measures already taken for prevention or treatment of the illness
- Develop mechanisms to increase communication, including the appropriate use of body language and personal space, along with the application of alternative teaching tools, such as audiovisual aids
- Consider transportation, community safety, and financial issues that relate to health care access
- Involve family support
- Emphasize advocacy and assertiveness for securing entitlements and services

SOURCES OF HELP IN THE COMMUNITY

Illness can render persons unable to function independently or perform their usual tasks. Likewise, persons may be left vulnerable or alone because of special problems or changed circumstances, such as crime, poverty, or widowhood. At these times help is needed. Because podiatrists may be important vehicles for identifying, evaluating, and accessing help for their patients, they should be familiar with the range available in the community.

This section begins with an overview on support networks and resource systems for persons in need. Throughout, particular attention is given to

■ Categorization of help
■ Resource limitations
■ Preference of help recipients
■ Role of health care professionals, especially podiatrists

The focus is placed on resources available for elderly persons. This focus is justified on three counts. First, the aged represent the fastest growing segment of American society.[23] Second, as a group they are the most likely to need and seek health care, along with social services and supportive housing.[24] Third, the resource system for the aged is more extensive than that available to any other special population; therefore, it represents a model of the diversity that is, or could be, available for other groups needing assistance.

There are three sources of help: (1) self-help, (2) informal network, and (3) formal network. Self-help was discussed earlier in the context of mutual aid and self-help groups. In general, self-help suggests personal resources (individual characteristics that facilitate competence). The most important of these in social interactions are communication skills, patience, adequate goal setting, and ego strength.[25] Collectively these characteristics enable persons to function well in most settings. Although their origins are found in both experience and temperament, the evolution of these characteristics is predicted on a person's track record of competence and incompetence.[26] Capacity for self-help also reflects self-concept and self-esteem. Those persons with altered self-concept and low self-esteem typically have reduced capacity for self-help.

Informal vs. Formal Networks

The informal network includes two sources of help. The first consists of family, friends, and neighbors. The second source includes other established community relationships, such as those held with persons in the workplace, at the beauty shop or bar, or through membership in religious, civic, social, or political associations.

The importance of the informal network as a source of help cannot be overstated. To illustrate, family and friends represent 80% of the help received by older persons.[27, 28] In this context, the spouse is the primary caregiver, followed by adult children (especially daughters and daughters-in-law). For those without children, siblings are important, and for those without family, friends and neighbors assume surrogate caregiving roles.[29] Older persons usually prefer the informal network as a source of help because of a belief in family responsibility, feelings of comfort with family and friends, and desire to keep private matters related to health and other areas of need.

The formal network consists of the vast array of agencies, institutions, professionals in private practice, and housing facilities that are organized to address human needs. There are many ways to categorize the resources of the formal network, some of which are indicated in Table 5–2.

Generally those who need help turn to the informal network first. Only when assistance is

TABLE 5–2. **Ways to Categorize the Formal Network**

Method	Illustration of Resulting Types
By clientele	Dependent and maltreated children
	Delinquents and offenders
	Unemployed
	Mentally impaired
	Physically handicapped
	Veterans
	Aged
By function	Income maintenance
	Housing
	Education
	Health care
	Employment
	Social services
By locale of the resource	Home
	Community setting
	Housing facility
	Communication media
By nature of the service provider	Public
	Voluntary
	Proprietary

unavailable or inadequate from this source do they turn to the formal network. Among the elderly needing help, for example, just 5% of those living in the community receive all of their help from paid sources.[30]

Reluctance to use the formal network in part reflects the traditional American value placed on independence. As humans, we are interdependent.[31] Our capacities and even survival depend on interaction with other persons. On the other hand, as Americans, we place heavy emphasis on self-reliance and "pulling oneself up by one's bootstraps." Hence, our formal network of resources for populations in need, except perhaps for the aged, is less developed than that found in Western Europe or many other industrialized countries.[32] Moreover, we seek assistance primarily only at the extremes of life or during illness.

There are notable differences between the informal network and formal network. They are identified in Table 5–3. Overall they suggest that the informal network is more personal and individually responsive, while the formal network is more professional and structured in service provision. Nonetheless, both play important roles in addressing the varied health and other needs of individuals.

Assisting Informal Caregivers

When members of the informal network provide assistance and support, they are called caregivers. Caregivers assume their role for many reasons:

■ Expression of affection
■ Sense of obligation
■ Return for past favors
■ Religious meaning

■ Fear of alternatives, such as self-neglect or institutionalization

No matter the reason behind the help extended, the caregiving role tends to be maintained even during periods of great stress and personal sacrifice.

According to national studies, the typical person providing unpaid assistance to a disabled older person living in the community spends about 4 hours daily on caregiving and has done so for 1 to 4 years. The typical caregiver is an adult daughter or wife, 57 years of age, who is married and has a middle-range income. Her caregiving tasks generally include shopping, transportation, housekeeping, handling finances, and some personal care. Furthermore, she provides emotional support and helps find professionals and community services to assist the older person as well. The major sources of caregiver stress for her are competing family obligations and work conflict. In addition, she finds the caregiving role especially difficult when the older person is socially impaired or exhibits difficult behaviors.[33-35]

Caregiving is not easy. It can be demanding, confusing, and costly. On the other hand, caregiving can offer a sense of purpose and competency for losses or failures. It can provide direct benefits, such as gifts of appreciation and an improved relationship with the person in need.

Podiatrists, and other health care professionals, are positioned to assist caregivers to better fulfill their role through information dissemination, reassurance, assessment, and resource referral.

Most caregivers assume their role without preparation or training. There is no job description for caregivers, and few ready sources of training exist. As a result, caregivers are

TABLE 5–3. **Differences Between Informal Network and Formal Network**

Characteristic	Informal Network	Formal Network
Relationship to help recipient	Personal	Professional
Help competency	Nontechnical	Technical
Adaptability of help extended	Flexible	Structured
Compatibility of help with personal need	Individually tailored	Standardized
Emphasis on emotional support	Primary importance	Secondary concern

often confused regarding role expectations, how much assistance to provide, and what feelings are appropriate.

Podiatrists can help fill these information gaps by explaining care needs, common behavior responses to illness, and potential reactions to treatment. They also can validate the caregiving experience. Comments such as "you are not alone" and "others share your frustrations" decrease the loneliness and guilt frequently associated with caregiving.

Podiatrists can help identify signs when caregiving is taking a toll on the caregiver's physical and emotional health. Signs of this may include

- Feeling irritable
- Having headaches or muscle strain
- Being tired but unable to sleep or rest
- Feeling depressed or overwhelmed
- Showing outbursts of anger or abuse

When such signs are indicated, podiatrists may suggest possible methods for coping or available community resources to help.

Methods for coping with a caregiving role include

- Establishing routines
- Concentrating on today
- Staying positive
- Being realistic
- Accepting compromise

Among the most important community resources targeting caregivers are self-help books, caregiver groups, courses on caregiving, counseling services, and respite. Together they offer information, support, and relief.

Many disease-specific organizations offer resources of interest to caregivers. For example, local chapters of the Alzheimer's Disease and Related Disorders Association have pamphlets on the caregiving role and fact sheets on dementia. Most offer information and service referral through telephone contact and stock books and videos for loan. In addition, many chapters sponsor educational programming for both caregivers and professionals along with caregiver groups of various types, including sometimes those for persons with newly diagnosed Alzheimer's disease. Nearly all of these services are available without cost.

Counseling services provide caregivers with emotional support and professional help in problem solving. Depending on the community, they may be available from mental health, family service, or specialized service agencies for the aged. Moreover, they are offered by psychiatrists, psychologists, social workers, and counselors in private practice. Fee is usually established through third-party sources, although agencies sometimes vary the amount by a client's ability to pay.

Finally, respite offers temporary relief from caregiving. It is available on an hourly basis from some agencies through volunteer or paraprofessional support in the home. It may also be available through nursing facilities or hospitals for extended stay. Payment varies by source.

The effective caregiver is one who accepts the role and appropriately manages related tasks, seeking help and relief when needed from both informal and formal support networks. The effective caregiver is able to understand and handle the transition from acute to chronic care needs and plans for the time when circumstances require someone else to assume the caregiving role. The effective caregiver is an ideal. Each person's ability to achieve the ideal relates to such factors as acquired competencies and adequate social supports.

Overview of the Formal Network

ACCESS

Help available through the formal network varies from community to community. The type of setting—whether rural or urban—is one reason for community difference in available help. In contrast to urban communities, rural ones tend to have fewer professionals, a smaller range of services, and fewer alternatives to choose from within any service type. Likewise, state and local funding can influence the resource base. Some locales are noted for high per-capita spending for resources benefiting vulnerable populations such as children, those with mental retardation or developmental disabilities, the mentally ill, and the elderly. Other locales do not have this distinction.

All communities, however, have a formal

network. Information on what is available and linkage to specific resources are facilitated through access programming. The most important of these are service guides, information and referral services, and outreach, case management, and educational programs. Service guides provide written lists of available resources, often arranged by locale or function. They tend to be provided by libraries, planning organizations, civic associations, and information and referral agencies. Since the providers typically do not evaluate the programs described in the guides, information on the quality of resources usually has to be gleaned from informal contact.

Information and referral services are scattered throughout the community. Almost every educational institution or health and social service organization offers a certain amount of information on, and linkage to, resources on request. However, one or two organizations in most locales have this as their major function. Many of these specialized information and referral services are operated either under the auspice of, or through funding from, United Way.

Outreach consists of actions taken by service providers to reach persons in need of assistance and to encourage their use of available resources. This access form has particular importance in certain fields, such as those serving the homeless, mentally ill, and elderly. Similarly, case management is broadly employed. Case management uses a human service professional to arrange and monitor an optimum package of services. It has various models—broker, service management, and managed care, which primarily differ from one another on the basis of resource allocation, financing, and case management authority.[36] Although case management has a long history, renewed interest in the concept has occurred with the deinstitutionalization movement, increased cost of care, and complexity of service needs in community settings.

Finally, educational programs can include lectures, workshops, and fairs as long as their intent is to highlight available resources and provide response to audience questions about them. Fairs are especially popular as a means for drawing attention to potential health problems or risk and available community re-

sources to address them. Hospitals and other health care providers frequently offer information, health screening, and inexpensive equipment at shopping malls and institutions that serve the elderly or disabled to attract potential consumers and fulfill perceived public service roles.

PROGRAM CATEGORIES AND ELIGIBILITY ISSUES

By and large, resources of the formal network can be categorized as benefits, goods, or services. What particular combination is appropriate for a person reflects assessed need and program eligibility criteria. For example, among those benefits most useful to low-income older persons are Supplemental Security Income, Medicaid, food stamps, homestead exemption, and energy or utility assistance. Respectively, these benefits augment income through cash transfer, medical assistance, vouchers for food purchase, property tax reduction, and utility or telephone bill discount.

Sometimes persons are eligible for such benefits but do not receive them. For instance, studies show that 48% of older persons eligible for Supplemental Security Income are not enrolled, and 65% of those who could receive food stamps do not.[37, 38] Reasons for low participation in these programs include lack of familiarity with program requirements, language barriers, the stigma of "welfare," and the complexity of the application process.

Podiatrists discussing these programs with patients should be aware of potential barriers to participation and have on hand strategies for overcoming them. For example, the podiatrist could help the older person in contacting the nearby senior center or municipal office on aging to access an outreach worker who could accompany the older person to the appropriate agency and assist the person through the application process. Also, the podiatrist could have a basic understanding of the application procedures himself or herself, so that general questions or concerns about them could be answered.

HOME CARE

A category of services that has special worth to persons who are ill or disabled and homebound is called home care. It offers social support in conjunction with medical care or instruction or assistance with daily tasks. Home care services found in most communities include the following:

■ Visiting nurses (medical care or instruction)
■ Homemakers (light housekeeping and errands)
■ Home health aides (personal care)
■ Chore services (minor repairs and grounds maintenance)
■ Home-delivered meals (hot noon meal)
■ Friendly visiting (regular companionship and activity)
■ Telephone reassurance (prearranged calls)

Like other categories of help, home care falls along a continuum. At one end is help, such as chore services, for those who function fairly independently. At the other end of the continuum is help, such as visiting nurses, for those who require extensive care. The physical and emotional health of persons determine the extent and type of home care required, with those who are very impaired needing much and varied assistance.

In selecting resources, patients should consider which ones best meet their needs while maintaining their independence as much as possible. Receiving more help than is required can foster dependency. Receiving less help than needed can be a health or safety risk.

COMMUNITY-BASED SERVICES

The range of community-based services is great. It includes congregate meal programs for the elderly, homeless persons, or school-aged children; recreational activities at senior centers and settlement houses; supervised day care for dependent adults and children; hospice for the terminally ill; legal services; and transportation and escort services aimed at the elderly or disabled persons.

HOUSING OPTIONS

Housing options vary by targeted populations. For the elderly, the array has increased in the past two decades in most communities. Although older persons typically live in housing arrangements like everyone else, about 5%

reside in nursing facilities or other institutions, and a similar percentage live in planned senior citizen housing or communities, such as assisted living or life care facilities.[14] Assisted living residents receive three meals daily and other services, including round-the-clock emergency response and some assistance with personal care. Life care facilities offer a range of housing options and supportive services to meet the needs of residents; they also require an entrance fee in addition to a monthly one.

Other housing options for the elderly include shared living, congregate care, and adult family care. Shared living consists of a group of independent older persons residing together, sharing common space, and pooling resources for household maintenance. Sometimes there are staff, and some shared living arrangements are intergenerational. Most are sponsored by a voluntary agency or government agency. It is estimated that there are 400 shared living homes nationally.[39]

Congregate care is housing with at least one meal daily provided in the rental fee. Congregate care facilities tend to be large, to include some services (although not nearly so many as assisted living), and to be divided into residential units rather than rooms. In some instances public subsidies enable residency at reduced cost for low income persons.

Finally, adult family or foster care offers room, board, supervision, and some personal care for elderly and disabled adults for a monthly fee. Usually state licensed and monitored, these homes fill a housing gap in the continuum from independent living to total care. They appeal to those who like a family style setting and whose personal care needs are limited.

BARRIERS TO OBTAINING SERVICES

Patients who require help may not want it. They may wish to be left alone. Pride may keep them from accepting assistance, even under extreme circumstances. They may have had unpleasant experiences with certain agencies or institutions and not want to bother with them again. Some may be unwilling to use their money to purchase needed services. Others may not trust service providers, whom they see as interfering and judgmental.

It is sometimes possible for podiatrists to

help patients overcome their reluctance to accept assistance. For instance, helping gain a clearer understanding of available income and assets may reduce unwillingness to purchase services. Nonetheless, adults, including elderly ones, have the right to refuse help, as long as they have the mental ability to make the decision and understand its consequences. When mental ability is impaired, legal interventions, such as guardianship and adult protective service law, in some cases can facilitate the involuntary extension of services. Since these interventions erode personal rights, caution must be exercised in their use.

Besides personal barriers to service, system level barriers can exist. Their classification is twofold: (1) problems of access and (2) problems of fragmentation. Access barriers include scarce resources, inconvenient service locations or hours, inefficient promotion of resources, high cost of care, and lack of transportation to reach services. System fragmentation results in service gaps, discontinuity of care, and inappropriate service linkage. The effect of system barriers can be that those in need of help may never receive it. Community planning agencies, government officials, and advocacy groups can be activated to remove system barriers if they are alerted to their existence by podiatrists and others in contact with vulnerable populations.

SUBSTANCE ABUSE

Substance abuse involves the excessive consumption of chemicals with resulting harm to the users or those around them. In its most severe form, there is dependence, evidenced by a reliance on the chemicals and withdrawal effects if they are discontinued. Categories of chemicals consumed in the United States are alcohol, barbiturates, cannabis, cocaine, opiates, psychedelics, stimulants, and volatile substances. In addition, over-the-counter drugs are sometimes abused. Because it is the major substance abuse problem, alcoholism will be used throughout this section for primary illustration.

Prevalence. The prevalence of substance abuse in the country is unknown. However, it is estimated that among adults who drink, 10% are alcoholics and as many as one third of late adolescents report that all or most of their friends drink regularly. Similarly 6 million American workers are believed to abuse drugs, and nearly two thirds of high-school seniors admit illegal drug use. Six million persons report at least weekly use of sleeping pills and more than 4 million Americans regularly use cocaine.[40, 41]

Over-the-counter drug use is primarily a problem for older persons, who consume seven times more of these drugs than younger adults.[42] Abuse of these substances generally occurs because persons fail to consult health care professionals about proper use, exceed recommended dosages, or do not consider potential interaction with other chemicals, such as a cough syrup containing alcohol.

Costs. The costs of substance abuse are significant. For the person, they can include physical illness and even death, psychological addiction, mental impairment, social dysfunction, and lost economic opportunities. For example, the ingestion of excessive amounts of alcohol in the body can irritate organ linings and disrupt chemical balance, with such resulting problems as cancer, ulcers, nephritis, and diabetes. For society, the costs of substance abuse include lost work productivity and increased expenses for health care, law enforcement, and social services. Again, focusing on alcohol abuse, four fifths of domestic violence and nearly one third of child abuse incidents involve drinking. Half of highway fatalities are alcohol-related, and alcoholics are 15 times more prone to suicide than the general population.[43]

Causes. There is no single or universally accepted explanation for substance abuse. Some believe that the origins are in personality traits, such as low self-esteem, which contribute to feelings of inadequacy and desire to escape problems. Others hold a physiologic perspective and propose genetic predisposition, body chemical abnormality, or metabolic defect etiologies for substance abuse. Still others point out social or cultural influences to chemical consumption. For instance, American culture permits and even encourages alcohol use at certain times, such as rites of passage, celebrating the new year, partying, and relaxing.[44–46] Most likely substance abuse results from the interplay of personality, physiology, and society rather than the dominance of any one explanation.

Signs. The signs of substance abuse vary by chemical. For example, cocaine users may have dilated pupils and seem agitated. In a drug-dependency state, they hallucinate, act suspicious, or seem depressed. Occasionally they may behave violently. In general, however, signs of substance abuse include some combination of the following:

- Flushed face
- Sleep disturbance and fatigue
- Loss of appetite and evidence of malnutrition
- Agitation
- Erratic behavior
- Deterioration of personal standards and social relationships

For some forms of substance abuse distinctive stages of addiction and abuser types have been identified. To illustrate, the Glatt chart suggests three stages of alcoholism: (1) prodromal, (2) crucial, and (3) chronic. Accordingly, the potential alcoholic begins as a social drinker who consumes more and more alcohol to relieve tensions and thereby develops increased tolerance to its effects. In the final stage, the alcoholic needs alcohol more than food or family and exhibits fears, deteriorated health, lengthy bouts of intoxication, and obsession with drinking.[47]

Three types of elderly alcoholics also have been identified: (1) early onset, (2) late onset, and (3) intermittent. Early-onset elderly alcoholics begin drinking in their teens and have long histories of chronic alcoholism but defied the odds and survived. On the other hand, they usually have developed medical problems, such as liver disorders or hypertension, as a result. Chronic brain syndrome may be evident. Furthermore, early-onset elderly alcoholics have such severe social relationship difficulties that they have pretty much limited social contact to friends who also drink or have long periods of isolation. Late-onset elderly alcoholics began drinking after age 50 usually in response to some loss, such as retirement or the death of a spouse. Because they have not built up a tolerance for alcohol, its toxic effects can result in serious health problems. Late-onset

elderly alcoholics also often feel guilt about their drinking and keep it well hidden. Finally, intermittent elderly alcoholics drink during early adulthood and have experienced periodic bouts of problem drinking followed by periods of abstinence. Events occurring in old age tend to precipitate drinking once again. The physical health and social relationship problems of intermittent elderly alcoholics are in direct proportion to the periods of problem drinking they have experienced.[48]

Persons who abuse chemical substances need help. Unfortunately, relatively few receive treatment. Sometimes this happens because health care professionals fail to identify the problem; or if the problem is professionally diagnosed, it is not confronted. At other times the abusers refuse to admit the problem or need for treatment.

Various defense mechanisms evident among substance abusers effectively serve to deter intervention. These defense mechanisms include denial, rationalization, and projection. With denial, abusers neither acknowledge nor accept responsibility for their substance-related problems; with rationalization, they minimize these problems; and with projection, they blame the problems on something or someone else.

Treatment. Podiatrists should be alert to the possible signs of substance abuse and aware of appropriate avenues for treatment. Moreover, they should recognize their own responsibilities and limitations for effecting behavior change.

Contact with patients about their substance abuse problems should be nonjudgmental and supportive. It should emphasize the need for further evaluation and encourage seeking help from qualified specialists. Intervention should focus on the development by the patient of a realistic rehabilitation plan and the involvement of significant others in the process. Setting limits is also important for substance abusers, whose addiction can render them manipulative, impulsive, and prone to anger.

Podiatrists also need to recognize when their response to substance abuse more reflects their own history or experience than the patient's symptoms or needs. Many health care providers are substance abusers or come from families with this problem. This background can color perception. On the other hand, each of us has a professional and ethical responsibility that our own and our colleagues' competencies are not impaired by alcohol or drug use.

Treating substance abuse requires multiple interventions. Because withdrawal can be life threatening, hospitalization, preferably in a special detoxification or drug unit, may be indicated. Inpatient rehabilitation usually requires 3 to 6 weeks. Following withdrawal, attention must be directed at changing behavior so that addictive patterns do not return. This will necessitate counseling or psychotherapy. For some persons, individual therapy is sufficient. Most, however, benefit from group support, through organizations such as Alcoholics Anonymous or Narcotics Anonymous. Alcoholic Anonymous groups, for example, set no fees and emphasize confidentiality. They are based on a 12-step process of recovery that relies on individual help from a higher power and interpersonal support from members. Beyond therapy, abusers may need help in establishing new relationships and returning to the labor force. Lastly, their families or significant others may require assistance in the form of education and support. In the latter regard, self-help groups focusing on substance abuse, such as Al-Anon and Alateen, are often invaluable.

FAMILY VIOLENCE

Until recently, interest in family violence in the United States was sporadic. During the mid 1600s, Massachusetts passed the first laws against "unnatural severity" to children. In the late 1800s, societies for the prevention of cruelty to children were formed. Additionally, smaller efforts were initiated to protect incest victims.

Modern interest in family violence began in the early 1960s with publication of an article in the *Journal of the American Medical Association* on the "battered child syndrome." During the early 1970s the women's liberation movement directed attention to wife battering and, later, to marital rape. Elder abuse became a public concern in the late 1970s, largely as a result of congressional hearings on the subject.

Other forms of family violence, such as sibling abuse and husband battering, although acknowledged problems, have never excited health care professionals or the public as much as abuse against children, women, and the elderly. In all likelihood, violence between siblings is ignored because the behavior is seen as natural. Husband battering only seems to engender sympathy when the husband is frail, impaired, or otherwise regarded as helpless.

This section will focus only on child abuse and elder abuse, because of the unique vulnerability of these populations and the special role health care professionals have in identifying these problems. Because abuse definitions, dynamics, and intervention strategies differ somewhat among these two aspects of family violence, they will be discussed separately.

Child Abuse

Infanticide was practiced among prehistoric groups, and violence against children was regarded as a parental right from ancient Rome to colonial America. Child abuse has a long history, but its recognition as a social problem in the United States probably cannot be dated until 1874, when church workers in New York City sought protection for a badly beaten foster child named Mary Ellen Wilson and could only find it in laws providing for the prevention of cruelty to animals. Arguing that Mary Ellen was part of the animal kingdom, the court granted her protection as well.

Interest in child abuse among physicians, notably John Caffey in 1946 and Henry Kempe in 1962, stimulated legislative activity requiring the mandated reporting of child abuse by health care professionals and others.[49, 50] By the end of the 1960s all 50 states had passed such laws. In 1974, the federal government offered its own support through enactment of the Child Abuse Prevention Act.

Child abuse can be defined as acts by an adult caregiver to a child younger than age 18 that are deemed harmful and inappropriate by community standards. The mistreatment of children tends to take four forms:

1. Physical abuse (such as beatings, shaking, and harming with a weapon)
2. Neglect (including abandonment, inade-

quate supervision, and lack of safe shelter or other essentials)

3. Emotional maltreatment (such as harsh criticism, scapegoating, and ridiculing)
4. Sexual abuse (such as incest, rape, and fondling)

Research on child abuse is more extensive than that available on other abused populations, but it, too, has notable methodologic and other limitations.[51] That said, from existing research and compiled abuse reports, it is estimated that perhaps 5% of children experience some form of child abuse during their first 18 years. In a single year about 6 in 1000 children are victims of physical abuse, emotional maltreatment, or sexual abuse, and 5 in 1000 endure neglect. Among the various forms of child abuse, physical abuse is most common, followed by neglect.[52–54]

Victim and perpetrator profiles vary by abuse form. For example, compared with physically abused children, sexually abused ones are more likely to be older, female, and white. In addition, the victim is less likely to be the perpetrator's child and the perpetrator is more likely to be unemployed. Finally, other forms of child abuse are less likely to be present in sexual abuse situations than in physical abuse ones.[52]

Explanations of child abuse vary by theoretical period and perspective. Early discussion of the subject, beginning in the 1960s, emphasized the psychopathology and emotional immaturity of abusers.[55, 56] This largely reflected the psychiatric backgrounds of many early researchers. Later, as sociologists and social workers entered the field, chronic stress, poverty, unemployment, single parenthood, and social isolation were emphasized correlates of abuse.[57–59] During this same time other researchers also suggested that certain characteristics on the part of the abuser (e.g., depression or anxiety) or abused child (e.g., mental retardation or hyperactivity) contributed to abuse occurrence.[60, 61] Murray Strauss and Richard Gelles have identified theoretical models for understanding these perspectives, categorizing them under the headings of intraindividual, social psychological, and sociocultural. Other theoretical models, such as evolutionary theory, also have been proposed that fall outside their framework.[62, 63]

Podiatrists and other health care professionals have several roles related to child abuse. These include

■ Problem identification and reporting
■ Help in assessment
■ Medical treatment for the consequences of child abuse
■ Possible court testimony in selected situations

These same roles apply to elder abuse, since most states have adult protective service or elder abuse reporting laws that are roughly comparable to state laws protecting children.

Medical indications of child abuse must be considered in light of the explanation given for their occurrence, the child's medical history, and the child's ability to inflict such harm on herself or himself. The possible medical indicators of physical abuse can be categorized as

■ Skin trauma (e.g., human bite marks, cigarette burns, and rope burns)
■ Internal or facial injuries (e.g., bald patches of hair, missing teeth, and tenderness in the abdomen)
■ Skeletal injuries (especially noting recurrent injury to the same spot, skull fracture, and multiple fractures at various stages of healing)

Indicators of neglect may include poor skin hygiene, pallor, failure to thrive, and untreated medical problems. Finally, although the indicators of emotional maltreatment tend to be less obvious, their long-term effect can be more damaging. Podiatrists should be alert to the possibility of emotional maltreatment in a child if they encounter antisocial behavior, low self-esteem, persistent and unrealistic fears, poor peer relations, indifference or listlessness.

If child abuse is suspected, state law requires podiatrists and other health care professionals to report it to law enforcement or child protective service agencies, which will take steps to investigate the situation and develop an intervention plan for addressing any child abuse that is uncovered, with an emphasis on protecting the child in the context of preserving the family, if at all possible. The mandate to report supersedes the sanctity of traditional professional–patient confidentiality. It may be possible to encourage the suspected abuser to self-refer. If this is not possible, the podiatrist should be ready to explain the legal provisions that require professional reporting and offer the patient support and guidance in the investigation that will follow.

Some health care professionals are reluctant to report child abuse. Despite the immunity provisions contained in state law, many fear civil or criminal liability for reporting. Sometimes, too, there is concern that the report may not be justified or the family will be stigmatized as a result. At other times professionals object to the time and paperwork involved in reporting or are hesitant to participate in related court proceedings. In the presence of all of these concerns, reporting child abuse is still a legal mandate. Moreover, a philosophical underpinning of society as a whole and of health care as a field is providing for the care and protection of vulnerable persons, such as children. On this basis, reporting suspected child abuse may be viewed as an ethical, civic, and professional responsibility.

Elder Abuse

Although elder abuse is referenced in early literature and recorded history, it was not recognized as a major aspect of family violence until 1975, when Robert Butler described "a battered old person syndrome" in his Pulitzer Prize–winning book *Why Survive? Being Old in America*.[64] Shortly thereafter, congressional hearings were held and research undertaken to explore the nature and scope of this problem.

Elder abuse is broadly defined as suffering or harm inflicted on an older person by self or significant others. It takes many forms:

- Physical abuse (e.g., hitting, shoving, or sexual assault)
- Physical neglect (when a caregiver deprives an older person of food, medical care, or other essentials)
- Psychological abuse (e.g., threats and belittling)

- Psychological neglect (including imposed social isolation or inadequate supervision)
- Exploitation (using the older person or his or her income or property for personal gain or profit)
- Violation of rights (such as denial of privacy or forced restraints)
- Self-neglect (when the older person deprives himself or herself of food, medical care, or other essentials)

Although research on this subject is limited, it is estimated that perhaps 5% of older Americans experience elder abuse. Physical abuse and exploitation are believed to be the most common forms. However, they are not reported to authorities as much as physical neglect and self-neglect. Actually only about one in eight situations of elder abuse are reported to authorities.[65-67] This is much less than for child abuse, which suggests the invisible nature of elder abuse as a problem because of older persons having fewer community contacts, public disbelief that the problem even exists, and ageism and a tendency to ignore the circumstances of older persons.

The etiology of elder abuse can be gleaned from profiles of the typical victim and perpetrator, which are thought to vary by abuse form. For example, the victim of physical abuse tends to be independent but emotionally impaired and the perpetrator tends to be pathologic and dependent on the victim. The victim of physical neglect tends to be physically or mentally impaired and socially isolated, and the perpetrator is stressed. Finally, the victim of exploitation tends to be single, socially isolated, and of advanced old age, with the perpetrator having financial and substance abuse problems.[68]

Identifying and assessing elder abuse can be difficult owing to confusion with the aging process, similarity with other problems or diseases, ambiguity of causes, and lack of cooperation by the victim. Identification and assessment, however, can be facilitated through use of a screening instrument. Several with a medical focus have been developed.[69, 70] In addition, it is important to be comprehensive in the evaluation, interview the victim and caregiver separately, and make collateral contacts.

Signs of elder abuse are many and varied,

with no single one clearly and consistently indicative of the problem. Possible signs of physical abuse include bruises in various stages of healing or clustered and forming patterns. Signs of physical neglect can include poor hygiene, fecal or urine smell, inadequate clothing, weakness, or underweight. Finally, evidence of possible psychological abuse can include fear, resignation, or embarrassment on the part of the older person.

Once elder abuse is suspected, most states require podiatrists and other health care professionals to report it to social service, aging, or other public agencies charged with investigating the problem and providing services to correct or discontinue it.

Unfortunately many elder abuse situations cannot be resolved. Studies suggest that as many as 45% to 70% are not effectively resolved.[71, 72] There are many reasons why, including the elder's right to live even in unhealthy or dangerous circumstances, unless legally judged incompetent or incapacitated; the lack of flexibility in intervention strategies to deal with elder abuse, given legal mandate, agency procedure, professional orientation, or personal preference; and the inadequacy of community resources in many locales, especially in the area of prevention and emergency intervention.

SUMMARY

The focus in this chapter is on psychosocial and behavioral problems that can affect the well-being of podiatric patients. Poor self-concept and low self-esteem are presented as potentially retarding ability to resist disease and inhibit treatment. Substance abuse and family violence are shown to cause both physical and emotional damage.

A wellness perspective is important in preventing illness, since it both energizes and empowers patients. Underlying this perspective is an understanding of illness and behavioral responses to it. Podiatrists need to be sensitive to these responses as well as to those health beliefs and practices exhibited by patients because of ethnic identity or minority status.

Effective podiatric care also requires the ability to identify, evaluate, and access the range of help available to patients. This includes self-help as well as assistance from informal and formal care networks in the community. Particularly significant in this regard are strategies podiatrists can employ to help patients overcome their reluctance to accept assistance.

REFERENCES

1. Kim MJ, McFarland GK, McLane AM: Pocket Guide to Nursing Diagnoses, ed 3. St. Louis, CV Mosby, 1989.
2. Stanwyck DJ: Self-esteem through the life span. Family Community Health 6:11–28, 1983.
3. Burns RB: The Self Concept in Theory, Measurement, Development, and Behavior. New York, Longman, 1979.
4. Erikson EH: Childhood and Society, ed 2. New York, WW Norton, 1963.
5. Krause N: Satisfaction with social support and self-related health in older adults. Gerontologist 27:301–308, 1987.
6. Muhlenkamp A, Sayles J: Self-esteem, social support and positive health practices. Nurs Res 35(6):334–338, 1986.
7. Healthy People: The Surgeon General's Report on Health Promotion and Disease Prevention. Washington, DC, US Public Health Service, 1979.
8. Healthy People 2000: National Health Promotion and Disease Prevention Objectives. Washington, DC, US Department of Health and Human Services, 1990.
9. Brill NI: Working With People: The Helping Process, ed 4. New York, Longman, 1990.
10. Leventhal H, Nering D, Steele D: Disease representations and coping with health threats. In Turk D, Kerns R (eds): Handbook of Psychology and Health. Hillsdale, NJ, Erlbaum, 1984.
11. Rose PI: They and We: Racial and Ethnic Relations in the United States, ed 2. New York, Random House, 1974.
12. Glazer N, Moynihan DP: Beyond the Melting Pot, ed 2. Cambridge, MA, Massachusetts Institute of Technology, 1970.
13. US Bureau of the Census: 1990 Census of Population. Washington, DC, US Department of Commerce, 1991.
14. Harwood A: Ethnicity and Medical Care. Cambridge, MA, Harvard University Press, 1981.
15. Nadar L, Maretzki TW (eds): Cultural Illness and Health. Washington, DC, American Anthropological Association, 1973.
16. Yap P: Culture-bound reactive syndromes. In Landy D (ed): Culture, Diseases and Healing. New York, Macmillan, 1977.
17. Leff J: Psychiatry Around the Globe. New York, Marcel Dekker, 1981.
18. Leininger M: Cultural care: An essential goal for nursing and health care. Am Assoc Nephrol Nurses Technicians J 10(5):11–17, 1983.
19. Leininger M: Transcultural Nursing: Concepts, Theories, and Practices. New York, John Wiley & Sons, 1978.
20. Tripp-Reimer T, Brink P, Saunders J: Culturological assessment: Content and process. Nurs Outlook 23(2):78–82, 1984.
21. Watson WH (ed): Black Folk Medicine. New Brunswick, NJ, Transaction, 1984.
22. Wilson UM: Nursing care of American Indian patients. In Orque MS, Block B, Monrroy LSA (eds): Ethnic

Nursing Care: A Multicultural Approach. St. Louis, CV Mosby, 1983.

23. US Senate Special Committee on Aging: Aging America: Trends and Projections. Washington, DC, US Department of Health and Human Services, 1991.

24. Montgomery RJV, Borgatta EF: Values, costs and health care policy. In Borgatta EF, Montgomery RJV (eds): Changing Issues in Aging Policy: Linking Research and Values. Newbury Park, CA, Sage, 1987.

25. McClelland DC: Testing for competence rather than for "intelligence." Am Psychologist 28:1–14, 1973.

26. Garbarino J: Social support networks: RX for the helping professions. In Whittaker JK, Garbarino J, et al (eds): Social Support Networks: Informal Helping in the Human Services. New York, Aldine, 1983.

27. US General Accounting Office: Report to the Congress: The Well-Being of the Older People in Cleveland, Ohio. Washington, DC, US Government Printing Office, 1977.

28. Brody EM: Older people, their families and social welfare. In The Social Welfare Forum, 1981. New York, Columbia University Press, 1982.

29. Cantor M, Little V: Aging and social care. In Binstock RH, Shanas E (eds): Handbook of Aging and the Social Sciences, ed 2. New York, Van Nostrand Reinhold, 1985.

30. Liu K, Manton K, Liu BM: Home care expenses for the disabled. Health Care Financing Rev 7(2):51–58, 1986.

31. Clark M: Culture values and dependency in later life. In Kalish R (ed): The Dependencies of Old People. Ann Arbor, University of Michigan/Wayne State University, Institute of Gerontology, 1969.

32. Hokenstad MC: Cross-national trends and issues in service provision and social work practice for the elderly. In Hokenstad MC, Kendall KA (eds): Gerontological Social Work: International Perspectives. New York, Haworth, 1988.

33. US House Select Committee on Aging: Exploding the Myths: Caregiving in America. Washington, DC, US Government Printing Office, 1987.

34. Stone R, Cafferta GL, Sangl J: Caregivers of the frail elderly: A national profile. Gerontologist 27(5):616–626, 1987.

35. Deimling GT, Bass DM: Symptoms of mental impairment among elderly adults and their effects on family caregivers. J Gerontol 41(6):778–784, 1986.

36. Applebaum R, Austin C: Long-Term Care Case Management: Design and Evaluation. New York, Springer, 1990.

37. 48% of eligible SSI recipients do not get benefits, study finds. Older Americans Reports, p 45, February 3, 1989.

38. US General Accounting Office: Food Stamps: Reasons for Nonparticipation. Washington, DC, US Government Printing Office, 1989.

39. Jaffe D: Shared Housing for the Elderly. Westport, CT, Greenwood Press, 1989.

40. Herington RE, Jacobson GR, Benzer DG (eds): Alcohol and Drug Abuse Handbook. St. Louis, Warren H. Green, 1987.

41. US Department of Health and Human Services: Drug Abuse and Drug Abuse Research, The Second Triennial Report to Congress from the Secretary, Department of Health and Human Resources. Rockville, MD, National Institute on Drug Abuse, 1987.

42. Kofoed LL: Over-the-counter drug overuse in the elderly: What to watch for. Geriatrics 40(10):55–60, 1985.

43. Estimating the economic cost of alcohol abuse. Alcohol Alert, pp 1–3, January 1991.

44. Barry H: Psychological perspective on development of alcoholism. In Pattison EH, Kaufman E (eds): Encyclopedic Handbook of Alcoholism. New York, Gardner, 1982.

45. Milkman H, Shaffer HJ: The Addictions: Multidisciplinary Perspectives and Treatments. Lexington, MA, Lexington Books, 1985.

46. Gottheil E, et al (eds): Etiologic Aspects of Alcoholism and Drug Abuse. Springfield, IL, Charles C Thomas, 1983.

47. Glatt MM: Group therapy in alcoholism: A chart of alcohol addiction and recovery. Br J Addiction 54(2):133, 1958.

48. Altpeter M, Schmall V: Late Onset Alcoholism: A Training Model for Formal and Informal Caregivers. Cleveland, OH, Case Western Reserve University, 1991.

49. Caffey J: Multiple fractures in the long bone of infants suffering from chronic subdural hematoma. Am J Roentgenol Radium Ther Nucl Med 46:163–173, 1946.

50. Kempe CH, Silverman FN, Steele BB, et al: The battered-child syndrome. JAMA 181:17–24, 1962.

51. Weis JG: Family violence research methodology and design. In Ohlin L, Tonry M (eds): Family Violence. Chicago, University of Chicago Press, 1989.

52. American Humane Association: National Analysis of Official Child Neglect and Abuse Reporting. Denver, American Humane Association, 1987.

53. Garbarino J: The incidence and prevalence of child maltreatment. In Ohlin L, Tonry M (eds): Family Violence. Chicago, University of Chicago Press, 1989.

54. Burgdorf K: Recognition and Reporting of Child Maltreatment: Findings from the National Study of the Incidence and Severity of Child Abuse and Neglect. Washington, DC, National Center on Child Abuse and Neglect, 1980.

55. Fischoff T, Whitton CF, Pettit MG: Psychiatric study of mothers of infants with growth failure secondary to maternal deprivation. J Pediatr 79:209–215, 1971.

56. Steele BF, Pollock CB: A psychiatric study of parents who abuse infants and small children. In Helfer RE, Kempe CH: The Battered Child. Chicago, University of Chicago Press, 1968.

57. Burgess RL, Youngblade LM: Social incompetence and the intergenerational transmission of abusive parental practices. In Gelles R, Hoteling G, Finkelher D, Straus M: Family Abuse and Its Consequences: New Directions in Family Violence Research. Beverly Hills, CA, Sage, 1988.

58. Gil DG: Violence Against Children: Physical Abuse in the United States. Cambridge, MA, Harvard University Press, 1970.

59. Garbarino J, Crouter A: Defining the community context of parent–child relations: The correlates of child maltreatment. Child Dev 49:604–616, 1978.

60. Reid JB, Patterson GR, Loeber R: The abused child: Victim, instigator, or innocent bystander? In Bernstein DJ (ed): Response Structure and Organization. Lincoln, University of Nebraska Press, 1982.

61. Wolfe DA: Behavioral Distinctions Between Abusive and Nonabusive Parents: A Review and Critique. Paper presented at the Second Family Violence Research Conference, Durham, University of New Hampshire, 1984.

62. Gelles RJ, Straus MA: Determinants of violence in the family: Toward a theoretical integration. In Burr WJ,

Hill R, Nye IK, Reiss IL (eds): Contemporary Theories About the Family. New York, Free Press, 1979.

63. Burgess RL, Draper P: The explanation of family violence: The role of biological, behavioral, and cultural selection. In Ohlin L, Tonry M (eds): Family Violence. Chicago, University of Chicago Press, 1989.

64. Butler RN: Why Survive? Being Old in America. New York, Harper & Row, 1975.

65. US House Select Committee on Aging: Elder Abuse: A Decade of Shame and Inaction. Washington, DC, US Government Printing Office, 1990.

66. Pillemer KA, Finkelhor D: The prevalence of elder abuse: A random sample survey. Gerontologist 28:51–57, 1988.

67. Tatara T: Summaries of National Elder Abuse Data: An Exploratory Study of State Statistics Based on a Survey of State Adult Protective Service and Aging Agencies. Washington, DC, National Aging Resource Center on Elder Abuse, 1990.

68. Wolf RS, Pillemer KA: Helping Elder Victims: The Reality of Elder Abuse. New York, Columbia University Press, 1989.

69. Fulmer TT, O'Malley TA: Inadequate Care of the Elderly: A Health Care Perspective on Abuse and Neglect. New York, Springer, 1987.

70. Hwalek MA, Sengstock MC: Assessing the probability of elder abuse: Toward the development of a clinical screening instrument. J Appl Gerontol 5:153–173, 1986.

71. Wolf RS, Godkin MA, Pillemer KA: Elder Abuse and Neglect: Final Report from Three Model Projects. Worcester, MA, University of Massachusetts Medical Center, 1984.

72. Chen PN, Bell SL, Dolinsky DL, et al: Elderly abuse in domestic settings: A pilot study. J Gerontol Soc Work 4(1):3–17, 1981.

CHAPTER 6

QUALITY ASSURANCE AND UTILIZATION REVIEW

Myron Boxer
Robert Marcus
Mark Caselli

Quality assurance and utilization review are rapidly expanding areas of administrative medicine that are having great impact. The effects of quality assurance and utilization review are felt in every hospital and in private practice.

Quality assurance refers to the process of patient-oriented quality care through continuous monitoring. This implies a standardized level of care over time. *Utilization review* is an evaluation of resources as they relate to the rendering of optimum care. The goals of quality assurance and utilization review are to provide the best and maximum patient care for the least cost.

Quality assurance encompasses physician review, chart analysis, volume indicators, and funding, to name but a few areas. In the private sector, utilization review has been associated primarily with postpayment review. In hospitals, utilization review includes drug usage evaluations, research, materials and methods, employee productivity, and many other areas.

The scope of quality assurance and utilization review is so tremendous that entire organizations such as the Joint Commission on Accreditation of Healthcare Organizations exist. Textbooks have been written and journals updated regarding the many complicated and sometimes tedious aspects of quality assurance and utilization review.

In this chapter we will not attempt to tackle topics such as volume indicators, vulnerability assessment, funding, risk management, problem assessment, and the JCAHO 10-step process. Much of this material can be gleaned from a quality assurance journal, JCAHO guidelines, or other administrative texts. It is our intention to significantly narrow the spectrum to three basic issues of concern to the podiatric physician: credentialing, resident supervision, and postpayment review.

PHYSICIAN CREDENTIALING

Physician credentialing is an integral part of quality assurance. The basic reason for credentialing individual physicians is to ensure good patient care. The JCAHO has long required peer review as part of its credentialing of physicians who apply for hospital privileges. As a part of the credentialing process, an applicant must prove current licensure, relevant training or experience in his or her field, current competence, and health status. The application process must have consistent rules that are evenly applied to all applicants through a hospital-specific mechanism. A hospital or other health care facility must conduct its own investigation and should not accept an applicant merely because he or she is on another hospital's staff. Care must be exercised to confirm all claims made by applicants.

Additional factors that should be taken into consideration at the time of credentialing an applicant include the following:

■ Continuing educational activities
■ Previous loss of staff membership or clinical privileges
■ Gaps in the history of the practitioner's previous activities
■ Attendance records at meetings and membership in committees and similar activities

To encourage peer review and credentialing activities, Congress passed the Health Care Quality Improvement Act of 1986. The purpose of this act is to provide those persons giving information to "professional review bodies" and those persons assisting in the review certified immunity from damages that may arise as a result of adverse decisions that affect a physician's medical staff privileges. Those entities covered by the immunity provision in the act include hospitals, medical groups, and professional societies in which formal peer review activities are intended to promote quality of care. The immunity provision only applies when the individual or entity satisfies the following requirements:

1. The challenged peer review action must have been taken "in the reasonable belief that the action was in the furtherance of quality health care."
2. The action must have been taken "after reasonable effort to obtain facts of the matter."

3. The entity must have afforded the affected physician "adequate notice and hearing procedures."
4. There must be a reasonable belief that the action was warranted.

A formal peer review process means the conduct of professional review activities through formally adopted written procedures would provide for adequate notice and an opportunity for a hearing. Immunity from civil damage actions attaches to the hospital and hospital medical staff members if certain minimum due process is afforded the physician as a part of the disciplinary hearing process. This due process should include written notice of the proposed discipline to the physician and a list of the reasons for the proposed action. The notice should also include the physician's right to request a hearing on the proposed action and a time limit of not less than 30 days in which to request such a hearing. If a hearing is requested, a second notice must be sent to the physician stating the place, time, and date for the hearing of not less than 30 days after the notice, as well as including a list of witnesses expected to testify at the hearing on behalf of the hospital. The hearing is to be held before a mutually acceptable arbitrator, before a hearing officer, or before a panel appointed by the hospital that is made up of persons who are not in direct economic competition with the physician involved. At the hearing, the physician has the right to be represented by an attorney. He or she also has the right to have a record made of the hearing; to call, examine, and cross-examine witnesses and present relevant evidence; and to submit a written statement at the close of the hearing. On completion of the hearing, the physician has the right to receive a written recommendation of the arbitrator or panel, including a statement of the basis for the recommendation, as well as receiving a written decision by the hospital that includes a statement of the basis for the decision.

A typical credentialing process of a physician to a medical staff usually requires that the current or aspiring physician submit an application including proof of medical education, training, or licensure, malpractice insurance, board eligibility or certification (if applicable), peer recommendations, sometimes proof of continuing medical education, statement of frequency of performance of certain procedures or treatment of specific pathologic processes, and a completed privileges delineation form to the clinical department chairman or service chief if he or she is seeking to attain or retain staff privileges. Following this, the applicant may be interviewed by the department chairman or service chief, who will then write a report and recommendation concerning staff appointment and clinical privileges to the hospital's credentials committee. The application or past service record of the physician is then reviewed by the hospital's credentials committee. The credentials committee then transmits a written report and recommendation concerning staff appointment, category of appointment, department assignment, and scope of clinical privileges to the medical board of the medical executive committee. This committee, which is mandated by the JCAHO, is often composed of the chairman or chiefs of the major clinical departments or services of the hospital. The medical board then forwards to the hospital director for transmittal to the governing body a written report and recommendation for clinical privileges to be granted with any special conditions or restrictions. Any physician who receives an adverse determination may then follow an appeals procedure as outlined in the hospital bylaws with various due process safeguards as previously discussed.

There are many defensible considerations for the acceptance or rejection of an applicant for staff privileges. The following are some general defensible criteria considered in the staff privileges decision-making process:

- Education, training, background, and experience of the applicant
- Needs of the department
- Ability of the applicant to work with others
- Ability to meet eligibility requirements specified in bylaws
- Freedom from conflict of interest
- Overburdening of the hospital's facilities
- Maintenance of adequate malpractice insurance
- Willingness to make a full-time commitment to the institution

- Use of the hospital as the physician's primary inpatient facility
- Medical record-keeping deficiencies
- Clinical performance profiles from available quality assurance records
- History of disciplinary actions by other hospitals or licensing boards

To assist the hospital credentialing committee in seeking information concerning the history of disciplinary actions taken against a physician by other hospitals or licensing boards, the Department of Health and Human Services has established a National Practitioner Data Bank. Each entity or individual who makes a payment on behalf of a physician as a judgment in a medical malpractice action must report the payment and related circumstances to the data bank. State licensing boards must report revocation, suspension or restriction of license, censure, reprimand, or placing a physician on probation to the data bank. In addition, each health care entity that takes a professional review action that adversely affects the clinical privileges of a physician for a period longer than 30 days must report that action to the appropriate state licensing board, which, in turn, must report the adverse reaction to the data bank.

Hospitals are required to request information from the data bank about any physician who is applying for a position on the medical staff or for clinical privileges. The hospital must also query the data bank about every physician who is on the medical staff every 2 years. Other entities that may request information from the data bank include state licensing boards, individual physicians about themselves, and individuals or their attorneys under certain circumstances during a malpractice action. The data bank became operational September 1, 1990. No retroactive reporting was required.

RESIDENT SUPERVISION

Resident supervision has become a complicated and often controversial issue in patient care. For years interns and residents were the "workhorses" for hospitals. Usually underpaid and overworked and assigned extremely long tours of duty, residents provided most of the initial contact with patients, as well as a vast majority of total patient contact. Surgical patients were (and still are) operated on by residents. This was quite beneficial to a hospital attempting to provide maximum service at the least expense. It also acted as an inducement for attending physicians to bring cases: the patients would receive coverage without the attending physician's having to be at the hospital.

However, many problems have arisen from the paucity of supervision. Residents eager to gain certain required skills sometimes perform unindicated procedures or new treatment regimens. Problems may arise when patients arrive at a hospital with signs and symptoms beyond the scope of the resident's expertise or with an atypical presentation. Residents are often reticent to consult the attending physician for fear of being berated, scolded, or looked down on. This naturally results in poor patient care.

Still other problems may occur when a resident is called on to perform a procedure beyond his or her expertise. For example, one resident, when asked to intubate a difficult patient, placed the tube in the esophagus by mistake.

In some states, regulating agencies have responded to such occurrences by enacting specific laws putting a "ceiling" on the number of hours a resident can work. In addition, the flood of lawsuits resulting from poor supervision has had a direct impact on the level of supervision. This has created a plethora of hospital regulations requiring varying degrees of supervision.

In podiatric medicine there are many types and levels of resident supervision:

■ Periodic notes by the attending physician in the patients' records
■ Notes by the attending physician that will countermand a resident's orders
■ Evidence of operating room supervision
■ Written resident evaluations
■ Conference discussion (morbidity and mortality)
■ Service level meetings

The major question is what level of supervision optimizes learning and adequately pro-

tects the patient. This is an individual decision made by each hospital residency program or staff consummate with each resident's fund of knowledge and training.

Certain institutions have policies that state the attending physician countersign every chart and be present on the clinic floor at all times. This is an effective form of supervision but is extremely problematic. Purely from a manpower perspective, clinics that have a single covering podiatric attending physician could be forced to close if the attending physician is absent and cannot be replaced. This policy may also be suffocating to a resident, limiting the ability of the resident to develop the clinical thought process required to be a good clinician.

At the other extreme, when there is no supervision, patient care suffers. Some institutions have vague policies to have an attending physician on call without a clear mission to supervise. Residents are heavily relied on to make what may be potentially important decisions without good consultation. This can be very destructive to patient care, as well as resident development.

Many institutions have policies stating that there is no reason to mandate on-site supervision at all times for podiatric medical and surgical procedures that do not necessarily require a medical license to practice. An example would be reduction of corns and calluses. Reduction of nails, radiography, injection therapy, prescription writing, and other medical procedures that may require a medical license are supervised in a competency-based fashion. More-invasive medical and surgical procedures that almost always require a license are also competency based. This can be an effective form of supervision, thus not always requiring an attending physician to be physically present if competency can be clearly documented.

The level of supervision that maximizes patient care and the level that maximizes resident learning are not the same. Assuming an ideal situation, the patient would receive the best care if that care was provided by the staff. However, the resident receives the best training if the staff serves only as a facilitator; allowing all decisions to be made by the resident and all procedures to be performed by the resident staff only facilitates resident decision making. The attending physician performs treatment only if the resident cannot, or as a demonstration if it is the first time the resident has been exposed to that procedure. For this reason we walk a fine line when defining appropriate levels of supervision. In addition, the level of supervision needed varies among residents depending on their level of training. Thus, the level of supervision needed on the first day of training is much different than that needed on the last day of training. These factors lead to a need for a flexible supervision standard that has minimum requirements to ensure good patient care.

From the standpoint of training, ideal supervision would include the ready availability of the staff in person, or by telephone for clinic patients, when complex or dangerous procedures are not being employed. The name of the attending physician along with a written document of the discussion should be placed in the patient's record and signed (by the attending physician within 24 to 72 hours when possible). Inpatient supervision should be performed by staff rounds not less than three times per week (ideally on a daily basis). The initial visitation should be within 24 hours of admission.

The supervision of invasive and dangerous procedures should be tailored to the level of training, with upper-year residents allowed to perform specifically defined procedures without the staff present but readily available by phone. The policy should clearly state the procedures allowed and should require documentation of the discussion held with the attending physician in the patient's record. Attending physicians should cosign the note containing the discussion or write a separate staff note within 24 hours and ideally in advance of an elective procedure. For all other procedures the staff should be present in the operating room and scrubbed as necessary. (The vast majority of podiatric and residency programs have an attending physician in the operating room. This may have contributed to the relatively low incidence of postoperative morbidity in podiatric residency programs.)

In summary, it appears that a competency-based supervision policy should exist in each podiatric department. This policy should allow residents to demonstrate their clinical skills and allow an attending physician to not necessarily be present during procedures for which the residents have clearly shown their competency and that the staff has documented the residents' ability to perform, especially procedures that do not require a medical or podiatric license.

POSTPAYMENT REVIEW FOR FRAUD AND ABUSE

Fraud is the willful intent to deceive to achieve material gain. It may involve complex machinations or can sometimes be as simple as upgrading a diagnosis. For instance, a practitioner may know that an insurance carrier is not going to pay for a particular diagnosis. The practitioner then falsely upgrades the diagnosis to one that he or she knows is reimbursable. When the diagnosis is upgraded, fraud is perpetrated by upgrading the treatment so that the bill for the uncovered diagnosis and treatment will be paid. The practitioner then files a false or fictitious insurance claim form, which then becomes a fraudulent document.

Another form of fraud is reporting a diagnosis that is nonexistent for reimbursement purposes. For example, a podiatrist may see a patient who has a normal, slight curvature of digits. The podiatrist will then fabricate a diagnosis of hammer toes and, for purposes of insurance reimbursement, may even go as far as to perform a surgical procedure to correct a hammer toe condition that did not really exist.

Some practitioners report treatments that they do not perform. For example, a physician may make a diagnosis of arthritis and report administering an injection when nothing was actually done except prescribing medication.

Practitioners who commit fraud are also abusive in some way. They may be abusing their license to practice, the patient's rights, or the insurance company's right to pay a legitimate claim. For example, a podiatrist may do a tenotomy on every patient who comes into the office, or bill for a tenotomy on every patient regardless of whether the surgical procedure is performed. When a reviewer looks at a number of claims from such a practitioner, a suspicious "pattern of practice" becomes quite obvious.

Billing patterns are frequently reviewed by insurance carriers. Some practitioners will bill extremely high fees when they know that a third party is going to be paying. These fees far exceed anything that they would bill to a patient. In addition, they will bill for more services than they actually perform and will fragment or "unbundle" procedures for billing purposes. A practitioner, for example, might bill for a bunion procedure and fragment it into four or five different procedures. This is done by billing separately for removal of the exostosis, capsulotomy, tenotomy, and osteotomy. A bunionectomy that would normally be priced at $1500 then costs $3500 or $4000.

Almost every insurance carrier has a utilization review department. This department will monitor several different areas of practice. For example, it will monitor the quality of care being rendered, billing practices, and patterns of practice.

Computers give an insurance company a greater ability to identify an abusive or fraudulent pattern of practice. Computers monitor fees, billing patterns, and patterns of practice. The computer will identify practices and practitioners who need to be scrutinized or audited. Thus, insurance company employees do not have to scrutinize every claim submitted.

What are some of the reasons a practitioner may be selected for an audit? One is high billing, that is, billing that is out of proportion to what is considered to be customary and prevailing in that area. Another is if a practitioner exceeds his or her peers in the number of procedures performed. Use of the same diagnosis repeatedly may cause an audit to be initiated. For example, Medicare has a parameter that only seven medical injections may be administered to a patient per year. Once a practitioner exceeds seven injections, the computer may alert the insurance carrier staff to look at this physician. The practitioner may not be doing anything wrong, but once the parameter is exceeded, he or she will be investigated.

Often, a patient will suspect that something is not legitimate. For example, the practitioner may perform a minor procedure, upgrade the diagnosis and treatment, and then bill an amount that is not consistent with what may have actually been done. Sooner or later, if a practitioner does it often enough, a patient is going to write a letter to an insurance carrier and advise the company of an irregularity. The patient may not know what is wrong but he or she knows "something is not right." The insurance carrier will then request copies of numerous office records, and an audit will be done.

Another practice that may precipitate an audit is serialization of surgery. Serialization is performance of multiple surgical procedures in a serial fashion rather than performance of the procedures at the same time. This is done to avoid insurance carriers' policies of full pay for a first procedure and lesser amounts for subsequent procedures done at the same time. By serializing surgical procedures, the practitioner has the potential of collecting a full fee for each procedure performed. Insurance carriers frown on this practice, and many consider it an abusive pattern. In an attempt to preclude this, Medicare has established an extended (90-day) after-care period in which no related care is payable.

Another form of abuse is the padding of fees. Insurance carriers almost always reimburse for less than the amount that a practitioner bills. Some practitioners, aware of this practice, pad a bill or increase their fees when accepting assignment. Instead of billing the normal fee, the practitioner may double or even triple his or her fee. The insurance carrier then looks at the inflated fee and cuts it back to what it believes it should be. However, the insurance carrier usually ends up overpaying for the service billed and the practitioner comes out ahead. On postpayment audits, these overcharges are frequently identified and reimbursement is sought.

Computer "screens" are turned on and turned off by insurance carriers. A carrier may have a policy of screening for a specific pattern of practice, diagnosis, or therapeutic procedure. However, when faced with a heavier than usual work load, the carrier may stop screening temporarily, and every claim that is billed for a period of time will be paid. When the screen is reinstated, practitioners who may have been exceeding parameters during the period of time that a particular screen was off may then get caught. The carrier may then look at the practitioner and declare that the care rendered was not medically necessary and request a refund of money paid for those services.

If a practitioner bills in a legitimate manner, the pattern of diagnosis and therapeutic procedures for the practice as a whole will evolve in a statistical sample that is consistent with what all other practitioners see and do. If the practitioner consistently upgrades diagnoses and treatments, it will rapidly become evident to reviewers. Suppose a podiatrist sees a patient with a mild incurvated nail and upgrades the diagnosis and treatment to paronychia with incision and drainage of an abscess. An auditor, reviewing the podiatrist's office records, will immediately suspect that the diagnosis and treatment are not being reported accurately if there are no follow-up visits, antibiotics prescribed, specimens obtained for culture and sensitivity studies, and other factors involved in the treatment of paronychia.

Frequency of visits very often is an indicator of what a practitioner is doing. For example, care of hyperkeratoses is usually monthly, whereas treatment of an ulcer is usually weekly. An infection may be treated every few days. If the frequency of visits does not conform to the pattern of a particular diagnosis, an auditor may become suspicious that a practitioner is fabricating the diagnosis. If the practitioner accurately reports and justifies the diagnosis and treatment, the practitioner will not have to be concerned that he or she might fail an audit.

Another area that has to be well documented is medical necessity. Medical necessity means documentation, in the medical record, of a subjective complaint and objective findings. The mere fact that a practitioner notes a problem in the record is not documentation of medical necessity. For medical necessity to be properly documented, one must clearly note all subjective complaints and objective findings with a relevant diagnosis or differential diagnosis. It is also important to document negative findings. Often practitioners only list positive findings. By noting negative findings, one has documented proof that certain areas were indeed examined. The use of instru-

ments that produce written records (e.g., recording Doppler instruments) is excellent supportive documentation of medical necessity as well as proof of a procedure having been performed. If medical necessity is not adequately documented, an insurance carrier has the right to deny payment or ask for a refund of any monies already paid.

A third area that is important in which to have a complete record is the *documentation of the services* that were performed. If each service rendered is not documented in the patient's chart, then an insurance carrier may assume it was not done and may request a refund of monies paid. If it is not in the record, there is no proof it was done.

It is imperative for reimbursement purposes to make sure that the services rendered were reasonable and necessary. For example, there are many things that practitioners do that insurance carriers, specifically Medicare, will deem not reasonable nor medically necessary. An example might be the use of vitamin B_{12} in the treatment of diabetic peripheral neuropathy. Podiatrists frequently use vitamin B_{12} as a treatment, but Medicare does not recognize it as valid therapy. It would, therefore, be denied for payment on the basis that the treatment is not reasonable or medically necessary. Another area in which payment might be denied as being not reasonably or medically necessary is in the use of physical therapy. Physical therapy must be administered at least twice weekly or preferably three times a week for it to be considered efficacious. If the therapy is not administered in an effective manner, the insurance carrier may request reimbursement or deny payment. Podiatrists commonly place patients in a whirlpool before rendering care and bill for physical therapy. Unless the patient is on a regular program of treatment, this form of treatment may be denied payment on the basis that it is not being administered in an efficacious manner and thus is not medically necessary.

When consultants review records for third-party fiscal intermediaries, there are many indicators in a record that may cause a reviewer to suspect fraud or abuse. For example, if in reviewing a chart, a reviewer finds different inks were used to keep one record or that different handwritings were noted in the production of a single entry, it suggests that all the records were not entered at the same time. A pen, when used on different dates, will produce different ink flows, and this, too, is quite noticeable. The same person, when writing on different dates, will have changes that are discernible in handwriting.

The use of preprinted records is often an indicator that there may be abuse or fraud. For example, some practitioners use preprinted operative reports. No two operative procedures are exactly alike. When a practitioner uses a preprinted record, the reviewer may suspect that the record is not an accurate description of what was performed.

In many instances, practitioners "prepare" records for submission when a request is made for office charts. Records become suspect when typed notes are perfectly aligned for various dates or service, errors in dating are made, and other mistakes tip off the reviewer that the record was prepared fraudulently. For example, a practitioner was asked to submit records for multiple dates of service. The practitioner had a beautiful record prepared and typed; however, the typist started the records for each patient on the top of a new page.

Since the dates of service requested were strictly at random, it was most unusual to find that the record for each patient started at the top of a fresh page.

In summary, altered records are easily identified and always highly suggestive of fraud. When a practitioner develops patterns in his or her notations, that is, all notes appear to be basically the same for all visits and for all patients, these are also highly suspicious. The use of preprinted records and reports is always highly suspect. Abusive billing patterns very often will be a flag for monitoring fraud and abuse.

REFERENCES

Bralliar F: Physician Credentialing and Profiling: Study Guide. Venice, FL, American College of Medical Quality, 1991.

Broader AI: The Health Care Quality Improvement Act of 1986: Study Guide. Venice, FL, Americal College of Medical Quality, 1991.

Couch JB: Emerging Medicolegal Issues in the Medical Specialty of Quality Assurance and Utilization Review: Study Guide. Venice, FL, American College of Medical Quality, 1991.

Demos, MP: What Every Physician Should Know About the National Practitioners Data Bank: Study Guide. Venice, FL, American College of Medical Quality, 1991.

Young G: Personal communication, January, 1993.

CHAPTER 7

SELF-DIRECTED LEARNING

Franklin J. Medio
Stephen J. Morewitz

As the podiatric profession enters the 21st century, podiatrists face significant challenges from the increasing complexity of the field. To meet these challenges, podiatrists need the skills and attitudes to be successful, independent lifelong learners. Development of these abilities should begin during the initial years of podiatric medical education and continue throughout one's career.

Therefore, it becomes imperative that podiatric medical educators examine current educational programs and ensure that instructional strategies are implemented that prepare podiatrists to be effective, self-directed learners. Self-directed learning is a process of active, independent inquiry that includes the ability to (1) acquire and utilize basic concepts and principles; (2) gather, assess, and analyze data; and (3) evaluate and apply information to the solution of problems.[1]

This chapter is designed to provide an overview of the self-directed, adult learner concept. In the first section, the theoretical framework of "andragogy," the adult learning model, is described. Andragogy is distinguished from the traditional model of pedagogy.[2–4] In the second section, applications of the adult learning model in professional education are presented. Two instructional methods are examined: (1) personalized self-instruction and (2) problem-based instruction. Also included in this section is a discussion of self-assessment techniques. In the final section, implications of the adult learning model for podiatric medical education and graduate training in podiatry are presented.

THE ADULT LEARNING MODEL

To appreciate the usefulness of an adult learning model as a tool to develop lifelong learners, one must recognize that we have come "full circle" in the evolution of educational systems. Despite the appearance of the "adult learner" as a development of contemporary education practice, it is based in ancient history.[5] In fact, the students of the great teachers (e.g., Confucius, Socrates, Plato, and Jesus) were adults.

Ironically, current educational practices that dominate our schools, universities, and professional schools can be traced back to the Middle Ages.[5] During this period, monks established centers of learning with the distinct purpose of training young men for the monastic life of obedience and servitude. Education of the learner, the child with the *tabula rasa* (blank slate) mind was the complete responsibility of an elite few. To accomplish their duties, the monks taught in a tightly controlled environment. As the concept of educating the public emerged from the Renaissance, spreading through Europe and the recently discovered America, this model of teaching, called "pedagogy" became the standard for education.[5] Literally translated from the Greek, it means "the leader of the child."

Within the dominant shadow of the pedagogic teaching model, the fields of psychology and sociology emerged and began to expand our understanding of the human developmental process. Research in the 1950s and 1960s began to challenge the centuries-old, monopolistic position of the pedagogic model. There was increasing evidence that physical maturation was accompanied by psychological and social maturation processes that included the means by which we learn and adapt to our environment.[6–10] Knowles[5] characterized these psychological and social changes in a person as, "an increasing *need* and *capacity* to be self-directing, to utilize his experience in learning, to identify his own readiness to learn and to organize his learning around life problems."

Andragogy vs. Pedagogy

Although Knowles did not create the term *andragogy* (Gk., "the leader of man"), he is recognized for establishing the theoretical foundation from which much of the contemporary work in adult learning has flourished. As delineated by Knowles, the andragogic model has four basic assumptions that differentiate adult learners from child learners:[11]

1. Self-concept
2. Life experiences
3. Readiness to learn

4. Orientation to problem solving

According to this model, adult learners perceive themselves as independently functioning beings who are responsible for making their own decisions. Each person possesses a unique set of needs and is motivated to participate in learning activities to meet these needs. Adult learners have a vast and rich reservoir of life experiences, including both positive and negative attitudes and behaviors. Learning is an ongoing activity throughout life.

Lifelong learning involves the process of assimilating each new experience into an existing scheme, as well as the process of unlearning old habits that have inhibited optimal growth and development. Each learner's life experiences are valued and utilized as learning resources to be shared. This diversity in past experiences among adult learners also means that each person possesses a different capacity or "readiness" to learn. Therefore, the identification of learning opportunities, the "teachable moment" is a critical factor in designing a successful learning experience. Acceptance of learners' diversity requires that teaching methods include individualized instruction to address each learner's needs.

Finally, it is recognized that the adult learner is motivated to learn by the immediate application of the knowledge and skills acquired. Cognitive knowledge, manual skills, and social awareness are integral parts of this learning process, but preference is given to those that have an *immediate use* in solving problems.

Table 7–1 illustrates the different characteristics of the pedagogic and andragogic models. Rather than consider these models as mutually exclusive, it is more appropriate to conceptualize them as opposite ends of a continuum. In much the same way that a child grows to become an adult, the model of teaching changes to match the learners' developmental needs. Therefore, the challenge facing educators is to select the most appropriate teaching model to meet the needs of learners. In a situation in which all the learners are inexperienced, the pedagogic model may be suitable. However, as the learners acquire knowledge and skill in the field, the teaching model should change to a more andragogic approach to optimize their

TABLE 7–1. **A Comparison of the Pedagogic and Andragogic Teaching Models**

	Characteristic	Pedagogy	Andragogy
I	Individual learner	"All the same"	"Each person is unique"
N	Needs of learner	Teacher determines	Determined together
S	Schedule of activities	Teacher establishes	Established together
T	Teacher's role	Expert or authority	Facilitator or guide
R	Role of learner	Dependent/passive	Independent/active
U	Understanding	Checked periodically	Checked continuously
C	Curriculum content	Factual knowledge	Problem-solving skills
T	Teaching methods	Didactic lectures	Learning contracts
O	Orientation	Toward "future use"	Toward "immediate use"
R	Responsibility for learning	Assumed by teacher	Assumed by learner

learning experiences. It is the inability to adapt different teaching models that creates problems for learners and instructors.

Educators in professional education often experience frustration when learners do not become more "independent and self-directed." Yet, on closer observation it is apparent that these educators employ a pedagogic approach to teaching that does not encourage the development of adult learning skills! The mismatch between the instructor's expectations and the teaching method is the source of the problem. Therefore, it is incumbent that each instructor examine his or her expectations and teaching methods and determine if they are appropriately matched. In fact, a hybrid model, combining elements of both andragogy and pedagogy, can be effective in some situations.

The Role of the Teacher

Implementing the andragogic model requires not only an understanding of the basic principles of adult learning but also a rethinking of the teacher's role. Adult learning thrives in a physical, psychological, and social atmosphere where each learner is treated as a unique member of a group (i.e., heterogeneity). The needs and experiences learners bring to the group contribute not only to their learning but also to others as well. The challenge each teacher faces is the dual task of creating an atmosphere that is conducive to learning in the group, while at the same time facilitating the fulfillment of each learner's needs. In the pedagogic model, all learners are assumed to have the same needs and level of prior experience (i.e., homogeneity).

In each model, the teacher plays a critical but vastly different role. The pedagogic model requires the teacher, as content expert, to address five questions:

1. What content needs to be covered?
2. How can the content be divided into manageable units?
3. What is the best sequence to present the material?
4. What is the most efficient method of transmitting this content?
5. What is the most efficient method of evaluating learning?

By contrast, the andragogic model requires the teacher, as both facilitator and content source, to address seven questions:

1. What are the needs of each learner?
2. How can I involve each learner in formulating his or her learning activities?
3. How can I assist each learner in planning his or her learning activities?
4. How can I create a physically comfortable environment?
5. How can I create a psychological and social atmosphere that is based on mutual respect, collaboration, trust, support, openness, and comfort?
6. How can I facilitate each learner's ability to conduct his or her learning activities?
7. How can I involve the learner in determining the best method for evaluating learning?

The Lifelong Learner

As the facilitator, the instructor assists the learner in acquiring new information and skills but, more importantly, engages the learner in the process of "how to learn." It is this second function that enables the learner to develop the critical skills and attitudes for self-directed learning.[12]

The skills that characterize the lifelong learner include the ability to

▪ Assess learning needs
▪ Establish learning goals and objectives
▪ Select relevant learning activities to achieve goals and objectives
▪ Identify resources and facilities to conduct learning activities
▪ Utilize self-discipline and time-management techniques to complete learning activities
▪ Select and conduct appropriate evaluation methods to measure learning

APPLICATIONS OF THE ANDRAGOGIC LEARNING MODEL: PROFESSIONAL EDUCATION

In the previous section, the origin and theoretical framework of the andragogic model of learning was described. The implications of this approach for teaching were discussed, highlighting the changes in the instructor's role. In this section, two instructional method-ologies are presented: personalized self-instruction and problem-based learning; both employ the principles of adult learning. The "learning contract" as a method of individualized instruction is discussed within the personalized self-instruction method. Finally, a portion of this section is devoted to the process of "self-assessment." Self-assessment is essential because self-improvement cannot occur without the recognition of one's deficiencies and the desire to change.

Two important technologic advances in medical education will not be discussed owing to space constraints. However, the importance of these educational tools, computer-based instruction and standardized (simulated) patients cannot be questioned. As computer technology advances, the applications of computer-based instruction will more closely simulate real-life clinical situations, similar to the uses in aviation training. Likewise, there have been significant improvements in the quality of "live," standardized patients for teaching and evaluating medical students. For more information, the reader is directed to the report by the Association of American Medical Colleges[13] for a review of medical infomatics and to the article by Stillman and colleagues[14] for a review of standardized patients.

Personalized Self-Instruction

In 1968, a psychologist named Fred Keller reported the successful implementation of a new teaching method called the Personalized System of Instruction (PSI).[15] This innovative teaching method was based on the behavioral learning principles of B. F. Skinner[16] and the principle of mastery learning espoused by the noted educator Benjamin Bloom.[17] PSI was based on the premise of individualized student learning. As such, this method was designed to accommodate the different abilities and needs of each learner. The cornerstone of this approach was the principle that persons learn at different *rates*. In contrast to the traditional teaching method in which the amount of learning varied (the "normal" grading curve), PSI requires all learners to attain the same level of learning (criterion-referenced grading).[18]

The five basic elements of the PSI or Keller method of teaching include the following:

1. *Emphasis on the written word.* Written study guide materials, which include specific "learning objectives," constitute the primary source of information to be learned. Relevant textbook and reference articles are included.
2. *Mastery requirement for advancement.* Criteria to demonstrate mastery of learning are determined for each unit of content material. Learners are required to achieve mastery before progressing to the next unit.
3. *Student-paced learning.* The rate of progress for learning is determined by the learner. As active participants, learners are responsible for managing their own learning activities.
4. *Lectures as motivational devices.* Using written materials as primary learning materials enables the instructor to use lecture time for motivational sessions. The information acquired through independent study could be applied to case studies or group problem-solving activities.
5. *Use of proctors.* Immediate feedback is provided to learners through the use of proctors or "peer-tutors." The personal interaction with proctors enhances the educational environment by meeting the unique needs of the learners. Also, the proctor bridges the gap of understanding that sometimes occurs between an experienced instructor and the learner.

In PSI, the instructor's role is more complex in comparison to the lecture method. Considerably more effort is required to prepare well-designed study guide materials than to prepare a lecture. To establish the mastery criteria, the entire course's content must be divided into units, must be properly sequenced, and must contain appropriate evaluation instruments. A method of selecting, training, and monitoring proctors needs to be established. Finally, the instructor assumes the responsibility for facilitating learning by creating and managing the educational environment. The image of the omnipotent speaker behind the lectern is eliminated in the PSI method.

The decade following Keller's report of PSI saw a widespread development and acceptance of this teaching technique among undergraduate education programs. Research studies comparing PSI with the traditional lecture method consistently demonstrated that students learned as well or better using the PSI method.[19, 20] Initial applications of the PSI method in medical, dental, and nursing education were also successful.[21–25]

Mager's work[26] helped to increase the understanding and use of "learning objectives" as an integral part of the educational process. Bloom's studies[27, 28] explained the hierarchical nature of learning in the cognitive and affective domains of knowledge, further challenging the one-dimensional teaching method of lecturing. Other techniques of individualized, independent learning, including "competency-based" instruction, were developed and implemented for adult education, especially in the field of continuing medical education.[29, 30]

Effective individualized, self-instruction teaching methods share a common set of educational principles despite variations in their structure and operation. These principles include the following:

- Emphasis on active participation by the learner
- Accommodation for individual differences in the *rate* of learning
- Adherence to a mastery criteria of performance as a measure of achievement
- Utilization of portable learning materials as the primary source of content
- Use of immediate feedback on performance by means of personal contact (i.e., tutor) or interactive programmed material
- Identification of the instructor's role as facilitator of learning rather than source of content information

As the content expert, the instructor is responsible for creating and managing the learning environment (e.g., study materials, learning resources, mastery criteria, testing/grading systems), but the learner is responsible for the learning that occurs.

Learners taught by an "individualized" method of instruction gain experience in "self-directed" learning skills. Time management and self-discipline are critical skills for success, since procrastination is a major obstacle to learning. The ability to use learning resources independently, and to seek assistance when necessary, is essential. As the learner progresses, internal motivation to learn and succeed becomes the controlling factor. The prescribed mastery level of performance teaches the learner perseverance. Goal achievement becomes valued as the measure of success. As a result, setting goals and objectives becomes an internalized process.

LEARNING CONTRACTS

Most of the individualized instructional programs reported in the literature are designed by the instructor. The term *self-instruction* may be misleading in these cases because it is the instructor who has arranged the instructional format. A more representative example of pure self-instruction is the learning contract. The learning contract is an agreement between instructor and learner that describes in detail what is to be learned (objectives), how it is to be learned (strategies and resources), what time period it will take (implementation), and how the learning will be measured (evaluation).[29–33] The learning contract exemplifies adult education by involving the learner in all facets of the educational process.

There are basically six steps in developing a learning contract:

1. Conduct an assessment of strengths and deficiencies in relation to a set of expected competencies.
2. Identify specific learning goals and objectives to correct deficiencies as noted in self-assessment.
3. Describe all learning resources available, including facilities, personnel, reading materials, and audiovisual/computer aids.
4. Establish the guidelines for the working relationship between instructor and learner, with particular attention to the purpose and structure of meetings.
5. Determine the suitable tools to measure attainment of the learning objectives and competencies.
6. Establish a timetable to monitor a learner's progress to ensure timely completion of the learning contract.

The advantages of a learning contract are that it

- Clarifies expectations for the learner by focusing on practical and attainable goals and objectives
- Builds greater responsibility for the learner by fostering a deeper sense of ownership of the goals and objectives
- Focuses the learner's attention on relevant and meaningful learning, leading to a stronger commitment
- Builds a more positive, personal relationship between the instructor and the learner
- Allows the instructor to serve as a personal tutor for the learner by accommodating different learning styles, educational backgrounds, and other learning characteristics
- Provides clear and fair documentation of a learner's accomplishments
- Improves the learner's self-discipline and independent learning skills through a learner-centered environment.

In a learning contract, the knowledge and skills learned are evaluated more critically than in conventional teaching methods. The final measures of success are the attainment of the learning objectives and the increased confidence toward learning. Successful completion of a learning contract leads a person to take more initiative in his or her own continuing self-development.

Problem-Based Learning

Problem-based learning (PBL) refers to a variety of methods that are used to enhance clinical problem-solving skills and foster self-directed learning through group learning methods. Instead of emphasizing the short-term memorization of facts and principles, PBL exposes students to educational triggers in real-life contexts. Using this format, students have an opportunity to solve a range of problems, including basic science, clinical, behavioral science, and community health issues.

According to Barrows[34] and other experts, PBL is designed to achieve a number of far-reaching and innovative educational objectives. First, PBL provides a relevant clinical context for learning to occur. Advocates of

PBL argue that traditional medical school teaching, with its focus on rote memory and standardized examinations, does not promote clinical learning. In contrast, PBL is designed to teach students to solve simulated problems that have a relevant clinical framework.[35] Because the simulated problem is placed in a context that will be relevant for future practice, students are better able to retain and apply this knowledge.

A second PBL objective is that students are offered ample opportunities to practice and receive feedback on their clinical reasoning skills.[34] An important strength of PBL is that it can offer students experience in the "how to" of solving clinical problems. Critics of conventional training point out that medical school teaching does not offer students extensive opportunities to practice clinical reasoning strategies.

The development of self-directed, independent learning skills is another PBL objective.[34, 35] Standard medical school teaching, according to its critics, has failed to nurture self-directed learning skills in students. To become life-time, independent professionals, students must be able to identify their own individual learning needs as well as available educational resources. Through PBL techniques, students have structured opportunities to identify their learning needs and utilize educational resources in solving simulated problems.

Stimulating students' motivation to learn is a fourth educational objective shared by many PBL proponents.[34, 36] Since PBL models the real clinical problem process, it can better motivate students to learn. The conventional medical education's focus on rote memory and excessive competition does not encourage students to engage in lifelong learning.

Others argue that PBL can be used to promote a community-based, primary care orientation to medical practice to better meet the needs of underserved urban and rural populations.[37–39] To achieve this objective, PBL techniques are designed to integrate basic science and broader primary care issues, such as the effects of demographic patterns on the patterns of community health.

Finally, medical educators assert that community-oriented PBL should give students ex-perience in working together as members of a community-based health care team.[39] According to this perspective, it will be easier for students to practice community-oriented, problem-based medicine as a member of a health care team if they have had experiences early in their medical education.

METHODS

Different PBL techniques can be employed in various ways to achieve the previously mentioned educational objectives (Table 7–2).[34] An important variable is the extent to which these techniques involve student-directed or teacher-directed learning activities.[40] Each PBL approach differs in terms of its potential success in achieving its objectives.[34]

Lecture-Based Cases. In lecture-based cases, the instructor gives a lecture and then presents one or two cases to illustrate the basic science or clinical issues.[34] This method is least likely to improve the students' problem-solving skills because their knowledge is not restructured in a clinically relevant context. In addition, students do not have chances to develop hypotheses, analyze data, test hypotheses, and develop treatment or management plans.

Case-Based Lectures. According to the case-based lecture approach, students are provided a fairly complete case presentation before the start of a lecture.[34] Unlike the previous technique, the case-based lecture method is stronger because it requires the student to restructure subsequent information obtained during the lecture. A flaw in this technique, however, is that students generally do not engage in self-directed learning unless their curiosity is sparked or if they are required to make use of educational resources outside the classroom.

TABLE 7–2. **Types of Problem-Based Methods**

Lecture-based cases
Case-based lectures
Case method
Modified case-based
Problem-based
Closed-loop, problem-based

From Barrows H: A taxonomy of problem-based learning methods. Med Educ 20:481–486, used with permission from Blackwell Scientific Publications.

Case Method. The case method has been a highly touted educational tool in business and law schools for many years.[34] Following this approach, students are assigned a complete case as homework. They are asked to analyze the case and do any research necessary in preparation for class discussion.

The case method offers greater opportunities for restructuring clinically relevant knowledge and promoting self-directed learning than the prior PBL methods. In addition, the subsequent class discussion can facilitate both student-directed and teacher-directed learning. A weakness in the case method is that the case is often already complete, so that students have few chances to develop or practice their clinical reasoning skills.

Modified Case-Based Method. The modified case-based tool has been employed in new medical schools that make use of PBL methods.[34] According to this method, students in small groups are exposed to a partially complete simulated case, such as a patient management problem or a standardized patient. This approach allows for more restructuring of knowledge than in the case method technique. In addition, students are better able to acquire clinical reasoning and self-directed learning skills than with the previously discussed methods.

A disadvantage of this technique is that students have limited chances to test hypotheses and gather additional information because of design flaws in most patient management problems or similar problem-based educational triggers. Moreover, patient management problems do not allow students to apply the results of learning to new clinical contexts.

Problem-Based Method. The problem-based method offers more restructuring of knowledge, promotion of clinical reasoning, and self-directed learning skills than the previously mentioned approaches.[34] Like the modified case-based technique, this method stimulates the students' motivation to learn.

Under the subtle guidance of a tutor, and with only general learning objectives provided, students work in a small group to critically assess and solve a simulated patient case, that is, a patient management problem, standardized patient, pathophysiologic issue, or other problem-based educational trigger. To accomplish

this task, a small group of students develops tentative hypotheses, determines their learning needs, and gathers additional data to test these hypotheses through the use of learning resources outside the classroom or laboratory setting.

In the problem-based method, it is critical that the instructor merely guide the students' clinical problem strategies and discussions and not provide content or attempt to dominate the group discussion. An inadequacy in this method is that students do not have an opportunity to apply the knowledge obtained in self-directed learning activities to simulated cases.

Closed-Loop or Reiterative Problem-Based Technique. The closed-loop or reiterative problem-based technique provides the most comprehensive approach to PBL because it enables students to apply knowledge that has been acquired in self-directed learning to the original simulated case.[34] This technique is easy to implement because it is simply an extension of the problem-based method.

After additional data have been collected and analyzed during the period of self-directed learning activities, the students report back to their group concerning their solutions to the original simulated case. Students are asked to evaluate their original reasoning strategies in light of their newly obtained information. In this way, students can improve their reasoning skills in similar simulated case situations and self-learning contexts.

THE USE OF PROBLEM-BASED LEARNING METHODS IN MEDICAL SCHOOLS: RESEARCH FINDINGS

PBL techniques were developed in the 1970s and 1980s in response to perceived inadequacies in traditional medical education. Originally, various forms of PBL were taught to medical students in the basic sciences.[38] At certain medical schools, PBL techniques also have been employed in both the preclinical and clinical years. PBL is a parallel curricular track at some medical schools, such as the University of New Mexico School of Medicine, Bowman Gray School of Medicine, and Rush Medical School.

Because of the vigorous efforts of highly regarded medical educators at medical schools such as McMaster University School of Medicine, University of Newcastle Medical School, and Harvard Medical School, PBL soon became the underlying philosophy and structure for entire medical school curricula. Yet, rarely have conventional medical schools changed completely into a total PBL program.

Is PBL more effective than conventional medical school training in teaching clinical problem-solving skills, enhancing student motivation, and facilitating self-directed learning? There are a number of obstacles to answering these evaluation questions. The goal of measuring clinical problem-solving skills has been difficult to achieve because of numerous methodologic problems.[41] Moreover, the tremendous variations in the types of PBL used, the quality and motivation of instructors, and the self-selection of students are other hurdles to assessing the efficacy of PBL. It is especially difficult to control for extraneous variables, contamination, or crossover effects of PBL and conventional curricula. Despite these methodologic difficulties, a number of investigations have yielded some findings on the effectiveness of PBL. Below are a summary of some of these results.

Does PBL Improve Clinical Problem-Solving Skills Better Than Traditional Methods?

Some experts have demonstrated that students tend to use one of three styles of learning: surface, deep level, or strategic.[12] The surface approach consists mainly of rote learning or memorization. Following the deep approach, students try to synthesize what they already know and try to understand the underlying explanations of a problem. In the strategic approach, students try to get the maximum learning results using minimum effort.

Students in a PBL curriculum may employ one or two deep approaches: the hypodeductive and forward approaches to solving medical problems.[38, 43] The hypodeductive method, or top-down or backward approach, refers to the process whereby a person develops general hypotheses after analyzing initial cues (i.e., patient history, clinical signs, and symptoms). These initial hypotheses then guide the person's formulation of additional lines of inquiry and subsequent acceptance or rejection of hy-

potheses under consideration. Researchers have found that once students acquire extensive knowledge in a subject area, they tend to bypass this somewhat inefficient method.[38] Instead, students with extensive prior knowledge may tend to rely on the forward method, which involves collecting all data first and then immediately developing a hypothesis.

Several medical educators argue that clinical problem-solving skills and strategies cannot be taught.[43–45] According to this perspective, most medical students possess essentially the same problem-solving skills and strategies. Students employ these skills and strategies in different ways, depending on their motivation or the external pressures of medical school. Instead of focusing on the unattainable goal of improving clinical problem-solving skills, Berkson[38] and others suggest that the focus of medical education should be on ensuring that students learn "content" areas.

Research reports have shown that PBL does not greatly enhance clinical problem-solving skills.[41, 45, 46] For example, Gordon[46] found substantial variability in how students solve simulated problems. Individual students have differed in their performance across different simulated situations, and there has been significant variability in problem-solving skills among groups of students with supposedly similar knowledge levels. This high variability in performance suggests that PBL may not be effective in improving clinical problem-solving skills.

In other research, Neufeld and colleagues[45] found that students in a PBL curriculum exhibited stable skills in clinical problem solving and were not substantially influenced by training in PBL. In this light, students' skills in generating and testing hypotheses were not correlated with educational level. However, the researchers did demonstrate that with PBL tutoring, students were able to improve the content and specificity in their hypotheses.

It is possible that current research methods, because of their insensitivity, have not captured adequately the true effects of PBL.[41, 47] Once these methods are perfected, researchers may be able to measure accurately the impact of PBL on clinical problem-solving skills.

In contrast to the previously mentioned findings, several research reports have demonstrated that PBL has a significant impact on medical students' clinical problem-solving skills. For example, Woodward[48] reported that graduates of PBL medical schools did consistently better than traditionally trained graduates on the patient management problems section of standardized Canadian medical examinations. However, some authorities question whether patient management problems are good indicators of clinical problem-solving skills.[49-51]

In a comparative study of one conventional medical school and one PBL school, Claessen and Boshuizen[52] reported that PBL-trained students were better able than traditionally trained students to recall and process information. Moreover, investigations by Coles[53] and Newble and Clarke[54] suggest that PBL curricula may be more likely to foster a deep approach to learning than conventional training.

Coles[53] noted that at the beginning of medical school training, students did not exhibit extensive differences in learning styles. Yet, throughout the students' training, the structure of the traditional medical school curricula seemed to encourage surface approaches to learning.

In summary, there is some tentative evidence to support the hypothesis that PBL can improve clinical problem-solving skills.

Does PBL Enhance Student Academic Achievement?

Overall, academic achievement appears to be essentially equivalent for students in either PBL or conventional curricula. For example, Baca[55] and Schmidt and colleagues[36] demonstrated that PBL-trained students perform equivalently to traditionally trained students on Part II of the National Board of Medical Examiners test.

Yet, other investigations have pinpointed some slight variations in academic achievement. On the one hand, several studies have revealed that PBL-trained students did slightly worse than conventionally trained students on standardized tests, such as Part I of the National Board of Medical Examiners test.[36, 48, 55]

Does PBL Increase Motivation to Learn and Encourage Self-Directed Learning?

Owing to the limits of research, evidence on the impact of PBL on students' level of moti-vation is lacking. However, there are a number of investigations that suggest that PBL-trained students have a more positive attitude toward their learning experiences in medical school than traditionally trained students. According to several surveys, many students in conventional medical schools are quite dissatisfied about their medical school training.[36] For example, one survey of more than 300 medical students at a traditional Dutch medical school reported significant dissatisfaction with their preclinical instruction.[36] Students frequently characterized their preclinical sciences training as "dull," "tough," "irrelevant," and "hardly adapted to the needs of practice."

The above survey was replicated by Schmidt and colleagues[36] using a randomly selected sample of 45 PBL-trained students at the University of Limburg. These researchers found that a large percentage (80%) of 147 evaluative comments from 45 PBL-trained students rated their problem-based curriculum as favorable.

The previous findings are partly consistent with the results obtained by Woodward and Ferrier.[56] They found that PBL-trained students considered the greatest strengths of PBL to be PBL experiences, electives, and self-directed learning. The greatest weaknesses of PBL were the evaluation system and instruction in clinical skills.

Does PBL Influence Careers in Community-Based Primary Care Settings?

According to several reports, the career preference of medical students is fairly stable throughout their medical school training. If changes do occur, they tend to be a shift from primary care to specialty and subspecialty practice.[57, 58] This trend in career choice makes the goal of many PBL advocates difficult to attain.

The effects of PBL on career choice have not been investigated extensively. One study was conducted at two newer medical schools in Finland, the University of Kuopio and the University of Tampere.[59] The results demonstrated that graduates of these two newer medical schools were more likely to choose primary care settings than graduates from the other medical school. However, the researchers could not determine if the career choices were affected by the PBL curricula or manpower needs during the period of the investigation.

In a study at the University of New Mexico School of Medicine, researchers measured the effects of two tracks, a PBL track and a conventional track, on career choices of students from the time of medical school admission to graduation.[55] At the time of admission, students from both tracks reported similar interests in primary care medicine. According to the study results, students in the PBL track were somewhat more likely than traditionally trained students to maintain their interest in primary care fields from the time of admission to medical school graduation.

Overall, there is weak evidence that PBL curricula does influence students to maintain their interest in primary care.

Self-Assessment

Valid self-assessment is an essential aspect of medical school training and continuing medical education.[60] Students as well as medical professionals must be able to identify and assess their own learning needs and take appropriate steps to meet those needs. Many medical educators consider effective self-assessment to be part of lifelong, self-directed learning. Unfortunately, self-assessment is *rarely* taught or practiced in undergraduate or graduate medical education.

To what degree can medical students assess their learning needs accurately? A related question is to what extent the process of self-assessment improves clinical problem-solving skills and motivation to learn. Below is a description of three methods for addressing these questions.

STUDENT SELF-ASSESSMENT VS. OBJECTIVE TESTS

Few experiments have been conducted to compare medical student self-assessment with formally tested objective knowledge. One type of research design in this area consists of measuring students' self-claimed knowledge using various self-ratings of course content. Student self-ratings are compared with objective measures of knowledge, such as final course examinations.

Some studies using samples of undergraduate and graduate students showed that self-assessed knowledge can be reliable or unreliable depending on a number of conditions.[60–62] It appeared that the greater familiarity with a given content area is associated with more accurate self-assessment.[61, 63]

USE OF VIDEOTAPES

Several experiments have been performed to compare student self-assessment ratings with faculty ratings using videotapes of students and residents performing histories and physical examinations. In a study of 187 second-year medical students, Calhoun and associates[64] correlated self-ratings of physical examinations with those of peers and experts. According to the results of this experiment, second-year students rated themselves 9.2 percentage points higher than did the experts.

Using standardized patients along with behavioral evaluation criteria, Stuart and coworkers[65] measured the interviewing skills of 56 family practice residents. The researchers found only low correlations between residents' self-ratings and faculty ratings. On the basis of follow-up interviews, the investigators found several sources of errors, including the fact that the residents did not rate themselves favorably even when their performance was good.

In addition to underestimating their performance, research demonstrates that students and health care professionals overestimate their clinical skills.[64]

GLOBAL SELF-ASSESSMENT DURING CLINICAL TRAINING

To obtain a broader perspective on the accuracy of self-assessment ratings, a number of investigators have compared end-of-clerkship self-evaluation ratings with faculty ratings and standardized examinations.[60] These self-ratings tap students' self-evaluation of clinical knowledge, skills, and professional behavior.

Arnold and associates[66] analyzed the self-ratings of 211 students in the internal medicine clerkship in the third through sixth years of the University of Missouri Combined Baccalaureate–Medical degree. The researchers found annual increases in students' self-assessment ratings, but these ratings were consistently below those of the faculty. By the end of the program, the positive correlation between students' self-ratings and faculty's ratings decreased to nonsignificance. The students' self-ratings at the end of the program were most likely to be positively correlated with their self-ratings in concurrent and recent courses.

In a study of 54 students in PBL group tutorials, Rezler[67] found that for six sequential units covering the first 2 years of medical training, there was a significant increase in students' self-ratings of knowledge and reasoning skills but no change in self-assessments for interpersonal and communication skills.

In summary, limited studies show that students tend to underestimate their performance, and the positive correlation between students' self-ratings and faculty's assessments actually declines over time. One explanation, according to Arnold and associates[66] is that students' self-ratings are based on noncognitive abilities related to performance, whereas faculty's ratings tend to be based on student grades and test scores. Studies demonstrate that when students are taught the self-assessment process, their self-assessment scores can better correlate with faculty ratings.[60, 68]

IMPLICATIONS FOR PODIATRIC MEDICAL EDUCATION

The evaluation data from other professional education programs convincingly indicate the limitations of the traditional lecture-based method of teaching. Use of the pedagogic teaching model and reliance on a theoretical "normal distribution" grading curve have created significant deficiencies in the training of professional students. However, recent developments have identified andragogic-oriented teaching methods that may better prepare learners to become lifelong, self-directed professionals.

By participating in educational activities that require active, independent learning, persons can effectively assimilate new knowledge and skills, as well as apply this information to the solution of problems. With varying degrees of guidance from experienced instructors, learners acquire the skills to assume greater control and responsibility for their own learning. Pre-

determined levels of competency described by learning objectives become the guideposts for achievement rather than arbitrarily selected periods of time. Both individualized and group-based formats can be used. These unconventional teaching methods have been successfully implemented within the time constraints of a multidisciplinary professional curriculum.

Preclinical Education

The preclinical curriculum of podiatric medical school shares many of the strengths and weaknesses apparent in other medical school curricula. Therefore, podiatric students may benefit from the adoption of individualized and problem-based learning methods. Although the responsibility for determining the content and criteria for acceptable performance still would reside with the faculty, the methods for teaching and learning would change.

Individualized learning methods could be designed for regular courses or remedial programs. The determination of clearly stated competencies and learning objectives ensures uniformity in the development of a basic science "foundation" among learners. It is reasonable to expect that learners can complete course requirements within the timetable of a curriculum schedule. Clinical opportunities or other relevant independent activities can be included as incentives for learners who progress rapidly through individualized, self-paced course content.

However, it is important to realize that utilization of individualized or personalized self-instruction methods does *not* guarantee that all learners will be successful. The responsibility for learning rests with the learner. Decisions and actions of the learner may lead to success or result in failure. Procrastination or other difficulties in time management can present obstacles to success. Nevertheless, the same standards for promotion and dismissal should apply for all students regardless of the teaching method used.

A major concern in the implementation of individualized teaching methods in the preclinical curriculum involves the ability of the instructors to adapt to their new role. As learners assume more responsibility for learning, the instructor's control over interactions with learners decreases. Instead of scheduled "lectures," much of the instructor–learner contact is unscheduled and widely distributed over time. Given the variability in learners' progress, instructors are required to quickly adjust to the needs of different learners. Monitoring tests and grading examinations require increased instructor time. One strategy may be to hire specially trained personnel to assist the faculty in managing these types of instructional programs.

Scheduling of laboratory and other "hands-on" learning activities must be considered in an instructional program in which learning occurs at different rates. If participation in these activities is based on mastery of cognitive information, there must be ample resources to accommodate the students who will master the material at different times.

Alternative-track curriculum programs can be designed for the preclinical education of podiatric medical students. The unique benefit of this method is an integrated approach to learning basic sciences and clinical sciences information.[69] To be successful, this model requires considerable cooperation and commitment among the faculty members involved. Negative attitudes or feelings directed toward either the conventional model or the problem-based model can only be destructive.

Comparisons of the curriculum models lead to competition for allegiances among learners and faculty. Unhealthy learner stress is created by competing loyalties and questions of competency. To avoid these problems, a curriculum model that includes elements of both conventional and problem-based teaching may be advantageous. Implementation of problem-based teaching may be more easily achieved by adopting a teacher-directed approach initially. Some studies have reported successful integration of components of PBL in traditional basic sciences courses.[70, 71]

The strategy of modifying existing courses rather than radically changing the entire curriculum's structure may reduce anxiety and resistance from both instructors and learners. As both gain confidence and skill using nontraditional teaching methods, the impetus to expand such teaching emanates from positive experiences. Teacher-directed methods gradually shift to learner-directed methods as learners demonstrate self-directed learning skills.

Clinical Education

Clinical education at both the undergraduate and graduate levels can be significantly improved by adoption of a "competency-based" system. The relevance of adult learner principles in clinical education is irrefutable. The most significant improvement in clinical education will occur by removing the shackles of pedagogy. Mastery of established competencies for clinical knowledge and skills should become the cornerstone of clinical training, replacing "blocks of time" in clinical disciplines. Efforts need to be directed toward the delineation of a "continuum" of training goals and objectives that increase in depth and expand in scope. These goals and objectives become the guidelines for teaching and learning, rather than the current method of random exposure to clinical problems that present during a rotation. In this way, learning requirements become standardized for all learners.

Self-instructional materials can be designed for learners to achieve cognitive objectives. These materials can be individualized, using written materials or computer-based programs, thereby allowing learners the opportunity to structure their learning around clinical activities. Learning contracts appear to be ideally suited to meeting the needs of students who require focused, remedial instruction during their clinical rotations.

Graduate Podiatric Medical Education

Progress through this continuum of clinical training should be accompanied by greater involvement of learners in designing their educational programs. Graduate training in podiatry provides an ideal opportunity to use learning contracts. Learners can participate in planning their training to achieve the professional requirements for competency, as well as to satisfy areas of personal interest. Self-assessment skills, which are woefully inadequate or nonexistent in most curricula, would be enhanced. Learners would have clear understanding of expectations through the descriptive competencies and objectives. In fact, the development of self-assessment skills could be improved throughout professional education if learners were given outcome measures to determine their level of achievement.

Faculty Development

The most critical and yet most difficult step to develop self-directed learning skills in students and residents is changing the teaching practices of the faculty. Most instructors, who are products of the pedagogic teaching model, have little or no experience using the andragogic model. Although recognizing the importance of developing self-directed learning skills, most instructors impede this process by using pedagogic techniques. Therefore, instructors must examine their educational environments and identify the "mixed" messages transmitted to professional students. Learners, encouraged to seek information through independent reading, are primarily rewarded for memorizing lecture material. Development of problem-solving skills is promoted as the goal of learning; yet learners who can recall textbook facts are highly regarded. Most importantly, learners are expected to learn a predetermined, voluminous amount of knowledge, but evaluation methods reveal that this is an unrealistic and unfulfilled expectation.[72]

Instructors need to expand their concepts of teaching and learning. To develop the future instructors, residents, who are responsible for teaching students, should receive training in educational methods during their residencies.[73, 74] Faculty need to assess their own teaching practices, noting effective and ineffective skills. As self-directed learners, those who need training can utilize existing resource materials as well as participate in seminars and workshops.[75–79] Through the improvement of their own teaching skills, instructors will model the very self-directed learning skills that they seek to instill in their learners. The result will be an improved educational environment in which podiatric medical students and residents can develop their skills for lifelong, self-directed learning.

REFERENCES

1. General Professional Education of the Physician: The GPEP Report. Washington, DC, Association of American Medical Colleges, 1984.
2. Knowles MS: The Modern Practice of Adult Education: From Pedagogy to Andragogy. Chicago, Associated Press, 1980.
3. Knowles MS: Andragogy in Action. San Francisco, Jossey-Bass, 1984.
4. Brookfield SD: Understanding and Facilitating Adult Learning. San Francisco, Jossey-Bass, 1986.
5. Knowles MS: The roots of andragogy—an interactive concept. In Knowles M: The Adult Learner: A Neglected Species. Houston, Gulf Publishing Co, 1978.
6. Erikson E: Childhood and Society. New York, WW Norton, 1950.
7. Piaget J: The Origins of Intelligence in Children. New York, International Linguistics, 1954.
8. Bruner JS: Toward a Theory of Instruction. New York, WW Norton, 1950.
9. Skinner BF: Contingencies of Reinforcement: A Theoretical Analysis. New York, Appleton-Century-Crofts, 1969.
10. Maslow A: Motivation and Personality, ed 2. New York, Harper & Row, 1970.
11. Knox AB: Adult Development and Learning. San Francisco, Jossey-Bass, 1978.
12. Knox AB: Lifelong Self-Directed Learning. San Francisco, Jossey-Bass, 1973.
13. Medical Education in the Information Age: Proceedings of the Symposium on Medical Infomatics. Washington DC, Association of American Medical Colleges, 1986.
14. Stillman PS, Regan MB, Philbin M, Heley HL: Results of a survey on the use of standardized patients to teach and evaluate clinical skills. Acad Med 65:288–292, 1990.
15. Keller FS: Goodbye teacher. J Appl Behav Anal 1:79–89, 1968.
16. Skinner BF: The Technology of Teaching. New York, Appleton-Century-Crofts, 1968.
17. Bloom BS: Learning for Mastery: Evaluation Comment. Los Angeles, UCLA Center for the Study of Evaluation of Instructional Programs, 1968.
18. Turnbull JM: What is normative versus criterion-referenced assessment? Med Teacher 11(2):145–150, 1989.
19. Johnson KR, Ruskin RS: Behavioral Instruction: An Evaluative Review. Washington, DC, American Psychological Association, 1978.
20. Robins AL: Behavioral instruction in the college classroom: A review. Rev Educ Res 46:313–354, 1976.
21. Cohen AJ, Slovin DL, Frazenblau C, Sinex FM: A self-paced biochemistry course for medical students. J Med Educ 48:289–290, 1973.
22. Stahl S, Hennes J, Fleischl G: Progress on self-learning in biostatistics. J Med Educ 50:294–296, 1975.
23. Weisman RA, Shapiro DM: PSI for medical school biochemistry. J Med Educ 48:934–938, 1973.
24. Schimpfhauser F, Richardson K: Medical education and personalized instruction. Educ Technol 17:31–36, 1977.
25. Bono SF, Medio FJ: PSI in the Health Sciences. Augusta, GA, Medical College of Georgia Press, 1979.
26. Mager RF: Preparing Instructional Objectives. Belmont, CA, Fearon Publishers, 1962.
27. Bloom BS: Taxonomy of Educational Objectives, Cognitive Domain. New York, David McKay Co, 1956.
28. Bloom BS: Taxonomy of Educational Objectives, Affective Domain. New York, David McKay Co, 1964.

29. Knowles, MS: Using Learning Contracts. San Francisco, Jossey-Bass, 1986.

30. Stein DS: The adult educator in the health profession: New roles and responsibilities. In: Lifelong Learning: The Adult Years, vol 4, pp 8–11, 1980.

31. Barlow RM: An experiment with learning contracts. J Higher Educ 45:441–449, 1974.

32. Stewart JW, Shank J: Student-teacher contracting: A vehicle for individualized instruction. Audiovis Instruct, pp 31–34, January 1973.

33. Mayville W: Contract learning. In ERIC Higher Education Research Currents. Washington, DC, ERIC Clearinghouse, 1973.

34. Barrows H: A taxonomy of problem-based learning methods. Med Educ 20:481–486, 1986.

35. Neame RLB: Problem-centered learning in medical education: The role of context in the development of process skills. In Schmidt HG, De Volder ML (eds): Tutorials in Problem-Based Learning, A New Direction. Assen, The Netherlands, Van Gorcum & Co, 1984.

36. Schmidt HG, Dauphinee WD, Patel VL: Comparing the effects of problem-based and conventional curricula in an international sample. J Med Educ 62:305–315, 1987.

37. Glick SM: Problem-based learning and community-oriented medical education. Med Ed 25:542–545, 1991.

38. Berkson L: Critique of Problem-Based Learning: A Review of the Literature, master's thesis. Health Professions Education, Graduate College, University of Illinois at Chicago, 1990.

39. Fulop T: Setting the stage: Problem-based learning in the mirror of social target—health for all. In Schmidt HG, et al (eds): Tutorials in Problem-Based Learning. Maastricht, The Netherlands, Van Gorcum & Co, 1984.

40. Wilkerson L, Hafler JP, Liu P: A case study of student-directed discussion in four problem-based tutorial groups. Acad Med 66(9):S79–S81, 1991.

41. Neufeld VR, Norman GR (eds): Assessing Clinical Competence. New York, Springer, 1985.

42. Marton F, Hounsell DJ, Entwistle NJ (eds): The Experience of Learning. Edinburgh, Scottish Academic Press, 1984.

43. Norman GR: Problem-solving skills, solving problems and problem-based learning. Med Educ 22:279–286, 1988.

44. Grant J, Marsden P: The structure of memorized knowledge in students and clinicians: An explanation for diagnostic expertise. Med Educ 21:92–98, 1987.

45. Neufeld VR, Norman GR, Feightner JW, Barrows HS: Clinical problem-solving by medical students: A cross-sectional and longitudinal analysis. Med Educ 15:315–322, 1981.

46. Gordon MJ: Use of heuristics in diagnostic problem-solving. In Elstein AS, et al (eds): Medical Problem Solving. Cambridge, MA, Harvard University Press, 1978.

47. McGuire CH: Medical problem solving: A critique of the literature. J Med Educ 60:587–597, 1985.

48. Woodward CA: Summary of McMaster medical graduates' performance on the Medical Council of Canada examination. Hamilton, Ontario, Canada, McMaster University Faculty of Health Sciences, 1984.

49. McGuire CH: Evaluation of student and practitioner competence. In McGuire CH, et al (eds): Handbook of Health Professions Education. San Francisco, Jossey-Bass, 1983.

50. Norman GR: Evaluation of problem-solving ability. In Hart, IR, et al (eds): Newer Developments in Assessing Clinical Competence. Montreal, Heal Publications, 1986.

51. Feightner JW: Patient management problems. In Neufeld VR, Norman GR (eds): Assessing Clinical Competence. New York, Springer, 1985.

52. Claessen HFA, Boshuizen HPA: Recall of medical information by students and doctors. Med Educ 19:61–67, 1985.

53. Coles CR: Differences between conventional and problem-based curricula in their students' approaches to studying. Med Educ 19:308–310, 1985.

54. Newble DI, Clarke RA: A comparison of the approaches to learning of students in a traditional and an innovative medical school. Med Educ 20:267–273, 1988.

55. Baca E, Mennin SP, Kaufman A, Moore-West M: A comparison between a problem-based, community-oriented track and a traditional track. In Khattab T, et al (eds): Innovations in Medical Education: An Evaluation of Its Present Status. New York, Springer, 1988.

56. Woodward CA, Ferrier BM: Perspectives of graduates two to five years after graduation from a three-year medical school. J Med Educ 57:294–303, 1982.

57. Rothman AI: Statements on career intentions as predictors of career choices. J Med Educ 60:511–516, 1985.

58. Glasser M, Sarnowski AA Jr, Sheth B: Career choices from medical school to practice: Findings from a regional clinical education site. J Med Educ 57:442–448, 1982.

59. Isokoski M: Innovative curriculum leads young doctors to primary health care. In Khattab T, et al (eds): Innovation in Medical Education: An Evaluation of Its Present Status. New York, Springer, 1988.

60. Gordon MJ: A review of the validity and accuracy of self-assessments in health professions training. Acad Med 66:762–769, 1991.

61. Berdie RF: Self-claimed and tested knowledge. J Educ Measurement 31:629–636, 1971.

62. Pohlmann JL, Beggs DLA: A study of the validity of self-reported measures of academic growth. J Educ Measurement 12:115–118, 1974.

63. Lichtenstein S, Fischoff B: Do those who know more also know more about how much they know? Organization Behav Hum Perform 20:159–183, 1977.

64. Calhoun JG, Wooliscroft JO, Ten Haken JD, et al: Evaluating medical student clinical skill performance: Relationships among self, peer and expert ratings. Eval Health Profess 11(2):201–212, 1988.

65. Stuart MR, Goldstein HS, Snope FC: Self-evaluation by residents in family medicine. J Fam Pract 10:639–642, 1980.

66. Arnold L, Willoughby TL, Calkins EV: Self-evaluation in undergraduate medical education: A longitudinal perspective. J Med Educ 60:21–28, 1985.

67. Rezler AG: Self-assessment in problem-based groups. Med Teach 11(2):151–156, 1989.

68. Henbest RJ, Fehrsen GS: Preliminary study at the University of Southern Africa on student self-assessment as a means of evaluation. J Med Educ 60:66–68, 1985.

69. Barrows H: How to Design a Problem-Based Curriculum for the Preclinical Years. New York, Springer, 1985.

70. Hollinger TG: Problem-based learning in the traditional curriculum. Proc Annu Conf Res Med Educ 28:40–45, 1989.

71. Farnsworth W, Medio F: Integrating clinical problem-solving workshops and lectures in a biochemistry course. Biochem Educ 16(4):196–200, 1988.

72. McKegney CP: Medical education: A neglectful and abusive family system. Fam Med 21(6):452–457, 1989.

73. Edwards J, Morier R (eds): Clinical Teaching for Residents: Roles, Techniques and Programs. New York, Springer, 1989.

74. Medio F, Wilkerson L, Lesky L, Borkan S: Integrating teaching and patient care. In Edwards J, Morier R (eds): Clinical Teaching for Residents: Roles, Techniques and Programs. New York, Springer, 1989.

75. Medio F, Greenberg L, Skeff F, Wilkerson L: Clinical teaching: Three perspectives on faculty development: Proceedings of the Annual Research in Medical Education Conference 24:329–336, 1985.

76. McGaghie WC, Frey JJ (eds): Handbook for the Academic Physician. New York, Springer-Verlag, 1986.

77. Foley R, Smilansky J: Teaching Techniques: A Handbook for Health Professionals. New York, McGraw-Hill Book Company, 1980.

78. Whitman N: Creative Medical Teaching. Salt Lake City, University of Utah School of Medicine, 1990.

79. Lowman J: Mastering the Techniques of Teaching. San Francisco, Jossey-Bass, 1984.

CHAPTER 8

COMMUNITY HEALTH

Leonard A. Levy

Community health, rather than focusing on the individual person, responds to larger groups of persons who have certain characteristics or interests in common. This may include a neighborhood or other geographic area, an ethnic group, an occupation, and other designations depending on how broadly one may wish to define *community*.

Because the term is often defined by the people involved, for the sake of discussion it may be best to accept whatever definition a group of people decide to use to delineate a community. In most instances, when the goal of those involved in community health is health promotion and disease prevention, that definition will be adequate and avoids controversies about political correctness.

EVOLUTION OF COMMUNITY HEALTH

For most of the 20th century much of the practice of public and community health was provided by individual health care providers who saw patients in a single or multidisciplinary private or group practice. Whatever health problems remained were of little concern to them and simply something in which the state or local health department was involved. Even if it was pointed out that community health activities directly affected the individual practitioner, it was still difficult to convince the practitioner to accept that conclusion with any degree of seriousness, in spite of what may have seemed to be the most rational of arguments.

Today, however, the nation faces a serious health care crisis, which is defined by the following:

- Rapidly escalating costs
- A growing older population
- A large segment of the population that is either without health insurance or underinsured
- A rural and inner city population who are underserved

- A growing technology further taxing health care costs
- The expanding acquired immunodeficiency syndrome (AIDS) epidemic
- Huge malpractice premiums
- Demand by the public that health care is a right
- Growth of specialization with a corresponding lack of interest in, and shortage of, primary care providers

The half century before the outbreak of World War II saw health as a cottage industry that featured the all-knowing family doctor who usually entered practice immediately after a 1-year internship. He (only a few were female) was both the provider of health care and functionally the center of community health for the neighborhood in which he was located. Since those years it has become no longer possible for one person to accumulate all the knowledge and skills and accept virtually all of the responsibilities required to provide health care.

AN AGING POPULATION

The introduction of penicillin during World War II and then into civilian health care practice resulted in the survival of countless persons who would otherwise not have survived infectious diseases that today we consider relatively minor. Other scientific and technologic advances allowed many persons with acute diseases to survive and many with chronic disease who would otherwise have died to live long enough to become part of the aged population. In 1940 about 7% of the population was older than age 65, rising by only 1%, or to 12.3 million, in 1950. By 1990 the number of persons older than age 65 increased more than 2.7 times to about 33 million, or about 12.7% of the total population. Between 1950 and 1990 the number of those older than age 85, the oldest of the old, grew more than three times to 3.3 million.

Most significant about the aging of the US population is the fact that while today they represent about 12% of the nation, about one third of the nation's health care expenditures are attributed to them. By the year 2000, there will be almost 15% of Americans older than

age 65 and an estimated 20% by 2020. All things being equal, the elderly then could be responsible for as much as 50% of the nation's health costs, an astounding amount of money considering estimates that today's 1 trillion dollar annual health budget will grow to about 1.6 trillion dollars at the start of the new millennium, more than 14% of the gross national product.

Older persons tend to be at higher risk for acquiring many health problems, including those affecting the feet. Such podiatric problems, for example, tend to cause or contribute to disability, contribute to loss of independence, and, in some instances, jeopardize their limbs as well as shorten their lives (e.g., the complications of diabetes).

Associated with this phenomenon of an aging America has been the growth of the long-term care industry. A combination of an older population, too frail to live independently, and a society in which increased mobility has led to the family's breaking up, leaving aging parents behind, has resulted in an expanding need for nursing home beds. The cost of these institutions in 1990 approached $25,000 yearly for each resident, far in excess of what the average American family can afford and, except for a relatively few persons with special coverage, not part of basic or major medical health insurance programs.

INNER CITY AND RURAL AMERICA

Inhabitants of rural and inner city America have another set of problems. Those health disciplines involved in providing primary health care are often absent or in very short supply in these communities. Throughout the nation, for example, there are rural communities without a single family physician. Similarly, in podiatric medicine, those completing podiatric medical residency programs are far less likely to practice in a rural or inner city community. Like their family medicine physician counterparts, they fear being isolated from colleagues, especially if they are the only podiatric physician in a town miles from another member of the profession. In addition, they are concerned that the potential for earning an income large enough to service school loans approaching or exceeding 100 thousand dollars could be difficult in rural practice. The unavailability of coverage necessary to be able to attend continuing education programs or assistance during the performance of podiatric surgical procedures also could be a concern in choosing a rural practice.

Poverty and socioeconomic deprivation in many inner city communities and the problems these generate often discourage the podiatric physician from practicing in these areas. This is further compounded by stressed state and federal budgets, which lead to cutbacks in government-funded health programs such as Medicaid, serving as a further disincentive to practice in such needy neighborhoods. The paradox of this situation is that most studies show that the poor are among the highest at risk for developing podiatric medical disorders, yet they often have less access to such care except when acute, sometimes limb-threatening conditions occur.

COMMUNITY HEALTH NEEDS: PUBLIC AGENCIES AND THE PRIVATE SECTOR

Too often the responsibility of meeting the needs of the community is perceived as being almost exclusively within the purview of some governmental entity, such as the local, state, or even federal public health agency. Certainly these public agencies have giant shares in such initiatives, but to assume that they are the exclusive protectors of the health of the community is both unrealistic and also not the case. The following discussion describes both the public agencies involved in the community health agenda as well as that which is and will probably continue to be the role of the private sector. Private sector institutions may be nongovernmental agencies that have accepted important roles in community health. However, the responsibility of the individual podiatric physician should also be considered within this context.

Over the years the attitude of the public has changed considerably concerning health care. Today health care is articulated as a right rather than a privilege reserved for the more affluent. In the late 1960s both Medicaid and Medicare legislation eliminated to a great extent financial barriers to health care for per-

haps the most at-risk populations in the nation, the poor and the elderly. Over the years, however, many changes have modified and reduced the extent of coverage that these programs provide. Medicaid, for example, in many states reimburses health care providers and institutions to a considerably lesser degree than it did in the past. This has driven many members of the health care community from the program, refusing to accept Medicaid recipients into their practice. Since neighborhoods with a large percentage of poor persons are also areas with the poorest health statistics or with the highest prevalence and incidence of health problems, it is these persons who are directly affected by the inadequacies of the Medicaid program. In addition, few health care providers choose to practice in the poor areas of the inner city, further compounding the problem of access to health care experienced by the poor. As a result, the poor are more likely to continue to neglect preventive health services, often seeking care only when their health problems are more acute and more expensive or utilizing already busy emergency departments for routine, nonemergency services. Although this may be due to a lack of sophistication in dealing with the health care system, it is also due to the lack of health care providers in their neighborhood.

For example, the podiatric medical problems that the poor experience tend to be further along in their natural history than what one would find among the middle class and more affluent groups. Diabetic foot ulcers and other serious complications found in podiatric patients are far more prevalent among the poor than segments of society that have access to preventive foot health services.

In addition, excessive costs, so-called defensive health care due to the fear of a malpractice action, and an increase of expensive technology as well as overutilization have been among the prominent factors leading to tighter and tighter restrictions and greater deductibles in the Medicare program. This becomes more obvious each year because of the rapidly growing population of older Americans. Failure to reimburse the podiatric practitioner and other health care providers also encourages the onset of problems, requiring more expensive care, which is also more complex.

For similar reasons, private insurance companies also have adopted more restrictions in reimbursement for podiatric and other health care services. Here, too, preventive services are either not covered or are highly restricted. In addition, the costs of health care have escalated premiums to the point that employers in smaller businesses in particular are unable to offer health insurance as a benefit and larger employers find that it has become one of the major contributing factors to the cost of their product or service. Today approximately 36 million Americans hold no health insurance.

COMPONENTS OF COMMUNITY HEALTH PROGRAMS

Components that could be included in community health programs are listed below:

■ Health promotion and disease prevention in schools, work sites, and churches or synagogues
■ Community-based screening and referral
■ Education of health care professionals
■ Community mobilization
■ Use of volunteers
■ Use of mass media

When such programs are developed they must be properly scaled to the level appropriate to the size of the community that is identified. This pragmatic approach is important to sustain funding, to monitor the effectiveness of the program, and to reach the populations that have been targeted.

Healthy People 2000

On a national scale, the Department of Health and Human Services issued what is referred to as Healthy People 2000: National Health Promotion and Disease Prevention Objectives. These objectives emphasize an increased focus on prevention of disability and morbidity; greater attention to improvements in the health status of definable population groups at highest risk of premature death, disease, and disability; and inclusion of more screening interventions to detect asymptomatic diseases and conditions early enough to

prevent early death or chronic illness. It is from these objectives that community health priorities could evolve both in general and to how they relate to the podiatric medical needs of the population.

Evolving from Healthy People 2000 objectives were a number of priorities categorized under health promotion, health protection, preventive services, and system improvement. Of the seven priorities listed under health promotion, three have obvious direct relationships to podiatric medicine. These include physical activity and fitness, tobacco use (i.e., the single most important cause of occlusive peripheral arterial disease), and vitality and independence of older persons. All three health protection priorities also have direct podiatric relationships, namely, environmental health, occupational safety and health, and unintentional injuries (e.g., hip fractures in the elderly). Preventive services priorities strongly relevant to podiatric medicine include maternal and child health, human immunodeficiency virus infection, high blood cholesterol levels, high blood pressure, cancer, and chronic disorders (e.g., diabetes, various arthritides, neurologic disorders).

PUBLIC AND PRIVATE COMMUNITY HEALTH AGENCIES

Among the private sector agencies concerned about certain aspects of community health are those that focus on various diseases or groups of health problems. Examples include the Arthritis Foundation, Juvenile Diabetes Foundation, American Diabetes Association, March of Dimes, and American Cancer Society. Their efforts frequently employ fund raising to support research and patient care activities. A number of fraternal and social groups may also have as part of their mission some aspect of community health concern. In addition to fund raising, private sector groups may also participate in developing health education activities aimed at making the community more aware of the prevention and early detection of a particular disease process.

Large and small foundations from time to time issue requests for proposals to educational institutions or other nonprofit groups designed to study or provide innovations to resolve or improve some community health concern. Current examples include requests for proposals in areas of primary care recently issued by the Robert Wood Johnson Foundation and the W.K. Kellogg Foundation.

More familiar are the various initiatives that come from the federal government. These grant programs emanate from community concerns that make their way to legislators in Congress through the political process. Examples include grants from the US Public Health Service designed to increase the number of podiatric physicians who enter primary care podiatric medicine (i.e., Podiatric Primary Care Residency Training Program).

PODIATRISTS AND COMMUNITY HEALTH

Community podiatrists from time to time find themselves addressing groups of lay persons or professionals to increase their awareness about such issues as good foot health, specific podiatric medical problems, and approaches to preventing and treating podiatric medical disorders. The focus may be on groups who are at risk, such as diabetics, the elderly, or even children. The outcome of the efforts of the podiatrist involved in such community-based activities is often an increase in the demand for podiatric medical services by those who need such care before a podiatric problem occurs or early in its natural history. These various at-risk groups are also made more aware of the role of podiatrists in the community.

BIBLIOGRAPHY

Health United States 1990. DHHS publication No. (PHS) 91-1232. Hyattsville, MD, US Department of Health and Human Services, Public Health Service, Centers for Disease Control and Prevention, National Center for Health Statistics, March 1991.

Healthy America: Practitioners for 2005, An Agenda for Action for U.S. Health Professional Schools: A Report of the Pew Health Professions Commission, October 1991.

Healthy People 2000: National Health Promotion and Disease Prevention Objectives. DHHS publication PHS 91-50213. Washington, DC, US Department of Health and Human Services, 1991.

Helfand AE: Public Health and Podiatric Medicine. Baltimore, Williams & Wilkins, 1987.

Levy LA: Prevalence of Chronic Podiatric Conditions in the U.S.: National Health Survey 1990. J Am Podiatr Med Assoc 82:221–223, 1991.

Rural Health Professions Facts. Supply and Distribution of Health Professionals in Rural America: Helping to Build a Healthier America. Rockville, MD, Bureau of Health Professions, Health Resources and Services Administration, US Department of Health and Human Services, 1991.

Seventh Report to the President and Congress on the Status of Health Personnel in the United States. DHHS publication No. HRS-P-OD-90-1. Rockville, MD, US Department of Health and Human Services, Public Health Service, Health Resources and Services Administration, Bureau of Health Professions, March 1990.

CHAPTER 9

DEVELOPMENT OF A FOOT HEALTH PROGRAM IN AN OCCUPATIONAL SETTING

Rock G. Positano

The foot is a biologic and engineering wonder. It consists of 26 bones and 19 intrinsic and 12 extrinsic muscles and is able to withstand tremendous force. [1] It permits the average human to ambulate thousands of miles during his or her lifetime.[2]

Nevertheless, the foot has only rarely been studied as compared with other body parts. There is no definitive explanation for this observation, except that the foot's anatomical relationship to the body's superstructure may be responsible for its not being a focal point of interest. It has however, been the focus of religious symbolism, as evidenced by the humble tradition of bathing the feet of kings, queens, magistrates, and theological figures. This ritual is commonly referred to in religious texts and was often performed by Christ and the apostles as an act of humility and goodwill. The foot is also well represented in artistic creations and paintings as an object of profound beauty and grace.

Anthropologists regard the human foot as being a unique anatomical and functional structure. The renowned anthropologist John Buettner-Janusch supports this statement about the human foot when he relates:

Man's foot is all his own. It is unlike any other foot. It is the most distinctly human part of his whole anatomical make-up. It is a human specialization and, whether he be proud of it or not, it is his hallmark. So long as man has been man, and so long as he remains man, it is by his feet that he will be known from all other members of the animal kingdom.[3]

The foot plays an integral role in maintaining quality of life, regardless of background or status. In the occupational setting, proper foot function is essential. Performance of work tasks requires ambulation, and any derangement of the ambulatory cycle may result in decreased worker productivity, function, and morale. In addition, painful feet may result in a worker's loss of concentration, leading to an increase in accidents.[4]

The prevalence of foot disorders is of great

magnitude, with at least 80% of the general population affected by age 65.[5] The foot is a mirror of some systemic diseases, as evidenced by the fact that approximately 500 disease processes may manifest in the feet.[6] This strongly indicates that an examination of the foot may assist an astute clinician in recognizing the presence of systemic disease that otherwise may have gone undetected.

The establishment of a corporate program in preventive and occupational podiatric health may assist in the recognition, evaluation, and treatment of foot disorders. The program utilizes many facets of professional intervention at the clinical, academic, and educational levels. Establishment of such a program may reduce the morbidity of foot disorders, decrease the number of accidents occurring in the workplace, increase worker productivity, and serve as a means of screening for systemic disease requiring subsequent referral.

The human foot deserves much more attention than it has received. In this chapter the importance of foot health in the performance of occupational tasks is discussed, and a program is suggested to improve and maintain that health.

HISTORY OF OCCUPATIONAL MEDICINE

Occupational medicine has evolved into a dynamic specialty during the past 20 years. Many reasons for this metamorphosis exist, with some being more self-evident than others.

Technology has played a significant role in the development of occupational medicine. As technology became more sophisticated there was an associated increase in workplace hazards. Although the specialty of occupational medicine is now well established, it traces its modest beginnings as far back as the Paleolithic Age.[7] Archaeologists Edwin, Smith, and Selier, while excavating a site, discovered ancient papyri that described in some detail what appears to be occupational hazards and injuries.[8] Most medical historians consider the year 1700 as the beginning of occupational medicine. In Italy, Bernardino Ramazzini published the first comprehensive work on occupational medicine, entitled *De Morbis Artificum Diatribe.*[9] This scholarly publication earned him the dis-

tinction of being considered the "father of occupational medicine." A sophisticated and detailed work, it was a description of diseases associated with specific occupations found during Ramazzini's time, such as corpse carrier, laundress, and porter. Ramazzini was equally devoted to the practice of medicine and the art of proper diagnosis. He was credited as being the first physician to ask the patient about his or her occupation and how the occupation was related to the patient's disease. Ramazzini stated:

When a doctor visits a working-class home he should be content to sit on a three-legged stool, if there isn't a gilded chair, and he should take time for his examination; and to the questions recommended by Hippocrates, he should add one more— What is your occupation?[9]

The important effect that a person's occupation had on health was also recognized in other parts of the world. In 1775, an English physician, Sir Percival Pott, discovered a link between exposure to soot deposits and cancer of the scrotum in chimney sweeps.[10] Some 50 years later, Charles Turner Thackrah published a book entitled *The Effects of Arts, Trades and Professions and All Civic States and Habit of Living on Life and Longevity.*[11] He authored this publication based on his experiences in the manufacturing district of Leeds, England.

Goldwater remarks that during a time span of 100 years after Ramazzini's publication there were no significant developments of a scientific nature in the specialty of occupational medicine.[10]

The 20th century presented different and unique challenges to the field of occupational health. The Industrial Revolution was underway, and with this came a variety of occupational injuries. In the early 1900s some attention was given to the prevention of occupational accidents and injuries. Workers' compensation became an important issue and, to meet this new challenge, programs dedicated to accident prevention were developed. During the 1930s the focus shifted from accident prevention and traumatology to the discipline of toxicology, the study of poisons. During World War II the fabrication of trinitrotoluene involved potentially hazardous steps that resulted in many casualties because of the toxicity of the ingredients used to compound this explosive.[10]

The 1950s marked the beginning of a sincere interest in atmospheric contaminants and pollution. Industrial hygienists were now faced with the monumental challenge of analyzing and evaluating outside air pollution.

Many variables complicate the problems confronting an occupational health practitioner. Industry has introduced thousands of new chemicals into the environment. Persons from all stations of life and occupations are exposed to these agents. Physical agents such as noise and radiation are ubiquitous and present unique problems to both the clinician and the patient.

Present-day occupational medicine addresses many of the areas just described and, in addition, emerging areas such as biomechanics, ergonomics, mental health, and rehabilitation, just to list a few. Occupational health practitioners must continue to meet these challenges by expanding research and clinical interventions at all levels of medical practice and care.

EPIDEMIOLOGY OF FOOT DISORDERS

As functional anatomic units, the feet may influence the performance and behavior of workers in an occupational setting.[12] In spite of this, there is relatively little information concerning the podiatric contributions to occupational medicine and epidemiology. Shore[13] examined the extent to which podiatry and occupational medicine have been interrelated. A computerized MEDLINE search reviewing the past 20 years revealed only 30 articles that addressed the relationship between epidemiology and podiatric medicine. One may conclude that many gray areas exist in our knowledge of the frequency and determinants of foot disorders in the population. Interestingly, of the articles found in this search, only 2 dealt with occupational health, indicating that the epidemiologic study of occupational foot disease is a relatively unexplored area.

In 1982, Rosenquist studied the prevalence of foot problems among diabetics.[1] In this cross-sectional study, diabetics were stratified by age to ensure that older and younger patients were equally represented. Some of the points of interest in the questionnaire were signs and symptoms of foot disease. Fifty-seven percent reported moderate foot pathology, and 33% were classified as having no foot disease. The study further yielded interesting information concerning the relationship between the respondents' domestic situation and the severity of disease. For example, respondents who were living alone or retired early were more prone to develop severe foot disease. This study was well conceived and executed with the exception of one weakness: the sampling frame was not representative of all diabetics but instead dealt exclusively with diabetics who were hospitalized. Shore[13] contends that the study provides excellent information about the impact of diabetes on foot disease and about how primary care and occupational health practitioners should monitor the podiatric health of diabetics who may present with foot disease.

Amputation of limbs and digits is a major problem in the diabetic population. Most and Sinnock,[14] in 1983, designed and conducted a surveillance-type descriptive study on amputees in the diabetic population utilizing the US Centers for Disease Control registers founded on state-based diabetes control programs. The researchers utilized these data to examine the incidence of lower-extremity amputation among diabetics. They found that the amputation rate increased with age. For example, the population of diabetics 45 years and younger had an amputation rate of 14 per year per 10,000 diabetics. In persons older than the age of 65 this rate increased dramatically to 101 per year per 10,000 diabetics. The site of amputation also was influenced by age. The most common amputation performed in the age group of 45 and younger was the toe, whereas leg amputation was commonly performed in the older diabetic age group. Some conclusions regarding gender and amputation were also formulated. Men had higher amputation rates than women in all age groups.

In 1963, Acheson and associates conducted a descriptive study in New Haven, Connecticut, entitled the New Haven Survey of Joint Diseases.[15] In this study, men and women were interviewed using a standardized form pertaining to the symptoms of diseases of joints. Some of the characteristics of joint diseases included in this interview were the presence of nocturnal pain, joint stiffness, and swelling. Morning stiffness in the feet and ankles was found in 1.7% and 1.5%, respectively, with 27% of participants reporting some degree of morning stiffness. A total of 14% of the respondents reported experiencing nocturnal pains. Approximately 1.6% involved the feet, and an equal percentage involved the ankles. A third symptom, joint swelling, was reported by 22% of the respondents. The foot and ankle swelling accounted for 4.8% and 7.9%, respectively.

The MEDLINE literature search found only two occupational epidemiology studies of foot disease. One study evaluated the prevalence of disorders of the lower extremities among 82 men employed in heavy industry.[16] This was a descriptive study in which 82 workers underwent a thorough podiatric examination. The researchers found that 73 of the respondents exhibited evidence of foot disease. This accounted for 238 diagnoses. Nine men were reported as having no signs of podiatric disorders. Static foot deformities were most prevalent among the 73 workers, occurring in 63% of the study population. Equally important were dermatologic disorders, which accounted for a prevalence rate of 59%. Shore comments that "taken as a whole, these data suggest there is a large burden of submerged problems of the lower extremities, which are not being detected adequately by the routine health examination in industry."[13]

The other cited occupational epidemiology study of foot disease focused on peripheral nervous system function among workers exposed to n-hexane.[13] These workers were employed in a factory that produced tungsten carbide alloys. Before this investigation the substance n-hexane was considered to be a nontoxic solvent used in industry. The American Conference of Government Industrial Hygienists standard for n-hexane is 100 ppm.[13] Personal monitoring for exposure showed an average exposure level of 58 ppm. The researchers were able to enlist the cooperation of 14 workers who conducted their occupational tasks in the exposed area. The investigators tested for the presence of 20 neurologic symptoms. The exposed group revealed a higher reported prevalence of headache, transient dysesthesia in the limbs, and transient muscle weakness. The exposed group performed poorly in the one-foot jump test, indicating decreased performance of the posterior tibial nerve, a major nerve supply to the foot. The investigators concluded that n-hexane had an adverse effect on lower-extremity function and physiology.

Occupational epidemiology is emerging as an invaluable addition to the scientific armamentarium as it explores and elucidates the determinants and distribution of disease in the workplace.[17, 18] There exists much information on worker exposure to various chemical compounds and their subsequent adverse effects. Hernberg[19] considers the workplace to be a community with specifically associated health problems. He further notes that although specific occupationally induced pathologic processes are the result of occupational exposure, the majority of health problems encountered in the occupational setting are part of a "general" morbidity.

Disease in any form is capable of interfering with the capacity of a worker to perform his or her tasks in an efficient and safe manner. Foot disorders may certainly be placed in this category since their presence may distract the worker and lead to an accident. Hernberg lists several important variables that should be identified to effectively assess the general state of health of the worker. A modification and adaptation of these variables to podiatric occupational medicine follows.

For example, persons at increased risk of contracting specific diseases should be identified. Preventive strategies may be implemented to avoid, curtail, or retard the occurrence of podiatric medical problems. This would include those workers who present with diabetes, peripheral vascular disease, and the biological and physical changes that occur with aging. These persons are more prone to developing serious and debilitating podiatric problems. Those workers who present with minor and treatable disorders constitute a large group. Nail disorders, hyperkeratotic lesions, biomechanical abnormalities, and nonthreatening dermatologic conditions would be included in this category. These conditions, although obviously not life threatening, may develop into painful and aggravating maladies.[2] An additional group includes employees whose suitability for certain occupational tasks is restricted or not recommended. Conditions such as flat feet, cavus feet, bunion, and hammer-toe deformities and obesity may be greatly aggravated and worsened by occupations that require prolonged standing and excessive ambulation.

PREVENTION OF OCCUPATIONAL INJURIES

A major objective of occupational health and medicine is prevention. Prevention of work-induced morbidity is achieved by the implementation of various measures, including preventive medical screening.[20–24]

Morbidity is an evolving process that may occur over a short or an extended period of time. The duration of time will determine whether the presenting pathologic process is reversible. Classically, prevention has been addressed in primary, secondary, and tertiary levels.[18, 21]

Primary Prevention

Primary prevention is the entry level of protective health intervention. Intervention at this level serves to prevent the onset and initiation of the disease process.[18] This implies that there is no disease or pathologic process present. It takes into account two specific types of health promotion. One is concerned with general health promotion,[18] which encourages the practice of desirable health habits in the home or place of business and school or any activity that promotes a healthy lifestyle. The other category is referred to as specific protective measures[18] and includes environmental control and immunization and in the occupational setting would encompass testing for dangerous chemicals, biologic monitoring, and implementation of protective engineering controls.[20, 23]

Podiatric medicine has much to offer at this primary level of prevention.[12] Health education is an important dimension of any health care system. The podiatrist serves a vital role as a health educator. Persons who benefit most from preventive podiatric education are those

in statistically high-risk groups for being disabled due to lower-extremity disease. These workers are generally afflicted with vascular and diabetic conditions and their associated complications.[14, 25]

Levine has written about the frequency of foot problems found in the diabetic population.[26] He reports that 20% of all diabetic patients admitted to a hospital are there because of podiatric problems. Byyny[27] reports that 50% of all diabetics will require surgical intervention for treatment of diabetic lesions sometime during their lifetime. There should be no question as to the value of podiatric health education for these medically high-risk groups. Primary preventive measures may play an integral role in reducing the significant morbidity that may occur in this population.

Gorecki[12] includes accident-prone persons and the handicapped in the high-risk category. Accident-prone persons have a greater propensity for traumatizing their feet. It is not uncommon for such persons to stub their toes or drop cartons heavy enough to cause metatarsal fracture. Wearing of appropriate shoes becomes an important preventive factor in such a situation. The podiatrist provides counseling on the proper shoes to be worn while performing various work tasks. Protecting and properly supporting the foot in the occupational setting should be an industrial hygiene priority. Bly et al.[28] support the merit of this strategy. They contend that the foot is the anatomical body part most susceptible to injury in industry and the workplace.

Secondary Prevention

When possible, the preventive and occupational medicine practitioner must prevent medical conditions before the disease process is initiated.[29] Unfortunately, it is not feasible for health care professionals to constantly monitor the personal activities of their patients. Realizing these limitations, however, compels the clinician to develop strategies that are able to detect disease at its earliest stage. This is the major focus of secondary prevention.[18, 21, 30]

The main advantage of secondary prevention is that it may permit prompt treatment of the disorder.[31] In many instances the disease may be completely cured or its progression retarded. This may prevent total disability and the development of more serious complications.

From a podiatric perspective secondary prevention is of paramount importance. The majority of patients seen by foot specialists are generally at the secondary level. They may present with a foot ailment that appears relatively benign, whereas it may ultimately develop into a serious problem. Levy contends that interrupting the progression of foot disease is of extreme importance.[32] There are various activities that may be employed to retard or interrupt the cycle leading to disability. Periodic screening examinations may reduce irreversible permanent disability. All too often persons frequent the offices of health care professionals during an acute medical crisis, not while asymptomatic. Screening at this level is effective and is a viable means for controlling the progression of foot deformity.

The podiatric practitioner is able to recognize, evaluate, and control foot problems at the secondary level. Podiatric problems that occur with greatest frequency include biomechanical abnormalities, dermatologic conditions, and osseous pain. Each of these entities is preventable. If such conditions progress to a more symptomatic stage, the practitioner can use numerous treatment modalities.

For example, nail problems constitute a major group of podiatric disorders that afflict the working population.[33] A nail condition may be extremely painful and result in disability. Many environmental etiologies exist for nail conditions, including trauma, biomechanical abnormality, physical and chemical agents, pharmaceuticals, heredity, and neoplastic lesions. The nail serves as an excellent indicator of underlying systemic disease and the proper examination of this unit may provide invaluable diagnostic information.[34] The nails are equally sensitive to environmental and physical stimuli and may provide clues that indicate toxic exposure and traumatic insult. Nail problems are manageable when recognized and treated promptly.

Tertiary Prevention

The main focus at this level addresses two major factors: (1) the limitation of disability

and (2) rehabilitation. For example, the application of physical therapy to an injured limb may enable the patient to resume ambulation and prevent additional adverse sequelae. Rehabilitation has evolved as a major force in patient care, especially in those cases in which the patient may be able to restore function to the injured part. Rehabilitation makes proper use of the person's residual capacities[18] and stresses the further development of the person's remaining abilities, not those abilities lost as a result of the illness.

Severe podiatric deformities may limit a person's ability to ambulate, thereby interfering with the quality of life. The tertiary level is of great importance to the podiatrist because it is a major priority to restore and or maintain the patient's ability to ambulate comfortably and effectively. Conditions such as diabetic ulcerations, hyperkeratotic lesions, and arthritis are maladies that may severely impair the patient's ability to walk. Major advances have been made in the field of rehabilitation medicine. Biomechanical and orthotic therapy, conservative medical therapeusis, and surgical intervention have been effectively utilized by the clinician to restore function of the diseased limb. There also exist two nonmedical components of the rehabilitation process. One is psychosocial, which integrates family counseling, spiritual counseling, recreation, social service, and psychological evaluation. Most clinicians will agree that a major influence on treatment and rehabilitation is the patient's attitude. The other component is vocational and concerns itself with placement, evaluation, and counseling. The employer plays a major role in assisting the employee to progress and recover from an injury or illness.

RATIONALE FOR AN OCCUPATIONAL FOOT HEALTH PROGRAM

Elderly in the Workplace

The growing elderly population is rapidly emerging as a major force that the health care system must deal with effectively, both now and in the future.[35] As a group, elderly persons are unique in many respects. Many are retired and live alone with or without the benefit of home caregivers and family. From a medical standpoint the geriatric patient is at great risk to develop systemic disease, which may be debilitating. For example, a geriatric patient may develop significant cardiovascular disease.[18] This may be the result of years of poor dietary habits, smoking, and the effects of the aging process on the arteriovenous system. Hypertension is another disease found with greater incidence in this population.[18] The arthritides commonly found in the aged population, secondary to joint wear and tear, may present a difficult challenge for geriatric patients by severely limiting their ability to walk and be productive.

A geriatric patient is confronted with social issues such as loneliness and depression that are often not addressed as legitimate problems. What remains as most striking, however, is the future demographic projections concerning this group. Medical technology, education, and genetic and environmental factors are influencing the life expectancy of the human race.[36]

Two terms commonly and incorrectly interchanged need to be clarified, namely, human *life span* and human *life expectancy*. Life span is concerned with the maximum amount of years that a human body may function. Schneider and Brody have reported this value to be within the range of 110 to 115 years.[37] Life expectancy, as defined by Mausner and Kramer,[18] is the average number of years a person is expected to be alive. Life expectancy is more germane to the topic of preventive and occupational podiatric medicine. As the life expectancy increases, so will the projected percentage of podiatric disease found within the population. It has been projected that by the year 2025, the number of persons aged 65 and older will escalate from 11.3% to 20% of the total population. This will constitute approximately 60 million persons.[35, 36] Additionally, the population of persons 85 years and older will increase from 2 million to 16 million.[35, 36, 38] Examination of projected figures concerning the year 1995 reveals that more than half of the persons presently 65 years and older will live to age 75 and older.[35, 36] Brody contends that at age 75 years and older the incidence of health problems increases sharply.[36] Why are these projections significant and related to po-

diatric medicine and the workplace? Approximately 80% of the United States population will be afflicted with a foot ailment at some point during their lifetime.[5] The anticipated increase in life expectancy will result in an older work force in greater need of foot care.[39] Studies of geriatric patients have demonstrated that 90% to 95% of this population present with foot disorders.[1] Programs of foot disease prevention must be initiated at an earlier age to retard the progression of foot pathology that occurs owing to the degenerative changes associated with the aging process and overuse of susceptible body parts. Foot health programs established at the work site by podiatric practitioners specifically trained in preventive and occupational health would prove to be very beneficial.

Projected statistics indicating a large increase in the elderly population are not being refuted. An older work force will be accompanied by increased incidence of pedal deformities and systemic disease. The present-day health care system is burdened by the obligation of providing medical services. Undoubtedly, this will become more complicated in the future.

In short, the recognition, evaluation, and control of foot deformities at the earliest possible stage will decrease the incidence of podiatric disease.

Ambulation and Performance of Occupational Tasks

The performance of many work tasks requires ambulation. This statement is well substantiated in the occupational setting. The doctor, nurse, salesman, engineer, and construction worker all require ambulation to execute their job responsibilities. Walking in the absence of pain and discomfort is a component of everyday life that many persons take for granted. The inability to ambulate comfortably presents a frustrating dilemma. In the workplace, therefore, maintaining the podiatric health of the worker by preventive means and/or acute care is essential to maintaining the well-being and productivity of the employee.

The most commonly reported employee complaints are foot pain and fatigue.[2, 4] The old adage "when your feet hurt, your entire body hurts" is generally well accepted. Foot complaints and conditions may not be disabling; however, their presence may cause distraction from the task at hand, resulting in carelessness and accidents. Machinists, for example, are at high risk for injuring their hands, extremities, and eyes. Performance of their occupational task requires standing and ambulation. A podiatric problem becomes increasingly painful considering the tremendous pressure exerted on the foot during walking or standing. Foot pain may distract the machinist's attention from the task and increase the risk of an accident.[6, 12, 40] Health care professionals with foot disorders present an equally threatening situation. Doctors and nurses, for example, are required to stand and ambulate for many hours during their work shifts. These occupations require tremendous mental and physical output and stamina. An annoying and painful foot problem poses a serious problem for professionals in these occupations and their patients. For example, a cardiology resident working in an urban hospital complained of an annoying, painful corn. She stated that her painful feet made it very difficult to concentrate, use good judgment, and subsequently render proper treatment.[41]

Biomechanical Foot Deformities

Biomechanically the foot plays an integral role in lower-extremity function.[42–45] The presence of foot pain and dysfunction, for example, may affect the function of other body parts, most notably the knee, hip, and lower back.[42] This may result in aggravation of a preexisting condition such as osteoarthritis and muscle spasm. There is a kinetic link between the knee, hip, lower back, and proper foot function.

Investigators[16] at the 1975 American Public Health Association meeting reported some significant findings associating abnormal foot biomechanics and pedal conditions. The majority of foot problems found in industry are biomechanically related. This study of information was procured in a retrospective study of physician referral patterns to podiatrists in a union clinic. The results revealed that approximately 35% of all workers were at risk for injury involving the feet. Pressure hyperkeratotic lesions were responsible for 15% of reported problems, while foot deformity accounted for 20%. An additional 14% of the complaints related to biomechanics were heel pain, heel spur syndrome, plantar fasciitis, and tenosynovitis. This study indicates that biomechanically induced foot pathology is prevalent in industry. The prognosis, however, is promising because abnormal biomechanics may be controlled by conservative therapeusis and orthotic appliance therapy.

The anatomical relationship of the foot to the body's superstructure renders it more susceptible to injury. It supports a great amount of body weight and is subject to large forces. The foot is distal to the superstructure and, therefore, is generally the first anatomical part to encounter an offending stimulus. For example, a metal weight when dropped will most likely strike the foot first. Johnson[46] studied the distribution of fractures in a retrospective study of 350 patients with forefoot fractures. The study found that approximately 50% of the fractures occurred in the first ray, 25% in the fifth ray, and 25% in the middle rays combined. These fractures, in addition to causing pain, resulted in significant absenteeism, ranging from 2 to 7½ weeks. The anatomical location of the fractures was important, with the phalanges accounting for 85% of the fracture sites. Phalangeal fractures, however, did not account for significant absenteeism.

Prevalence of Foot Disorders in Industry

Americans in the workforce are exposed to numerous environmental influences and physical agents.[30] Included in this category are chemicals, radiation, vibration, and ergonomic stresses. In spite of these environmental stresses, few professionals appreciate the effects these agents have on the foot and how often the foot is involved in occupational accidents and compensation.

In 1971, the National Safety Council published a report that illustrated the strong relationship between the foot and occupational injury.[47] It revealed that nearly 600 million dollars was paid in compensation for work-related injuries of the feet. Approximately 16% of the injuries were compensable, resulting in more than 484 million dollars in payments; approximately 50% of all foot injuries and related conditions resulted in compensation, whereas almost all leg injuries were compensable. The council further reported that in 1985 lower-extremity medical conditions accounted for 19% of the 900,000 work-related injuries in the United States.[48]

Statistically, of the total number of compensation cases settled during 1984 in New York, 20.6% of the 22,951 cases involved the lower extremity.[49] These cases accounted for 170,322 weeks of lost time from the workplace. Only the lower back, which accounted for 21.9% of cases, was more prevalent in compensation cases. These statistics illustrate the relationship between foot injury and compensation in the occupational setting. Preventive measures in this setting would help to decrease the occurrence of such injuries.

OCCUPATIONAL MEDICAL SERVICES AND FOOT HEALTH PROGRAMS

In recent times there has been a great effort to establish health services for workers in the occupational setting. Many authors have defined the occupational health service and how it should function.[50–54] All such services share a common objective: maintenance and improvement of employee health.

Current figures indicate that of the total workforce in the United States, approximately 34% of workers undergo a periodic health examination.[23] No mention is made as to whether foot function is evaluated in this examination. Ramazzini was the first to recognize the significance of the foot and leg in occupational medicine. In his classic work published in 1700, he referred to Agricola's recording of "hands and feet eaten away to the bone" and substances "which eat away the feet of the workmen when they have become wet. . . ."[9]

The importance of preplacement and periodic screenings cannot be overemphasized. The Occupational Safety and Health Administration (OSHA) believes that such activities are effective preventive measures.[20–22, 31, 55, 56] To safeguard against the development and progression of occupation-related disease, health care professionals implement numerous preventive measures, which include medical intervention, engineering controls, education, and awareness.[21]

The concept of worksite health promotion is desirable and gaining momentum.[28, 57–66] Companies are increasingly becoming aware of the benefits such programs reap. These programs have gained widespread acceptance and the interest of corporate managers. Some of the reasons for this interest are because the company has a genuine interest in improving the health of the employee, in preventing accidents and associated costs, in decreasing health care and absenteeism costs, in improving employee morale, and in increasing worker job satisfaction.

These programs have achieved amazing success in encouraging positive changes in employee health behavior and health status. Examples of targeted behavior include increases in physical activity and exercise, weight control, smoking cessation, and decreasing serum cholesterol levels.[28, 67]

One study that has been established as a milestone is the Johnson and Johnson Live for Life (LFL) program, the primary objective of which is to provide a means by which employees "become the healthiest in the world," in addition to decreasing accident costs and illnesses in the corporation.[28] The components of this program consist of voluntary screening for employees and a seminar sponsored by the company that introduce employees to the program and target areas addressed. The programs were offered free of charge and conducted at the employees' place of business. This encouraged increased employee participation. As of 1986, Johnson and Johnson reported that the LFL program was in operation at 50 Johnson and Johnson companies. It was estimated that 28,000 employees participated. The results of this study indicate that the LFL group savings was $245,079 per year, or a total of $980,316 for the study period. This increase in savings, however, contradicts the findings of another health promotion program study conducted by Shepard and associates,[64] who compared two companies on the basis of health care costs and utilization. One company was evaluated a year before and a year after the introduction of a fitness program. The other company served as a control. The study found projected medical cost savings of $84.50 per employee in the company that implemented the fitness program but that "costs stabilized at the test company, while costs significantly increased at the control company." In general, these programs have a positive effect on employee health; however, more information is needed to assess their overall influence on health care costs.

An additional illustration examines the Japanese "quality of work life" ethic and its effect on labor relations. Tepper[54] remarks that the Japanese believe that "a successful business in not simply a financial machine. It is a human institution that needs nurturing if it is to survive and prosper." Many companies, similar to those operated by the Japanese, are becoming aware of the importance of environmental health issues. These issues are becoming central to the success of the enterprise. This trend continues to grow, as illustrated by a program designed by the National Institute for Occupational Safety and Health (NIOSH) entitled Project Minerva. This program, as described by NIOSH, is "to assist business schools in incorporating occupational safety and health concepts and principles into existing curricula." Lack of familiarity with occupational health and safety issues leads to poor decision making. Poor decision making may lead to litigation, loss of advantage in a competitive market, and possible bankruptcy.

Health promotion should exist at all levels. The foot is an important tool, responsible for efficient functioning in industry. Consider once again how many of the tasks performed during business hours require ambulation. This fact prompted renowned occupational physician Dr. Leonard J. Goldwater to state that "programs of health promotion and physical fitness conducted by employers for their employees saw phenomenal growth in the 1980s. The prevention of and care for injuries of the feet find a logical place in these programs."[10]

Podiatric Evaluation

The podiatric practitioner evaluating employees in the workplace should be thoroughly familiar with the work tasks being performed. This requires keen observational skills. In addition, other essential information should be ascertained. Included in this category are foot injury and disorder data that may be found in medical records, workers' compensation claims, and accident reports.[68] This valuable information enables the practitioner to focus on podiatric problems occurring with the greatest frequency. It would be advisable to review the medical records of workers who demonstrate an increased rate of absenteeism from the job due to podiatric complaints. It would be interesting to note how many of such workers had prior foot surgery.

Many occupational tasks require excessive standing and ambulation. The podiatrist may evaluate the physical stresses applied to the feet from the performance of various occupational tasks. Evaluating the physical stress of an occupational task will enable the practitioner to determine whether a particular job may be too physically demanding for the employee in question. Various ergonomic and temporal relationships should be analyzed. For example, the duration of time spent standing or walking, the types of motion and range of joint motion required to complete the work task, and coordination and muscular strength requirements are important considerations. Careful analysis of this information may assist the practitioner in modifying work stresses and thus place a susceptible employee in a safer work environment that is physically less demanding of the feet.

BIOMECHANICS AND ERGONOMICS

The foot is located at the distalmost aspect of the human body. Because of its location the foot sustains tremendous forces, particularly during weight bearing and ambulation.[42, 69] Locomotion is a series of steps that requires a concerted effort from various body parts. Motion of the foot and ankle is related to motion at the knee, which in turn affects hip motion and ultimately the function of the biomechanical superstructure. Derangement of one of these anatomical sites may cause a clinical problem elsewhere. The foot is the first structure to contact the ground. Hence, it has received much attention in measurement of biomechanical pressures and stresses. Several studies measure and evaluate peak foot pressure while subjects are both barefoot and wearing shoes.[69, 70] Interestingly, the greatest peak pressures occur during activities such as walking, jogging, and running.[70] The pressures are greatest at the medial aspect of the metatarsal heads.[70] Great variability in pressure exists owing to the person's intrinsic biomechanics, body weight, heel height, weight of the shoe, and variations in length of the first and second rays.[70] While a person is standing, loads are distributed equally between the heel and ball of the foot; however, the first metatarsal sustains double the load of any other metatarsal.[44] Biomechanics plays a major role in proper foot function. The discipline of foot biomechanics is very complex, and a comprehensive description is beyond the scope of this discussion. When evaluating foot disorders, however, the clinician must always consider the possibility of a biomechanical etiology.

PREPLACEMENT AND PERIODIC EXAMINATIONS

The preplacement examination serves as an important health strategy and should be performed before assigning a recently hired employee to a particular task.[12, 31, 55] A podiatric preplacement examination will identify any existing foot deformity that may progress to increased deformity and pain.[12] Common podiatric problems that are easily recognized include flat feet, bunions, hammer toes, interdigital maceration, and ulceration. Flat feet and cavus feet may progress to painful conditions.[44] Recognition of these foot types at an early stage leads to early intervention and appropriate treatment, thus decreasing further development of potentially disabling foot disorders. These pathologic foot types may cause great discomfort and pain when the worker is placed in a physically demanding environment. For example, it is not advisable to assign a person with flat feet or a severe bunion deformity to a job that requires excessive ambulation and standing. It is also not prudent to place an employee who presents with venous insufficiency in an occupational capacity that requires static standing for great lengths of time. The occupational foot health program should focus on periodic evaluation of employees to screen for the presence of new podiatric

disorders and to monitor the progression of previously identified foot problems. Bunion and hammer-toe deformities tend to progress in severity over time, especially when they are not treated properly.[44] Interestingly, when recognized and treated at an early stage, the majority of podiatric disorders need not result in costly surgical correction. This is particularly relevant when treating employees in the high-risk groups for the development of serious and disabling podiatric problems.

The foot may reveal information about the general health status of the person because it has vascular, dermatologic, osseous, and nervous system components. Many systemic disorders may be recognized after examination of the foot and lower extremity. The foot health clinic functions as an additional portal into the health care network. The podiatrist is uniquely trained to recognize the pedal signs of an underlying systemic problem. The patient may be referred to the appropriate specialist for further evaluation and treatment. An employee may be more inclined to frequent the corporate medical service for a painful heel than for undetected, serious medical conditions such as hypertension and diabetes. In situations in which the podiatric problem requires surgical intervention, the podiatrist may consider surgical therapeusis or refer the employee to an appropriate specialist.

History

The complete history is an important component of the occupational examination.[71] The podiatrist should ask the employee about previous employment and work tasks. The medical history assists the practitioner in making diagnoses and serves as an authentic record. It serves a legal function as well, particularly for documentation of insurance and compensation claims. The scope of the occupational podiatric history is very similar to that of the general history.

Evaluation of Footwear

The clinician must know the type of work the employee does. Many occupations have inherent hazards. The podiatrist should determine the type and fit of the shoes being worn by the employee.[72] For example, some shoes have steel innersoles to protect against crush injuries. The footwear should be appropriate for the type of task being performed. The practitioner should observe that the shoes fit properly and check for the presence of areas of excessive wear.

Physical Examination

Podiatric Orthopedic Examination and Gait Analysis. The podiatric orthopedic examination assists the clinician to determine the cause of mechanically induced foot disorders and permits the practitioner to treat the cause and the symptom of the podiatric complaint. A gait evaluation should be included in this assessment since it provides further information about the locomotive and neurologic status of the patient.[38, 73]

Dermatologic Examination. The skin and nail are prone to contracting disease.[74] De-Lauro[75] points out that the "foot's daily working environment plays a major role in predisposing it toward occupational skin disease." The nail and skin are frequently the sources of podiatric complaints and are also excellent indicators of systemic disease.

The practitioner has useful clinical and diagnostic aids available to arrive at the proper diagnosis of skin and nail pathology. Included are potassium hydroxide and dermatophyte test medium for fungal studies, culture and sensitivity for suspected infection, and skin biopsy to rule out benign and malignant lesions.[75]

Vascular and Neurologic Examination. Vascular disease remains the number one cause of death in the United States.[76] The vascular assessment should never be deferred during a podiatric examination. Evaluation of vascular status is particularly important for diabetic patients, who are more prone to compromise of vascular supply to digits, which may progress to gangrene, necessitating amputation. To further evaluate the vascular status of the patient, the clinician may utilize noninvasive vascular testing such as Doppler studies, photoplethysmography, and plethysmography. The neurologic examination is essential and must be evaluated in all patients. At a minimum, a monofilament (Semmes-Weinstein) test should be performed on diabetic patients.

Radiographic Evaluation. Radiographic evaluation of the employee's feet may indicate the presence of osseous deformities, exostoses, hammer toes, bunions, calcaneal spurs, tumors, and abnormal foot types. Diseases that are progressive, such as arthritis, bunion deformity, and contracted digits, may be monitored, and original baseline views may be compared with the most current radiographs.[77]

Rehabilitation

Many podiatric conditions require rehabilitative treatment. Rehabilitation of foot problems may require long periods of time. The podiatrist should work in conjunction with other health care specialists to design and implement a rehabilitation program for the physically impaired employee. An effective rehabilitation program assists the patient in restoring the functional capability of the foot, decreases absenteeism, and ultimately improves the patient's quality of life. Surgical correction of a podiatric problem should require subsequent rehabilitative treatment. The podiatrist may participate in this care and determine a maximum time period that the employee may remain in the rehabilitation program. Ultimately, the practitioner may establish criteria used to safely terminate the participation of employees in the program.

Consultative Services

An astute health care professional practicing in the occupational setting should consider the possibility that a presenting podiatric complaint is occupationally related. The podiatrist in the foot health program may evaluate the etiology of the disorder and provide treatment. The podiatrist may then employ fundamental principles of occupational hygiene to control the problem. Included in this category of control are appropriate footwear (e.g., safety shoes), protective clothing and socks, instruction in general foot care, and explanation of general safety measures.[72]

Practitioners of general medicine in the occupational setting may recognize podiatric disease. In this situation, referral of the employee to the podiatric health clinic for consultation would be recommended. The employee who complains of severe back pain serves as an illustrative point. The physician may suspect abnormal foot biomechanics as the cause of the problem and subsequently request a consultation with the podiatrist trained in occupational medicine, occupational hygiene, and ergonomics. Additional areas in which the occupational health podiatrist may make significant contributions are workers' compensation and disability evaluation. These two areas pose unique problems for both the employee and management. A podiatrist who is well trained in occupational medicine and in the evaluation of foot disorders and injuries is invaluable in resolving such controversies in a fair and equitable manner.

Educational Services

The podiatrist participating in an occupational foot health program is in an excellent position to disseminate information concerning the importance of foot health. Seminars to educate employees on the importance of foot safety and proper hygiene and their relationship to healthy foot function are of great benefit. Employees are made aware of the strong correlation between quality of life, proper foot function, and good health. It should be emphasized that the ability to ambulate comfortably is considered to be a major constituent of a desirable quality of life.

The podiatrist should particularly focus attention on those employees who are in high-risk groups for developing podiatric disorders. Diabetics are a major constituent of this group. The employee who participates in athletics is also at great risk for pedal injury and should be instructed in proper footwear, in stretching exercises, and in good foot hygiene.

In the medical center occupational setting, the design and implementation of a professional teaching track directed at corporate physicians, occupational health nurses, and medical students is of tremendous value. All too often the foot is overlooked in the evaluation of a person's health status. Professional instruction would focus on a comprehensive examination of the foot, including gait analysis, biomechanical factors, and vascular, orthopedic, and dermatologic systems. The major objective of a teaching program is to alert

health care practitioners to the importance of the foot in disease recognition. In addition, health care practitioners would better understand and appreciate the role of podiatrists in providing foot care.

Research Opportunities

The concept of occupational podiatric health is relatively new. Many viable and important topics of interest to occupational health care professionals require investigation. Further development of the concept and its relevance to mainstream occupational medicine is dependent on the conduct of clinical research in collaboration with other health care disciplines and specialists. The establishment of occupational foot health programs will yield many benefits. Data collected in the foot health program may initiate the establishment of a quantitative statistical base concentrating on occupationally related foot disorders and injuries. This would be of great value to many agencies, both medical and nonscientific. Unfortunately, many foot disorders and ailments that are occupationally related are not reported. In addition, such information would be invaluable in assessing the relationship between abnormal foot function and a number of occupational medical problems, such as lower back pain.[78, 79] These data would be used by insurance companies, workers' compensation boards, and professionals who design preventive medicine strategy programs.

SUMMARY

The disciplines of occupational and preventive medicine, although well-established specialties, are flexible in their ability to expand the scope of practice and assimilate new disciplines. Podiatry serves as a vital entry point into the medical care network, is an excellent screening tool for systemic disease, and, when practiced competently, may enhance the quality of life of these persons in need of such care.

It is evident from the statistics presented that the foot deserves greater attention in the areas of preventive medicine and occupational health. The podiatrist, to be effective and credible in this environment, must follow an academic and training path similar to that for the doctor of medicine who specializes in these disciplines. Advanced training in occupational hygiene, toxicology, epidemiology, and biostatistics must be undertaken.

Establishing a foot health program in the occupational setting is not a difficult task. The focus of the program is nonsurgical, and the program does not require substantial revenues to initiate. The podiatrist may use the specialized equipment already found in the occupational medicine clinic. Such equipment includes x-ray units, examination tables, a laboratory, and consultation rooms.

The potential benefits to be reaped from an occupational foot health program are self-evident. Improving the podiatric health of the employee is the major benefit; however, industry will benefit equally. Proper foot care and hygiene will improve worker morale, decrease the number of accidents and absenteeism, and lead to a reduction in expenditures due to surgical correction. In addition, industry will prepare for the projected increase in the population older than 60 years of age who will comprise an increasingly large proportion of manpower in the workplace. This age group is presently the one most afflicted with podiatric disorders.[1]

The majority of podiatric complaints may be addressed in the foot clinic and treated with therapeutic modalities most commonly employed by podiatric practitioners. This will result in decreased utilization of external podiatric care. It follows that one may expect a decrease in corporate podiatric expenditures for these treatments.

Foot health programs that serve the podiatric needs of employees will also serve their preventive and general medical needs. Painful feet will bring persons who may have never presented to the medical clinic into the health care network. During evaluation of the podiatric complaint an underlying systemic problem may be recognized.

In terms of research investigation, the establishment of such a program will enable practitioners to collect valuable data about podiatric health and injuries in the workplace that are not currently available. This knowledge may serve as the basis for designing preventive strategies and ultimately abet the establishment of an occupational podiatric epidemiology profile. In addition, important research issues such as biomechanics, traumatology, and mycology may be investigated and provide additional valuable information.

A foot health program and clinic are needed in the occupational setting. They merit the consideration of corporate executives, health planners, and medical directors in controlling and reducing morbidity associated with foot disorders. The program is cost effective, requires minimal start-up costs and personnel to operate, and addresses an essential prerequisite of a quality working life: the ability to ambulate comfortably and efficiently.

REFERENCES

1. Helfand AA: At the foot of South Mountain. J Am Podiatr Med Assoc 63:512–521, 1973.
2. Polakoff PL: Proper care minimizes risk of developing foot problems. Occup Health Safety 16:57–58, 1984.
3. Buettner-Janusch J: Origins of Man, Physical Anthropology. New York, John Wiley & Sons, 1966.
4. Occupational Health Bulletin: Foot Health, vol 6, No. 1. New Jersey State Department of Health, Bureau of Adult and Occupational Health, 1981.
5. Health Planning Kit. Washington, DC, American Podiatry Association, 1979.
6. Gorecki GA, Brzyski TP: Podiatric Medicine: A new threshold in health manpower. Am J Public Health 65:1212–1216, 1975.
7. Teleky L: History of Factory and Mine Hygiene. New York, Columbia University Press, 1948.
8. International Labor Office: Health and Occupation. Geneva, World Health Organization, 1926–1933.
9. Ramazzini B: In Wright W (trans): The Diseases of Workers (Reprint of 1717 edition). Chicago, University of Chicago Press, 1940.
10. Goldwater LG: The history of occupational medicine. J Clin Podiatr Med Surg 4:523–527, 1987.
11. Hunter D: The Diseases of Occupation, ed 5. London, English Universities Press, 1974.
12. Gorecki GA: Sufficient challenge—podiatric occupational medicine. J Am Podiatr Assoc 67:481–483, 1977.
13. Shore RE: Applications of epidemiologic methods to podiatric medicine. J Clin Podiatr Med Surg 4:593–604, 1987.
14. Most R, Sinnock R: The epidemiology of lower extremity amputations in diabetic individuals. Diabetic Care 6:87–91, 1983.
15. Acheson R, Chan Y, Payne M: New Haven survey of joint disease. J Chronic Dis 21:533–542, 1969.
16. Gorecki GA: Preliminary investigation of lower extremity impairment among men in heavy industry. J Am Podiatr Assoc 63:47–56, 1973.
17. MacMahon B, Push TF: Epidemiology: Principles and Methods. Boston, Little, Brown & Co, 1970.
18. Mausner JS, Kramer S: Epidemiology: An Introductory Text. Philadelphia, WB Saunders, 1985.
19. Hernberg S: Epidemiologic methods in occupational health research. Scand J Work Environ Health 11:59, 1974.
20. Environmental and health monitoring in occupational

health. Technical Report Series, No. 535. Geneva, World Health Organization, 1973.
21. Halperin WE, Ratcliffe J, Frazier TM, et al: Medical screening in the workplace: Proposed principles. J Occup Med 28:547–552, 1986.
22. Millar JD: Screening and monitoring: Tools for prevention. J Occup Med 28:544–546, 1986.
23. National Occupational Hazards Survey I. Volume II: Survey analysis and supplemental tables. Bethesda, MD, National Institute for Occupational Safety and Health. DHEW (NIOSH) publication No. 78–114, 1978.
24. Shilling RM: Prevention of occupational disease. In Shilling R, Hall S (eds): Occupational Health Practice, London, Butterworth, 1973.
25. National Diabetes Advisory Board: The Prevention and Treatment of Five Complications of Diabetes, 1980.
26. Levine ME: Saving the diabetic foot. Prob Prim Care 27:65–185, 1981.
27. Byyny RL: Management of diabetes during surgery. Postgrad Med 68:191–202, 1980.
28. Bly JL, Jones RC, Richardson JE: Impact of worksite health promotion on health care costs and utilization. JAMA 256:3235–3240, 1986.
29. Rom WN (ed): Environmental and Occupational Medicine. Boston, Little, Brown & Co, 1983.
30. Upton AC: The physician in industry. Clin Podiatr Med Surg 4:529–549, 1987.
31. Reiser SJ: The emergence of the concept of screening for disease. Millbank Mem Fund Q 56:403–425, 1978.
32. Levy LA: Epidemiology of podiatric medical diseases and disorders. In Levy LA (ed): Public Health and Podiatric Medicine, pp 91–101. Baltimore, Williams & Wilkins, 1987.
33. Positano RG, George D, Miller AK: A systemic approach to examining the patient with nail disease. Clin Podiatr Med Surg 6:247–251, 1989.
34. Kosinski MA, Stewart D: Nail changes associated with systemic disease and vascular insufficiency. Clin Podiatr Med Surg 6:295–318, 1989.
35. Brody JA: Prospects for an aging population. Nature 315:463–467, 1985.
36. Brody JA, Brock DD: In Handbook of the Biology of Aging, ed 2. New York, Van Nostrand, 1984.
37. Schneider EL, Brody JA: Aging, natural death, and the compression of morbidity: Another view. N Engl J Med 309:854–856, 1983.
38. Rzonca EC, Fitzgerald T: Gait analysis examination. New York College of Podiatric Medicine, Department of Orthopedics, 1987.
39. Spencer G: Current Population Report Series P-25, No. 952. Washington, DC, US Government Printing Office, 1984.
40. Gorringe JAL, Sproston EM: The influence of particle size upon the absorption of drugs from the gastrointestinal tract. In Binns TB (ed): Absorption and Distribution of Drugs. Baltimore, Williams & Wilkins, 1964.
41. Burgess N: Personal communication, 1984.
42. Bejjani FJ: Occupational biomechanics of athletes and dancers. Clin Podiatr Med Surg 4:671–711, 1987.
43. Mann RA: Biomechanical approach to the treatment of foot problems. Foot Ankle 2:205, 1982.
44. Root M, Orien W, Weed J: Normal and Abnormal Function of the Foot. Los Angeles, Clinical Biomechanics Corp, 1977.
45. Snijders CJ: Biomechanics of footwear. Clin Podiatr Med Surg 4:629–644, 1987.
46. Johnson US: Treatment of fractures of the forefoot in industry. In Bateman JE (ed): Footscience, pp 257–265. Philadelphia, WB Saunders, 1976.
47. Accident Facts. Chicago, National Safety Council, 1971.
48. Accident Facts. Chicago, National Safety Council, 1985.
49. Gleason TW, Dunne AJ (eds): Compensated Cases Closed. Albany, The State of New York Workers Compensation Board, 1984.
50. Collings GH: Managing the health of the employee. Occup Med 24:15–17, 1982.
51. Felton JS: The scope of occupational health services. Semin Occup Med 1:11–21, 1986.
52. Freedman SA: Megacorporate health care: A choice for the future. N Engl J Med 312:579–582, 1985.
53. McCunney RJ: A hospital-based occupational health service. J Occup Med 26:375–380, 1984.
54. Tepper LB: The strategic dimensions of occupational medicine. J Occup Med 29:325–329, 1987.
55. Charap MH: The periodic health examination: Genesis of a myth. Ann Intern Med 95:733–735, 1981.
56. Russell LB: Is prevention better than cure? Washington, DC, Brookings Institute, 1986.
57. Blair SN, Smith M, Collingwood TR, et al: Health promotion for educators: Impact on absenteeism. Presented to the InterAmerican Symposium on Health Education, Mexico City, November 1984.
58. Cox M, Shepard R, Corey P: Influence of an employee fitness program upon fitness, productivity and absenteeism. Ergonomics 24:795–806, 1981.
59. Fielding JE: Effectiveness of employee health improvement programs. J Occup Med 24:907–916, 1982.
60. Fielding JE, Piserchia PV: Frequency of worksite health promotion activities. Am J Public Health 79:16–20, 1989.
61. Gibbs JO, Mulvaney D, et al: Work-site health promotion: Five-year trend in employee health care costs. J Occup Med 27:826–830, 1985.
62. Heinzelman F, Bagley R: Response to physical activity programs and their effects on health behavior. Public Health Rep 85:905–911, 1970.
63. Hurst R, Khall TM: Universities need adequate employee safety, health programs. Occup Health Safety 6:39–42, 1986.
64. Shepard RJ, Corey P, Renzland P, et al: The impact of changes in fitness and lifestyle upon health care utilization. Can Public Health 74:51–54, 1983.
65. Warner KE: Selling health promotion to corporate America: Uses and abuses of the economic argument. Health Educ Q 14:39–55, 1987.
66. Warner KE, Wickizer TM, Wolfe RA, et al: Economic implications of workplace health promotion programs: Review of the literature. J Occup Med 30:106–112, 1988.
67. Bowne DW, Russell ML, Morgan JL, et al: Reduced disability and health care costs in an industrial fitness program. J Occup Med 26:809–816, 1984.
68. Langmuir AD: The surveillance of communicable diseases of national importance. N Engl J Med 268:182–192, 1963.
69. Manter JT: Distribution of compression forces in the joints of the human foot. Anat Rec 96:313, 1946.
70. Blank IH, Scheuplein RJ: Transport into and within the skin. Br J Dermatol 81(suppl 4):4–10, 1969.
71. Goldman RM, Peters JM: The occupational and environmental health history. JAMA 246:2831, 1981.
72. Bateman JE: Foot Science, pp 272–283. Philadelphia, WB Saunders, 1976.
73. Rzonca EC, Fitzgerald T: Lower extremity biomechanical examination. New York College of Podiatric Medicine, Department of Orthopedics, 1987.
74. Maibach HI, Gelbin OS: Occupational and Industrial

Dermatology. Chicago, Year Book Medical Publishers, 1952.

75. DeLauro TM: Occupational skin diseases of the feet. Clin Podiatr Med Surg 4:571–579, 1987.

76. Trainor FS, Cole D: Noninvasive vascular testing in occupational medicine. Clin Podiatr Med Surg 4:529–549, 1987.

77. Weissman SK: Radiology of the Foot. Baltimore, Williams & Wilkins, 1983.

78. McVeigh E: Occupational low back pain: An introduction. August 1989, pp 9–16. OSHA.

79. Snook SH: Back and other musculoskeletal disorders. In Levy BS, Wegman DH (eds): Occupational Health, pp 341–356. Boston, Little, Brown & Co, 1983.

CHAPTER 10

ETHICAL CONSIDERATIONS

Martin L. Smith
Jacquelyn Slomka

Discussions in clinical ethics focus frequently on end-of-life decisions (e.g., removing life supports) and beginning-of-life questions (e.g., use of reproductive technologies and neonatal intensive care resources). Any tendency to reduce clinical ethics to these major individual and societal concerns should be avoided. In fact, such a tendency is dangerous because it ignores the moral and ethical issues that are part of primary care and routine encounters between patients and health care professionals. Pursuing foot comfort and the restoration of health, especially through routine appointments and practices, involves a moral relationship between patient and podiatrist and has its own set of ethical and moral issues and concerns.

In this chapter the focus is on the podiatrist and the ethical values, duties, and issues that arise during routine interactions with patients. Special attention is given to the podiatrist as moral agent; to interprofessional and intraprofessional relationships; to practitioner–patient communication; and to the care of specific patient populations, which can raise special issues. Ethical resources are recommended for handling more difficult and complex cases.

The topics to be developed here are characterized more by a *relational ethic* than a *decisional ethic*.[1] A decisional ethic is the approach most often found in the tertiary care facility and the intensive care unit. Decisions must be made by participants who often have no prior history with each other and who will not see each other again once decisions are made and carried out. In contrast, a relational ethic is more appropriate for the office of primary care practitioners who engage patients and families in longer-term relationships. The development and maintenance of these relationships may be just as important or even more so than the individual decisions and behaviors of the participants. The ultimate purpose of the relationships is to create a favorable context for health care practitioners as moral agents to respond to patients' needs and their experiences of illness and discomfort.

THE PODIATRIST AS A MORAL AGENT

The moral agency of the podiatrist is multifaceted, but in its simplest expression it refers to an ability to act on the patient's behalf and for his or her best interests. The medical need of the patient calls the "agency" into existence; the interpersonal nature of the practitioner–patient relationship gives the agency its "moral" dimension. Although a frequently cited maxim is "above all, or first, do no harm," moral agency affirms a positive responsibility to promote the patient's good and to weigh possible benefit against possible harm to maximize the benefit and minimize the harm.

Technical Proficiency and Competence

A foundation and even presupposition of the moral agency of the podiatrist is technical proficiency and competence, which is usually understood as the general knowledge and skills that correspond to the diagnostic and therapeutic acts performed for the patient's good. For the patient's physical comfort and personal well-being, skill and dexterity are needed to perform highly individualized tasks, such as trimming of corns, calluses, and thickened, deformed toenails[2] or the "high tech" incision and vaporization of soft tissues with a carbon dioxide laser.[3] Knowledge of recurrence rates for patients with healed plantar ulcers who use normal footwear versus those who use modified shoes and orthoses[4] can lead to good patient outcomes and satisfaction.

The scientific knowledge, technical competence, and skill of the podiatrist require continuing education, training, updating, and collaboration with colleagues. This is not peripheral to the podiatrist's moral agency but is essential to its proper exercise. As stated in the *Code of Ethics* of the American Podiatry Association (Section 2), "Podiatrists should strive continually to improve their knowledge and skill, and should make available to their patients and colleagues the benefits of their professional attainments."[5] However, possessing and developing expertise to restore and enhance a patient's health and comfort does not negate the honest acknowledgment of personal, professional, and scientific limitations, uncertainties, and fallibility.

Personal Character Traits and Virtues

The exercise of one's moral agency on behalf of patients is not conterminus with having a command of, and being able to apply, the body of systematic scientific knowledge and technical skills required for the practice of podiatry. Podiatrists must integrate their technical expertise with personal character traits such as honesty, respect, compassion, friendliness, and fairness. What is being proposed here is the ancient concept of "virtue," that is, acting habitually in good ways with a commitment to being a good person in private, professional, and communal life.[6]

One way of operationalizing this humanistic side of podiatric practice is to focus on those character traits and habits that correspond to the specific needs of sick persons. The way illness is experienced by patients and the needs it creates in them serves as an objective guide for the practitioner's character development.[7] Persons with foot ailments, like others with different medical problems, seek relief and the restoration of health through proficient, but also personal, diagnosis and treatment. They need, expect, and should be given honest, clear, and caring communication, including understanding of their doubts and answers to their questions. They desire respect for the sometimes difficult choices they must make, according to their own reasons, values, and purposes. They want to be partners in their own health care and the prevention of future problems and hope for patience with their efforts to understand medical information and to be educated. They desire to be regarded as moral equals in the practitioner–patient relationship, bringing to the relationship their own indispensable kind of knowledge about their histories and hopes. They expect courtesy and friendliness and confidentiality regarding disclosed information. They seek unprejudiced, equal access to health care resources.

Occasionally, because of acute, life-threatening, or chronic debilities and diseases that assault their self-image and identity, patients may even raise with the trusted and caring podiatrist questions about the meaning of their lives, their pain and suffering, or their losses and debilities. The moral agency of the podiatrist does not necessarily include expertise in such spiritual issues but does require sensitivity, understanding, and referral when needed.

The humanistic elements of virtues and character traits that correspond to patient needs should be given continuous attention and development. Long hours, stress, critical and cantankerous patients, and lack of appreciation are a few factors that can erode virtuous patterns of behavior. The practitioner periodically may need to be reminded about the experiences of illness from the patient's perspective.

One current proposal for health care professionals to participate imaginatively in the experiences of patients and to be sensitized to their needs and perspectives is the reading of contemporary literature (e.g., short stories, poetry, novels) with medical themes.[8-10] The reading of artfully told renditions about the inherent drama of sickness and its deprivations and lessons can offer a fresh way of looking at the medical encounter.[11]

The achievements and exercise of proper moral agency thus proceed along two paths: (1) an outer-directed process of study, instruction, and the development of technical skills and scientific knowledge and (2) an inner-directed process of personal insight and the development of chosen attitudes, character traits, and patterns of behavior. The direction of both paths is toward the promotion of the patient's good and the restoration of the patient's health.

PRACTITIONER–PATIENT COMMUNICATION

In the latter half of the 20th century, a radical revolution in understanding has transformed the clinical encounter between health care professional and patient.[12] The ''parentalism'' or paternalism that characterized the relationship in former days has been rejected. The new model that has emerged emphasizes and recognizes the health care practitioner and the patient as partners in a process of shared decision making. In general, patients expect to participate in their pursuit of health as equal and full moral agents. No longer are patients to be childlike, passive, obedient recipients of care. The new model involves patients to be seen and heard as adults.

For this new model to be actualized, clear and open communication between practitioner and patient is essential. Patients have a personal knowledge about themselves and their experience of illness that must be joined with the general scientific knowledge of human health and disease that the practitioner can be expected to possess. The meeting of these two worlds of expertise can occur only in the context of respectful and mutual communication.

The Patient-Centered Interview

In the provision of primary care, one of the first opportunities for communication between podiatrist and patient is the clinical interview, which has three general functions: (1) data gathering, (2) establishing a therapeutic relationship, and (3) implementing a treatment plan.[13] Especially with initial and early encounters, the interview process should be patient centered and patient led.[14] Frequently this is difficult because patients experience themselves in a ''foreign territory,'' may be intimidated by the podiatrist's authority and status, and may only have vague and imprecise language to describe their symptoms and their reasons for seeking medical assistance. But the podiatrist, motivated by the goals of discovering and relieving the patient's concerns and discomforts, as well as establishing a relationship with the patient, can facilitate a setting and an atmosphere that is conducive for the patient to reveal his or her story. Ordinary courtesies contribute to this patient-centered context, such as introducing oneself, welcoming the patient, using the patient's name, ensuring privacy and comfort, and putting the patient at ease with conversation about non–health-related topics.

A significant skill of the podiatrist in this context is the ability to ask open-ended questions that will encourage patients to reveal personal perspectives on their goals and values. The podiatrist will often need to use imagination, metaphors, and images to evoke patient responses. Placed in the larger context of relational ethics, these and other interview suggestions and skills are more than simply proper or creative techniques; they are affirmations of and encouragements to the patient as a partner in the health care enterprise.

The Podiatrist as Patient Educator

Implicit in the role of the practitioner as communicator is the responsibility to be a patient educator. To educate patients is to contribute to their empowerment as equal and active participants in the treatment program. For example, education of the patient in proper foot hygiene procedures can potentially lead to good outcomes, patient satisfaction, and prevention of future ailments.

The podiatrist's teaching role requires the skill of translating medical information and concepts into language and images that will be understandable to patients. In most situations the education process will include reinforcement of ideas through a variety of oral, written and readable, visual, and even tactile means.

The role of patient educator should be embraced with confidence; if it is done well, it will bear positive results. In one study in which comprehensive podiatric care was integrated with inpatient and outpatient services, along with clinical nurses and an extensive educational program, the amputation rate declined by almost 50%.[15] Another example relates to diabetic patients who smoke and who are therefore at a higher risk for amputation. The advice of physicians and the reiteration of a stop-smoking message has been found to be a key element in motivating smokers to attempt to quit smoking, eventually leading them to successful abstinence from smoking.[16]

One of the challenges of the patient-educator role is to encourage and motivate patients while avoiding any semblance of coercion (either subtle or overt) as well as manipulation and deception. The temptation to manipulate, deceive, or coerce to attain a good end may be strongest when patients are noncompliant, are medically unsophisticated, or require more time than allotted in a busy schedule.

Despite good intentions by all participants, however, barriers to the process of communi-

cation and education can be present.[17, 18] Differing educational levels, the acuteness of the medical condition, the care with which information is exchanged, cognitive or emotional disabilities affecting comprehension, deficits in memory and attention span, fatigue, anxiety, and passivity can all hinder effective communication. When barriers are identified, repetitive and creative educational efforts directed at basic categories of information may be necessary. The goal is to maximize as much as possible patient participation in the collaborative effort of health care decision making.

Not all patients respond to educational efforts. Physicians fulfill their obligation after genuine attempts are made to educate patients. In a partnership model each party is expected to contribute to the process. Even when one party does not contribute or respond, the other party can fulfill the responsibilities of being a partner.

Informed Consent

Repeated clinical encounters between patient and podiatrist can be interpreted as the cumulative steps in a process of informed consent to treatment and the health care plan.[19, 20] A presupposition here is that informed consent should not be reduced to a discrete act occurring in a circumscribed time period, characterized by a one-way giving of information from practitioner to patient and symbolized by the patient's witnessed signature at the end of a consent form. Rather, informed consent should be understood as a process of shared decision making, achieved by multiple encounters over time in a context of communication, collaboration, and negotiation.[21]

The care sought and received for many foot disorders and ailments corresponds well to this model of informed consent. After initial examination and diagnostic workups, and possibly even surgery, routine visits occur to examine and adjust footwear, to evaluate degree of discomfort, and to discuss treatment impact on issues of quality of life such as employment and social interactions. During these routine appointments, patients can come to a better understanding of their treatment plan, self-care and preventive techniques, prognosis, and even financial obligations. Ordinary visits are also opportunities for podiatrists to learn about patients' goals, values, expectations, frustrations, and any reasons for failure in compliance with medical recommendations. Acute complications, whether handled over the telephone or in person, can also contribute to this mutually respectful and fiduciary process of informed consent and communication.

Informed consent is usually easier when patients themselves are in partnership with their podiatrist. However, on occasion the decisional capacity of the patient may be in doubt owing to immaturity, age, dementia, mental retardation, or severe emotional distress. Assessment of the patient's capacity to make health care decisions and to carry out the treatment plan may therefore be needed.[22] If a patient clearly cannot communicate a choice, understand relevant information, appreciate the current situation and its consequences, and manipulate information rationally, an alternative or surrogate decision maker (usually a family member or friend) must be identified to speak on behalf of the patient's best interest or previously expressed wishes. Even in those situations when a surrogate or guardian must be involved, the patient's best interests seem better served when both patient and family member or friend are viewed together as the decision makers. Conflicts may arise between patient and surrogate, but they are frequently resolvable through continued efforts at communication.

Advance Directives

The best efforts and achievements in primary and additional levels of care ultimately cannot prevent irreversible conditions and death. This unavoidable reality that someday will overtake all patients (and their podiatrists) points to an additional area of communication between patient and practitioner. Primary care practitioners should consider initiating conversations with patients about their wishes regarding end-of-life decisions and educating patients about advance directives (i.e., living wills and durable powers of attorney for health care)[23, 24] in the event that patients lose the ability to make their own health care decisions.

The Patient Self-Determination Act[25–27] man-dates, as part of a provider's agreement with Medicare, that during the admission process hospitals, health maintenance organizations, skilled nursing facilities, home health agencies, and hospice programs provide written information to patients about advance directives and inquire whether a patient has executed such directives. This federal act undoubtedly has increased public awareness about patients' rights for informed consent and refusal and their role in end-of-life decision making. However, there is a general perception that the time of hospital or nursing home admission is a less than optimum moment for appropriate and substantive discussion about such issues.[28] During the admission process patients are often seriously or acutely ill, mentally debilitated, or even unconscious. Many of these discussions on admission are performed as an administrative task (e.g., between admissions clerk and the patient) rather than as a part of a clinical process (e.g., in the context of a practitioner–patient relationship).

The context of a practitioner–patient dialogue and identification of general health care goals, values, and quality of life (usually in the outpatient setting) is better suited for soliciting a patient's wishes about life-supporting or death-prolonging therapies should these become necessary. In this less stressful setting patients can be educated about various options and therapies if they should suffer a loss of decisional capacity in the circumstances of a life-threatening illness. Over a series of office visits patients will have time to reflect on these issues and ask their questions. Confusion, fears, and misunderstandings can be addressed. Actual documents (according to specific state statute) can be reviewed or provided, discussed, and incorporated into the patient's medical record.

Practitioners may have a tendency to reserve conversations about advance directives for geriatric patients or those with degenerative diseases. This is not a realistic approach. The young and the old, the healthy and the sick, can experience life-threatening illness, trauma, and loss of mental capacity. If patient partnership is a value to be honored, then all patients should be given the opportunity to express their wishes, values, and directives in advance of when end-of-life choices must be made for them.

Some practitioners may be reluctant to initiate such conversations with patients, especially those who are young and the healthy, for fear of scaring or upsetting patients needlessly. The question is still open and should be pursued in a scientific manner. However, the reverse may be true: many patients wait for their doctors to initiate these discussions and welcome and are even relieved when such discussions occur.

SPECIAL PATIENT POPULATIONS

Podiatrists should be alert to the ethical dimensions of treating certain special populations of patients. A partial listing of these groups includes children, the mentally impaired, the indigent, the homeless, the elderly, and those infected with the human immunodeficiency virus (HIV).

Children and the Mentally Impaired

Regarding young children as well as the severely mentally impaired, the podiatrist may find it necessary to deal with surrogate decision makers, that is, the parents or guardians of the patient who can be presumed to act in the best interests of the patient. In dealing with both children and the mentally handicapped, the podiatrist should offer explanations of treatment in accordance with the patient's level of understanding. Even though minor children may not have a legal right to participate in decisions regarding their health care, podiatrists, parents, and guardians should allow children and mentally handicapped persons who exhibit some degree of comprehension to participate in decisions that affect their well-being.

In treating children, the mentally handicapped, or elderly demented patients, the podiatrist should be alert for suspicious lesions and bruises that might indicate physical abuse or neglect. The podiatrist shoulders a serious responsibility in cases of suspected abuse: failure to report abuse may have legal ramifications for the practitioner, while a mistaken diagnosis could have severe social, psychological, and legal consequences for the family or caregivers.[29]

The Elderly

As the aging population of our country has continued to increase, much emphasis has been placed on the health care concerns of the geriatric patient. The great need of elderly patients for foot care and the special problems brought on by aging have led to the development of the specialty of podogeriatrics. Care of the feet is an essential part of keeping elderly patients mobile, independent, and free from institutional care, while foot care for the institutionalized elderly can improve their quality of life.[2, 30, 31]

Ethical treatment of the elderly involves a respect for the individual and a holistic knowledge of the geriatric patient's special needs. In a society where a high value is placed on youth, the elderly patient may be taken less seriously than a younger person. Our society tends to believe that elderly persons want to remain independent and self-sufficient. This assumption may be only partially true. Elderly patients may experience detrimental effects on their health if they are not allowed to exercise control over their activities. On the other hand, they may also experience stress if they are encouraged and empowered to take more control of their lives than they desire.[32–34] The podiatrist, in providing essential primary care services to elderly patients, should be sensitive to individual differences in patients and recognize those who desire a great amount of control over health care decisions and those who would prefer to turn over some decision making to significant others.

The Indigent and Homeless

Indigent and homeless patients may also present special ethical challenges to the podiatrist. Specific foot problems related to poverty and homelessness may include lack of nail care due to a lack of instruments, tinea pedis, tissue injury from cold weather, and skin and foot trauma due to inadequate shoes.[35] Although respect for poor or homeless persons is a major ethical consideration, the treatment of indigent patients also raises the issue of societal allocation of scarce health care resources. Informal rationing of health care is already occurring since many medical services remain available only to those who can pay and are restricted for those who are unable to purchase health care insurance or to pay out of pocket. Furthermore, bureaucratic procedures related to insurance payments may work to discourage patients from seeking care and professionals from providing it, a situation that results in a form of health care "rationing through inconvenience."[36]

Currently, health care insurance in our society is geared toward payment for curative rather than preventive services. The result of this focus is often a seemingly irrational payment system; for example, an insurance plan may pay for treatment of a mycotic toe of a diabetic patient but may not pay for treatment of the mycotic toe of a nondiabetic patient until an abscess has formed.

Podiatrists may find that ethical concerns often coincide with social problems of patients. For example, a diabetic patient with a partial foot amputation may be forced to walk up nine floors to his apartment because the elevator in his housing project is frequently out of order. Or an indigent patient could benefit from the use of a cane for walking but has neither money nor insurance to pay for it. Podiatrists by themselves do not have the ability or the obligation to solve the myriad of patient problems brought on by poverty and homelessness, either at the individual or societal level. However, as caring professionals, they do have an ethical responsibility to learn about social service referral resources for patients. And as primary health care providers, they also have an ethical and professional responsibility to become familiar with and actively involved in the larger political and social issues involved in the equitable delivery of health care. Podiatrists in private practice and those who work at clinics should also give consideration to providing a certain percentage of their service at no cost to indigent patients.[35]

HIV-Positive Patients

Podiatric care of the HIV-infected patient presents special issues because of the nature of the disease and because the potential for HIV infection exists in all age groups and at all socioeconomic levels. The podiatrist as a primary care provider may be the first to recog-

nize signs and symptoms of HIV infection.[37] Furthermore, podiatric diagnosis of diseases such as gonococcal arthritis[38] may suggest evidence that the patient may be at risk for HIV infection and in need of education regarding high-risk behaviors.

The debate over whether health care providers are ethically obligated to care for HIV-infected patients may be overshadowed by a legal concern that refusal to treat these patients may constitute illegal discrimination against the handicapped.[39] Although some health care professionals will refuse to treat HIV-infected patients, many will continue to care for these patients because of personal virtues and a belief in a professional obligation to care for all patients.[40, 41]

Disclosure of HIV test results may present ethical dilemmas for the podiatrist. The acquired immunodeficiency syndrome (AIDS) is a highly stigmatized disease because of its association with homosexuality and illicit intravenous drug abuse. AIDS may take on a religious meaning for some persons, who may view the disease as a punishment for sins, just as venereal disease historically was believed to be a punishment for promiscuity. Because of the potentially disastrous social consequences resulting from disclosure of HIV infection, the podiatrist has a strong obligation to maintain confidentiality in regard to the patient's infection. Improper disclosure of test results could result in legal liability for the practitioner or for the institution.[42] However, the obligation to respect the patient's confidentiality may need to be weighed against conflicting obligations, such as a duty to warn an identified innocent third party (e.g., a spouse) if the patient refuses to disclose a positive test result to a sexual partner; an obligation to protect the patient (e.g., if a patient threatens suicide on learning of a positive test result); and an obligation to protect society (e.g., if the patient engages in irresponsible actions that are a threat to public health).[43]

COLLEGIAL AND ORGANIZATIONAL CONFLICTS

Relationships with professional colleagues, other coworkers, and institutions may involve circumstances that create ethical concerns for the podiatrist. Furthermore, the commercialization of health care raises new ethical questions for practitioners. Frequently these concerns and questions involve several kinds of conflicts of obligations and interests.

Intraprofessional Conflicts

Some conflicts of obligations and interests are related to the "esprit de corps" that develops as part of any professional socialization[44] and the fact that colleagues are often friends. The podiatrist may observe that a colleague's personal problems interfere with proper care of patients (e.g., substance abuse, mental health problems such as stress or depression); or incompetence, either gross or in regard to specific procedures, may be observed. The podiatrist's sense of loyalty to colleagues and the desire to help them may conflict with the professional responsibility to benefit patients and protect them from harm.

Questions for guiding ethical action in such conflictual situations include the following: How can the patient be protected from harm? Does the questionable action have the potential for harming the patient? Are professional values at stake? Is there actual or potential harm to the integrity of the podiatric profession? Are personal moral values of the professional at stake? Privately confronting the professional may induce a change in behavior; but in cases of substance abuse or emotional problems, the colleague may need referral and professional assistance. Confidentially sharing the dilemma with a trusted colleague or superior may lead to the formulation of a plan of action that will uphold as many values as possible. The state podiatry association may serve as a resource for dealing with the impaired or incompetent podiatrist.

Interprofessional Conflicts

The podiatrist is in a powerful position vis-à-vis other health care workers. Educational level, social class, and sometimes cultural and religious background separate the podiatrist from fellow health care workers. Such social distance can lead to an irresponsible use of power in medicine. Verbal and even physical abuse of medical students[45] and nurses[46] can occur as a result of traditional hierarchical relationships in medicine. The socialization of the podiatrist into the medical climate where traditional hierarchical values dominate relationships can lead to the tolerance of unethical behavior if care is not taken to recognize such behavior as unethical.

The realities of good management of a busy podiatry clinic require that patients move through the system efficiently. Some patients, because of unexpected or complicated problems, may require a longer period of time with the podiatrist, time that must then be made up by shorter visits with patients with more routine problems. Clinic professionals may become stressed when patients arrive late for appointments or present with "trivial" complaints on a busy afternoon or when patients become angry because of a long wait. During high-stress periods, the temptation is often to blame subordinates or to direct one's feelings of anger and frustration at them.

In such situations the ethical response can be supported not only by a sense of humor but also by creative solutions to the actual causes of the anger. Patients may have a reasonable excuse for tardiness or simply may not share the same cultural values of the podiatrist that dictate promptness regarding appointments. An acceptance of human frailty that stems from human nature or from a person's illness is essential for an ethical response. The ethical concept of respect for persons should be primary, and problems in relationships with co-workers that routinely cause stress due to expressed or repressed emotions should be dealt with directly by the persons involved or by using an outside consultant.

Business Concerns and Conflicts

In the current entrepreneurial climate of health care, the podiatrist may encounter a variety of situations in which conflicts of interest can occur owing to financial or business concerns. How such situations are handled may depend on the organizational ethos and policies of the podiatrist's clinic or hospital, in addition to the individual podiatrist's sense of ethics and responsibility.

The podiatrist should be aware that accepting gifts from pharmaceutical companies may have ethical repercussions, such as increasing the cost of drugs for patients and influencing the professional to prescribe a drug that may not be in the patient's best interests.[47] The marketing of health care services such as podiatry is becoming an acceptable practice and may serve to promote collegial relationships with allopathic and osteopathic physicians.[48] However, the podiatrist as entrepreneur should recognize conflicts of interest such as referring patients to health care facilities in which the podiatrist has ownership, a situation that is receiving increasing scrutiny in health care today.[49, 50]

Organizational Conflicts

The individual is usually viewed as the locus of moral agency. At the same time, the morality of the organization of which the individual is a part can influence a person's moral actions. Although much of the research on ethics in organizational culture has dealt with corporate morality, the clinic and hospital setting can be seen as parallel to the corporation, especially as medicine moves toward acceptance of "managed care" models and other business metaphors. Organizational barriers to a person's ethical behavior[51, 52] can occur in the health care setting where a growing profit motive, socialization into the professional model, and an acceptance of the status quo coexist.

Organizational barriers to ethical behavior by the individual have been identified.[53] The orientation of the newly employed podiatrist into the work setting of a clinic or group practice will involve the socialization of the podiatrist into the norms of the group. If unethical practices already occur and are tolerated by peers in the workplace, then the new persons may be unable to disengage from such practices in performing his or her responsibilities and may conclude that nothing can be done about the situation. A strict "chain of command" in an organization may inhibit the reporting of unethical actions to top management authorities and insulate executives from learning about unethical practices. Loyalty to the working group is valued in terms of "being a team player" and acts against internal or external "whistleblowing." In addition, whis-

tleblowing may involve great personal and professional risk.[54]

The difficulty in dealing with organizational blocks to ethical action by a person is partly due to lack of knowledge of an efficient language for dealing with moral and ethical issues. Medical language and corporate language is brief, concise, and efficient. Lack of knowledge of an efficient vocabulary for moral and ethical issues may inhibit such discussions from taking place.[53] This underscores the need for ethics education not only during the training period for podiatrists and other health care professionals but also on a continuing basis for practicing professionals and as a continuing interest of podiatric professional societies.

ETHICAL RESOURCES

Extraordinary ethical situations can arise during the provision of routine, primary care. Against medical advice a diabetic patient could refuse amputation and hospitalization and express a desire to die. Should the refusal be honored? A young adult male, presenting with foot ulcers and lesions, might reveal when interviewed that he is homosexual and has had multiple sexual partners and then dismiss a recommendation for HIV testing. What is the podiatrist's responsibility to the patient? to any identified sexual partners? to society? The podiatrist need not struggle alone and without guidance for solutions to such dilemmas. Ethical resources are available.

Casuistry, a Model for Decision Making

Ethically supportable options for ethical dilemmas can often be identified by using a systematic, practical process of decision making. Casuistry,[55] analogous to clinical judgments and decision making, is a workable and valuable model for finding solutions for ethically troubling situations. The method of casuistry includes the following elements[56]: attention to the circumstances and details of the case or situation; discovery and consideration of analogous cases; determining which moral maxims (i.e., commonly accepted rules for good conduct) should prevail in the case and to what extent; and weighing accumulated arguments and considerations for the identified options. The goal of this method is not to discover or create a perfect, unchallengeable answer but to arrive at a reasonable, prudential moral judgment leading to action. Familiarity with this (or some other) practical decision-making model can give some initial direction to the podiatrist for reflection, analysis, and action.

Ethics Consultants and Committees

In the burgeoning field of clinical ethics, clinical ethics consultants and institutional ethics committees are available to assist health care professionals in making decisions when duties and values seem contradictory.

Clinical ethics consultants[57–60] generally have received professional training in philosophy, theology, law, medicine, ethics, religion, or nursing, with specialized education and experience in clinical ethics. Two primary areas of their involvement are ethics education and case consultation. In the latter instance, the role of the ethics consultant is not to make decisions for the parties involved but to analyze the case at hand, using knowledge of a moral reasoning process and of relevant cases from the literature, and to recommend appropriate, ethically supportable courses of action.

Ethics consultants can provide timely, reasoned insight, guidance, and advice. For health care professionals interested in pursuing a greater understanding of ethical issues (e.g., patient confidentiality, informed consent or refusal), ethics consultants can provide bibliographies and facilitate educational experiences.

The institutional ethics committee,[61–63] with a diverse and multidisciplinary membership, ordinarily has three basic purposes: (1) promoting and providing educational efforts; (2) case consultation, both prospective and retrospective; and (3) policy formulation, recommendation, and review.

When consulted on a particular issue, the institutional ethics committee can provide a broad range of viewpoints. Frequently, a clinical ethics consultant is a member of the institutional ethics committee. Access to the institutional ethics committee and its availability are usually determined by a committee's mandate from the administration of a particular institution.

The 1992 *Accreditation Manual for Hospitals* of the Joint Commission on the Accreditation of Healthcare Organizations specifies that institutions must have a mechanism in place to consider ethical issues arising in the care of patients and to educate caregivers and patients on bioethical issues.[64] Even before this regulation, the presence of someone trained in bioethics, or a bioethics program that included an ethics committee, had become more common in health care facilities such as hospitals and nursing homes. The requirement from the Joint Commission will increase the likelihood that podiatrists will have access to these ethics resources through association with such institutions.

Ethics Literature

Professional health care journals regularly publish articles on clinical ethics and case studies. Attention to this literature can provide creative approaches to problems and enhance and enrich encounters with patients.

Journals, newsletters, and publications entirely devoted to clinical ethics now exist. Ethics consultants or members of institutional ethics committees who are familiar with this literature can direct podiatrists regarding subscription choices according to interests and needs.

SUMMARY

In contemporary ethical analysis and decision making, respect for persons is the primary value that underlies ethical injunctions to respect autonomy, to do good, to do no harm, and to promote justice. Respect for persons is also the foundation for the relational ethic proposed here for the primary care podiatrist.

The podiatric profession renders valuable service to patients and therefore is due the respect and compensation that individuals and society offer. At the same time, because of the moral nature of the profession, the podiatrist has the added responsibility to provide health care in a humane and caring fashion. Obligations to individual patients and coworkers, to oneself and one's family, and to society may sometimes overlap or conflict. A focus on the development of human relationships in podiatric practice can provide the caring environment for the humane management of conflicts of obligations. Development of human relationships implies not only a clinical knowledge of podiatry and theoretical concern with respect for persons but also a sincere interest in the welfare of others, a practical knowledge of communication techniques, and a willingness to reflect on the meanings underlying human behavior and illness.

The relatively recent growth of interest in clinical ethical issues and the development of bioethics as a discipline need not create a sense of insecurity regarding the podiatrist's ability to deal with ethical issues. The individual's moral upbringing and the process of professional training provide the podiatrist with a wealth of moral knowledge that one may not realize one has. The podiatrist may not be familiar with particular issues or with the language of ethics. However, reading, attending conferences, or consulting with a trained bioethicist can expand one's interests, knowledge base, and comfort in recognizing and addressing ethical issues in the everyday practice of clinical podiatry. Such knowledge, together with the focus on a relational ethic of practice, will serve to promote the humanistic practice of podiatry.

REFERENCES

1. Brody H: Stories of Sickness. New Haven, CT, Yale University Press, 1987.
2. Conforti JA: On humanistic podogeriatrics. J Am Podiatr Med Assoc 72:102–103, 1982.
3. Frykberg RG: Lasers in podiatry. Clin Podiatr Med Surg 4:767–776, 1987.
4. Dyck PJ, Thomas PK, Asbury AK, et al (eds): Diabetic Neuropathy. Philadelphia, WB Saunders, 1987.
5. Kanat IO: President's message. J Am Podiatr Med Assoc 64:841–844, 1974.
6. Pellegrino ED: The virtuous physician and the ethics of medicine. In Shelp EE (ed): Virtue and Medicine, Explorations in the Character of Medicine. Dordrecht, The Netherlands, D. Reidel, 1985.
7. Drane FJ: Becoming a Good Doctor, The Place of Virtue and Character in Medical Ethics. Kansas City, MO, Sheed & Ward, 1988.
8. Downie RS: Literature and medicine. J Med Ethics 17:93–96, 98, 1991.
9. Radwany SM, Adelson BH: The use of literary classics in teaching medical ethics to physicians. JAMA 257:1629–1631, 1987.
10. Nixon LL: Patients are more than their ilnesses: The use of story in medical education. Law Med Health Care 18:419–421, 1990.
11. Radey C: Telling stories: Creative literature and ethics. Hastings Cent Rep 20(6):25, 1990.
12. Bartholome WG: A revolution in understanding: How ethics has transformed health care decision making. QRB 18:6–11, 1992.
13. Quill TE: Recognizing and adjusting to barriers in doctor–patient communication. Ann Intern Med 111:51–57, 1989.
14. Smith RC, Hoppe RB: The patient's story: Integrating the patient- and physician-centered approaches to interviewing. Ann Intern Med 115:470–477, 1991.
15. Bild ED, Selby JV, Sinnock P, et al: Lower extremity amputations in people with diabetes: Epidemiology and prevention. Diabetes Care 12:1, 1989.
16. Glynn TJ: Methods of smoking cessation—finally, some answers. JAMA 263:2795–2796, 1990.
17. Cassileth BR, Zupkis RV, Sutton-Smith K, et al: Informed consent: Why are its goals imperfectly realized? N Engl J Med 302:896–900, 1980.
18. Lidz CW, Meisel A, Osterweis M, et al: Barriers to informed consent. Ann Intern Med 99:539–543, 1983.
19. Connelly JE: Informed consent, an improved perspective. Arch Intern Med 148:1266–1268, 1988.
20. Faden RR, Beauchamp R, King NMP: A History and Theory of Informed Consent. New York, Oxford University Press, 1986.
21. Lidz CW, Appelbaum PS, Meisel A: Two models of implementing informed consent. Arch Intern Med 148:1385–1389, 1988.
22. Appelbaum PS, Grisso T: Assessing patients' capacities to consent to treatment. N Engl J Med 319:1635–1638, 1988.
23. Annas GJ: The health care proxy and the living will. N Engl J Med 324:1210–1213, 1991.
24. Emanuel EJ, Emanuel LL: Living wills: Past, present, and future. J Clin Ethics 1:9–19, 1990.
25. LaPuma J, Orentlicher D, Moss RJ: Advance directives on admission, clinical implications and analysis of the Patient Self-Determination Act of 1990. JAMA 266:402–405, 1991.
26. McCloskey EL: The Patient Self-Determination Act. Kennedy Inst Ethics J 1:163–169, 1991.
27. Greco PJ, Schulman KA, LaVizzo-Mourey R, et al: The Patient Self-Determination Act and the future of advance directives. Ann Intern Med 115:639–643, 1991.
28. Emanuel L: PSDA in the clinic. Hastings Cent Rep 21(5):S6–S7, 1991.
29. Weiner I, Gastwirth, CM: The abused child: A primer for podiatric physicians. J Am Podiatr Med Assoc 78:452–454, 1988.
30. Helfand AE: Our responsibility to our aging patients. J Am Podiatr Med Assoc 73:50–51, 1983.
31. Helfand AE: Guidelines for podiatric services in long-term care facilities. J Am Podiatr Med Assoc 80:448–450, 1990.
32. Foner N: Old and frail and everywhere unequal. Hastings Cent Rep 15(2):27–31, 1985.
33. Rodin J: Aging and health: Effects of the sense of control. Science 233:1271–1276, 1986.
34. Kapp MB: Medical empowerment of the elderly. Hastings Cent Rep 19:5–7, 1989.
35. Jones CL: Foot care for the homeless. J Am Podiatr Med Assoc 80:41–44, 1990.
36. Grumet GW: Health care rationing through inconven-

ience: The third party's secret weapon. N Engl J Med 321:607–611, 1989.

37. Cohen, EJ, Cole E, Stewart DM, et al: Kaposi's sarcoma of the lower extremity as the first sign of AIDS. J Am Podiatr Med Assoc 80:127–133, 1990.

38. Hirsch E, Sherman M, Lenet MD: Gonococcal arthritis: Case report. J Am Podiatr Med Assoc 79:190–194, 1989.

39. Lo B: Ethical dilemmas in HIV infection. J Am Podiatr Med Assoc 80:26–30, 1990.

40. Zuger A, Miles SH: Physicians, AIDS, and occupational risk: Historic traditions and ethical obligations. JAMA 258:1924–1928, 1987.

41. Emanuel EJ: Do physicians have an obligation to treat patients with AIDS? N Engl J Med 318:1686–1690, 1988.

42. Restaino JM Jr: AIDS: Professional liability implications for the podiatrist. J Am Podiatr Med Assoc 78:92–97, 1988.

43. Walters L: The principle of medical confidentiality. In Beauchamp TL, Walters L (eds): Contemporary Issues in Bioethics. Encino, CA, Dickenson Publishing Co, 1978.

44. Freidson E: Profession of Medicine: A Study of the Sociology of Applied Knowledge. Chicago, University of Chicago Press, 1988.

45. Silver HK, Glicken AD: Medical student abuse: Incidence, severity and significance. JAMA 263:527–532, 1990.

46. Cox HC: Verbal abuse in nursing: Report of a study. Nurs Manage 18:47–50, 1987.

47. Chren MM, Landefeld CS, Murray TH: Doctors, drug companies and gifts. JAMA 262:3448–3451, 1989.

48. Hubbard ER: Personal professional marketing. J Am Podiatr Med Assoc 80:55–56, 1990.

49. Hyman DA, Williamson JV: Fraud and abuse: Setting the limits on physicians' entrepreneurship. N Engl J Med 320:1275–1278, 1989.

50. Iglehart JK: Health policy report: Efforts to address the problem of physician self-referral. N Engl J Med 325:1820–1824, 1991.

51. Argyris C, Schon DA: Reciprocal integrity: Creating conditions that encourage personal and organizational integrity. In Executive Integrity: The Search for Higher Human Values in Organizational Life. San Francisco, Jossey-Bass, 1988.

52. Victor B, Cullen JB: The organizational bases of ethical work climates. Admin Sci Q 33:101–125, 1988.

53. Waters JA: Catch 20.5: Corporate morality as an organizational phenomenon. Organ Dynam, Spring 1978; 6:3–19.

54. Blowing the whistle on incompetence: One nurse's story. Nursing 89:47–50, 1989.

55. Jonsen AR, Toulmin S: The Abuse of Casuistry. Berkeley, CA, University of California Press, 1988.

56. Jonsen AR: Casuistry as methodology in clinical ethics. Theoret Med 12:295–307, 1991.

57. Fletcher JC, Quist N, Jonsen AR: Ethics Consultation in Health Care. Ann Arbor, MI, Health Administration Press, 1989.

58. Glover JJ, Ozar DT, Thomasma DC: Teaching ethics on rounds: The ethicist as teacher, consultant, and decision-maker. Theoret Med 7:13–32, 1986.

59. Pellegrino ED: Clinical ethics: Biomedical ethics at the bedside. JAMA 260:837–839, 1988.

60. Purtilo RB: Ethics consultations in the hospital. N Engl J Med 311:983–986, 1984.

61. Fleetwood JE, Arnold RM, Baron RJ: Giving answers or raising questions? The problematic role of institutional ethics committees. J Med Ethics 15:137–142, 1989.

62. LaPuma J, Toulmin S: Ethics consultants and ethics committees. Arch Intern Med 149:1109–1112, 1989.

63. Ross JW, Bayley C, Michel V, et al: Handbook for Hospital Ethics Committees. Chicago, American Hospital Publishing, 1986.

64. Joint Commission on the Accreditation of Healthcare Organizations: Accreditation Manual for Hospitals. Chicago, JCAHO, 1992.

CHAPTER 11

THE MEDICAL LITERATURE: EPIDEMIOLOGY AND BIOSTATISTICS

Marvin H. Waldman

As the technologic revolution in the world of medicine winds its way into the next century, the ability to assimilate new clinical information is paramount. Primary care podiatrists practice in the midst of these changes and, accordingly, must be prepared to meet the challenge. With thousands of medical journals reporting more thousands of articles, the need to comprehend the basics of biostatistics, epidemiology, and clinical study design is a task faced by all practitioners. The purpose of this chapter is to provide basic information so that one may read and critique the medical literature in a manner that is timely and provides access to that new information deemed most valuable in the care of patients. This can be accomplished best by presenting the material in the chapter without emphasis on mathematical calculation. Although a basic course in biostatistics would be helpful, its absence will not preclude gaining valuable information from the material presented here.

Many practitioners are inadequately informed about the importance of quantitative methods as they relate to ascertaining the importance of medical articles. This issue is addressed in this chapter in an attempt to persuade readers that those podiatrists who best serve the health of their patients, as well as their communities, are those who stay current with new information. More importantly, it is hoped that after completing this chapter, busy practitioners will be better able to decide which articles are germane to their needs and be able to critique the validity and importance of these articles. This is particularly important in podiatric medicine, in which information is often obtained from the review of various non-podiatric journals. Each podiatrist, therefore, must be prepared to invest in the self-study of biostatistics, epidemiology, and clinical research design.

Figure 11–1 shows the use of a uniform framework for review of a clinical study and how this is applied to case-control, cohort, and experimental studies. Figure 11–2A provides useful guidelines for reviewing medical jour-

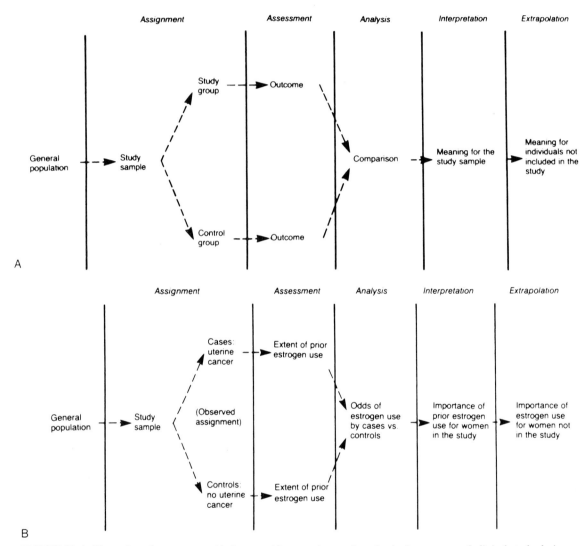

FIGURE 11–1. These flow charts are provided as a guide to understanding the basic concepts of clinical study design. They emphasize the structure of case-control, cohort, and experimental studies. *(A)* Uniform framework for studying a study. *(B)* Application of the uniform framework to a case-control or retrospective study.

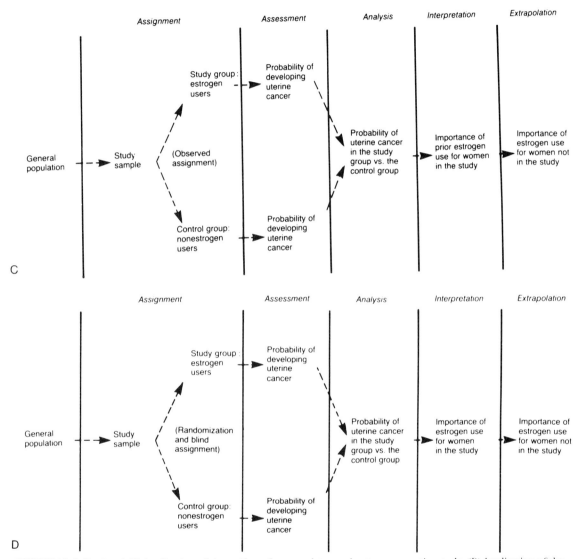

FIGURE 11-1 *Continued (C)* Application of the uniform framework to a cohort or prospective study. *(D)* Application of the uniform framework to an experimental study. (From Riegelman RK, Hirsch RP: Studying a Study and Testing a Test: How to Read the Medical Literature, ed 2, pp 10–13. Boston, Little, Brown & Co, 1989.)

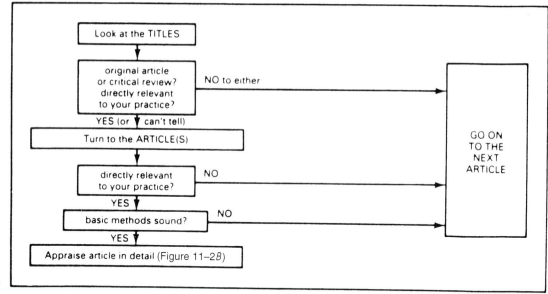

FIGURE 11–2. *(A)* This algorithm is useful in reviewing medical journals, particularly when time is short or the reading list is long. It provides a context for shortening the time-consuming task of choosing which journal(s) to read.

nals, and Figure 11–2*B* is a detailed continuation of this review algorithm. The reader should review these figures before proceeding with the rest of the chapter.

TYPES OF CLINICAL STUDIES

Medical studies may be anecdotal case reports, case series, literature reviews, case-control studies, cohort studies, surveys, or clinical trials. The need to appreciate the differences and varied usefulness of each type of study is of obvious importance. This chapter focuses on the case-control, cohort, and clinical trial types of studies. This in no way is meant to minimize the value of case reports, surveys, or literature reviews. Indeed, many important breakthroughs in diagnosis and therapy were initiated from these types of reports. As an example, the initial reports of unusually high numbers of cases of Kaposi's sarcomas in homosexual men led to the recognition of the acquired immunodeficiency syndrome epidemic. Literature reviews often provide timely review to podiatrists concerning subjects of universal interest—reviews that otherwise might be impossible for the busy practitioner to accomplish individually. Later in this chapter, meta-analysis, a relatively new statistical

method used to review the results of many studies on a given subject, is discussed. Lastly, surveys are a well-recognized way of obtaining useful scientific information from samples or large populations.

Most clinical studies can be subdivided into the categories of prospective, retrospective, descriptive, observational, and interventional. There is some overlap with the use of these terms, and they are subject to a certain degree of semantic conflict within the epidemiologic and statistical professions. Nevertheless, they are useful ways of accurately defining the type of study being reviewed. *Prospective studies* are those that follow a group of patients forward in time, to ascertain either the occurrence of disease or other incidents of interest. *Retrospective studies* are those that, beginning at the present, look backward in time to identify data of interest. *Descriptive studies* are those that provide a specific snapshot of various demographic and clinical data in a sample or population. *Observational studies* refer to clinical studies in which the observer is unable to manipulate the primary variables of interest. Instead, data are obtained from the observation of reality per se. Charles Darwin's work on the theory of evolution is a universal example of observational science. *Interventional studies,* sometimes known as experiments, exist where

Following from Figure 11–2A, is the article a report of an original study or a critical review that is directly relevent to your own clinical practice? NO ──────────────────────▶ GO ON TO NEXT ARTICLE

YES ──────

Purpose of study?

Therapy	Diagnosis	Screening	Prognosis	Causation	Quality of Care	Economics Analysis	Review
Was the assignment of patients to treatments really randomized?	Was the test compared blindly with a gold standard?	Was the study a randomized trial? If YES, see Therapy If NO:	Was an inception cohort assembled?	Was the type of study strong? (RCT · cohort · case control ·survey)	Did the study focus on what clinicians actually do?	Did the economic question include alternatives to be compared and viewpoint?	Were the questions clearly stated?
Were clinically important outcomes assessed objectively?	Was there an adequate spectrum of disease among patients tested?	Are there efficacious treatments for the disorder?	Were baseline features measured reproducibly?	Was the assessment of exposure and outcome free of bias? (e.g., blinded assessors)	Have the clinical acts under study been shown to do more good than harm? If not, did the study compare process to outcome?	Were the alternative programs adequately described?	Were the criteria for selecting articles for review explicit?
Was the treatment feasible to use in your practice?	Was the referral pattern described?	Does the current burden of suffering warrant screening?	Were the outcome criteria clinically important and reproducibly measured?	Was the association both significant and clinically important? If not, was power considered?	Were the clinical processes or acts measured in a clinically sensible and valid way?	Have the programs' effectiveness been described?	Was the validity of the primary studies assessed?
Was there at least 80% follow-up of subjects?	Was the description of the test clear enough to reproduce it?	Does the screening test have high sensitivity and specificity?	Was follow-up at least 80%?	Was the association consistent across studies?	Were both clinical and statistical significance considered?	Were all relevant costs and effects identified?	Was the assessment of primary studies reproducible?
Were both statistical and clinical significance considered?	Was the test reproducible (observer variation)?	Can the health system cope with the screening program?	Was there adjustment for extraneous prognostic factors?	Was the "cause" shown to precede the "effect"?		Were the measurements credible?	Was variability in the results of studies analyzed?
If the study was negative, was power assessed?	Was the contribution of the test to the overall diagnosis assessed?	Will positive screenees comply with further assessment and intervention?		Was there a dose-response relationship?		Was a sensitivity analysis performed to assess the effect of assumptions?	Were the findings of the primary studies combined appropriately?

B

FIGURE 11–2 *Continued (B)* Following the lead suggested in *A*, this flow chart provides specific guidelines for the critical appraisal of a journal article. The reader must have the skills to decide whether published information is clear, logical, valid, and applicable to the practice. (From Sackett DL, Haynes RB, Guyatt GH, Tugwell P: Clinical Epidemiology: A Basic Science for Clinical Medicine, ed 2, pp 364, 366, 367. Boston, Little, Brown & Co, 1991.)

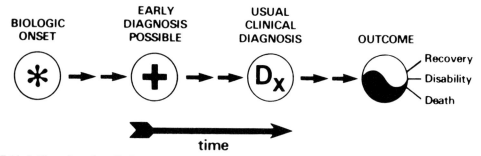

FIGURE 11–3. The value of medical care depends on a sound understanding of the natural history of each disease. The validity of diagnostic, prognostic, and therapeutic information is greatly influenced by the temporal relationship of this information to the natural history. (From Sackett DL, Haynes RB, Guyatt GH, Tugwell P: Clinical Epidemiology: A Basic Science for Clinical Medicine, ed 2, p 155. Boston, Little, Brown & Co, 1991.)

the observer is able to manipulate variables of interest to test specific hypotheses. Clinical trials are prospective and interventional; case-control studies are retrospective and observational; cohort studies may be retrospective or prospective, descriptive, observational, or interventional.

All medical studies share the purpose of improving diagnosis, prognosis, or treatment. *Clinical studies* emphasize the elicitation of data primarily from small groups of unhealthy or diseased individuals. *Epidemiologic studies,* however, emphasize studying populations that include sick as well as healthy persons. Both clinical and epidemiologic studies use sampling techniques to make assumptions about individual or community health. Because the principles of epidemiology are generally unfamiliar to many physicians, this area of research design is emphasized in this chapter. Figure 11–3 is an illustration of the natural history of disease.

EPIDEMIOLOGY

Epidemiology is the medical discipline that is concerned with defining the determinants of disease in populations. By describing, measuring, and comparing the extent of disease and its risk factors by time, place, and person, it is possible to investigate the causal mechanisms in disease. Thus, etiology can be determined and preventive measures instituted. Epidemiologic studies are often descriptive, correlating the geographic occurrence of disease to other common group attributes. Epidemiologic studies are also interventional; a

prime example is the trial of poliomyelitis vaccine in the 1950s. This large, population-based study proved the efficacy of the new vaccine in preventing cases of disease. Thus, there exists a spectrum of types of studies that begin with basic description of disease patterns and that extend to interventional studies. The most well known of the latter is the randomized clinical trial. This is discussed later in the text. The use of the epidemiologic method in medical studies adds much to the logic of care for individual patients, helps in the evaluation of community health status, and provides a basis for the formulation of public health policy. Data gathering for epidemiologic purposes depends on resources such as medical records, hospital admission and discharge summaries, government vital statistics, census and other survey data, insurance data banks, and the reporting of state and local public health agencies.

BIOSTATISTICS

Biostatistics bridges the gaps between formulation of clinical hypotheses, study design, and study analysis. Appreciation of its basic principles allows for the design of reliable studies and the best interpretation of study outcomes. Quantitative methods in epidemiology are the backbone of the discipline, and thus most epidemiologists have an intimate working knowledge of the area of statistics. Most clinical medical research involves the gathering of data from a sample drawn from a population at large, and the use of statistical principles allows for confident extrapolation from sample back to population. The major medical journals now place great emphasis on

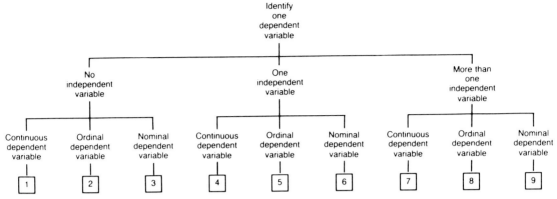

FIGURE 11-4. Master flow chart to determine which of the subsequent flow charts are applicable to a particular data set. The numbers at the bottom of the flow chart refer to subsequent flow charts (Figs. 11-5 through 11-13). (From Riegelman RK, Hirsch RP: Studying a Study and Testing a Test: How to Read the Medical Literature, ed 2. Boston, Little, Brown & Co, 1989.)

the design and analysis of data in the articles they publish. Familiarity with these concepts is of great advantage to the clinician reading the medical literature. Figures 11–4 through 11–13 include a master flow chart and also more detailed flow charts to help the reader of medical literature determine which statistical methods are appropriate.

Since improved patient care and prevention of illness in the community are the goals of medical research, confidence must rest in the quantitative methods used. In epidemiology, comparisons between groups are made with the use of rates and ratios; this allows description of the extent of disease and exposure factors and any associations that may exist between them. The use of rates and ratios allows for surveillance of temporal trends so that changes in disease occurrence may be noted and appropriate action taken if necessary. In the area of infectious disease, continuing surveillance allows for the control of many illnesses; in the area of chronic disease, surveillance has allowed for the development of preventive interventions in the area of cardiovascular disease, as an example.

Text continued on page 126

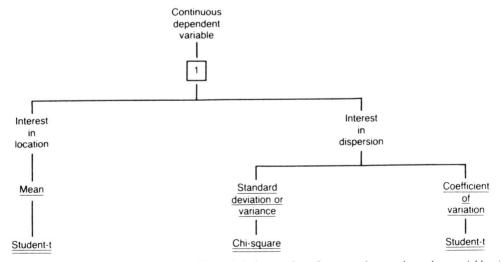

FIGURE 11-5. Flow chart to select a univariable statistical procedure for a continuous dependent variable. (From Riegelman RK, Hirsch RP: Studying a Study and Testing a Test: How to Read the Medical Literature, ed 2. Boston, Little, Brown & Co, 1989.)

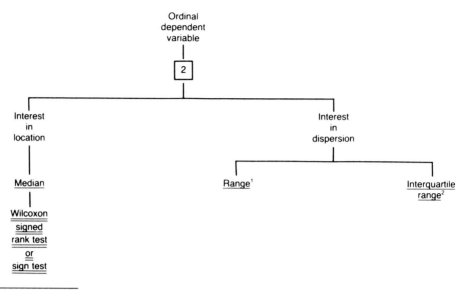

¹The range is included here only because of its widespread use. It is, however, difficult to interpret as discussed in Chapter 27.
²Statistical significance testing and calculation of confidence intervals are not obtained for the interquartile range unless it is used to approximate the standard deviation.

FIGURE 11–6. Flow chart to select a univariable statistical procedure for an ordinal dependent variable. (From Riegelman RK, Hirsch RP: Studying a Study and Testing a Test: How to Read the Medical Literature, ed 2. Boston, Little, Brown & Co, 1989.)

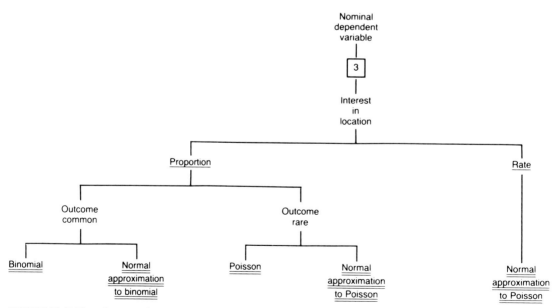

FIGURE 11–7. Flow chart to select a univariable statistical procedure for a nominal dependent variable. (From Riegelman RK, Hirsch RP: Studying a Study and Testing a Test: How to Read the Medical Literature, ed 2. Boston, Little, Brown & Co, 1989.)

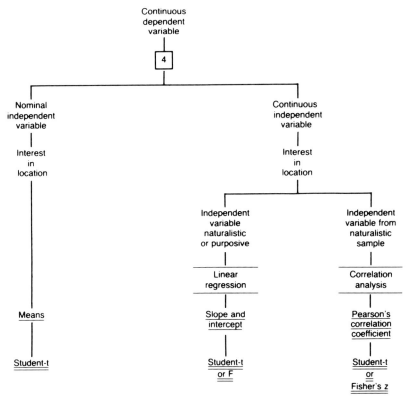

FIGURE 11–8. Flow chart to select a bivariable statistical procedure for a continuous dependent variable. (From Riegelman RK, Hirsch RP: Studying a Study and Testing a Test: How to Read the Medical Literature, ed 2. Boston, Little, Brown & Co, 1989.)

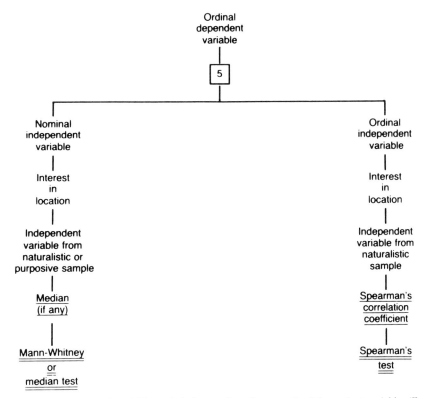

FIGURE 11–9. Flow chart to select a bivariable statistical procedure for an ordinal dependent variable. (From Riegelman RK, Hirsch RP: Studying a Study and Testing a Test: How to Read the Medical Literature, ed 2. Boston, Little, Brown & Co, 1989.)

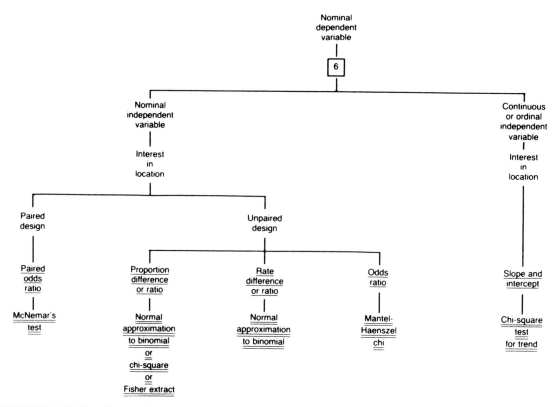

FIGURE 11–10. Flow chart to select a bivariable statistical procedure for a nominal dependent variable. (From Riegelman RK, Hirsch RP: Studying a Study and Testing a Test: How to Read the Medical Literature, ed 2. Boston, Little, Brown & Co, 1989.)

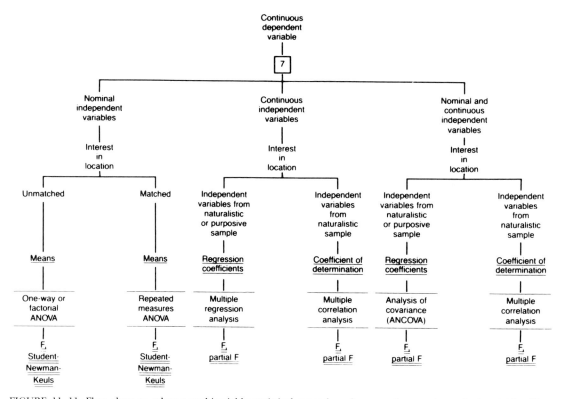

FIGURE 11–11. Flow chart to select a multivariable statistical procedure for a continuous dependent variable. (From Riegelman RK, Hirsch RP: Studying a Study and Testing a Test: How to Read the Medical Literature, ed 2. Boston, Little, Brown & Co, 1989.)

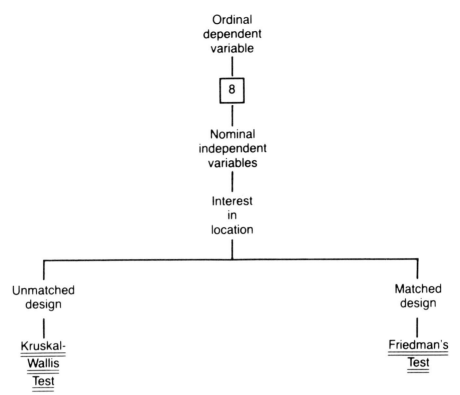

FIGURE 11–12. Flow chart to select a multivariable statistical procedure for an ordinal dependent variable. (From Riegelman RK, Hirsch RP: Studying a Study and Testing a Test: How to Read the Medical Literature, ed 2. Boston, Little, Brown & Co, 1989.)

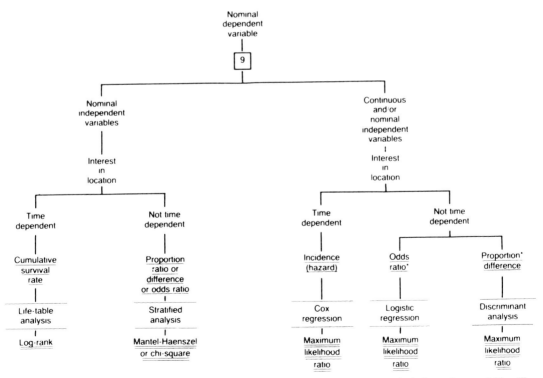

FIGURE 11–13. Flow chart to select a multivariable statistical procedure for a nominal dependent variable. (From Riegelman RK, Hirsch RP: Studying a Study and Testing a Test: How to Read the Medical Literature, ed 2. Boston, Little, Brown & Co, 1989.)

Measurement Scales

To understand the statistical analysis of a clinical study, one needs to understand which measurement scales are used. This is important because the measurement scale often dictates which statistical test is needed. A statistic is the mathematical representation of a characteristic of data (e.g., the mean and the standard deviation). Some statistics are calculated from sample data, and these statistics are extrapolated from the sample to the population from which the data were drawn (inferential statistics). Data can be measured using a *continuous* scale, exemplified by the reading of blood pressure in millimeters of mercury. Here there is an infinite array of readings that can be attained. *Categorical* data, on the other hand, are typified by their mutually exclusive character. They may be nominal or ordinal: that is, a person may be male or female, but not both; or one can be taller than 6 feet but not at the same time shorter than 4 feet tall. Data, whether continuous or categorical, may fit the so-called normal curve (which indicates a certain distribution of data) or other statistical distributions. This is important because the type of statistical test used is often dependent on the distribution of the data.

The Gaussian Curve

Since it is commonly used, the normal or *gaussian curve* is described here. Table 11–1

gives six definitions of normal in common clinical use. The curve is a distribution of continuous data that when plotted on a graph is bell shaped with two "tails" extending to either side. Since it uses continuous data, the tails of the curve do not meet the x-axis; instead, they are assumed to continue in an infinite fashion. The importance of the normal curve is its ability to allow us to characterize a data set as to measures of central tendency and dispersion, as shown in Figure 11–14. In this case the mean is found at the apex of this bell-shaped curve; this represents the measure of central tendency. Other measures also used (but not typically when referred to the normal curve) are median and mode. Also, the mathematical construct of the normal curve allows for a measure of the dispersion of the data about the mean, known as the standard deviation. If further information concerning the normal curve or other statistical distributions is desired, please see the bibliography at the end of this chapter. The word "parametric" refers to those statistical methods that can be applied to continuous data, with "nonparametric" being used for non-normal categorical data.

Hypothesis Testing

Medical science, whether basic or clinical, seeks to learn the "truth" about a subject through the use of *hypothesis testing*. This oc-

TABLE 11–1. **Six Definitions of Normal in Common Clinical Use**

Property	Term	Consequences of Its Clinical Application
The distribution of diagnostic test results has a certain shape	Gaussian	Ought to occasionally obtain minus values for hemoglobin, etc.
Lies within a preset percentile of previous diagnostic test results	Percentile	All diseases have the same prevalence. Patients are normal only until they are worked up
Carries no additional risk of morbidity or mortality	Risk factor	Assumes that altering a risk factor alters risk
Socially or politically aspired to	Culturally desirable	Confusion over the role of medicine in society
Range of test results beyond which a specific disease is, with known probability, present or absent	Diagnostic	Need to know predictive values that apply in your practice
Range of test results beyond which therapy does more good than harm	Therapeutic	Need to keep up with new knowledge about therapy

From Sackett DL, Haynes RB, Guyatt GH, Tugwell P (eds): The selection of diagnostic tests. In Clinical Epidemiology: A Basic Science for Clinical Medicine, ed 2, p 58. Boston, Little, Brown & Co, 1991.

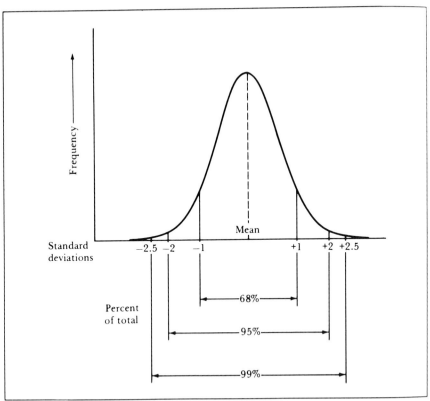

FIGURE 11–14. The normal curve is used with continuous data. Notice that it is bell shaped and divisible on either side of the mean into areas of dispersion known as standard deviations. Although the mean is the commonly used measure of central tendency, the mode, median, and range are also used. (From Hennekens CH, Buring JE: Presentation and summarization of data. In Mayrent SL [ed]: Epidemiology in Medicine. Boston, Little, Brown & Co, 1987.)

curs as new ideas evolve from accepted concepts or, in some cases, de novo. Nevertheless, it is through the acceptance or rejection of hypotheses that medical advances are made. This is important when reviewing the literature because hypotheses are not easily accepted; often many studies are published for and against a given hypothesis. The enlightened reader of the medical literature is able to make sense of the often-conflicting results and decide whether to accept or reject the new idea. What then is a hypothesis and how is it tested? Once a hypothesis is tested, how do we interpret the results?

A hypothesis is a type of theory, related to a very specific issue, that proposes some element of truth about that issue. The issue in medicine could be the effect of an antibiotic on bacterial metabolism, the suspected cause of osteonecrosis, or even the effect of screening programs on the occurrence of diabetic lower-extremity amputations. A new hypothesis (H_1)

is carefully scrutinized before being fully accepted and is subject to continuous debate and revision. Almost without exception hypotheses are "tested" by comparing them with a so-called null hypothesis (H_0), which is the assumption that no difference exists between the two hypotheses. The testing takes the form of statistical comparisons. Table 11–2 shows the framework with four possible outcomes in hypothesis testing.

As is true with most things in medicine, there is never absolute certainty about the results in hypothesis testing. It is important that there not be type I or type II errors, because this would allow for the incorrect inference to be drawn. The type I, or alpha, error occurs when a true null hypothesis is rejected; a type II, or beta, error occurs when a false null hypothesis is accepted. Alpha and beta are represented as probabilities of the occurrence of the error in question. The *P value*, which appears in medical journals, is related to these

TABLE 11–2. **Four Possible Outcomes of Hypothesis Testing**

Conclusion of Test of Significance	Truth	
	H_0 *True*	H_1 *True*
Do not reject H_0 (not statistically significant)	Correct: H_0 is true, and we do not reject H_0	Type II or beta error: H_1 is true, but we do not reject H_0
Reject H_0 (statistically significant)	Type I or alpha error: H_0 is true, but we reject H_0	Correct: H_1 is true, and we reject H_0

From Hennekens CH, Buring JE: Evaluating the role of chance. In Mayrent SL (ed): Epidemiology in Medicine, p 259. Boston, Little, Brown & Co, 1987.

errors. It is the probability that the results obtained, or those more extreme, could have been due to chance and may not be reflective of a true difference between groups. If the *P* value is low enough, we say that the results are statistically "significant" and we will accept the data as reflecting the truth. Later in the chapter the difference between statistical significance and clinical significance is discussed.

Another way of assessing experimental data for significance is through the use of *confidence intervals*. Indeed, the medical world has seen considerable debate over the pros and cons of *P* values versus confidence intervals, to the extent that some journals use only one or the other while others report both. The basic difference is that the use of the confidence interval gives the reader a somewhat more vivid idea as to where the experimental results lie within a probability range.

CASE-CONTROL AND COHORT STUDIES

The case-control and cohort studies are common in the medical literature. There are basic differences in the design of these studies. *Case-control investigations* are retrospective; that is, they involve the collection of data after disease has occurred in cases and use matched controls to compare the difference in exposure between the diseased and nondiseased groups. By matched control we mean that persons without the disease in question are selected so that they are as similar as possible to the cases, who are persons with disease. Then it is relatively simple to compare the exposure frequency between the two groups, arriving at

an odds ratio for exposure, which is a measure of the degree of disease risk associated with the exposure variable. The larger the odds ratio compared to 1.0 (unity), the more likely that the putative risk factor is causally related to the disease. Case-control studies are useful when investigating rare diseases or those with small prevalence rates. It was through the mechanism of case-control studies that the association between diethylstilbestrol use by pregnant women and vaginal cancer in their daughters was recognized. Toxic shock syndrome was likewise identified as being causally related to tampon use. Case-control studies are also important because they help with the generation of new hypotheses.

Cohort studies are considerably different from case-control designs. First, they are most often prospective; that is, they have a fixed starting point in the present and accumulate data as time moves forward. Sometimes a design known as a historical prospective study may be used; in this case a retrospective determination of the cohort is made and then followed forward in time. For our purposes, however, the discussion will be only of the usual cohort design. Here a group or groups of persons who are free of the disease are identified and categorized according to the level of exposure to the risk factor being studied. The groups are then followed forward, as time passes, and the rate of occurrence of disease is noted. At the end of the study these rates are compared, resulting in a relative risk measure, which is the ratio of incidence rates of disease in each group. This tells the investigator the magnitude of the difference in disease occurrence between the exposed and nonexposed groups. Relative risk is a measure of the increased (or decreased) risk incurred with exposure to an exposure factor. Relative risk figures in excess of unity indicate an increasing quantitative relationship between the exposure and outcome variables. Thus, if the relative risk of lung cancer for those who smoke is 3.2, then smokers have a 3.2 greater chance of getting cancer than nonsmokers. The reverse can also be true: numbers less than unity can suggest a protective, rather than an etiologic, relationship.

Cohort designs have the advantage of following large groups for extended periods of time but, compared with case-control studies, are more expensive and complicated to design and analyze. A prospective cohort study including 6 years of follow-up to examine prospectively the association between regular aspirin use and the risk of first myocardial infarction in women concluded that "the use of one through six aspirin per week appears to be associated with a reduced risk of a first myocardial infarction among women."[1] This study suggests the need for a clinical trial. Figure 11–15 illustrates the temporal differences among case-control, prospective cohort, and retrospective cohort. Although the nomenclature here is different from in other texts, it still provides a good description of the differences. Table 11–3 shows the pros and cons of case-control studies. Table 11–4 shows the pros and cons of cohort studies.

THE CLINICAL TRIAL

The last major clinical design is the *randomized clinical trial*. This is a major contribution to the world of research in medicine in the 20th century. It allows accurate testing of new diagnostic and treatment regimens through the use of randomization techniques that control for the many types of bias that can occur. Even so, bias can occur, and this design is not without the potential for misinterpretation. It is, however, the best model we now have to ensure that clinical outcomes reflect the truth of treatment effects. Figure 11–16 shows a new and important finding concerning increasing risk for myocardial infarction in treated patients with hypertension whose diastolic blood

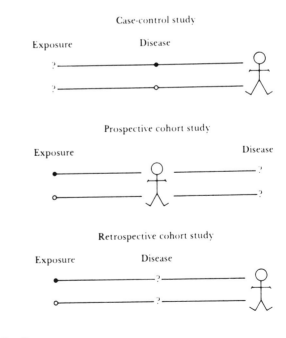

FIGURE 11–15. This figure graphically shows the temporal differences among case-control, prospective cohort, and retrospective cohort studies. (From Hennekens CH, Buring JE: Design strategies in epidemiologic research. In Mayrent SL [ed]: Epidemiology in Medicine. Boston, Little, Brown & Co, 1987.)

● = Present
○ = Absent
⎫ basis on which groups are selected at beginning of study

? = To be determined

☆ = Investigator at beginning of study

TABLE 11–3. **Strengths and Limitations of the Case-control Study Design**

Strengths

Is relatively quick and inexpensive compared with other analytic designs

Is particularly well-suited to the evaluation of diseases with long latent periods

Is optimal for the evaluation of rare diseases

Can examine multiple etiologic factors for a single disease

Limitations

Is inefficient for the evaluation of rare exposures, unless the attributable-risk percent is high

Cannot directly compute incidence rates of disease in exposed and nonexposed persons, unless study is population based

May be difficult to establish the temporal relationship between exposure and disease in some situations

Is particularly prone to bias compared with other analytic designs, in particular selection and recall bias

From Hennekens CH, Buring JE: Case-control studies. In Mayrent SL (ed): Epidemiology in Medicine, p 259. Boston, Little, Brown & Co, 1987.

TABLE 11–4. **Strengths and Limitations of the Cohort Study Design**

Strengths

Is of particular value when the exposure is rare

Can examine multiple effects of a single exposure

Can elucidate temporal relationship between exposure and disease

If prospective, minimizes bias in the ascertainment of exposure

Allows direct measurement of incidence of disease in the exposed and nonexposed groups

Limitations

Is inefficient for the evaluation of rare diseases, unless the attributable-risk percent is high

If prospective, can be extremely expensive and time consuming

If retrospective, requires the availability of adequate records

Validity of the results may be seriously affected by losses to follow-up

From Hennekens CH, Buring JE: Cohort studies. In Mayrent SL (ed): Epidemiology in Medicine, p 259. Boston, Little, Brown & Co, 1987.

pressure falls below 84 mm Hg. Tables 11–5 through 11–8 show crude vs. adjusted data, odds ratios with confidence intervals, likelihood ratios, and relative risk. It is important to remember when reading clinical trial reports that the method is not foolproof; some logical skepticism is usually warranted. There are numerous examples of large clinical trials that proved to have been flawed in design or analysis.

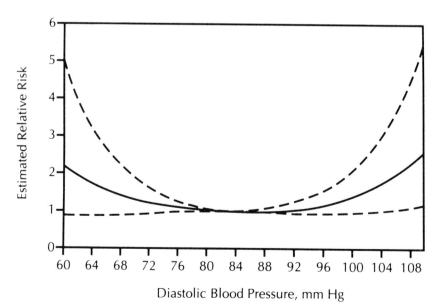

FIGURE 11–16. There has been some debate in the medical community about what minimum level of blood pressure reduction should be attained. This graph illustrates that as diastolic blood pressure is reduced below 84 mm Hg, the relative risk of myocardial infarction stops its decline and actually increases. (From McCloskey LW, Psaty BM, Koepsell TD, et al: Level of blood pressure and risk of myocardial infarction among treated hypertensive patients. Arch Intern Med 152:516, 1992. Copyright © 1992, American Medical Association.)

TABLE 11–5. **Blood Pressures and Medical Interventions in Cases and Controls**

	Cases	Controls
Blood pressure, mm Hg (n), mean ± SD (n)		
Pretreatment*		
Systolic	169.5 ± 19.6 (125)	166.4 ± 21.3 (531)
Diastolic	104.0 ± 12.5 (125)	103.4 ± 10.5 (533)
Last†		
Systolic	147.1 ± 20.1 (175)	142.5 ± 17.6 (737)
Diastolic	86.8 ± 10.6 (175)	86.4 ± 8.8 (737)
Duration of treatment, y, No. (%)		
≤5	64 (36.5)	296 (40.2)
6–10	47 (26.9)	232 (31.5)
11–15	29 (16.6)	105 (14.2)
16–20	15 (8.6)	43 (5.8)
≥21	4 (2.3)	20 (2.7)
Unknown	16 (9.1)	41 (5.6)
No. of pharmacy visits, mean ± SD (n)‡	4.7 ± 3.0 (175)	5.8 ± 2.9 (737)
No. of antihypertensives, mean ± SD (n)§	1.2 ± 0.75 (175)	1.4 ± 0.7 (737)

*Recorded on the day that antihypertensive therapy was initiated.

†Level of treated blood pressure most recently recorded before the index date (last during treatment).

‡Number of pharmacy visits during the past year at which one or more prescriptions for an antihypertensive medication were filled.

§Total number of medications being used for the treatment of hypertension.

Note: Here we see the descriptive data obtained from the study on diastolic blood pressures relationship to the risk for myocardial infarction. This crude data has been subjected to only basis analysis (i.e., the number of patients, the means, and standard deviations).

From McCloskey LW, Psaty BM, Koepsell TD, et al: Level of blood pressure and risk of myocardial infarction among treated hypertensive patients. Arch Intern Med 152:516, 1992. Copyright © 1992, American Medical Association.

BIAS

When reading the medical literature, one must remember that, no matter how well planned a study may be, there is always the problem of potential *bias*. A bias is a characteristic of the design or analysis of the study that in some way distorts the truth as reflected in the data. Bias can occur for numerous reasons. Some of the most common are selection bias, recall bias, observer bias, sampling bias, confounding, effect modification, misclassification, and publication bias. For our purposes we mean conceptual rather than simple mathematical error. Figures 11–17 through 11–19 and Tables 11–9 and 11–10 provide an excellent example of new information that could greatly affect podiatric decision making. They show increased sensitivity for the diagnosis of osteomyelitis through the use of indium-111 isotope scanning. When compared with current diagnostic indicators these data make an appealing case for the use of indium scans. However, the use of this test cannot be relied on completely because, while its sensitivity, specificity, and accuracy are high, the test, as the data show, is not completely foolproof. This is a good example of the importance of informed, critical reading of the literature.

Selection bias occurs when those subjects who participate in a study are not representative of the target population. *Recall bias* occurs when subjects are asked questions concerning past illnesses or other events: in many cases they may remember more or less than other participants, or their memory may be distorted by the passage of time. *Observer bias* occurs when the observer or data recorder is unable to perform objectively. *Sampling bias* results when the

TABLE 11–6. **Estimated Relative Risk of Myocardial Infarction by Strata of Diastolic Blood Pressure**

Last Diastolic Blood Pressure (mm Hg)	No. (%)		Odds Ratios for Various Models (95% Confidence Intervals)		
	Cases (n = 175)	Controls (n = 737)	Crude	Adjusted*	Adjusted†
≤74	21 (12)	62 (8.4)	1.60 (0.90–2.84)	1.56 (0.87–2.8)	1.49 (0.80–2.77)
75–84	55 (31.4)	260 (35.3)	1.00 (Reference)	1.00 (Reference)	1.00 (Reference)
85–94	67 (38.3)	303 (41.1)	1.04 (0.71–1.55)	1.08 (0.72–1.61)	1.10 (0.72–1.67)
95–104	22 (12.6)	98 (13.3)	1.06 (0.61–1.83)	1.14 (0.65–1.99)	1.20 (0.66–2.16)
≥105	10 (5.7)	14 (1.9)	3.38 (1.43–8.00)	3.57 (1.47–8.65)	3.20 (1.27–8.09)

*Controlled for pharmacy visits, age, sex, and index year.

†Controlled for pharmacy visits, age, sex, index year, smoking, cholesterol level, previous diastolic blood pressure, duration of treatment, congestive heart failure, and diabetes.

Note: Inspection of this table will show that for the crude and adjusted data the odds ratios for myocardial infarction increased once diastolic blood pressure dropped below 84 mm Hg. The figures in parentheses in these columns are the confidence intervals.

From McCloskey LW, Psaty BM, Koepsell TD, et al: Level of blood pressure and risk of myocardial infarction among treated hypertensive patients. Arch Intern Med 152:517, 1992. Copyright © 1992, American Medical Association.

TABLE 11–7. **Estimated Relative Risk of Myocardial Infarction by Strata of Diastolic Blood Pressure**

	Model							
	1	*2*	*3*	*4*	*5*	*6*	*7*	*8*
Odds Ratio (95% Confidence Interval)								
Last diastolic blood pressure (mm Hg)								
≤74	1.60 (0.90–2.84)	1.65 (0.92–2.95)	1.56 (0.87–2.8)	1.53 (0.84–2.78)	1.58 (0.87–2.89)	1.56 (0.85–2.87)	1.64 (0.89–3.03)	1.49 (0.80–2.77)
75–84 (reference level)	1.00	1.00	1.00	1.00	1.00	1.00	1.00	1.00
85–94	1.04 (0.71–1.55)	1.07 (0.72–1.59)	1.08 (0.72–1.61)	1.08 (0.72–1.63)	1.10 (0.73–1.66)	1.10 (0.73–1.66)	1.08 (0.71–1.64)	1.10 (0.72–1.67)
95–104	1.06 (0.61–1.83)	1.09 (0.63–1.89)	1.14 (0.65–1.99)	1.10 (0.62–1.95)	1.10 (0.62–1.96)	1.12 (0.62–2.00)	1.10 (0.61–1.99)	1.20 (0.66–2.16)
≥105	3.38 (1.43–8.00)	3.45 (1.43–8.29)	3.57 (1.47–8.65)	3.15 (1.27–7.78)	3.19 (1.28–7.94)	3.14 (1.26–7.85)	3.06 (1.22–7.65)	3.20 (1.27–8.09)
Factors Controlled								
Pharmacy visits		x	x	x	x	x	x	x
Age			x	x	x	x	x	x
Sex			x	x	x	x	x	x
Index year			x	x	x	x	x	x
Smoking				x	x	x	x	x
Cholesterol level					x	x	x	x
Previous diastolic blood pressure						x	x	x
Duration of treatment							x	x
Congestive heart failure								x
Diabetes								x

Note: This table expands on the information in Table 11–8B and graphically shows that as more factors are controlled for there continues to be a significant increased risk. To control for a factor in a statistical analysis means that the independent effects of that factor on the outcome in question, in this case myocardial infarction, are removed from the analysis. Thus, after the effects of all the listed factors were removed, the increasing risk with a reduction below 84 mm Hg continued.

From McCloskey LW, Psaty BM, Koepsell TD, et al: Level of blood pressure and risk of myocardial infarction among treated hypertensive patients. Arch Intern Med 152:517, 1992. Copyright © 1992, American Medical Association.

TABLE 11–8A. **Likelihood Ratio Tests of Significance (*P* Values)**

For Analysis of	Terms Added to Logistic Model*		
	x	**x²**	**(x + x²)**
Last diastolic blood pressure			
Unadjusted	.59	.008	.03
Adjusted for PCFs†	.33	.02	.04‡
Last systolic blood pressure			
Unadjusted	.003	.25	. . .
Adjusted for PCFs†	.05§	.11	. . .
Adjusted for PCFs and last diastolic blood pressure	.12‖	.22	. . .

*Tests of significance for the addition to the logistic model of variables that characterize the exposure in three ways; ie, the use of x alone as the exposure variable; the addition of x^2 to a model already containing x; and the simultaneous addition of $(x + x^2)$ to the model.

†Potentially confounding factors (PCFs) include number of pharmacy visits, age, sex, index year, smoking status, serum cholesterol level, pretreatment diastolic blood pressure, duration of treatment, congestive heart failure, and diabetes.

‡$\hat{\beta}_1 = -0.2232$; $\hat{\beta}_2 = 0.001339$; $v\hat{a}r(\hat{\beta}_1) = 0.00936$; $v\hat{a}r(\hat{\beta}_2) = 0.3093 \times 10^{-6}$; $cov\hat{a}riance\ (\hat{\beta}_1, \hat{\beta}_2) = 0.5355 \times 10^{-1}$.

§$\hat{\beta} = 0.01031$; SE $(\hat{\beta}) = 0.00525$.

‖$\beta = 0.009089$; SE $(\hat{\beta}) = 0.00583$.

TABLE 11–8B. **Estimated Relative Risk of Myocardial Infarction by Levels of Treated Diastolic Blood Pressure***

Diastolic Blood Pressure (mm Hg)	Adjusted Odds Ratio†	Confidence Interval	SE
60	2.07	0.86–5.01	0.4498
70	1.27	0.86–1.87	0.1990
80	1.01	0.93–1.10	0.0428
84	1.00‡	. . .	0
90	1.06	0.95–1.18	0.0566
100	1.45	1.02–2.06	0.1791
110	2.59	1.21–5.54	0.3886

*$\hat{\beta}_1 = -0.2232$; $\hat{\beta}_2 = 0.001339$; $v\hat{a}r(\hat{\beta}_1) = 0.00936$; $v\hat{a}r(\hat{\beta}_2) = 0.3093 \times 10^{-6}$; $cov\hat{a}riance\ (\hat{\beta}_1, \hat{\beta}_2) = -0.5355 \times 10^{-1}$.

†Adjusted for number of pharmacy visits, age, sex, index year, smoking history, serum cholesterol level, pretreatment diastolic blood pressure, duration of treatment, congestive heart failure, and diabetes.

‡Reference level.

Note: These tables show the estimated relative risk for myocardial infarction after the data were subjected to logistic regression. This method of analysis is commonly used in medical research. A review of texts on biostatistics is recommended for those wishing to pursue the subject.

From McCloskey LW, Psaty BM, Koepsell TD, et al: Level of blood pressure and risk of myocardial infarction among treated hypertensive patients. Arch Intern Med 152:518, 1992. Copyright © 1992, American Medical Association.

BONE BIOPSY-PROVEN OSTEOMYELITIS
(n=28)

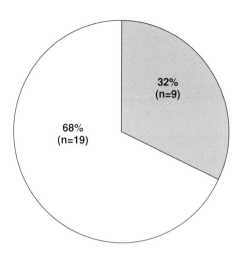

☐ Clinically Suspected Osteomyelitis
☐ Clinically Unsuspected Osteomyelitis

FIGURE 11–17. This figure shows how graphics can be used to summarize and convey information. It shows that, of 28 bone biopsy–confirmed cases of osteomyelitis, 68% (19 patients) showed clinically unsuspected disease. (From Newman, LG, Waller J, Palestro CJ, et al: Unsuspected osteomyelitis in diabetic foot ulcers: Diagnosis and monitoring by leukocyte scanning with indium 111 oxyquinoline. JAMA 266:1248, 1991. Copyright © 1991, American Medical Association.)

sample chosen for the study either overrepresents or underrepresents the population at large. *Confounding* is a type of bias that is particularly common in basic epidemiologic studies, although it can also occur in clinical trials. In this case there exists an unrecognized third variable that is associated with the exposure factor under study and is also causally related to the outcome variable of interest. *Effect modification* occurs when the impact of an effector on outcome varies across differing levels of a third variable. Unlike with confounding, there is no direct relationship among the modifier, the exposure factor, and the outcome variable. *Misclassification* occurs when data are wrongly categorized in relation to exposure or outcome. Figure 11–20 shows the relationship among exposure, confounding factor, and disease. *Publication bias* refers to the propensity of many journals to report only those studies with "positive" outcomes. A study of publication

bias showed that positive studies are more likely to be published regardless of quality of design. Those studies most susceptible to publication bias are also those known to be more prone to the problems of bias and confounding, which can threaten the validity of conclusions.[2] The importance of this bias relates to its effect on literature reviews and meta-analysis. This should be kept in mind when reading the literature because the true state of reality is often insufficiently reported when negative studies are not reported for consideration. As an example, an unexpected weak relationship between body mass and peak plantar pressure has been found in diabetic males.[3] This finding was particularly well analyzed by the authors and new hypotheses generated, even in view of an unexpected experimental outcome.

A new type of study known as *meta-analysis* has become more popular as an attempt to condense the results of many clinical studies. New statistical methods have been developed to reach a consensus from the combined data

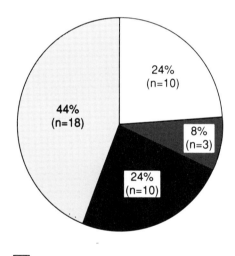

☐ Noninflamed Ulcers With Osteomyelitis
☐ Noninflamed Ulcers Without Osteomyelitis
■ Inflamed Ulcers Without Osteomyelitis
■ Inflamed Ulcers With Osteomyelitis

FIGURE 11–18. This graph shows the relationship between inflamed ulcers and osteomyelitis. (From Newman LG, Waller J, Palestro CJ, et al: Unsuspected osteomyelitis in diabetic foot ulcers: Diagnosis and monitoring by leukocyte scanning with indium 111 oxyquinoline. JAMA 266:1248, 1991. Copyright © 1991, American Medical Association.)

TABLE 11–9. **Results of Clinical and Laboratory Characteristics Used to Diagnose Osteomyelitis**

	Sensitivity	Specificity	Accuracy*
	No. (%)	*No. (%)*	*No. (%)*
Clinical judgment	9/28 (32)	13/13 (100)	22/41 (54)
Ulcer area, >2 cm²	15/27 (56)	12/13 (92)	27/40 (68)
Ulcer inflammation	10/28 (36)	10/13 (77)	20/41 (49)
Bone exposure	9/28 (32)	13/13 (100)	22/41 (54)
Erythrocyte sedimentation rate			
>70 mm/h, noninflamed ulcers	5/18 (28)	10/10 (100)	15/28 (54)
>100 mm/h, all ulcers	6/26 (23)	13/13 (100)	19/39 (49)

*Accuracy is defined as the number of correct predictions divided by total predictions.

From Newman LG, Waller J, Palestro CJ, et al: Unsuspected osteomyelitis in diabetic foot ulcers: Diagnosis and monitoring by leukocyte scanning with indium-111 oxyquinoline. JAMA 266:1248, 1991. Copyright © 1991, American Medical Association.

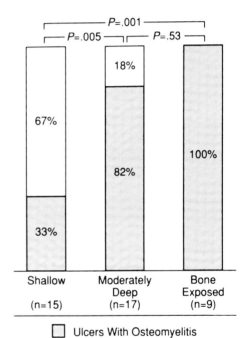

FIGURE 11–19. In this case the summary of data is expanded by using histograms to correlate ulcer depth with the occurrence of disease. (From Newman LG, Waller J, Palestro CJ, et al: Unsuspected osteomyelitis in diabetic foot ulcers: Diagnosis and monitoring by leukocyte scanning with indium 111 oxyquinoline. JAMA 266:1248, 1991. Copyright © 1991, American Medical Association.)

TABLE 11–10. **Results of Noninvasive Imaging Techniques Used to Diagnose Osteomyelitis**

Test	Sensitivity	Specificity	Accuracy*
	No. (%)	*No. (%)*	*No. (%)*
Radiograph	7/25 (28)	11/12 (92)	18/37 (49)
Bone scan	18/26 (69)	5/13 (39)	23/39 (59)
Leukocyte scan			
At 4 h	17/22 (77)	10/13 (77)	27/35 (77)
At 24 h	23/26 (89)	9/13 (69)	32/39 (82)

*Accuracy is defined as the number of correct predictions divided by total predictions.

From Newman LG, Waller J, Palestro CJ, et al: Unsuspected osteomyelitis in diabetic foot ulcers: Diagnosis and monitoring by leukocyte scanning with indium-111 oxyquinoline. JAMA 266:1248, 1991. Copyright © 1991, American Medical Association.

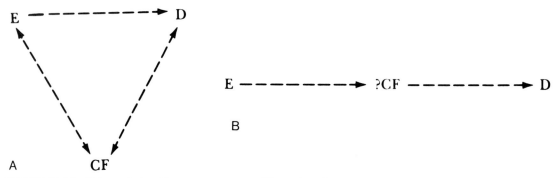

FIGURE 11–20. *(A)* Interrelationships among exposure (E), confounding factor (CF), and disease (D). *(B)* Interrelationships among exposure (E), disease (D), and a potential confounding factor (?CF), which is in the causal pathway and thus *not* a confounder. These figures illustrate the problem of confounding, a common bias that occurs in clinical studies. This occurs when the factor is associated with the exposure factor but can be independently causal to the disease. An effect modifier, on the other hand, is a third variable that distorts the magnitude of association between exposure and outcome—as the level of the modifier changes. (From Hennekens CH, Buring JE: Analysis of epidemiologic studies: evaluating the role of confounding. In Mayrent SL [ed]: Epidemiology in Medicine. Boston, Little, Brown & Co, 1987.)

of numerous studies of the same subject. In so doing it is hoped that the reader can gain some feel for the uniformity, or lack thereof, of often disparate results, thus alleviating the confusion that often results from conflicting study outcomes.

QUANTITATIVE DATA ANALYSIS

Whether a study is epidemiologic or clinical, recognition of the importance of quantitative data analysis is critical to the appreciation of articles that appear in the medical literature. Epidemiologic data are used to assay the prevalence or incidence of disease (i.e., occurrence assay), to seek relationships between disease and risk factors (association and risk assay), to map the causal mechanisms of disease, to establish etiology, to determine the accuracy of diagnostic tests, to aid in the process of clinical decision making, to plot the natural history of a disease, to better prognosticate the outcome of disease, to test the efficacy of treatment, to structure public health preventive programs, and to investigate the cost-benefit consequences of medical care. Different quantitative measures may be used. Those used in epidemiology will be discussed in this chapter. First, however, it is necessary to discuss the dependability of data.

Validity, Precision, Reproducibility

Data reported in the medical literature are reliable to the extent that they are valid, precise, and reproducible. Whether the data are gathered from a review of hospital records, from a survey, or from the outcomes of a diagnostic test, faith in their usefulness must depend on these three factors. This is critically important when reading the literature: to accept at face value all reported data is to invite problems. A measurement is considered valid if it measures what it claims to measure. Although there are many direct valid measures, there are also many indirect measures. As an example, a sphygmomanometer actually measures the rise and fall of a column of mercury directly, but this has been proven to be a valid indirect measure of blood pressure. Precision, or accuracy, refers to the quality of a measurement that reflects how close the measure is to the true value. This is why measurement technique and instrument calibration are so important: an error in either of these could severely bias the result from the truth. Reproducibility is that quality of a measure related to whether repeated measurements are the same or within an acceptable range of deviation.

Rates, Ratios, Risks

Epidemiologic measures deserve further comment. To compare the impact of risk factors on disease occurrence, great emphasis is placed on the use of rates and ratios. A rate is a count of events occurring within a specified group over a defined period of time. Ratios are derived by comparing rates of two different

TABLE 11–11. **Various Forms of Incidence and Prevalence Measures**

Rate	Type	Numerator	Denominator
Morbidity rate	Incidence	New cases of nonfatal disease	Total population at risk
Mortality rate	Incidence	Number of deaths from a disease (or all causes)	Total population
Case-fatality rate	Incidence	Number of deaths from a disease	Number of cases of that disease
Attack rate	Incidence	Number of cases of a disease	Total population at risk, for a limited period of observation
Disease rate at autopsy	Prevalence	Number of cases of a disease	Number of persons autopsied
Birth defect rate	Prevalence	Number of babies with a given abnormality	Number of live births
Period prevalence	Prevalence	Number of existing cases plus new cases diagnosed during a given time period	Total population

From Hennekens CH, Buring JE: Measures of disease frequency and association. In Mayrent SL (ed): Epidemiology in Medicine, p 62. Boston, Little, Brown & Co, 1987.

groups or time periods. The commonly used rates and ratios are used to measure occurrence, association, and risk. The use of rate and risk descriptors provides a convenient summary of the dynamics of exposure impact and disease occurrence, makes interpopulation and intrapopulation studies possible, establishes causal pathways, helps decipher the variable contribution of multiple risk factors, and allows the monitoring of intervention strategies over time.

The most commonly used occurrence measures are prevalence and incidence. Prevalence measures the extant cases of disease at a given moment in time in a specific population. Incidence measures the occurrence of new cases in a defined population over a given time interval. Prevalence thus includes a count of new and existing cases. Table 11–11 defines the various forms of incidence and prevalence measures. In all of these forms reference is made to the denominator. This is critical because the use of a denominator provides a reference base for the measure: if the denominator is not precisely defined, no conclusions can be drawn! Table 11–12 provides information that summarizes the differences between prevalence and incidence. It also defines cumulative incidence as a function of the population at risk and incidence density as a function of person–time observation. The bibliography at the end of this chapter can be consulted to further expand on this area.

Measures of association are used to quantify the relationship between degree of exposure to risk factors and the occurrence of disease. As Tables 11–13 and 11–14 show, there are a number of these measures used in case-control as well as cohort studies, the purpose of which is to fine-tune the association between exposure and disease. Association of a disease with a risk factor does not imply a finite causal connection but narrows the focus so that suspected etiologic agents can be pursued.

TABLE 11–12. **Measures of Disease Frequency**

$$\text{Prevalence (P)} = \frac{\text{Number of persons with disease at a point in time}}{\text{Number of persons in population}}$$

$$\text{Cumulative incidence (CI)} = \frac{\text{Number of new cases of disease in a given time period}}{\text{Total population at risk}}$$

$$\text{Incidence density (ID)} = \frac{\text{Number of new cases of disease in a given time period}}{\text{Total person-time of observation}}$$

From Hennekens CH, Buring JE: Measures of disease frequency and association. In Mayrent SL (ed): Epidemiology in Medicine, p 94. Boston, Little, Brown & Co, 1987.

TABLE 11–13. **Measures of Association: Case-control Studies**

Relative risk (RR), calculated as odds ratio (OR)	$= \dfrac{ad}{bc}$
Attributable-risk percent (AR%)	$= \dfrac{RR - 1}{RR} \times 100$
Population attributable-risk percent (PAR%)	$= \dfrac{P_e\,(RR - 1)}{P_e\,(RR - 1) + 1} \times 100$ or AR% × proportion of exposed cases
Attributable risk (AR)*	$=$ Incidence rate among exposed (I_e) − Incidence rate among nonexposed (I_0)
Population attributable risk (PAR)*	$=$ AR × proportion of exposed (P_e)

*If the study is population based or if incidence rates can be estimated.
From Hennekens CH, Buring JE: Measures of disease frequency and association. In Mayrent SL (ed): Epidemiology in Medicine, p. 96. Boston, Little, Brown & Co, 1987.
Case-control data are entered into a 2 x 2 table, with exposure listed in rows and outcome listed in columns. Thus, *ad/bc* is derived by multiplying the number of exposed persons with disease *(a)* by the number of unexposed persons without disease *(d)*, and dividing by the number of exposed persons without disease *(b)* multiplied by the number of persons not exposed but with disease *(c)*. The odds ratio (OR) is an approximation of the relative risk (RR); both of these measures quantify the association between risk factor exposure and the development of disease, but using different study designs.

TABLE 11–14. **Measures of Association: Cohort Studies**

Relative risk (RR)	1. Cumulative incidence (risk) ratio = $\dfrac{\text{Cumulative incidence in exposed (CI}_e)}{\text{Cumulative incidence in nonexposed (CI}_0)}$ 2. Incidence density (rate) ratio = $\dfrac{\text{Incidence rate among exposed (I}_e)}{\text{Incidence rate among nonexposed (I}_0)}$
Attributable risk (AR)	$= I_e - I_0$
Attributable-risk percent (AR%)	$= \dfrac{AR}{I_e} \times 100$
Population attributable risk (PAR)	$= I_T - I_0$ or AR × prevalence of exposure (P_e)
Population attributable-risk percent (PAR%)	$= \dfrac{PAR}{\text{Incidence rate of disease in population (I}_T)} \times 100$

From Hennekens CH, Buring JE: Measures of disease frequency and association. In Mayrent SL (ed): Epidemiology in Medicine, p. 95. Boston, Little, Brown & Co, 1987.
Relative risk (RR) is a measure of the increased (or decreased) risk incurred with exposure to an exposure factor. Relative risk figures in excess of unity indicate an increasing quantitative relationship between the exposure and outcome variables.
This table shows how to calculate relative risk for cumulative incidence and incidence density measures. The attributable risk (AR) further extends the impact of a risk factor by quantifying the difference in rates between those exposed and those not exposed. The population attributable risk (PAR) quantifies the impact of exposure on the population by relating incidence to prevalence.

SUMMARIZATION OF DATA

Clinical and epidemiologic data are often best appreciated by the use of graphic summaries, including histograms, charts, and maps. This can be appreciated by inspection of the material shown in Figure 11–21, which represents the incidence rates of Lyme disease, by county, in New York from 1986 through 1989. These maps dramatically illustrate the increasing incidence of the disease and its geographic spread from the New York City area. Figure 11–22 again illustrates the summary value of graphs and histograms as they related to changes in infant mortality among a Native American population. The reader is also invited to inspect Tables 11–15 and 11–16 and compare the differences between the tabular presentation of data and the graphic format of the same material as presented in Figure 11–23.

CAUSALITY

What then is the relationship among causality, association, etiology, risk factors, and natural history? How do they relate to intelligent review of the medical literature? Because it is the purpose of medicine to cure disease and alleviate pain and suffering, knowledge of the cause of disease is of obvious importance. It is not easy to determine the cause of a disease in a simple and straightforward manner. Indeed, the world's medical literature is filled with a continuous stream of sometimes corroborative, and often conflicting, theories, hypotheses, and arguments concerning the cause of disease (and effectiveness of treatment).

Causality refers to the rational link between the occurrence of an event (an exposure) and the subsequent appearance of an altered natural state (a disease or predisease state). At first glance it might seem to be a simple issue

Text continued on page 144

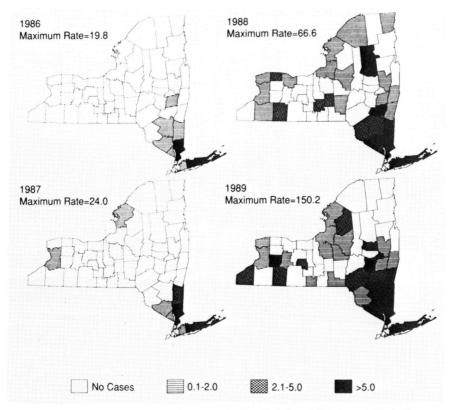

FIGURE 11–21. Incidence rates of Lyme disease, by county, in New York from 1986 through 1989. Maps are exquisite in their impact of illustrating the extent of disease by place and time. In this example a picture is worth a thousand bits of raw data. (From White DJ, Chang HG, Benach JL, et al: The geographic spread and temporal increase of the Lyme disease epidemic. JAMA 266:1232, 1991. Copyright © 1991, American Medical Association.)

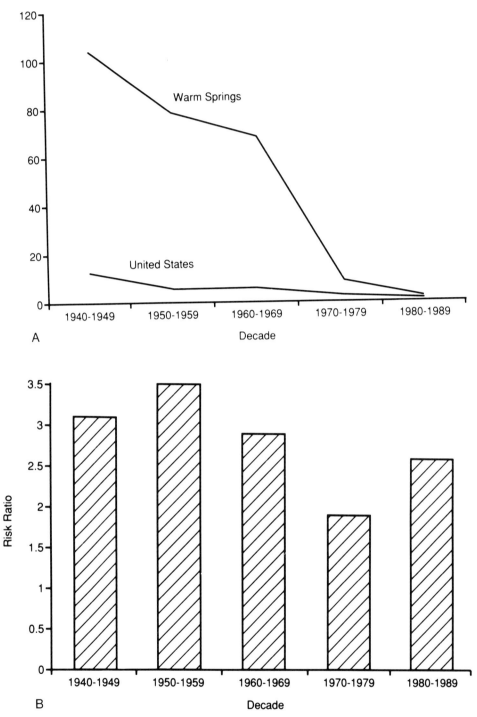

FIGURE 11–22. These graphs show the comparisons between infant mortality among Native Americans and the US population as a whole. *(A)* The first graph compares infant mortality per 1000 live births between the US population and that of the Warm Springs Indian Reservation. *(B)* Histograms can be used to represent the risk ratios between the two populations. Thus, we can see that for each decade there is a greater risk of infant mortality for the Native American infants, ranging from a high of 3.5 to a low of 2.0.

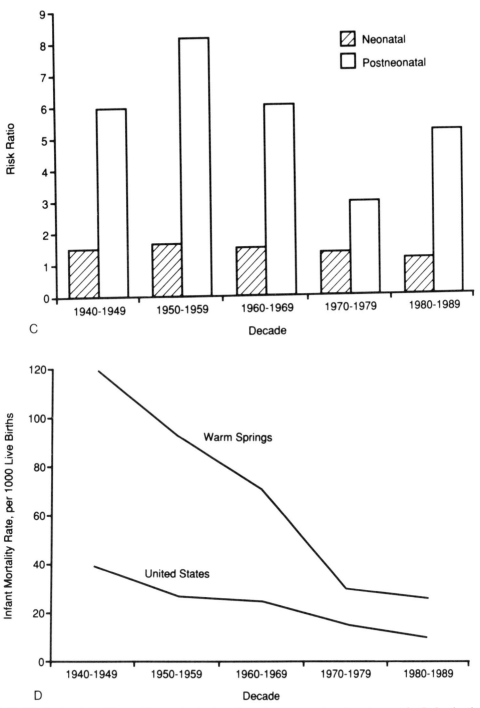

FIGURE 11–22 *Continued (C)* These risks can be broken down into neonatal and postneonatal. *(D)* Lastly, the infant mortality rates resulting from infectious disease are compared. When comparing this last figure to the previous ones, what conclusions might one draw? (From Nakamura RM, King R, Kimball EH, et al: Excess infant mortality in an American Indian population, 1940 to 1990. JAMA 266:2245, 1991. Copyright © 1991, American Medical Association.)

TABLE 11-15. **Incidence of Amputations and Sores or Ulcers by Characteristics of the Population in Younger-Onset Diabetic Persons***

Characteristic Value	No. of Participants	Incidence of Amputations		P†	No. of Participants	Incidence of Sores/Ulcers		P†
		N	%			N	%	
Systolic BP (mm Hg)								
78–110	218	1	0.5		196	11	5.6	
111–120	241	3	1.2	<.001	219	17	7.8	<.005
121–134	224	3	1.3		199	21	10.6	
135–221	190	12	6.3		159	24	15.1	
Diastolic BP (mm Hg)								
42–71	228	1	0.4		206	11	5.3	
72–78	223	3	1.3	<.01	198	23	11.6	<.05
79–85	203	5	2.5		183	15	8.2	
86–117	217	10	4.6		184	24	13.0	
Pulse pressure (mm Hg)								
8–33	217	3	1.4		196	17	8.7	.26
34–41	219	3	1.4	.07	188	13	6.9	
42–52	220	3	1.4		202	21	10.4	
53–125	215	10	4.7		185	22	11.9	
Body mass (kg/m²)								
14.4–20.9	225	5	2.2		205	27	13.2	
21.0–23.0	215	5	2.3	.96	194	19	9.8	<.05
23.1–25.5	222	4	1.8		189	13	6.9	
25.6–50.8	215	5	2.3		188	14	7.4	
Glycosylated hemoglobin (%)								
6.0–10.8	211	2	0.9		192	10	5.2	
10.9–12.2	207	5	2.4	.13	186	11	5.9	<.0005
12.3–14.1	215	6	2.8		180	17	9.4	
14.2–23.3	201	6	3.0		180	31	17.2	
Sex								
Male	442	14	3.2	<.05	386	40	10.4	.42
Female	437	5	1.1		392	34	8.7	
Proteinuria								
Absent	688	9	1.3	<.05	625	50	8.0	<.01
Present	156	6	3.8		123	20	16.3	
History of sores/ulcers								
No	783	7	0.9	<.0001	...	...	...	
Yes	96	12	12.5		...	...	...	
Retinopathy								
None	273	0	0.0		259	15	5.8	
Mild	298	5	1.7	<.0001	261	13	5.0	<.0001
Moderate	142	1	0.7		127	22	17.3	
PDR	166	13	7.8		131	24	18.3	
Smoking status‡								
Nonsmoker	384	6	1.6		347	28	8.1	
Ex-smoker	115	5	4.3	.06	98	9	9.2	<.005
Current smoker	197	8	4.1		160	28	17.5	
Pack-years smoked‡								
0	385	6	1.6		348	28	8.0	
<5	97	3	3.1	<.0005	87	9	10.3	<.005
5–14	90	0	0.0		77	11	14.3	
≥15	122	10	8.2		91	17	18.7	

*BP indicates blood pressure; PDR, proliferative diabetic retinopathy.
†Based on the Mantel-Haenszel test for trend or the χ^2 test with 1 df (sex, proteinuria, history of sores/ulcers).
‡Restricted to age 18 years or more.
From Moss SE, Klein R, Klein BEK: The prevalence and incidence of lower extremity amputation in a diabetic population. Arch Intern Med 152:611–613, 1992. Copyright © 1992, American Medical Association.

TABLE 11–16. **Incidence of Amputations and Sores or Ulcers by Characteristics of the Population in Older-Onset Diabetic Persons***

Characteristic Value	No. of Participants	Incidence of Amputations		P†	No. of Participants	Incidence of Sores/Ulcers		P†
		N	%			N	%	
Systolic BP (mm Hg)								
80–130	243	7	2.9		220	21	9.5	
131–144	266	3	1.1	.86	237	23	9.7	.35
145–160	239	2	0.8		221	23	10.4	
161–263	207	9	4.3		177	23	13.0	
Diastolic BP (mm Hg)								
45–70	213	8	3.8		179	23	12.8	
71–78	254	4	1.6	.07	230	24	10.4	.12
79–87	254	7	2.8		232	25	10.8	
88–129	231	2	0.9		211	16	7.6	
Pulse pressure (mm Hg)								
19–50	239	4	1.7		218	18	8.3	
51–64	235	4	1.7	.25	216	20	9.3	.08
65–79	243	5	2.1		218	22	10.1	
80–153	235	8	3.4		200	28	14.0	
Body mass (kg/m²)								
17.1–24.6	206	4	1.9		179	19	10.6	
24.7–28.1	241	7	2.9	.90	215	25	11.6	.64
28.2–31.7	245	5	2.0		221	24	10.9	
31.8–56.8	264	5	1.9		241	22	9.1	
Glycosylated hemoglobin (%)								
6.2–9.2	230	2	0.9		212	9	4.2	
9.3–10.8	220	5	2.3	<.05	198	16	8.1	<.0001
10.9–12.6	214	5	2.3		193	20	10.4	
12.7–23.6	214	8	3.7		182	34	18.7	
Sex								
Male	423	14	3.3	<.05	379	46	12.1	.17
Female	533	7	1.3		477	44	9.2	
Proteinuria								
Absent	821	13	1.6	<.0001	742	69	9.3	<.005
Present	101	8	7.9		84	17	20.2	
History of sores/ulcers								
No	857	12	1.4	<.0001	...	...	...	
Yes	98	9	9.2		...	...	...	
Retinopathy								
None	477	3	0.6		447	32	7.2	
Mild	291	9	3.1	<.001	256	29	11.3	<.0001
Moderate	129	5	3.9		109	19	17.4	
PDR	59	4	6.8		44	10	22.7	
Smoking status								
Nonsmoker	537	11	2.0		480	51	10.6	
Ex-smoker	286	5	1.7	.38	256	24	9.4	.78
Current smoker	133	5	3.8		120	15	12.5	
Pack-years smoked								
0	538	11	2.0		480	51	10.3	
<5	77	3	3.9		69	10	14.5	
5–14	58	0	0.0	.77	52	5	9.6	.77
15–29	85	2	2.4		79	5	6.3	
≥30	196	5	2.6		174	19	10.9	
Taking insulin								
No	497	10	2.0	.68	463	35	7.6	<.005
Yes	459	11	2.4		393	55	14.0	

*BP indicates blood pressure; PDR, proliferative diabetic retinopathy.

†Based on the Mantel-Haenszel test for trend or the χ^2 test with 1 df (sex, proteinuria, history of sores/ulcers, insulin-taking status).

From Moss SE, Klein R, Klein BEK: The prevalence and incidence of lower extremity amputation in a diabetic population. Arch Intern Med 152:613, 1992. Copyright © 1992, American Medical Association.

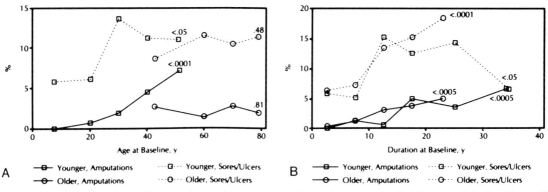

FIGURE 11–23. *(A)* Incidence of amputations and sores or ulcers by age in younger- and older-onset diabetic patients. *(B)* Incidence of amputations and sores or ulcers by duration of diabetes in younger- and older-onset diabetics. In both graphs, annotated numbers are *P* values for a test of trend. These graphs summarize data from Tables 11–15 and 11–16. Inspect the tables, then the graphs, and try to correlate the findings. (From Moss SE, Klein R, Klein BEK: The prevalence and incidence of lower extremity amputation in a diabetic population. Arch Intern Med 15:611–613, 1992. Copyright © 1992, American Medical Association.)

to establish the connection, but this is not so. Indeed, issues of causality have intrigued philosophers and scientists for the entire span of human history. Issues of causality in medicine have a philosophical basis; they are continuing processes that seek to answer the question, "What is truth?"

A prospective study of 51,529 male health care professionals supported the hypothesis that the inverse relationship between alcohol and the risk of coronary disease is causal.[4] This study did not claim that alcohol is the sole agent responsible for a decrease in heart disease. Rather, it established that the hypothesis concerning the relationship between the two is supported by the data and, furthermore, that this support strongly suggests an association between the two. To further test this theory, clinical trials will be necessary.

The Causal Web

It is important to remember that issues of causality are rarely straightforward. Indeed, the use of the term *causal web* perhaps best describes the intricacies of etiology, risk, and natural history that form the basis for causal relationships. A good example of this is the dilemma of the etiology of diabetic foot disease. Results of a study, as shown in Figure 11–24, present a conceptual causal pathway to

integrate which risk factors lead to lower-extremity amputation in diabetics. One can easily appreciate the complexity of trying to dissect the interactions among risk factors. The scheme shown does not, however, complete the etiologic picture, nor does it quantify the relative degree of risk contributed by peripheral vascular disease, neuropathy, inadequate foot care, or infection. To do this we must consider the important contemporary concept of the sufficient-component model of causality, an important contribution of late 20th century epidemiology.

Sufficient-Component Causality

The sufficient-component model of causality takes into account, conceptually and quantitatively, the interrelationship of multiple factors in the development of disease. Figure 11–25 illustrates this. Sufficient causes inevitably produce pathologic change. Component causes, while sufficient themselves to produce change, must be present for the sufficient cause to have an impact. Figures 11–26 and 11–27 apply this concept to the dilemma of diabetic amputation. It can be seen that there is improved specificity of the events that lead to amputation, the importance of which is to allow for more effective preventive and treatment measures to be used.

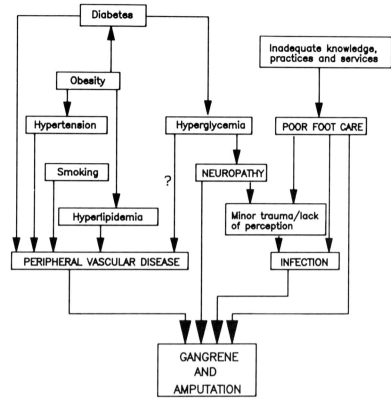

FIGURE 11–24. This information represents one author's representation of the causal web in diabetic foot disease. After reviewing the scheme, try to determine whether it is all-inclusive. Does it establish a logical causal pathway? Are the associations between the various factors in etiologic sequence? (Reprinted with permission from Bild DE, Selby JV, Sinnock P, et al: Lower extremity amputation in people with diabetes: Epidemiology and prevention. Diabetes Care 12:25, 1989. Copyright © 1989. American Diabetes Association, Inc.)

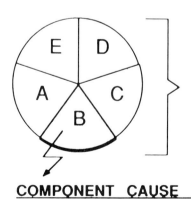

SUFFICIENT CAUSE :

— INEVITABLY PRODUCES THE EFFECT

— RESTRICTED TO THE MINIMAL NUMBER OF COMPONENT CAUSES REQUIRED FOR CAUSATION

COMPONENT CAUSE :

— NOT SUFFICIENT IN ITSELF

— REMOVAL OR BLOCKING RENDERS ACTION OF OTHER COMPONENTS INSUFFICIENT

FIGURE 11–25. Use this information to bridge the differences between the scheme in Figure 11–24 and those in Figures 11–26 and 11–27. (Reprinted with permission from Pecoraro RE, Reiber GE, Burgess EM: Pathways to diabetic limb amputation: Basis for prevention. Diabetes Care 13:515, 517, 1990. Copyright © 1990 by the American Diabetes Association, Inc.)

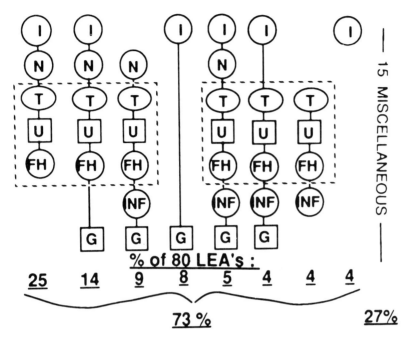

FIGURE 11-26. Most unique causal pathways required interaction of pathophysiologic components (ischemia [I], neuropathy [N], infection [INF], faulty wound healing [FH]), pathologic conditions (ulceration [U], gangrene [G]), and environmental events (minor trauma [T]). Prevalent triad of factors *(dashed boxes)* leading to amputation included trauma, causing ulceration, which was subsequently complicated by faulty wound healing. There are 23 causal pathways and 80 lower-extremity amputations (LEAs). (Reprinted with permission from Pecoraro RE, Reiber GE, Burgess EM: Pathways to diabetic limb amputation: Basis for prevention. Diabetes Care 13:515, 517, 1990. Copyright © 1990 by the American Diabetes Association, Inc.)

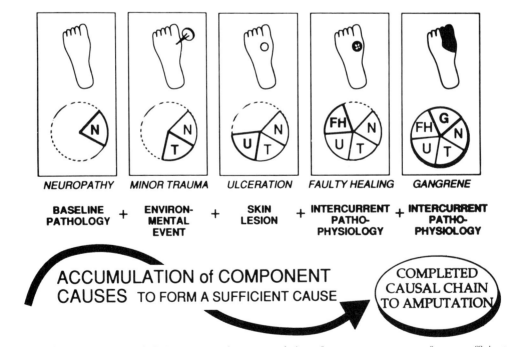

FIGURE 11-27. Completed causal chain to amputation: accumulation of component causes to form a sufficient cause. (Reprinted with permission from Pecoraro RE, Reiber GE, Burgess EM: Pathways to diabetic limb amputation: Basis for prevention. Diabetes Care 13:515, 517, 1990. Copyright © 1990 by the American Diabetes Association, Inc.)

Determinism vs. Probabilism

Determinism is based on the assumption of the specificity of cause and effect; that is, A always causes B. It is a paradigm that does not fit easily with the fact of imperfect knowledge that exists in the real world. Also, it does not work well with cases of multifactorial etiology or when there are multiple treatment effects. Thus, it finds limited usefulness in medicine. Probabilism, on the other hand, is more consonant with the reality of the scientific world. This is based on the laws of probability. Probabilism is used widely in medicine, it relies heavily on the principles of statistical significance, and it provides a rationale for the principles of causal association.

An example of the often-conflicting messages found in the literature and how they relate to the determination of etiology and treatment is the subject of the relationship between thiazide use and the risk for hip fracture. Tables 11–17 through 11–22 show the results of two studies on the subject. Both were case-control studies, and they reached opposing conclusions. The Framingham study suggested that recent pure thiazide use protected women against hip fracture. The report from the state of Washington concluded the opposite. What is the reader of the literature to believe? Perhaps more important is the issue of trying to interpret study design and analysis in such a

TABLE 11–17. **Washington State Study: Medical Factors Affecting the Risk for Hip Fracture**

Factor*	Relative Risk (95% CI)†
Current alcoholism (24)	7.4 (3.3 to 16.4)
The organic brain syndrome (101)	7.3 (4.2 to 12.5)
Leg paralysis (14)	3.7 (1.1 to 12.1)
History of cerebrovascular accident (83)	3.6 (2.1 to 6.0)
Phenobarbital use (71)	3.2 (1.9 to 5.4)
History of syncope (29)	2.9 (1.3 to 6.5)
Corticosteroid use (48)	1.8 (1.0 to 3.2)
Obesity	0.4 (0.3 to 0.6)

*In parentheses is the number of patients with the factor.
†Calculated using the Mantel-Haenszel method while controlling only for matched pairs.
Reproduced with permission from Heidrich FE, Stergachis A, Gross KM: Diuretic drug use and the risk of hip fracture. Ann Intern Med 115:4, 1991.

TABLE 11–18. **Washington State Study: Risk for Hip Fracture Among Users of Thiazide Diuretics**

Characteristic	Relative Risk (95% CI)*	Adjusted Relative Risk (95% CI)†
Gender		
Men	1.1 (0.7 to 1.8)	1.2 (0.5 to 2.9)
Women	1.6 (1.2 to 2.3)	1.7 (1.1 to 2.6)
Use‡		
Current	1.1 (0.8 to 1.6)	1.6 (1.0 to 2.5)
Former	1.9 (1.2 to 3.1)	1.2 (0.6 to 2.4)
Duration of use (y)‡		
<2	1.5 (0.8 to 2.8)	2.2 (1.0 to 4.7)
2–5	1.5 (1.0 to 2.4)	1.5 (0.9 to 2.5)
>5	1.8 (1.2 to 3.0)	1.7 (1.0 to 2.9)
Daily dosage (mg)‡		
25	2.1 (1.1 to 3.8)	1.2 (0.6 to 2.4)
50	1.3 (0.9 to 1.9)	1.5 (0.9 to 2.3)
≥ 75	1.1 (0.5 to 2.6)	1.9 (0.8 to 4.7)
Total	1.5 (1.1 to 1.9)	1.5 (1.0 to 2.2)

*Calculated using the Mantel-Haenszel method while controlling for matched pairs. Nonusers were the reference category for the analyses of each subgroup of use and dosage.
†Conditional logistic regression analysis controlling for alcoholism, the organic brain syndrome, leg paralysis, history of stroke, days of hospitalization in the preceding year, nursing home residence, body mass index, use of phenobarbital, corticosteroids, and furosemide.
‡There were 195 current and 112 former users of thiazide. Analysis by duration of use categories involved 412 matched pairs; analysis by dosage categories involved 385 matched pairs.
Reproduced with permission from Heidrich FE, Stergachis A, Gross KM: Diuretic drug use and the risk of hip fracture. Ann Intern Med 115:4, 1991.

way as to be able to make intelligent comparisons. This, of course, is the purpose of this chapter.

Once statistical significance is attained, the following criteria must be met to establish a causal link. First, the data must follow the proper temporal sequence; that is, if A causes B, then A must always precede the occurrence of B. The data, no matter how statistically significant, must be consistent with current scientific theory. The statistical strength of association must be strong; an odds ratio of 1:6 is far less convincing than one of 2:3. When applicable, there must be evidence of a dose–response relationship. The data must withstand scrutiny for plausible confounding factors and other potential bias. Finally, the strength of the association must be replicable.

The importance of the critical place of causal theory when reading and evaluating the

TABLE 11–19. Framingham Study: Risk Factors for Hip Fracture at Most Recent Biennial Examination: Comparison of Cases and Controls

Risk Factors	Cases (n = 176)	Controls (n = 672)	P
Age (y), mean ± SD	77.2 ± 9.4	78.0 ± 9.2	.27
Most recent alcohol consumption (oz/wk)	1.8 ± 3.3	1.7 ± 2.9	.84
Age at cessation of menses (y)	47.5 ± 5.3	47.4 ± 5.5	.89
Most recent body mass index (kg/m²)	23.3 ± 3.9	24.5 ± 4.3	.0006
Most recent caffeine consumption (mean number of cups of coffee equivalents/d)	2.2 ± 1.5	1.9 ± 1.3	.02
Most recent number of cigarettes smoked (mean ± SD)	2.8 ± 7.3	1.8 ± 5.7	.06
Ever took estrogen replacement (%)	20.7	30.9	.008
Recently designated as hypertensive (%)*	38.6	40.4	.67
Recently received nondiuretic antihypertensive therapy (%)	15.9	18.8	.38
Poor vision (%)†	44.2	28.8	.003
Mobility limitation (%)	58.1	54.6	.78

*Subjects were designated as hypertensive if they were receiving antihypertensive therapy or if blood pressure was greater than 160/95 mm Hg.

†Vision worse than 20/25 in at least one eye.

From Felson DT, Sloutkis D, Anderson JJ, et al: Thiazide diuretics and the risk of hip fracture: Results from the Framingham study. JAMA 265:370–373, 1991. Copyright © 1991, American Medical Association.

TABLE 11–20. Framingham Study: Association Between All Thiazide-Containing Medications and Hip Fracture

	Frequency of Use, No. (%)		Adjusted* Matched Odds Ratio
	Cases	Controls	
Ever used thiazides	46/176 (26.1)	172/672 (25.6)	1.33 (0.86, 2.05)
Recent use, all thiazides	19/107 (17.8)	90/430 (20.9)	0.69 (0.34, 1.40)
Recent use only	2/77 (2.6)	7/309 (2.3)	2.10 (0.12, 35.76)
Recent and past use	17/92 (18.5)	83/385 (21.6)	0.75 (0.35, 1.61)
Past use during one examination	4/79 (5.1)	24/326 (7.4)	0.43 (0.09, 2.15)
Past use during more than two examinations	13/88 (12.8)	59/361 (16.3)	0.87 (0.37, 2.04)
Past use only	11/86 (12.8)	28/330 (8.5)	3.37 (1.14, 9.95)

*Adjusted for body mass index, estrogen use, number of cigarettes smoked, alcohol consumption, and age at menopause. Additional adjustments for caffeine consumption, vision, and mobility dysfunction did not affect the odds ratio.

From Felson DT, Sloutkis D, Anderson JJ, et al: Thiazide diuretics and the risk of hip fracture: Results from the Framingham study. JAMA 265:370–373, 1991. Copyright © 1991, American Medical Association.

TABLE 11–21. Framingham Study: Association Between Pure Thiazide Medications* and Hip Fracture

	Frequency of Use, No. (%)		Adjusted† Matched Odds Ratio
	Cases	Controls	
Ever used thiazides	27/171 (15.8)	119/650 (18.3)	0.91 (0.56, 1.49)
Recent use, all thiazides	9/97 (9.3)	51/390 (13.4)	0.31 (0.11, 0.88)
Recent use only	1/81 (1.2)	5/313 (1.6)	• • •
Recent and past use	8/88 (9.1)	46/354 (13.0)	0.38 (0.14, 1.09)
Past use during one examination	3/83 (3.6)	13/321 (4.1)	0.80‡ (0.14, 4.52)
Past use during more than two examinations	5/85 (5.9)	33/341 (8.5)	0.27‡ (0.07, 1.01)
Past use only	6/86 (7.0)	21/329 (6.4)	1.86 (0.53, 6.51)

*Excludes thiazide-containing combinations.

†Adjusted for body mass index, estrogen use, number of cigarettes smoked, alcohol consumption, and age at menopause. Additional adjustments for caffeine consumption, vision, and mobility dysfunction did not affect the odds ratio.

‡Increasing duration of recent and past use significant (P<.05) by Mantel-Haenszel test for trend.

From Felson DT, Sloukis D, Anderson JJ, et al: Thiazide diuretics and the risk of hip fracture: Results from the Framingham study. JAMA 265:370–373, 1991. Copyright © 1991, American Medical Association.

TABLE 11–22. **Framingham Study: Association Between Thiazide-Containing Combination Medications and Hip Fracture**

	Frequency of Use, No. (%)		Adjusted* Matched Odds Ratio
	Cases	*Controls*	
Ever used thiazides	27/169 (16.0)	73/627 (11.6)	2.23 (1.26, 3.94)
Recent use, all thiazides	10/95 (17.8)	41/375 (10.9)	1.16 (0.44, 3.05)
Recent use only	2/79† (2.5)	9/327† (2.8)	0.96 (0.09, 10.46)
Recent and past use	8/85 (9.4)	32/350 (9.1)	1.30 (0.44, 3.83)
Past use during one examination	0/77 (0.0)	10/328 (3.1)	•••
Past use during more than two examinations	8/85 (9.4)	22/340 (6.5)	2.86 (0.75, 10.88)
Past use only	6/83 (7.2)	6/324 (1.9)	14.23 (1.14, 138.00)

*Adjusted for body mass index, estrogen use, number of cigarettes smoked, alcohol consumption, and age at menopause. Additional adjustments for caffeine consumption, vision, and mobility dysfunction did not affect the odds ratio.

†For some exposure categories, adding up pure users (Table 11–21) and combination users (Table 11–22) does not equal all users (Table 11–20). This occurs because, for example, a subject with recent use only of pure thiazides may have used combination drugs in the past (past use only). For all thiazides (Table 11–20), this person would be characterized as a recent and past user and the recent use only exposure would be missing.

From Felson DT, Sloutkis D, Anderson JJ, et al: Thiazide diuretics and the risk of hip fracture: Results from the Framingham study. JAMA 265:370–373, 1991. Copyright © 1991, American Medical Association.

medical literature cannot be overemphasized. The issue of tobacco smoke and the occurrence of lung cancer is a prime example. Repeated studies have demonstrated the strong association between smoking and the disease, but there is still not positive proof as to what specifically causes the disease. Nevertheless, the association is so strong that there is no doubt that intervention programs can result in a decreased incidence of disease. This example represents the intricacies of the epidemiologic triad, that is, the interactions among host, agent, and environment that colors all disease. It is also a good example of a statistically significant event that is clinically important.

DIAGNOSTIC TESTS

Lastly, the enlightened reader must be able to judge the value of diagnostic tests. This is of no small concern when we realize the rapid advances occurring in medical technology and the increasing reliance placed on them. To assist the reader with this, Table 11–23 and Figure 11–28 are included. The first lists ways of deciding on the usefulness of a test; the second diagrams the concepts of sensitivity, specificity, positive predictive value, and negative predictive value. Remember that useful tests are those with high sensitivity and speci-

ficity but that an increase in one is always associated with a decrease in the other. Sensitivity is the proportion of persons who test positive who actually have the disease, and specificity is that proportion who test negative and are actually free of the disease. Positive

TABLE 11–23. **Eight Guides for Deciding the Clinical Usefulness of a Diagnostic Test**

1. Has there been an independent, "blind" comparison with a "gold standard" of diagnosis?
2. Has the diagnostic test been evaluated in a patient sample that included an appropriate spectrum of mild and severe and treated and untreated disease, plus patients with different but commonly confused disorders?
3. Was the setting for this evaluation, as well as the filter through which study patients passed, adequately described?
4. Have the reproducibility of the test result (precision) and its interpretation (observer variation) been determined?
5. Has the term *normal* been defined sensibly as it applies to this test?
6. If the test is advocated as part of a cluster or sequence of tests, has its individual contribution to the overall validity of the cluster or sequence been determined?
7. Have the tactics for carrying out the test been described in sufficient detail to permit their exact replication?
8. Has the utility of the test been determined?

From Sackett DL, Haynes RB, Guyatt GH, Tugwell P (eds): Clinical Epidemiology: A Basic Science for Clinical Medicine, ed 2, p 52. Boston, Little, Brown & Co, 1991.

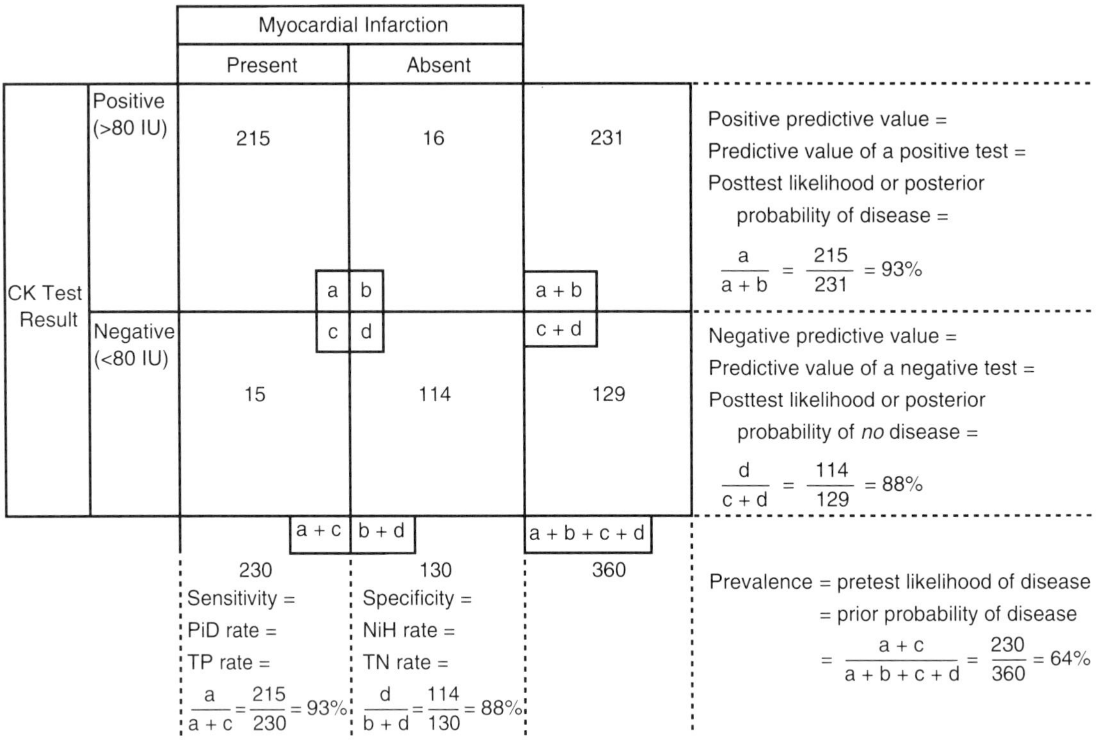

		Myocardial Infarction			
		Present	Absent		
CK Test Result	Positive (>80 IU)	215	16	231	Positive predictive value = Predictive value of a positive test = Posttest likelihood or posterior probability of disease = $\dfrac{a}{a+b} = \dfrac{215}{231} = 93\%$
		a | b	c+d | a+b		
	Negative (<80 IU)	15	114	129	Negative predictive value = Predictive value of a negative test = Posttest likelihood or posterior probability of *no* disease = $\dfrac{d}{c+d} = \dfrac{114}{129} = 88\%$
		a+c | b+d	a+b+c+d		
		230	130	360	Prevalence = pretest likelihood of disease = prior probability of disease $= \dfrac{a+c}{a+b+c+d} = \dfrac{230}{360} = 64\%$

Sensitivity = PiD rate = TP rate = $\dfrac{a}{a+c} = \dfrac{215}{230} = 93\%$

Specificity = NiH rate = TN rate = $\dfrac{d}{b+d} = \dfrac{114}{130} = 88\%$

FIGURE 11–28. The sensitivity, specificity, and predictive values of the creatine kinase (CK) test in myocardial infarction among patients admitted to the coronary care unit (positive in health [PiD], true positives [TP], negative in health [NiH], true negatives [TN]). (Redrawn from Sackett DL, Haynes RB, Guyatt GH, Tugwell P [eds]: Clinical Epidemiology: A Basic Science for Clinical Medicine, ed 2, p 87. Boston, Little, Brown & Co, 1991.)

and negative predictive values relate to the probability of a true diagnosis given a positive or negative test result.

REFERENCES

1. Monson JE, Stampfer MJ, Colditz GA, et al: A prospective study of aspirin use and primary prevention of cardiovascular disease in women. JAMA 266:521–527, 1991.
2. Easterbrook PJ, Berlin JA, Gopalan R, et al: Publication bias in clinical research. Lancet 337:867–872, 1991.
3. Cavanagh PR, Sims DS, Sanders LJ: Body mass is a poor predictor of peak plantar pressure in diabetic men. Diabetes Care 14:750–755, 1991.
4. Rinn EB, Giovannuchi EL, Willett WC, et al: Prospective study of alcohol consumption and risk of coronary disease in men. Lancet 338:464–468, 1991.

BIBLIOGRAPHY

Altman DG: Practical Statistics for Medical Research. London, Chapman and Hall, 1991.

Bailar JC III, Mosteller F (eds): Medical Uses of Statistics. Boston, New England Journal of Medicine Books, 1986.

Fletcher RH, Fletcher SW, Wagner EH: Clinical Epidemiology: The Essentials, ed 2. Baltimore, Williams & Wilkins, 1988.

Hennekens CH, Buring JE: In Mayrest SL (ed): Epidemiology in Medicine. Boston, Little, Brown & Co, 1987.

Last JM (ed): A Dictionary Of Epidemiology, ed 2. New York, Oxford University Press, 1988.

Riegelman RK, Hirsch RP: Studying a Study and Testing a Test: How to Read the Medical Literature, ed 2. Boston, Little, Brown & Co, 1989.

Sackett DL, Haynes RB, Guyatt GH, Tugwell P (eds): Clinical Epidemiology: A Basic Science for Clinical Medicine, ed 2. Boston, Little, Brown & Co, 1991.

PART TWO

Practice of Podiatric Primary Care

CHAPTER 12

TEACHING AND LEARNING CLINICAL PROBLEM SOLVING

Rodney Tomczak

By definition, podiatry is a primary medical practice,[1] in that it has the following features: its practitioners see patterns of illness that approximate the patterns of illness within the community; the illness has not been previously assessed by another physician; illnesses are frequently a complex mixture of physical, emotional, and social elements; diseases are often seen early, before the full clinical picture has developed; and the relationship of the podiatrist with patients is continuous and transcends individual episodes of illness. The special features of clinical problem solving and decision making are a direct result of these characteristics.

At some point in the educational process, the skills of problem solving and clinical decision making must be taught. Residents may graduate from a program quite adept at performing a base wedge osteotomy on a first metatarsal when the intermetatarsal angle is 18°. They assume they have solved the patient's problem, but actually they may have failed to take into account other physical, emotional, and social factors that caused a treatment failure and should have altered the choice of therapies. The problem may not be the increased intermetatarsal angle. Unless the podiatrist is taught the skills of clinical problem solving, he or she is functioning as a technician and merely treating symptoms. Podiatry has evolved into an art and science so complicated that practitioners can no longer follow simple algorithms for treatment without making a careful diagnosis and considering all the factors that may influence the illness, the patient, and the success of the treatment. It is precisely this change in perspective that will empower podiatry and place it soundly in the group of medical specialties designated as primary care.

MOTIVATION

Motivation has always been an issue for educators at all levels, giving rise to a number of educational theories.

In accordance with the *behaviorist theory* of

motivation,[2, 3] residents will be prepared to perform a base wedge osteotomy of the first metatarsal if they know they will actually be doing it the next day. The resident is motivated to complete the task of preparation by being promised the reward of performing the surgery.

Consistent with *social learning theory*,[4] the resident imitates every nuance of the residency director and often retains these characteristics after residency. Surgeons are products of their training.

Residents may also possess an inherent desire to maintain a sense of organization and balance in their conceptions of podiatry. New experiences must be assimilated into existing schemes. This is in line with the *cognitive theory* of motivation.[5] Finding an answer or mastering a skill is its own reward; motivation is intrinsic.

The cognitive theory of motivation does not always hold, especially in students. *Maslow's theory*[6] explains the differences between learners and their levels of motivation. Humans initially have lower, or deficiency, needs consisting of physiologic needs, safety needs, belongingness and love needs, and esteem needs. When these have been satisfied, a person will be motivated to satisfy growth or being needs, not because of deficit but because of a desire to gratify higher needs. These include a need for self-actualization, a desire to know and understand, and aesthetic needs. Unfortunately, the medical school experience often puts students into a survival mode in which they must be concerned with deficiency needs. This may also be the situation at times in some residency programs. There is no motivation to understand and become self-actualizing, but rather the motivation is to escape punishment.[3]

Barrows[7] postulates that the perceived relevance of work with real medical problems and the challenge of solving problems provide strong motivation for learning. By being initiated as residents and students into the intellectual culture of the profession, learners view the task of learning within a useful context that can be educationally humanistic and profitable. The motivation is to fulfill growth needs rather than survival needs.

INTRODUCTION TO LEARNING THEORIES

Learning is a change in behavior, or the ability to behave, that is the result of experience and not simply the result of maturation or fatigue. Behaviorists have focused on overt behavior while the cognitivists have emphasized the mind. An actual visible change in behavior is the essence of learning for the behaviorists. For the cognitivists, learning is a nonvisible change in the mental state, resulting in a potential behavior.

Pavlov, a behaviorist, was the first to describe classical conditioning.[2] Pavlov noticed that dogs with which he was experimenting began to salivate when meat powder was placed in their mouths. By repeatedly hearing a bell a few seconds before the meat powder was placed in their mouths, the animals became "conditioned" to the bell and would begin salivating when they heard the bell. Classical conditioning has been applied in the classroom in the form of contiguous association of a stimulus and a response that results in a change of behavior. Constant repetition is the avenue to classical conditioning; however, this can bring on negative affects and attitude problems.

Skinner expanded on these principles and originated operant conditioning, which emphasized the laws of effect and reinforcement. In short, behavior that is followed by positive reinforcement tends to be repeated. Forgetting, or extinction, according to Skinner, resulted from a lack of reinforcement or reinforcement of competing behaviors.

Skinner became interested in his daughter's education and was appalled by it. He believed that most students learned in order to avoid negative consequence such as punishment and embarrassment. It was impossible in a large class for the teacher to give frequent, immediate, positive reinforcement to all the students. As a consequence of this perception Skinner wrote *Technology of Teaching*.[3] The basic technique he recommended became known as programmed instruction, in which there are two basic considerations: (1) the gradual elaboration of extremely complex patterns of behavior and (2) the maintenance of the behavior in strength at each stage. The whole process of becoming competent in any field must be divided into a very large number of very small steps. These ideas have been recently expanded into linear (one path) and branched (multiple path) computer-assisted instruction. Forgetting, or extinction, according to Skinner results from a lack of reinforcement or reinforcement of competing behaviors.

The last of the behaviorists germane to this discussion is Bandura, who actually bridges the gap between the behaviorists and cognitivists. His *Social Learning Theory*[4] developed a schema describing observational learning, which consists of four phases. In the attention phase, certain models receive more attention than others. In the retention phase, vivid, concise, familiar symbols facilitate retention. The third phase is the reproduction phase, in which there is overt enactment and imitation facilitating learning. The last phase is reinforcement of the action, which may be direct, that is, from another person; vicarious, meaning it is anticipated; or from self, when a person strives to meet personal standards and does not depend on or care about the reactions of others.

To the behaviorist, learning is essentially passive and reactive, not active. Conditioning and social learning happen *to* a person. It is possible to differentiate this passive learning from the active mental processes called thinking or cognition, in which terms such as *insight, creativity,* and *problem solving* exist.

The gestalt view of education is an example of cognitive learning theory. The gestalt view calls attention to the fact that many things are learned when they are arranged into patterns. Impressions are not added together arithmetically, but rather relationships are perceived. Bigge was the first to base teaching techniques on gestalt principles.[5] He believed that instruction should be arranged so that there was active student participation and student insight while solving a problem. This could be accomplished in discussions involving the students and teacher if the teacher switched subject matter, introduced disturbing data, and permitted the students to make mistakes.

Piaget believed that humans possessed an innate tendency to make sense of their perceptions of the world. When a person cannot make sense, he or she is in a state of "disequilibrium" and must rectify this by developing stable conceptions of the world. These stable conceptions develop as humans incorporate (assimilate) experiences into their cognitive structure and modify (accommodate) their conceptions as they encounter new experiences.[8] In summary, students have a built-in desire to learn and make sense of what they observe and experience.

Bruner's conceptions of cognitive development were similar to Piaget's. Bruner's basic technique is often called the discovery approach.[9] He suggested that students grasp an overall pattern of what they are studying. By solving problems, the conceptions that students arrive at are more meaningful than those prepared and merely presented by others. When given a substantial amount of practice in finding solutions to problems, students not only develop problem-solving skills but also acquire confidence in their own learning abilities. They learn how to learn as they learn.

ORIGINS OF PROBLEM-BASED LEARNING

The behaviorists and cognitivists continue to disagree over basic concepts. The behaviorists stress learning, while the cognitivists emphasize techniques that allow teaching for intelligence. Hunt[10] and Sternberg[11] believe that intelligence really should be thought of as an analysis of cognitive and metacognitive skills rather than simply a correlation between scores on tests. Baron[12] thinks that a general theory of intelligence ought to say what it means to think intelligently. By thinking intelligently, a person can learn to manage his or her own limitations as if they were problems to overcome. Thinking then sits at the heart of intelligence, while teaching and learning of thinking skills essentially amounts to education that fosters intelligence.

Dewey[13] attempted to define a type of thinking he called reflective thinking. It involved a state of doubt or perplexity (a problem) and an active search of previous experiences and knowledge for materials that would resolve the problem. This is akin to Piaget's state of disequilibrium, the essential ingredient in his cognitive theory. Many persons, in an attempt to be relieved from this uneasy state of disequilibrium that they may regard as mental inferiority, assimilate the situation into well-rehearsed schemata and mindlessly bring to bear inappropriate knowledge and skills.[6]

The state of doubt must be sustained and

protracted and itself become a stimulus to inquiry. It is neither impulsive nor routine but enables one to act in a deliberate fashion. Dewey[13] listed five steps to accomplish this:

1. Suggestion of an initial action that is not carried out because of doubt
2. Intellectualization of the difficulty into a problem to be solved
3. Hypothesis formation to further guide reasoning
4. Mental elaboration of the idea
5. The testing of the hypothesis

These five steps are a form of hypothetical-deductive reasoning, problem-solving heuristics, or general strategy. Teaching to intelligence would then mean that it is reasoning that should be taught if one wishes to enhance students' cognitive skills.

The problem (which will now be recognized, some divergent thoughts offered, theories assimilated, and deductive conclusions reached in the finest sense of the problem-solving tradition) is that reasoning cannot in and of itself be taught. Thorndike[15] believed that there were no inferential rules but only highly domain-specific empiric rules dealing with concrete, specific types of events. In other words, the problem-solving process for quadratic equations is specific only to the domain of quadratic equations and of no value to any other domain. It is therefore, according to this theory, impossible to transfer the skill to anything else. Another view is that humans use abstract inferential rules but that these rules cannot be taught. Rather, these rules are induced by every person in the normal course of development and cannot be improved by instruction.[16]

The contraposition of the above theories was first voiced by Polya,[17] who argued that the formalities of mathematical proof and derivation had little to do with the real work of problem solving in mathematics. He discussed such heuristics as breaking problem solving into subproblems, solving simpler problems that actually reflected some aspect of the main problem, using diagrams to represent the problem in different ways, and examining special cases to get a feel for the problem.

A computer program developed in 1957 by Newell, Shaw, and Simon utilized a flexible heuristic that relied on "means-end analysis." This program worked by comparing a present state with a desired goal and seeking an operation that would bring the present state closer to the goal. It appeared that the problem-solving power lay in general principles. The knowledge of the specific domain in which the problem took place was not deemed to be important. It was just that the problem had to exist in *some* domain. The real ability to think was the important thing and not what one was thinking about.

The arguments against the teaching of general heuristics fall into three categories. These are (1) the argument from expertise, (2) the argument from weak methods, and (3) the argument from transfer.[18]

DeGroot[19] showed that the knowledge base of chess grandmasters was what separated them from the novice chess players. A novice who knew the rules of chess but who reasoned well in another domain did not have a chance of beating the master. The reason was that the masters could memorize at a glance the layouts of pieces on a chessboard if the pieces had gained their positions in the normal, logical course of a game. The novice could not do this. However, if the pieces were randomly placed on the board, the novices did as well as the masters in remembering the positions of the pieces. The conclusion was that the masters knew something powerful and specific to chess or they would have done well on the random layouts also.

According to Chase and Simon,[20] a master possesses about 50 thousand chess-specific configurations or schemata with which he thinks. A generalization of expertise began to develop and it entailed a large knowledge base of domain-specific patterns, rapid recognition of situations in which these patterns apply, and reasoning that moves from such recognition directly toward a solution. Novices did not see *patterns* but based their reasoning on superficial problem content and worked in reverse order rather than forward.[21] This would be analogous to interviewing a patient with an unknown condition, assuming the diagnosis was tarsal tunnel syndrome, then asking the patient if he or she had a symptom complex consisting of all the symptoms of tarsal tunnel syndrome and performing all the physical and laboratory tests for this syndrome. When the evidence gained did not fit the disease, the clinician would move to the next disease, perhaps a septic joint. Obviously, no logic is involved.

The argument from weak methods refers to the fact that when solving a problem in a new domain, a computer could use only weak methods that turned out weak results.[22] The result was that artificial intelligence researchers switched to developing expert powerful systems that were domain specific.

The argument from transfer was initiated by Thorndike,[15] who reached the conclusion that the degree of transfer from one domain to another was a function of the number of elements identical to the target domain and the trained domain. Therefore, teaching general context independent strategies has little value outside the domain in which they are taught. When transfer does occur, it must be cued, primed, and guided. It seldom occurs spontaneously.

These arguments are the strongest against teaching general heuristics or general problem-solving skills. Perkins and Salomon,[18] however, offer counter examples to refute these arguments from expertise, weak methods, and transfer.

Experts do not frequently solve problems in their specific domain. They usually recognize *patterns*. What may be a difficult diagnostic problem for a podiatric medical student could be a simple task of pattern recognition for the experienced podiatric practitioner. When an expert is faced, however, with an atypical problem in his or her domain, how is it solved? Johnson and colleagues[23] suggest that the expert resorts to analogies with systems he or she understands better, searches for potential misanalogies in the analogy, refers to intuitive mental models to understand how the target system works, investigates the target system with no preconceived limitations, and constructs simpler problems of the same sort. Experts are usually more than technicians limited by the known. Rather, they search for new problems to solve that advance the particular field.

Schoenfeld[24] did much to refute the argument from weak methods. Using general heuristics and metacognitive questions to monitor the progress of problem solving, he found that students were able to improve mathematical problem solving.

It has been shown that graduate students in psychology and medicine were able to show clear transfer of probabilistic and methodologic reasoning to everyday problems.[25] Transfer can occur if certain conditions are met. One type of transfer is called "low road" transfer and occurs when practice in a certain skill exists to such a high degree that it becomes automatic. The second method of transfer is called "high road" transfer and refers to the deliberate abstraction of principles. The learner actually takes a context-bound principle, decontextualizes it, and then synthesizes a new principle applicable to another domain.

It seems that rather than arguing for context-specific knowledge and against general heuristics (which would serve to foster rote memorization), or arguing for general heuristics and against context-specific knowledge (which falls to the three arguments), the podiatric medical teacher should seek a marriage of heuristics and the specific domain of podiatry.

The Psychological Origins of Medical Problem-Based Learning

In 1890, Chamberlin published a paper in *Science* entitled "The Method of Multiple Working Hypotheses."[26] This seemed to be the first mention of problem solving as a method of learning. Chamberlin thought that if the intellectual method used by the student in learning was the "ruling theory," then a certain intellectual affection would exist. Learning should be dominated by impartial intellectual rectitude. When this did not occur, the learner was buying into a paradigm of the teacher without questioning or being allowed to question.

When one worked with just one hypothesis, the inquiry that was made was done not for the sake of the hypothesis but for the sake of facts. Under the method of the "ruling theory," the stimulus was directed to the finding of facts for the support of the theory. Under the one-hypothesis theory, the facts were sought for the purpose of ultimate induction and demonstration, the hypothesis being but a means for the development of facts and their relations and for the arrangement and preservation of material for the final induction.

To guard against this, Chamberlin recommended the method of multiple working hypotheses. This method was directed against the most radical defect of the other two methods—intellectual parenting. By intellectual parenting, Chamberlin meant that once an idea or diagnosis was conceived it became part of the author, who tried everything to prove that idea or diagnosis correct. All objectivity was lost. By using the multiple working hypotheses method, one entertained every possible explanation of a phenomenon and developed every tenable hypothesis.

Chamberlin believed that education was largely a doctrine of what he called "pedagogical uniformitarianism," a synonym for "educational paradigm." Education according to Chamberlin should use the same multiple working hypotheses for teaching and learning that science should use for new discoveries.

Miller[27] reviewed much of what was known at that time about receiving, processing, and remembering information. He believed that there were severe limitations on the amount one could actually put into long-term memory at any one time and later recall. It appeared that no matter who performed the study or where it was done, most humans were limited to the magical number seven, plus or minus two bits of information.

Bruner, who was a colleague of Miller at Harvard University, thought that the major problem with the memory process was not the amount that could be stored, but rather it was the retrieval.[28] The key to retrieval was knowing where to find information and how to get there. Looked at from the retrieval side, the process of memory then became a process of problem solving. Material that was organized in terms of a person's own interests and cognitive structures was material that had the best chance of being accessible in memory. Therefore, the very activities that characterized "figuring out" or "discovering" things for oneself would seem to have the effect of making material more readily accessible in memory.

This ability to "figure out," or as Bruner

called it "learning the heuristics of discovery," probably occurred initially through the use of analogies. It was Bruner's hypothesis that only through the exercise of problem solving and the efforts of discovery and practice was one more likely to generalize what one had learned into a style of problem solving or inquiry that served for any task encountered. Bruner was not sure that the technique could actually be taught as such, but he was convinced that the only way to improve was to engage in the inquiry.

Katona[29] did not think that the learning and teaching of problem-solving skills were that much of an unknown. By stating higher-order rules along with the expected goal for the problem, the problems could be solved. More impressive, however, was the use of illustrations to stimulate the learners to discover the rules for themselves.

Gagne[30] summarized the conditions needed for effective problem solving to occur. They fell into two categories: (1) conditions within the learner and (2) conditions in the learning situation. The learner had to be able to call on his or her own previous experiences, specifically, previously learned rules. The learner also had to be able to use the cognitive strategies that were previously learned. These basically consisted of divergent thought, assimilation of theories, and deductive or convergent conclusions. The conditions in the learning situation consisted of verbal instructions that may be stimulated by the recall of relevant experiences. Initial guidance or channeling of thinking was important to inform the problem solver of the goal of the activity.

Problem solving as a method of learning then required that the learners discover certain higher-order rules without specific help. These higher-order rules could be effectively generalized to many situations and were highly resistant to forgetting.[31] The newly learned higher-order rules then became simpler rules to be used in the discovery of new higher-order rules.

TEACHING CLINICAL PROBLEM SOLVING

Knowles[32] coined the term *andragogy*. It refers to the teaching of adults, whereas *pedagogy* refers to the teaching of children. There are foundational and philosophical differences between the two concepts. As a person grows and matures, his or her self-concept moves from one of total dependency to one of increased self-directedness. Treating the learner as a child impedes the learning process. As a person matures he or she accumulates an expanding reservoir of experience that causes the learner to become an increasingly rich resource for learning. There is a decrease in teacher-centered information transmittal and an increasing emphasis on experiential learning. As persons mature, their readiness to learn increases. Children are conditioned to have a teacher- or subject-centered orientation to most learning experiences, whereas adults tend to have a problem- or learner-centered orientation to learning. The difference results from the child's perspective of postponed application. The adult, conversely, seeks out an educational setting or activity in large part because of some inadequacy in coping with current problems. The adult wants to apply "today" what is learned "today"—thus the perspective is one concerned with the immediacy of application. If this does not actually occur, it can at least occur vicariously through simulated patients, as in the case of a problem-based curriculum.

Practitioners, of course, must continue to learn. Perhaps the students should watch the faculty learn rather than watch them teach. It has been suggested that to ensure that learning to learn receives appropriate emphasis, the curriculum must include educational exercises designed specifically for that purpose.[33] There really are so many medical facts to learn that students cannot learn them all, and since the database is changing and expanding so rapidly, students must be prepared to learn on their own.

For students, medicine is a lot of problem solving. By solving a problem assigned by an instructor, the student learns to learn, and independent study is fostered. The learning is active, as opposed to the passive learning of the lecture, from which students can only process a few bits of information.[27] Even with a lot of information assimilated, students, when placed in a clinical situation where they have to use this information, cannot utilize higher-order thinking skills of the cognitive domain. Clinicians see students and residents with very high podiatry school grades in a clinical setting and are amazed at how little they appear to know. These students have been exposed to the academic content, and they have passed their examinations.

Well-structured problems that have specific objectives that are hidden from the student offer the opportunity to practice the heuristics needed for medical problem solving and at the same time allow for active learning and the opportunity for independent study in the specific domain of medicine. The major argument against problem-based medical education is that students will not be exposed to all the content. It is impossible to remember all the content of 4 years of podiatric medical school. The human mind simply cannot process all those facts into long-term memory.

Miller[34] showed that examinations in medical school rarely went beyond the comprehension level of Bloom's taxonomy. Even then, the concern should not be what the student has at the end of the course but rather what is kept and becomes part of the student for life. Miller asked sophomores, juniors, and seniors to retake the examinations they had passed as freshmen. No student passed gross anatomy, and only a few passed histology and physiology. Whether the student had come from the upper or lower quarter of the class made no difference. The members of the clinical faculty were asked to take the same examinations. A board-certified internist scored a 30% in biochemistry and an associate professor of surgery received a similar score in anatomy. Retention of classroom learning and subsequent transfer to a clinical situation seemed to be a significant problem.

Shortly after Miller's study, Barrows, a clinical neurologist in Canada, developed simulated neurology patients who were standardized so that faculty evaluations could provide more helpful data to the student.[35] It revealed that students had a paucity of basic knowledge that they could apply to patient problems. The findings seemed paradoxical since Barrows was closely associated with the preclinical curriculum and was sure that the students had been exposed to and passed courses in neuroanatomy, neurophysiology, and clinical neurology.

Many shared the feeling that students were coming to the clinical years ill prepared.[36] Some suggested an "inverted curriculum" in which students would have 2 years of patient exposure and then 2 years of basic science. Miller[37] also showed that the retention of basic science information decreased at the same rate as nonsense syllables. West[38] summarized the fallacies of the traditional approach to medical education and pointed out that logic and research proved that the traditional educational approach was ineffective and inefficient.

TEACHING FUTURE CLINICIANS TO SOLVE CLINICAL PROBLEMS

It must be remembered that for the neophyte practitioner, almost every patient presents with a significantly difficult problem that requires solving. A diabetic with troublesome calluses has a significant problem that needs solving; the diagnosis of calluses is not the problem; the problem is what needs to be done in light of the fact that the limb may be at risk. Diagnosing does not solve the problem. It is only an initial step. For example, if the reader is hiking through the woods on a warm summer day and almost steps on a 3-foot long, 2 inch in diameter, coiled, tubular animal that has exposed fangs and is making a rattling noise, merely making the diagnosis of "rattlesnake" does not solve the hiker's problem.

The actual behavior or clinical reasoning process used in problem solving contains the following steps and is summarized in Figure 12–1.[39] Initially, the student or practitioner confronts the patient, perceives cues, and assembles an initial mental picture of the problem. Multiple hypotheses are generated as possible explanations of the problem. Next an inquiry strategy is engaged that uses clinical skills to build a database with which the initial problem is refined. This refined problem formulation is then compared to the hypotheses generated. These hypotheses are retained, discarded, or enlarged to fit the revised problem. This process is continued until a particular hypothesis is deemed appropriate and decisions concerning management can be implemented.

There are three goals in clinical problem solving: (1) acquisition of retrievable and usable knowledge, (2) self-directed learning, and (3) acquisition of clinical reasoning skills. Within the context of a well-constructed problem, all these can be met. The first task in problem solving is to make the diagnosis; the second is to choose the appropriate treatment. On treating a patient, either the problem can be resolved or new problems arise from the treatment (i.e., complications) and a new problem surfaces.

It is important to realize that teaching and learning through clinical problem solving is not the same as the case method of learning. First, in the case method, made famous in law schools, the entire case is presented to the students and then discussed. In clinical problem solving, the student or resident must build the case just as the practitioner would do in the office. The clinical picture of the patient is presented to the problem-based learners just as the patient would or did present. In simulation format, students then proceed through the clinical reasoning process, history taking, and physical examination. The clinician serves as the patient, answering inquiries from the learners. The clinician may also switch roles to question the student.

The second difference between problem-based learning and the case study method concerns the questioning process. Brancati wrote an article in 1989 entitled "The Art of Pimping."[40] In it he states that it is always possible to ask questions dealing with arcane points of history, metaphysical "why" questions, exceedingly broad questions that cannot be answered, the origin of eponyms, and technical points of laboratory research. These types of questions often occur in the case study approach. The clinician, in problem-based learning, who is called a coach, facilitator, or tutor, should be asking "metacognitive questions."[41] These are questions such as, "Why do you need to know that about this patient?" "What do you mean by that?" "How do you know that is true?" "What does this lab result mean in light of your thoughts about this problem?"

The tutor functions as a coach who must *guide* the students through the clinical reasoning process. This is situated learning, and the student is being put into the culture of the profession. The method is a cognitive apprenticeship. The tutor models the behavior, and

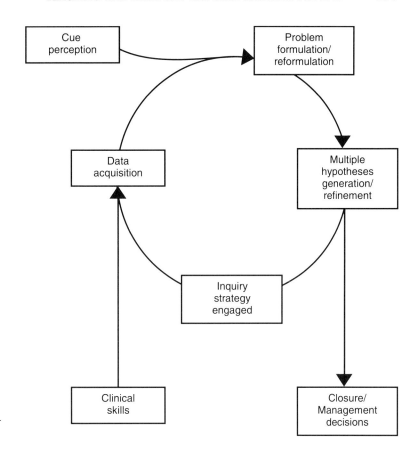

FIGURE 12–1. The clinical reasoning process.

according to Bandura[4] and the social learning theory, students will learn by what they see. In the beginning, the tutor builds a scaffold to support the learners where needed, then ideally fades out of the picture to return only when necessary.

The tutor should avoid expressing an opinion concerning the correctness of any decision. If the student chooses an action that results in the death of the patient, it is better that it occurs vicariously than in reality. The tutor should also refrain from answering academic questions. Usually problems are constructed so that certain objectives or learning issues will be encountered. When the group does not know the answer to a question or cannot identify a term, these become group learning issues and must be researched.

Clinical problem solving is a group process. The group should reach a consensus through discussion and research. The tutor must facilitate this through whatever means necessary. It is important that all the participants become involved so that no one either is silent or assumes the role of lecturer. The tutor must also

ensure that the students do not go too far down a blind alley. This can be done through the use of metacognitive questions such as "What are you thinking about now?" "What are you expecting to see with what you already know about this patient?" This skillful redirecting will ensure that all objectives of the problem will be satisfied.

When students leave the group meeting, they must research the learning issues that have been encountered. Tutors must be sure that students know how to use resources efficiently. To assume that they already have acquired this skill is not wise. The quality of material to be read for the next meeting must also be assessed. For the most part, textbooks are not a primary source of knowledge but generally a review of the literature. As a result, the use of textbooks is discouraged and students are asked to bring original articles to group meetings. These articles are also critiqued, especially concerning such validity issues as maturation, regression, random selection, mortality, instrumentation, testing, history, and generalizability. In this manner, students learn to recognize good research from less stringently prepared articles. It is not uncommon for students to spend 4 hours a day reading.

To illustrate the process, a problem outside of the realm of podiatry is offered. In this way, the reader can experience Piaget's[8] disequilibrium, which is felt by podiatry students trying to solve a podiatry problem.

Assume you are a general practitioner in rural Iowa. A 73-year-old farmer is brought to your office by his 43-year-old son. The farmer has a large bruise on the left side of his face. The son says he came to the farm today and found this on his father. The older gentleman says it happened yesterday. He was in the barn pitching hay yesterday morning. The next thing he knew he was waking up on the floor and the side of his face was sore. The bruise began to develop yesterday afternoon. Solve the problem!

Students and clinicians alike have been conditioned in the traditions of both Pavlov[2] and Skinner[3] to have immediate ideas about what could be ailing this patient. First, the problem solver makes a list of ideas or possible causes. For this patient the list may include, but not be limited to, diabetes mellitus, hypoglycemia, brain tumor, arrhythmia, myocardial infarction, transient ischemic attack, orthostatic hypotension, epilepsy, chemical intoxication, or a lie (the father may not have fallen, but was struck by the son—elder abuse). These ideas are listed on the blackboard by a student under a column headed ''Ideas.'' This list may be modified at any time during the process. The ideas listed involve numerous organ systems, forcing the student to view the patient and the problem as a whole, in a fashion similar to that used by the ''gestalt'' theorists.[5]

The next step is to employ the problem-solving hypotheses of Bruner[9] and Dewey[13] and begin the problem-solving sequence. Having had some divergent thoughts that have resulted in a list of ideas, the learner must somehow exclude certain ideas or include one or more into a final diagnosis. This is initially done by history and physical examination. It is important that the novice clinician follow an established protocol for gleaning this information. It is inappropriate to ask for a computed tomographic scan of the skull, even if the student knows it may rule out or rule in a brain tumor. The students must be conditioned[2, 3] to ask for a complete history and perform a complete physical examination.

In the course of history taking and the physical examination, it is important that the coach not respond to inquiries with ''normal,'' ''within normal limits,'' or ''negative.'' The coach should respond with what the examiner would actually see, hear, palpate, smell, or read, in the case of radiographs or laboratory results. When possible, the actual radiographs or laboratory slips should be given to the group if that particular examination is requested. Care is also taken to ensure that students know how to perform the elements of a complete physical examination and that the results can be properly interpreted. The mechanics of heart auscultation are simple to perform, and in the majority of cases a response of S_3, S_4, no murmurs, no gallops, no rubs will be true, but the student must be able to identify these abnormal sounds when they occur. Again, by judicious questioning, competency in identifying and interpreting heart sounds can be ensured. After a few problems have been solved, the time allotted to determining expertise in these areas can be shortened and new learning issues can be encountered.

On completion of the history and physical examination, the students should continue to gather more data through alternative forms of examination. These may include, but are not limited to, radiographs, blood studies, urinalysis, cerebrospinal fluid analysis, electromyography, electrocardiography, or electroencephalography. It is important to bear in mind that if a student asks for a test, a positive or negative result must have some influence on the diagnostic process. After a definitive diagnosis has been achieved, if additional tests are requested, they can only be justified if a positive result will result in an alternative treatment choice. When test results are handed to the students, this will ordinarily signal new learning issues of such consequence that it is impossible to proceed further with the problem until these issues have been researched and interpreted. At this point, the group adjourns and the next meeting time is set. This should occur in 24 to 48 hours, depending on the complexity and number of the learning issues. Before meeting with the tutor, students normally meet by themselves to discuss results and interpretations. Resources may include anything or anyone except the tutor. Resources are, of course, critiqued at the next meeting.

Returning to the farmer, it has been discovered that he has not been to a physician in 12 years. At that time, his physician told him he had high blood pressure and gave him some pills. He finished those pills as he was told, but the doctor died soon afterward and he had not seen another physician since. About a year ago he was ill for 5 days. He was doing heavy manual work on the farm and his chest began to hurt. It really "knocked him for a loop" and he spent the next 5 days in bed because his chest hurt so much. Since that time, he has passed out twice, once 2 weeks ago and yesterday. When being questioned, the father seems concerned that the son wants to put him in a "rest home" and take over the farm.

The physical examination (it would be impossible to list all normal and abnormal findings of the physical examination for the reader at this time; it is assumed that the experienced clinician reader is familiar with normal findings) reveals a holosystolic precordial pulsation at the cardiac apex and an S_4 gallop rhythm when the heart is auscultated. At this point the significance of these findings is discussed and learning issues derived. If appropriate, the group can continue with suitable laboratory tests. In an attempt to re-create life situations, should a student wish a computed tomographic scan, the student is informed that it would take a day to schedule it at the hospital and no results are readily available. In the case of a magnetic resonance image, the patient would have to go to the closest city where this clinical examination can be performed. A test that is both available to the patient while in the physician's office and also relevant is an electrocardiogram. When this is requested, the students are handed a 12-lead electrocardiogram, which should take some time to interpret. Students will find significant ST-segment elevation on the precordial leads as the only abnormality. They would be expected to return to the next group meeting knowing the significance of this finding. The results of any other tests that might be done in the office, such as electrolytes, glucose level, and urinalysis, can be given to the student if the student can justify that particular test.

After the assimilation of pertinent data, the clinician must guide the students through focused convergent thought that will result in a precise theory of illness accounting for all signs and symptoms of the disease and stating concise pathophysiologic reasons. At this point in the problem-solving sequence, metacognitive questions are essential to evaluate the higher-order thinking skills of the students.[25, 29, 38] If there is no evidence that there is hypothetical-deductive reasoning based on facts revealed during the history and physical examination, on other examinations, and on tests that are grounded in sound physiologic principles, the synthesis and evaluations levels of Bloom's[42] taxonomy of the cognitive domain cannot be reached.

For this patient, the syncopal episodes are consistent with ventricular tachycardia secondary to a ventricular aneurysm caused by a myocardial infarction. The causes of syncopal episodes should have been explored. Auscultation of the heart revealed abnormalities consistent with aneurysm, and prolonged ST-segment elevation on the electrocardiogram can be found with ventricular aneurysm secondary to myocardial infarction, which in this case might have been the 5-day episode of chest pain a year ago that left the farmer in bed. If students have a strong suspicion that this patient really has a ventricular aneurysm, it needs to be determined if this a real emergency, if there is a likelihood that the aneurysm could rupture, and what is the standard test that should be used to confirm the diagnosis.

Confirmation of the diagnosis of ventricular aneurysm is analogous to discovering the rattlesnake in the woods. Students must still decide if anything needs to be done, and if so what it should be. In this case, the aneurysm is sufficiently large to warrant surgery rather than treating symptomatology medically. Discussion of the surgical procedure of choice should ensue, and at this point the problem might end, or complications such as an infection or a postoperative arrhythmia might be discovered. These may be a continuation of the same problem or the source of a new problem. The results of the treatment must be evaluated in light of what effect it had on the patient. Should the students pick an incorrect treatment, the coach does not intervene to tell the students that the choice is inappropriate but rather informs the students of the results, and the success of that treatment choice is evaluated.

Students are tested over the problems encountered at the end of a rotation by completing an essay examination that requires higher-order thinking skills rather than by a multiple choice examination that stresses recognition of terms.

CONSTRUCTING PROBLEMS FOR CLINICAL PROBLEM SOLVING

There are four basic criteria that should be applied to the construction of problems[43]:

1. A problem should match the students' level of knowledge. There are differences between problems presented to a student in the first year of a podiatry school that uses complete problem-based learning, a problem presented to a third-year student at a podiatry school that uses problem-based learning for the clinical sciences, and a problem presented to a resident.

2. A problem should motivate students for further study activities. It is important that students and residents grasp the applicability of the problem to their future practice of podiatry.

3. A problem should be suitable for the process of analysis to be applied. The problems must be formulated so that they are open enough to sustain discussion about possible solutions.

4. A problem should direct the students inevitably to confrontation with the predetermined objectives.

Problems are constructed to fill a need. To teach the clinical sciences in a podiatry school, problems can be constructed to meet the needs (objectives) set forth in the *Terminal Objectives and Competency Task Index for Podiatric Medicine*,[44] also called the CELE document after the Committee for Entry Level Expectations for Podiatric Medicine. In a residency program, problems can be constructed to fill a deficit in a program. A patient with severe osteoarthritis of the ankle requiring fusion is not

seen by every resident during a residency experience. This deficit can be overcome by finding radiographs of a patient with the condition and constructing a problem around the condition seen on the radiographs. Teaching files are radiographs of real persons who have had this condition. All that remains is for the residency director, clinician, or chief resident either to find the history and physical examination for this patient or to construct a history and physical examination that is consistent with the diagnosis. In this case, the problem constructor, after defining objectives, works inductively[21] rather than deductively as a problem solver would. There are certain variations on this theme. Should the diagnosis of the problem lie heavily on especially esoteric information discovered in the course of a physical examination, simulated patients may be used.[45] Simulated patients are persons without a disease who are taught to act as if they have a certain problem and are instructed in the appropriate answers in the history that would be consistent with the condition. A simple example would be a patient who presents with sudden onset of shortness of breath. This is a patient with a spontaneous unilateral pneumothorax. When the lungs are auscultated on the unaffected side, the simulated patient breathes normally. When the affected side is auscultated, the simulated patient lifts the chest just as one does with deep inspiration but does not breathe in any air.

An ankle fusion could also be performed on a cadaver or plastic bones. Postoperative radiographs can be taken when appropriate and critiqued. If postoperative radiographs exist from the original case, they can be reviewed when consent of the surgeon is acquired or when anonymity can be preserved. The problem-solving process is limited only by the person creating the educational experience. It is important, however, to issue a caveat concerning problem construction. Creation of problems within a residency program or institution should not evolve into a "look how smart I am for making this incredible diagnosis and performing this almost impossible surgery" contest. Problem-based learning is student centered, while this "contest" is both teacher centered and self-serving.

Another option is to employ the use of videotapes in actual patient encounters. After consent from the patient is given, the initial encounter between student/resident and patient is videotaped. This tape is then reviewed by both clinician and student/resident to determine not only proficiency but also efficiency in the problem-solving sequence. If the clinician is present in the examining room, it is only human nature to interrupt the learner at the first perception of an incorrect action. If assets permit, examining rooms can be constructed with one-way windows so that simulated patients may be examined by learners in a situation approximating reality while being observed by classmates and clinicians.

SUMMARY

Problem-based learning is used in some form in the majority of American and Canadian medical schools. It does not appear to be a passing pedagogic fantasy but is obviously founded in solid educational and cognitive psychological principles. Recent publications have shown that problem-based learning does not result in any improvement in general, content-free problem-solving skills; that learning in a problem-based format may initially reduce levels of learning but may foster, over periods of years, increased retention of knowledge; that some evidence suggests that problem-based curricula may enhance both transfer of concepts to new problems and integration of basic science concepts into clinical problems; that problem-based learning enhances intrinsic interest in the subject matter; and that problem-based learning appears to enhance self-directed learning skills, which may be maintained.[46]

REFERENCES

1. McWhinney IR: Problem-solving and decision-making in primary medical practice. Proc R Soc Med 65:34–38, 1972.
2. Pavlov IP: Conditioned Reflexes. New York, Oxford University Press, 1927.
3. Skinner BF: Technology of Teaching. New York, Appleton-Century-Crofts, 1968.
4. Bandura A: Social Learning Theory. Englewood Cliffs, NJ, Prentice-Hall, 1977.
5. Bigge ML: Learning Theories for Teachers, ed 4. New York, Harper & Row, 1982.
6. Maslow AH: A theory of human motivation. Psychol Rev 50:370–396, 1943.
7. Barrows HS: A taxonomy of problem-based learning methods. Med Educ 20:481–486, 1986.
8. Piaget J: The Origins of Intelligence in Children. New York, International University Press, 1952.
9. Bruner JS: Toward a Theory of Instruction. New York, WW Norton, 1966.
10. Hunt E: Mechanics of verbal ability. Psychol Rev 85:271–283, 1978.
11. Sternberg RJ: The nature of mental abilities. Am Psychol 38:214–230, 1979.
12. Baron J: Reflective thinking as a goal of education. Intelligence 5:291–309, 1981.
13. Dewey J: How We Think: A Restatement of the Relation of Reflective Thinking to the Education Process. Boston, DC Heath, 1933.
14. Langer E: Mindfulness. Reading, MA, Addison-Wesley, 1989.
15. Thorndike E: The Psychology of Learning, New York, Mason-Henry, 1913.
16. Nisbett RE, Fong GT, Lehman DR, Cheng PW: Teaching reasoning. Science 238:625–631, 1987.
17. Polya G: How to Solve It: A New Aspect of Mathematical Method, ed 2. Garden City, NY, Doubleday, 1957.
18. Perkins DN, Salomon G: Are cognitive skills context-bound. Educ Res 18:16–25, 1989.
19. DeGroot AD: Thought and Choice in Chess. The Hague, Mouton, 1965.
20. Chase WC, Simon HA: Perceptions in chess. Cogn Psychol 4:55–81, 1983.
21. Rabinowitz M, Glaser R: Cognitive structure and process in highly competent performance. In Horowitz FD, O'Brien M. (eds): The Gifted and Talented: Developmental Perspectives, pp 75–98. Washington, DC, American Psychological Association, 1985.
22. Rich E: Artificial Intelligence. New York, McGraw-Hill Book Company, 1983.
23. Johnson PE, Ahlgren A, Blount JP, Petit NJ: Scientific reasoning: Garden paths and blind alleys. In Robins J (ed): Research in Science Education: New Questions, New Directions. Colorado Springs, CO, Biological Sciences Curriculum Study, 1980.
24. Schoenfeld AH: Mathematical Problem Solving. New York, Academic Press, 1985.
25. Lehman DR, Tempert RO, Nissbett RE: The effects of graduate training on reasoning: Formal discipline and thinking about everyday life problems. Am Psychol 43:431–442, 1988.
26. Chamberlin TC: The method of multiple working hypotheses. Science 15:92–97, 1890.
27. Miller GA: The magical number seven, plus or minus two: Some limits on our capacity for processing information. Psychol Rev 63:81–97, 1956.
28. Bruner JS: The act of discovery. Harvard Educ Rev 31(1):21–32, 1961.
29. Katona G: Organizing and Memorizing. New York, Columbia University Press, 1940.
30. Gagne RM: The Conditions of Learning. New York, Holt, Rinehart & Winston, 1977.
31. Worthen BR: Discovery and expository task presentation in elementary mathematics. J Educ Psychol Monogr Suppl 59 (No. 1, part 2), 1968.
32. Knowles MS: The Adult Learner: A Neglected Species. Houston, Gulf Publishing, 1973.
33. West KM: The role of the library in learning to learn clinical medicine. J Med Educ 39:910–917, 1964.
34. Miller GE: An inquiry into medical teaching. J Med Educ 37:185–191, 1962.
35. Barrows HS, Abrahamson S: The programmed patient: A technique for appraising student performance in clinical neurology. J Med Educ 39:802–805, 1964.

36. Barrows HS, Tamblyn RM: Problem-Based Learning: An Approach to Medical Education. New York, Springer, 1980.

37. Miller GE: The contributions of research in the learning process. Med Educ 12:28, 1978.

38. West KM: The case against teaching. J Med Educ 41:766–771, 1966.

39. Coulson RC: Problem-based student-centered learning of the cardiovascular system using the problem-based learning module (P.B.L.M.). Physiologist 26:220–224, 1983.

40. Brancati FL: The art of pimping. JAMA 262:89–90, 1989.

41. Barrows HS: The Tutorial Process. Springfield, IL, Southern Illinois University School of Medicine, 1988.

42. Bloom BS: Taxonomy of Educational Objectives: Handbook I: Cognitive Domain. New York, McKay, 1956.

43. Major GD, Schmidt HG, Snellen-Balendong HA, et al: Construction of problems for problem-based learning. In Nooman ZM, Schmidt HG, Ezzat ES (eds): Innovations in Medical Education: An Evaluation of its Present Status. New York, Springer, 1990.

44. Burnham S (chairman): Terminal Objectives and Competency Task Index for Podiatric Medicine. Washington, DC, American Association of Colleges of Podiatric Medicine, 1984.

45. Barrows HS: Simulated Patients. Springfield, IL, Charles C Thomas, 1971.

46. Norman RN, Schmidt HG: The psychological basis of problem-based learning: A review of the evidence. Acad Med 67:557–565, 1992.

CHAPTER 13

PALLIATIVE CARE

Steven L. Friedman

NAIL CARE

Debridement of Normal Nails

Normal nails are those that are not thickened, deformed, or discolored. A patient may seek a podiatrist's help with debriding these nails because of a physical inability to reach the toes or a medical condition such as diabetes or peripheral vascular disease that requires professional care. The instruments necessary to debride these nails are a nail nipper of the practitioner's choice, a nail curette, and a nail rasp or power rasp (Fig. 13–1).

The free edge of the nail extending from the hyponychium should be reduced as much as the patient can tolerate. The nail should be shaped to the contour of the distal aspect of the digit. It is not necessary to debride down into the corners of the nail unless the patient is experiencing discomfort in this area. Patients should be counseled to cut their own nails straight across, to file the edges to follow the contour of the toe, and never to cut into the corners.

When debriding normal nails, the practitioner should grasp the nail nipper comfortably. The opposite hand should be used to grasp the patient's toe, placing the thumb under the nail on the distal end of the toe (Fig. 13–2A). The distal end of the toe should be pulled down to free the hyponychium from the free edge of the nail. The lower jaw of the nail nipper is placed between the hyponychium and the nail, and the thumb is then moved over to cover the jaws of the nail nipper (Fig. 13–2B). This is to protect the eyes and face from nail fragments that can fly off the nail nipper at high velocity. The nail is then cut, using as many cuts as are necessary to cut across the nail plate.

The nail folds of the hallux nails should then be curetted to remove any debris. A double-ended nail curette can be used, utilizing the size of curette that the nail fold will accommodate. The curette is a cutting instrument and should be used with care. The open end

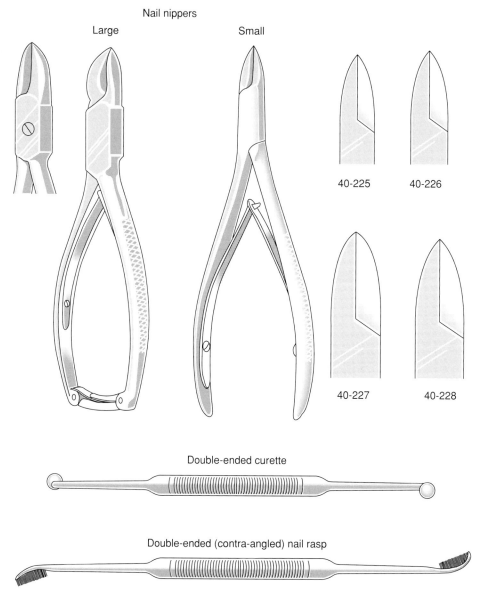

FIGURE 13–1. Instruments used for nail debridement: small and large nail nippers, curette, and nail rasp.

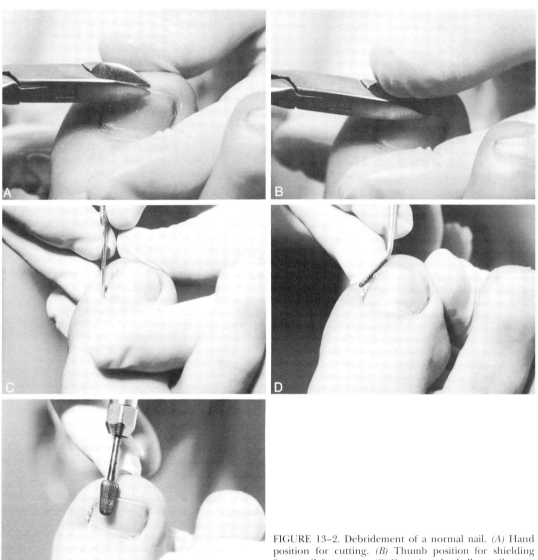

FIGURE 13–2. Debridement of a normal nail. *(A)* Hand position for cutting. *(B)* Thumb position for shielding from nail fragments. *(C)* Curetting the hallux nail to remove debris. *(D)* Hand rasp position. *(E)* Power rasp position.

or cutting edge of the curette should be placed against the nail and pulled distally (Fig. 13–2C). All loose debris should be removed from the nail grooves. The cut ends of the nail plate have sharp edges and should be smoothed. This can be accomplished with a hand nail rasp or a power nail rasp or moto-tool (Fig. 13–2D and E). The choice of rasp or bur is left up to the practitioner.

Debridement of Deformed or Mycotic Nails

Trauma or other disturbance to the nail matrix may cause the nail to become extremely hard and may require a great deal of force to cut the nail. It is best to cut these nails with a large (either curved or straight) nail nipper. Those who do not have sufficient strength in their hands to cut large sections of nails may find it easier to use only the tips of the nippers and cut small sections at a time (Fig. 13–3A). These nails frequently will crack down the nail plate past the tips of the nail nipper. Care must be taken when cutting the corners of the nail plate not to crack the nail too far down into the nail folds. This will be very uncomfortable for the patient. A power rasp should be used to reduce the thickness of the nails as well as to smooth the rough cut edges (see Fig. 13–2E).

Mycotic toenails are generally thickened, deformed, discolored, and sometimes crumbling. Debris collects under the nails, lifting them up off the nail bed. It is sometimes difficult to distinguish the mycotic debris from the nail bed. The nail plate will conform to the shape of the underlying nail bed, and often the nail bed and nail plate will be peaked owing to an underlying bony deformity or shoe pressure.

The nail plate should be cut in sections corresponding to the sides of the "peak." The edge of the nail nipper should be placed under the edge of the nail plate, between the mycotic debris and the nail plate if possible.

Most mycotic nail plates are brittle but not hard, and some are soft and crumbling. Mycotic nails generally become thickened and do not grow out over the distal end of the toe as do normal nails. When not debrided regularly, mycotic nails will grow dorsally, resembling a horn.

Instruments for debridement of mycotic toenails include a small or large nail nipper, depending on the thickness of the nail and the preference of the practitioner; a nail curette; and a power rasp. Mildly thickened or soft and crumbling nails can usually be debrided using a small nail nipper. The normal contour and shape of the nail should be followed when debriding. Cutting straight across should be avoided, particularly if the nail plate is deformed, since this may trap the soft tissue of the nail bed in the jaws of the nipper, causing discomfort for the patient. The division of the nail bed from the nail plate should be identified when possible. The shape of many mycotic toenails and the debris that collects subungually make it difficult to distinguish the nail

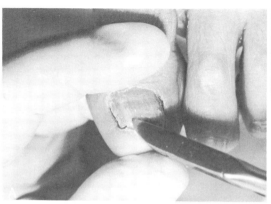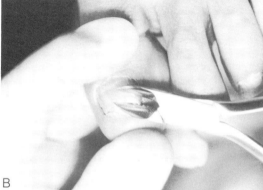

B

FIGURE 13–3. Methods for debridement of a deformed nail. *(A)* If the nail is too hard to cut in one piece, one may "bite" the nail into smaller sections for cutting. *(B)* Severely thickened mycotic toenails should be reduced in thickness as much as possible before grinding by using a large nail nipper held at a 45° angle.

plate from the nail bed. When these types of nails are debrided, small sections are cut at a time until the nail bed can be identified. Watching the patient's face when closing the jaws of the nail nipper may give a clue as to whether the nail bed has been trapped. Small nicks to the nail bed may be unavoidable on some nails and should be treated properly with hemostatic and/or antibiotic medication.

Severely thickened mycotic toenails should be debrided using a large nail nipper either with straight or curved jaws. The shape of the jaws of the nail nipper to be used depends on the personal preference of the practitioner. When a nipper with curved jaws is used, care must be taken to be aware of the position of the tips of the nipper at all times. When debriding with a curved-jaw nail nipper it is easy to be concentrating on the central position of the jaws and forget the position of the tips of the nippers. The tips of the nippers are lower than the central portion of the jaws and may inadvertently lacerate soft tissue.

As much of the diseased nail plate as possible should be reduced before grinding with the power rasp. A goal should be to create as little nail dust by grinding as possible. A thickened and deformed nail plate can be reduced in thickness by holding the nail nipper at an approximately 45° angle to the nail plate (Fig. 13–3B). Pressure is applied downward while closing the jaws of the nail nipper. The nipper may slip off the nail plate if the plate is extremely hard. Several attempts should be made to cut the nail in this manner. The tips of the nipper may be used to "bite" into the nail plate by digging them into the nail plate. At this point the thickened nail plate may crack almost in layers or may be cut across in layers. Care must be taken not to cut into the nail bed under the nail plate. Debriding the thickened nail plate at an approximate 45° angle reduces the length and thickness of the nail.

Once the nail plate has been reduced with the nail nipper, the power rasp is used to smooth and further reduce the thickness. There are several attachments for the power rasp to accomplish this, including a sanding disk, cross-cut burs, and diamond burs of several shapes. The disk or bur attachment on the power rasp must not be allowed to remain in one position on the nail plate for an extended period of time. The attachment will build up heat and may burn the nail bed or nail plate if it is not moved rapidly across the nail plate.

Removing mycotic debris from beneath the nail plate after debriding and rasping the nail may loosen the remaining nail plate, necessitating further debridement. A painful condition may be created owing to exposure of an excessive amount of nail bed to trauma from shoes if too much nail plate is removed.

Onychocryptosis

Onychocryptosis, or ingrown toenail, is one of the most common conditions that a podiatrist sees. The nail plate may be curved into the skin of the nail fold, or the tissue of the nail fold may be hypertrophied.

Shoe pressure plays a major role in the formation of onychocryptosis. The outside pressure forces the soft tissue into the nail plate, creating discomfort. If the nail plate punctures the skin of the nail fold, an infection may result. A normal-appearing nail plate may cause discomfort from outside pressure.

Onychocryptosis generally presents as pain in one or both of the hallux nail borders, but it may also occur in the lesser digits. The pain may be at the distal aspect of the nail plate or more proximally toward the eponychium.

The instruments needed to treat onychocryptosis are a small nail nipper, preferably with narrow jaws, a No. 61 or 62 blade on a long or short handle, and a nail curette. The discomfort is generally at the distal one third of the nail edge. The impinging nail edge should be removed in a large enough section to render relief. This can generally be accomplished by angling the nail nipper toward the nail fold and cutting out a small section (Fig. 13–4A). This section should be triangular and extend from the distal nail edge to approximately one third down the nail fold (Fig. 13–4B). The nail should be cut completely through to the nail fold so as not to leave a sharp hook, which may cause future problems. If the nail fold continues to be painful, the nail plate may need to be cut farther down the nail edge. This can be accomplished with a straight nail splitter blade such as a No. 61 or 62 blade on a handle (Fig. 13–4C). The initial

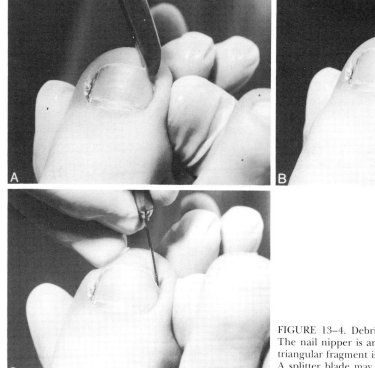

FIGURE 13–4. Debridement of an ingrown toenail. *(A)* The nail nipper is angled toward the nail fold and *(B)* a triangular fragment is cut completely to the nail fold. *(C)* A splitter blade may be needed to cut farther down the nail edge.

cut is carried farther down the nail fold at a similar angle with the blade, taking care not to leave a hooked nail. The nail curette is used to remove any debris in the nail fold and to probe the nail fold, checking for remaining nail spicules. These rough or partially cut areas may be removed using the cutting edge of the nail curette pulled from proximal to distal.

When this condition becomes chronic, permanent surgical removal of the offending nail border should be considered.

Onychia and Paronychia

Onychia is an inflammation of the nail bed caused by infection. The infection is generally bacterial and may or may not be accompanied by a purulent exudate. The usual signs of infection are erythema, edema, and, at times, increased local temperature. There is generally a halo of white or yellow tissue surrounding the eponychium representing the purulent drainage collecting at this point.

Treatment of this condition consists of incision and drainage of the infection, which re-

quires removal of the entire nail plate. The infection and purulent drainage becomes trapped under the nail plate and can spread to underlying and surrounding tissue if the nail plate is not removed. Topical antibiotics and soaks in an astringent solution are all that are usually necessary after removing the nail plate. Soaks should not be prescribed for patients with diabetes or peripheral arterial disease or when any neuropathy is present. Oral antibiotics may be necessary for those patients with impaired immune response or in any situation the practitioner deems appropriate.

Paronychia is an inflammation of one or both nail folds usually caused by infection. Onychocryptosis may also cause paronychia. The signs of inflammation or infection are erythema, edema, and possible increase in local temperature. Often the nail folds will be hypertrophied when the inflammation or infection has been chronic or recurring.

The source of the infection at the nail fold is puncture of the skin of the nail fold by the edge of the nail plate. Once the skin has been punctured it is susceptible to infection. Puncture of the skin by the nail edge may occur owing to outside pressure forcing the nail fold into the nail edge or by improper trimming of the nails. When the corner of the nail is cut back incompletely, a "hook" of nail grows out as the nail plate grows and punctures the skin at the distal nail fold. Purulent drainage may be seen at the distal nail fold, and at times a white or yellow area may be seen at the distal nail fold. This area is an abscess caused by the nail plate puncturing the skin at this point.

Treatment of paronychia consists of removal of the offending nail edge to incise and drain any infection. The distal abscess must be incised and drained, with debridement of all affected tissue. When the infection is localized to the distal nail fold, the nail plate may be cut with a technique similar to that used for onychocryptosis, without anesthesia. When the infection affects more than the distal one third of the nail fold, the entire nail edge must be removed. This requires anesthesia of the digit, using a local anesthetic injected at the base of the digit. A greater amount of anesthetic may be necessary when dealing with a chronic or severe infection owing to pH changes to the local tissues. Topical antibiotics and astringent soaks are all that are generally necessary once the offending nail edge has been removed. Remember that foot soaks are contraindicated in patients with insensitive feet. Again, oral antibiotics are necessary in patients with impaired immune response or in any situation the practitioner deems appropriate.

Onychophosis

Onychophosis, or calloused nail grooves, is a very painful condition that may accompany onychocryptosis. The chronic impingement of the nail edge on the nail fold creates hyperkeratotic tissue in the nail fold of some patients. This condition is recognized by the extreme pain felt by the patient and by the presence of yellow hard hyperkeratotic tissue in the nail fold.

Treatment of onychophosis consists of removal of the offending nail edge and reduction of the hyperkeratotic tissue. The hard tissue in the nail fold should be removed by debridement with a sharp blade and not a nail curette (Fig. 13–5). Debriding this tissue with

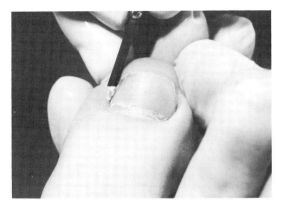

FIGURE 13–5. Debridement of a calloused nail groove.

a curette causes discomfort and is usually ineffective. The hyperkeratotic tissue in the nail fold may be treated with a softening agent (e.g., 3WEA, Amphil, or potassium hydroxide) to aid in debridement.

When a patient is extremely sensitive, debridement may not be possible. A dressing of salicylic acid may be packed into the nail groove with cotton for 3 to 5 days. When this dressing is removed, the hyperkeratotic tissue may be easily removed with a curette or sharp blade. Chronic onychophosis may require permanent removal of the nail edge.

Subungual Exostosis

Subungual exostosis is a growth of bone on the dorsal distal aspect of the distal phalanx. This exostosis may cause the nail plate to become deformed and rounded or "peaked" dorsally. The nail deformity may create onychocryptosis at one or both nail folds and may be painful to direct pressure on the nail plate.

Conservative treatment consists of reduction of the nail edges and of the thickness of the nail plate with the power rasp. Padding such as a tube foam shield placed on the digit or padding of the shoe may provide relief. Failure of the conservative treatment may necessitate permanent removal of the complete nail plate. The exostosis should be resected when extremely large or when it causes discomfort after the nail plate has been removed. Severely deformed and "peaked" nail plates should not be treated with permanent removal of the nail edges only. The remaining nail plate is deformed and may create future difficulty. The entire nail plate should be removed.

HYPERKERATOTIC DIGITAL LESIONS

Heloma Durum

Hyperkeratotic tissue forms in response to excessive friction and pressure on the skin. The skin forms this hard tissue to protect against the outside friction and pressure. When the friction and pressure continues, the skin continues to manufacture the hyperkeratotic tissue to the point where the thickness causes pain.

Heloma durum is a hyperkeratotic lesion on the dorsal aspect of a digit. Heloma durum

means "hard corn" and is generally located at the dorsal aspect of the distal or proximal interphalangeal joint. The digit is usually contracted with one or both interphalangeal joints prominent dorsally and subject to excessive friction and pressure from shoes. The hyperkeratotic lesion has distinct borders and covers the prominent skin over the head of the proximal or distal phalanx. A deep-seated "core" may be noticed within the lesion, usually corresponding to the area of most friction and pressure. The "core" may be recognized as an area darker in color and more painful than the surrounding hyperkeratotic tissue.

Treatment of heloma durum consists of debridement of the hyperkeratotic tissue along with padding of the digit or shoe. Instruments necessary for debridement are the scalpel handle and corresponding blades or the chisel

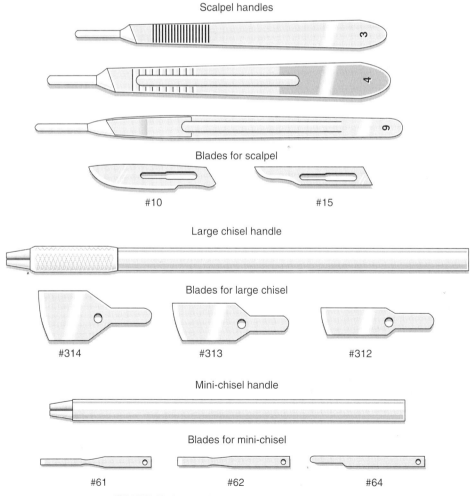

FIGURE 13–6. Handles and blades for debriding lesions.

handle and corresponding blades. The choice of instrument is the personal preference of the practitioner. A No. 3 scalpel handle with a No. 15 blade or a long or short chisel handle with a No. 312 of 313 blade is generally used (Fig. 13–6). Other scalpel and chisel blades are available and again are the personal preference of the practitioner.

When heloma durum is debrided with a scalpel, the instrument is held in the hand like a pencil with the blade parallel to the lesion (Fig. 13–7A). The fingers on the opposite hand are used to hold the digit, with the index finger under the digit and the thumb on the top pulling the skin on the dorsum of the digit. Holding the digit in this manner will stabilize the digit and the skin for debriding. The blade is moved distal to proximal, i.e., toward the patient, during debridement (Fig. 13–7B). Cutting with the blade from proximal to distal or toward the practitioner increases the risk of lacerating the fingers of the practitioner. The blade is moved in small smooth strokes, cutting only thin layers of hyperkeratotic tissue with each stroke. Small increases in

the angle at which the blade is held to the lesion result in progressively thicker layers of tissue removed. The lesion is debrided to the contour of the digit and not flat on the dorsal surface. Debriding the lesion flat on the dorsal surface will leave thick edges on the lesion that may cause the patient discomfort. The hyperkeratotic tissue should be removed until pink normal tissue is seen. The hyperkeratotic tissue is yellow and waxy and feels different than the normal surrounding tissue. During debridement the lesion should be felt to determine if the edges are too high and if an adequate amount of hyperkeratotic tissue has been removed. Periodically during debridement the digit should be released and the color checked. When stabilizing the digit, some blanching may occur, making the presence of pink normal tissue difficult to determine.

When a deep-seated "core" is present, it has a greater depth than the surrounding hyperkeratotic lesion. The tip of the blade is held at a 20° or 30° angle to the lesion, and the "core" is circumscribed and removed. When the

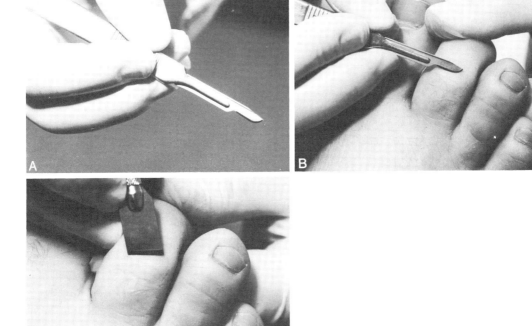

FIGURE 13–7. Heloma durum debridement. *(A)* Hand position for debridement with a scalpel. *(B)* Scalpel blade position on the skin. *(C)* Chisel blade position on the skin.

"core" still appears dark, the preceding procedure is repeated until sufficient tissue is removed to provide relief to the patient.

When heloma durum is debrided with the chisel, the instrument is held like a pencil with the blade parallel to the lesion. The digit is held with the opposite hand as in the previously described technique. The blade is moved in small, smooth, side-to-side strokes, cutting from distal to proximal, toward the patient (Fig. 13–7C). Thin layers of hyperkeratotic tissue should be removed until the lesion is reduced. Debridement is done to the contour of the digit to avoid leaving edges on the lesion. Deep-seated "cores" may be removed by using the corner of the chisel blade in a similar manner as with the scalpel blade.

Heloma Molle

Heloma molle, or soft corn, is an interdigital lesion that has absorbed moisture. The moisture macerates the hyperkeratotic lesion, generally causing the lesion to be more painful than a hard corn. Heloma molle may occur at any point interdigitally from the web space to the distal aspect of the digit, wherever there is increased friction and pressure from adjacent bony prominences or other sources such as an adjacent nail plate. Interdigital hyperkeratotic lesions are not always soft and macerated. Often these lesions appear the same as heloma durum.

Treatment of heloma molle consists of debridement of the hyperkeratotic skin and padding. Debridement may be with the scalpel or chisel. The technique is similar to that used for heloma durum with the exception of the hand position. When debriding an interdigital lesion the digits must be spread to allow access, while at the same time holding the skin tight to stabilize. The blade is moved in whatever direction space and digit position will allow. As much hyperkeratotic tissue as possible should be removed.

Distal Clavus

Distal clavus is a hard corn on the distal pulp of the digit. A severely contracted or overly long digit may develop a hyperkeratotic lesion on the distal aspect of the digit. Distal clavus may occur on one digit or on multiple digits. Multiple lesions are referred to as distal clavi.

Treatment of distal clavus consists of debridement of the hyperkeratotic tissue and use of padding. Instrumentation and technique are as previously discussed. The plantar skin of the toe is pulled tight to stabilize the toe. The blade is moved dorsal to plantar to remove as much hyperkeratotic tissue as possible.

Padding for Digital Lesions

When the hyperkeratotic tissue is removed from a heloma, the area may be sensitive until the hard tissue re-forms to protect it. Padding should be used to reduce any discomfort after debridement and to prevent the rapid return of the painful lesion. Felt and foam rubber pads are manufactured for heloma durum in ¹⁄₁₆- and ⅛-inch thickness. These pads are oblong with an aperture and have an adhesive backing (Fig. 13–8). The choice of felt or foam rubber is decided, with foam being for cushioning and felt being for reduction of friction and pressure. The pad is placed with the aperture centered over the lesion, being sure that the aperture is large enough to completely surround the lesion. The pad should not extend onto the medial or lateral sides of the digits or

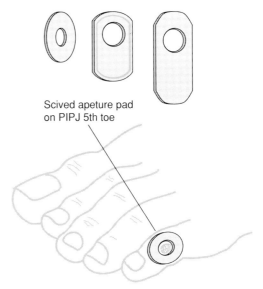

Scived apeture pad
on PIPJ 5th toe

FIGURE 13–8. Types of pads and their placement on the fifth toe.

cross any joints, and the edges should be skived at approximately a 45° angle. The skived edges direct the pressure away from the lesion.

The heloma durum pads may be used for heloma molle by cutting them in half, making a horseshoe-shaped pad. The pad is placed interdigitally with the open end of the horseshoe oriented proximally (Fig. 13–9). The pad should not extend onto the dorsal or plantar surface of the digit.

The precut heloma durum pads may be used to pad for distal clavus. The pad is cut into a round shape and placed onto the distal end of the digit with the aperture surrounding the lesion.

All of these pads may be covered with a self-adherent gauze, adhesive tape, or other covering made for this purpose to allow the pad to remain in place for a longer period of time. These pads are temporary, lasting on average from 1 to 3 days. Adhesive pads should not be allowed to remain in place for longer than 5 to 7 days or damage may occur to the underlying skin.

Patients with uncontrolled diabetes, peripheral vascular disease, or any skin lesions should not have adhesive pads placed on their skin. An alternative might be a pad fabricated with foam rubber tubing or tube foam. This tubing can be cut to the length of the digit and worn over the digit. The pad can then be removed when not needed by the patient. This type of pad may last for weeks and should not irritate the skin if worn properly. Tube foam pads may be used for heloma durum, heloma molle, and distal clavus. For distal clavus, a flap may be formed at one end of the tube foam by folding it and then taping it to form a toe cap.

Another alternative is the use of lamb's wool to cover and cushion heloma durum or heloma molle. A strand of lamb's wool is wound around the digit with little to no tension. The lamb's wool should be tight enough not to unravel easily but not tight enough to impair circulation. The lamb's wool may also be used to cover felt or foam pads. This padding can be made water resistant by applying flexible collodion over the lamb's wool. Flexible collodion is a viscous liquid that renders the lamb's wool water resistant when the lamb's wool is saturated with the collodion. Lamb's wool and flexible collodion may remain in place for long periods of time but should be removed in approximately 1 month.

A specialized type of pad for distal clavus is the buttress pad. The buttress pad slips around the digit or digits with bulk under the digit in the toe sulcus. This bulk under the digit lifts the digit during gait, removing friction and pressure from the distal pulp of the digit. The buttress pad may be fabricated from 3-inch elastic tape folded over a roll of soft material used for bulk. The roll of soft material should be cut to the size of the plantar aspect of the digit or digits to be lifted. The 3-inch elastic tape is pinched around the roll and then cut around the roll, leaving the elastic tape above the roll. An aperture is then cut in the tape to allow the pad to slip over the digits. Another method is to slip the bulk roll into tube gauze, wrap the tube gauze around the digit or digits, and then tape the ends together dorsally with moleskin or adhesive tape. Either method is satisfactory and allows the pad to be worn when necessary (Fig. 13–10).

A more permanent type of pad may be fabricated from silicone rubber, which can be shaped to accommodate several different deformities. There are several different commercially available types of silicone rubber material.

Lateral PIPJ 4th toe

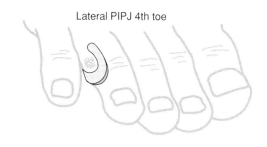

Foam corn pads

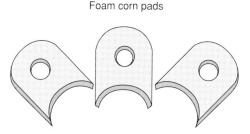

FIGURE 13–9. Pads and their placement on fourth toe for heloma molle.

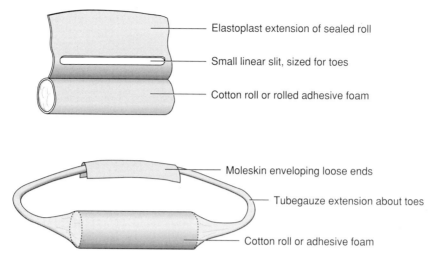

FIGURE 13–10. Buttress pads for distal clavus.

When padding of the foot is not possible, the shoes may be modified to render relief. Shoes may be stretched if not fabricated from man-made materials. A contracted digit may press on the toe box of the shoe. When appropriate, the shoe may be cut at this point by making an X over the deformity. The X cut allows the digit to raise above the level of the toe box without creating an unsightly hole in the shoe.

HYPERKERATOTIC PLANTAR LESIONS

Tyloma

Tyloma is a hyperkeratotic plantar lesion without distinct borders that occurs under weight-bearing surfaces. A tyloma is generally diffuse, extending under multiple metatarsal heads owing to the excessive friction and pressure of abnormal biomechanics. Treatment for tyloma consists of debridement of the hyperkeratotic tissue and padding. Instruments to be used depend on the personal preference of the practitioner and include a No. 3 scalpel handle with a No. 10 blade, a No. 4 scalpel handle with a No. 20 blade, and a chisel handle with a No. 312, 313, or other blade made for that handle (see Fig. 13–6). A diffuse tyloma is best debrided with a blade that has a large surface cutting area, such as a No. 10, 20, 312, or 313. A blade with a small surface cut-

ting area will require more effort and is more difficult to control.

The scalpel handle is held across the fingers on the palmar surface with the index finger on the bottom surface of the blade and the thumb on the top surface of the blade (Fig. 13–11A). The hand is then closed, and the fingers hold the handle to the palm of the hand (Fig. 13–11B). The end of the handle opposite the blade may be held between the forth and fifth fingers or left in the palm of the hand, whichever is more comfortable for the practitioner. The scalpel is held with the blade parallel to the lesion, the index finger on top of the blade, and the thumb on the side of the blade. The front one third of the blade is used to debride the lesion. The distal tip of the index finger and the distal interphalangeal joint of the second finger are placed on the plantar aspect of the foot and act as a fulcrum or pivot point (Fig. 13–11C). The blade is moved in long smooth arcs from distal to proximal, debriding thin layers of hyperkeratotic tissue. Slight increases in the angle at which the blade is held to the lesion will result in progressively thicker layers of tissue debrided. The thumb of the opposite hand is used to stabilize the skin. The thumb should be placed distal to the lesion and the skin pulled tight to stabilize. Care must be taken not to lacerate the stabilizing thumb during debridement. As much hyperkeratotic tissue as possible should be removed from the lesion. An adequate amount of hyperkeratotic tissue has been removed

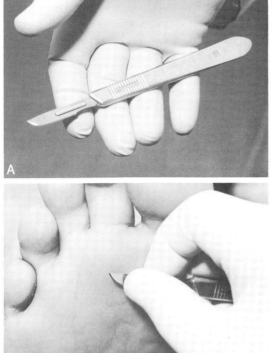
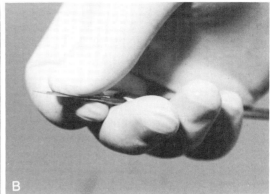

FIGURE 13–11. Tyloma debridement using a scalpel. (*A* and *B*) Hand positions for scalpel. (*C*) Blade position on the skin.

when pink healthy tissue is seen, and the skin surface no longer feels waxy or raised above the level of the surrounding skin.

The chisel handle is held like a pencil between the fingers just above the blade (Fig. 13–12*A*). The dorsal surfaces of the fingers are rested on the plantar surface of the foot with the blade parallel to the skin surface (Fig. 13–12*B*). The blade is moved in a smooth cutting motion from side to side, debriding thin layers of hyperkeratotic tissue at a time. The thumb

of the opposite hand is used to stabilize the skin, as previously described.

Intractable Plantar Keratosis

Intractable plantar keratosis is sometimes described differently by different sources. "Intractable" means difficult to cure, and this is a lesion that seems to defy all treatment. An intractable plantar keratosis is a discrete hyper-

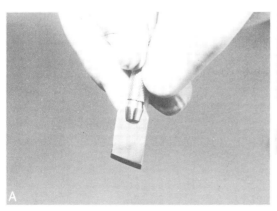
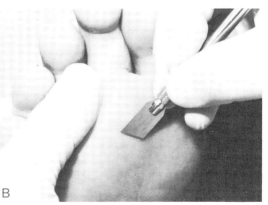

FIGURE 13–12. Tyloma debridement using a chisel. (*A*) Hand position. (*B*) Blade position on the skin.

keratotic lesion that is usually located under a single weight-bearing surface, such as a metatarsal head. This lesion generally has a deep-seated "core," which creates a great deal of discomfort for the patient.

Treatment of intractable plantar keratosis consists of debridement of hyperkeratotic tissue and padding. A softening agent may be used to ease debridement. Instrumentation and debridement techniques are similar to those described for tyloma. The deep-seated "core" must be removed to render relief to the patient. After removing the most superficial layers of hyperkeratotic tissue, the "core" is observed as a darker area within the keratosis. The tip of the scalpel or a corner of a chisel blade is used to remove the "core" area. The blade is held at a 20° or 30° angle to the skin surface. At this low angle the blade is used to circumscribe the "core" area. A section of hyperkeratotic tissue almost in the shape of an inverted cone is removed. The area is then inspected and palpated for any remaining discomfort. Any remaining dark or uncomfortable tissue may be removed, using the previous technique. The area may then be padded.

Porokeratosis Plantaris Discreta

Porokeratosis plantaris discreta is generally a small well-defined hyperkeratotic lesion that may have a white halo surrounding the lesion observed on debridement. The lesion is usually located beneath weight-bearing surfaces but may be found in non–weight-bearing areas. Treatment for porokeratosis plantaris discreta consists of debridement and padding but may include chemical or surgical techniques as well. Debridement is performed using the instrumentation and techniques previously described. Chemical treatment consists of salicylic acid applied to the lesion for 5 to 7 days in an attempt to soften the horny plug. The area is debrided after removing the salicylic acid dressing. Surgical treatment consists of excising the lesion.

Verruca Plantaris

Verrucae plantaris, or plantar warts, are caused by the human papillomavirus and consist of abnormal growths within the outer layers of the skin. Verrucae do not penetrate into the dermis. Verrucae on the plantar aspect of the foot form hyperkeratotic tissue owing to weight bearing and may resemble tylomas. The normal plantar skin lines will travel through a tyloma but travel around and not through a verruca. Verrucae are discrete lesions of varying sizes and may be solitary or occur in multiple patches known as mosaic verrucae.

Treatment consists of debridement and chemical or surgical removal. The lesion may be treated with various types and strengths of acid, freezing, hyfrecation, laser, and surgical excision. Verrucae tend to recur frequently and are difficult to cure.

Padding for Plantar Lesions

Pads for plantar lesions are generally manufactured of felt or foam rubber in ⅛- or ¼-inch thicknesses. Plantar pads may be individually cut from sheets of material or purchased precut to shape. Plantar pads are usually square to rectangular with a U-shaped aperture at one end. The pad is placed with the aperture surrounding the lesion and with the bulk of the pad extending proximally down the shafts of the metatarsals (Fig. 13–13). The pad should extend approximately to the base of the metatarsals. All edges of the pad except the aperture should be skived at an approximately 45° angle to distribute the weight, friction, and pressure away from the lesion. The choice of felt or foam rubber is the personal preference of the practitioner. The felt pad will distribute the pressure away from the lesion more effectively than the foam rubber, which will cushion. The plantar pads may be covered with adhesive tape or moleskin to increase wearing time. Moleskin may be used to cover plantar lesions after debridement. The moleskin will aid in reducing friction to the area and will protect freshly debrided skin.

Pads placed on the skin are a temporary solution since they will remain in place for only a few days. An alternative might be insoles worn in the shoes on a daily basis. This type of device is referred to as a chairside orthotic and can be easily produced in an office setting. There are numerous materials of various thick-

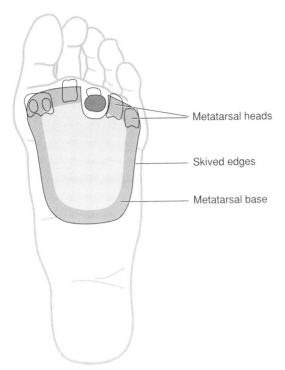

FIGURE 13–13. Pad for plantar lesions.

nesses and cushioning ability available. Some materials are heat moldable and can be heated, placed on a block of foam rubber, and molded to the patient's foot in a semi–weight-bearing position. The material may then be ground to fit into the shoe. An insole may also be cut to the shape of the foot and placed in the shoe. After wearing the insole for 1 to 2 weeks, the patient is asked to return, and areas of increased friction and pressure are identified. These areas may then be padded on the top or bottom of the insole.

BUNION DEFORMITIES

Hallux valgus deformity may have an associated bunion or enlarged dorsomedial aspect of the first metatarsal head. The prominent bunion deformity may be irritated by shoes and become painful. Patients may develop hyperkeratosis of the skin overlying the bunion or may develop an adventitious bursae. Treatment for painful bunion consists of debridement of any hyperkeratotic tissue and padding. Adventitious bursae may be treated with injectable corticosteroids and padding. Shoes

may be modified by cutting the side of the toe box adjacent to the bunion just above the sole of the shoe. This will create a flap that will allow the bunion extra room without an unsightly hole in the shoe. A ball and ring stretcher may also be used to stretch the shoe in the area of the bunion. Surgery may be necessary to correct the deformity when conservative measures have failed.

Tailor's bunion deformity is an enlargement of the dorsolateral aspect of the fifth metatarsal head. The prominent bunion may be irritated by shoes, forming a hyperkeratotic lesion on the dorsolateral aspect of the fifth metatarsal head with possible plantar hyperkeratotic lesion beneath the fifth metatarsal head. Treatment consists of debridement of the hyperkeratotic lesions and padding.

Pads for bunion deformities may be cut from sheets of material or precut felt or foam rubber of $1/16$- or $1/8$-inch thickness. Hallux valgus pads are oval with an aperture at one end. The aperture is placed surrounding the bunion with the longer end of the pad oriented proximally (Fig. 13–14). The edges of the pad are skived to distribute the friction and pressure away from the bunion. Tailor's bunion pads are similar to hallux valgus pads scaled down to the size of the tailor's bunion. The pads may be covered with tape or moleskin to increase wearing time.

Foam rubber tube pads may be used for those patients in whom adhesive is contraindicated or for convenience and increased wearing time. A section of tube foam is cut long

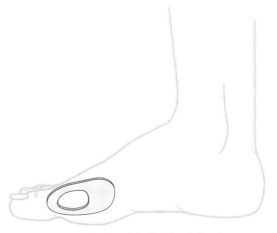

FIGURE 13–14. Pad for bunion deformity.

enough to extend from the distal aspect of the digit to just proximal to the bunion. A section extending from the toe sulcus to the proximal end of the tube, equal to approximately one half of the tube's circumference, is removed. This creates a flap that extends over the bunion deformity when the tube is worn on the toe. This type of pad may be used for hallux valgus as well as tailor's bunion deformities.

A latex shield is a more permanent type of pad for bunion deformities. A cast is made of the first or fifth metatarsophalangeal joints, and a positive mold is made from that cast. The positive mold is covered with latex, and padding material is placed surrounding the bunion deformity. The latex shield is worn on the foot to protect the bunion area.

Custom-molded shoes are also an effective therapy for deformed feet. Patients with severe hallux valgus, contracted digits, or other deformities may have their feet and ankles cast and shoes manufactured from these casts.

CHAPTER 14

PEDAL MANIFESTATIONS OF SYSTEMIC DISEASE

Jeffrey M. Robbins
James L. Canterbury

The focus of this section is on the manifestations of various diseases in the lower extremity, with emphasis placed on problems arising in the foot. Physicians caring for the lower extremity will frequently observe these manifestations in patients affected by systemic disease.

The podiatrist is often in a long-term relationship with his or her patient. This affords a vantage point to the physician, enabling early detection of disease states and a framework for the monitoring of chronic illness. Most important in this long-term relationship is the proactive preventive care afforded by primary care. Therefore, the physician must look at the evaluation of systemic disease as merely a part of the podiatric diagnosis. It cannot be separated from the workup of a patient. The principles remain the same, a good history being essential, followed by a thorough organized physical examination.

Special attention should be paid to the patient as a whole person, disregarding many preconceived opinions of age-related disabilities. It is extremely important to consider in all patients a few simple, but frequently forgotten, health risks. Possibly the most destructive of these risks to health is the use of tobacco. The smoking of cigarettes by or around a patient is sometimes ignored by the podiatric physician. This significant environmental poison will produce untoward effects in all patients.

Another significant health risk is substance abuse. This may encompass outright illicit drug abuse in the form of marijuana or heroin, or it could be the abuse of the "legal" drugs prescribed by one or more physicians, including the podiatrist. Questioning of the elderly patient regarding substance abuse is often avoided or simply forgotten.

The single most important drug of abuse, alcohol, is a legal drug that requires no prescription. The abuse of alcohol may be a lifelong problem hidden since early adulthood or may be a newer-onset abuse that began at retirement age.

NAIL PATHOLOGY

In podiatric medicine a great deal of time is spent in the care of nails. The nail in its normal state is a clear thin plate that appears to fit precisely within the nail folds on either side. It is composed of layers of dead compact keratinocytes that are nonnucleated. At the proximal end of the nail there is a pale white area that is crescent shaped. This area is actually projecting from beneath the proximal nail fold. Known as the lunula, it is an extension of the nail root. Its white color is produced by juvenile keratinocytes.

The distal tip of the digit just below the nail plate is called the hyponychium. It is a thickened mass of skin that also is created by keratinocytes. The onychial dermal band is found near the distal end of the nail plate. This area is about 1 mm wide and is situated transversely on the nail. It is an important landmark for systemic disease.

In the nondiseased state the nail is very adherent to the nail bed, being fully anchored in vertical fibers projected from bone and fibers from the tendon of extensor digitorum longus.

It is also valuable to note the rate of nail growth, shape, and thickness. Observations such as grooving of the nail, pitting, and nail loss can also be very significant. The nail acts as an historical record of past disturbances in diet, metabolism, and environmental exposure. This makes the nail an important tool in the investigation of systemic illness.

AUTOIMMUNE DISORDERS

Many diseases and syndromes are included in the category of autoimmune disorders. Some of these have a very high probability of being caused by autoimmunity, while others are strongly associated with autoimmunity but have no easily demonstrable link to autoimmunity.

Autoimmune diseases are the result of the immune system's misidentification of endogenous tissue as foreign. The production of antibodies to these tissues ensues. Sometimes this occurs because the tissue or fluid is usually not presented to the immune system for identification. These tissues are often intracellular or are in some other way normally hidden from the immune system by virtue of their locations in the body.

Progressive Systemic Sclerosis

Progressive systemic sclerosis is a connective tissue disorder of unknown etiology. The disease causes the body to lay down collagen in tissues abnormally. There are significant inflammatory, fibrotic, and degenerative changes associated with this illness. Frequently involved areas are the esophagus, intestines, heart, lungs, and kidneys. There are also vascular lesions of the skin, hence the commonly used term *scleroderma*. A significant number of affected persons are found to have antinuclear antibodies. Those that do not will generally have anticentromeric antibodies.

This disease usually follows a slow course, with symptoms appearing gradually. Women are affected two to three times more frequently than men. The disease is rarely seen in childhood and is considered to be an illness of the third to fifth decades of life. There are, however, more rapidly progressing forms of the disease. Some of these forms may yield fulminating hypertensive renal disease, cardiac failure, pulmonary disease, or severe intestinal malabsorption.

The suspicion of progressive systemic sclerosis is markedly increased with the presence of diminished gastric motility along with Raynaud's symptoms. Thus, the pedal manifestations of this entity may contribute to the final diagnosis. Confirmation of the disease must be by biopsy of affected skin, deep fascia, and adjacent muscle. The specimen, if positive, will yield histiocytes, plasma cells, lymphocytes, and eosinophils in some cases.

The pedal manifestations of progressive systemic sclerosis are primarily those of Raynaud's phenomenon. Patients may present with insidious swelling of the distal extremity, thick tightening skin, myalgia-arthralgia, or sensitivity to cold. The nail in patients with long-standing disease exhibits ridging longitudinally and becomes very thin. The thinning of the nail may lead to splitting and lysis as well as to lucency. The nail bed can then be seen to cause the nails to have a red hue. The digits may also have ulcerations at the distal tip that are small but exquisitely painful. The skin will be shiny and smooth. Other nail manifestations may include pterygium formation, with the cuticle overgrowing and fusing to the dorsal nail fold, as well as Beau's lines (transverse ridging of nails).

Noninvasive testing such as bidirectional Doppler studies and photoplethysmography can be very useful. Post cold exposure photoplethysmography is highly reliable and easily accomplished in the office setting.

Raynaud's Syndrome

Raynaud's syndrome can be either a primary disease entity or a phenomenon secondary to another disease entity, such as the connective tissue diseases. Therefore, treatment and prognosis are linked to the distinction between Raynaud's disease and Raynaud's phenomenon secondary to progressive systemic sclerosis. Raynaud's disease is usually bilateral and demonstrates no progression of symptoms over 2 or more years. To further illucidate this distinction, the practitioner should keep in mind that in idiopathic Raynaud's disease there are usually no gangrenous areas.

Treatment of the disease in its mild forms can be as simple as avoidance of cold temperatures and the total cessation of all nicotine drugs in any form. Many other treatments have been tried with varying degrees of success. Relaxation-type activity such as biofeedback has been used. Various drugs have been tried, but success seems more patient dependent. Drugs such as calcium channel blockers (nifedipine), and pentoxifylline are reported to be beneficial. Sympathectomy is a last resort and appears to be of benefit for several years.

Acrocyanosis is frequently confused with the symptoms of Raynaud's syndrome. This benign disease should be placed in any differential list with Raynaud's syndrome because of its association with cold exposure. Acrocyanosis also produces vasospasm in the extremities. The superficial arterioles are affected and yield a persistent cyanotic appearance. No ulceration, pain, or ischemic trophic changes occur with acrocyanosis, and there is usually no need for treatment. These symptoms are generally found to be symmetric and are seen in the hands or the feet. Hyperhidrosis may also be present. Like many of the processes in the

autoimmune category the disease occurs more often in females.

Polymyositis and Dermatomyositis

Polymyositis and dermatomyositis are two closely associated disorders of the striated muscle. The etiology is unclear, and these disorders will most frequently appear to be asymmetric in their presentation of muscular weakness and atrophy. Usually affected are the limb girdle, neck, and pharynx. This disorder is found more frequently in females in a ratio of 2:1. When symptoms are found in the skin it is termed dermatomyositis.

This process can be seen at any time in life from infancy to old age. It is frequently described as a mixed connective tissue disease. Accompanying gastrointestinal and esophageal symptomatology as well as the dermal component makes it possible to argue that this is actually progressive systemic sclerosis. The cutaneous manifestations also resemble systemic lupus erythematosus.

The pedal manifestations may include lower-extremity muscle weakness in 95% of the cases. Distal muscle weakness is seen in 27% of the documented cases. Rash may be distributed over the lower extremity over the dorsum of the feet and the medial malleoli and will be similar in appearance to the rash seen on the trunk, elbows, and arms. It will appear slightly elevated, scaly, and erythematous, just as in systemic lupus erythematosus. There will be arthritic complaints in approximately 24% of those afflicted, and 30% will have associated Raynaud's phenomenon.

The presenting complaint is most often difficulty climbing stairs, getting up from a chair, or changes in gait. The evaluation of the gait cycle will reveal progressive clumsiness and waddling. In the acute phase, severe constitutional symptoms and rapid weight loss may be seen.

Systemic Lupus Erythematosus

Systemic lupus erythematosus is a chronic inflammatory disease of unknown origin. Frequently patients present to their family doctor after an exposure to sunlight with the complaint of a rash or "burn." Many of these patients will have complained about problems with sunbathing in the past. This disease is seen more often in females than males in a ratio of 10:1. Young adults, older than age 30, are more likely to be afflicted.

As previously described, the rash is a red, papular scaly rash. The term *butterfly rash* is used when the rash occurs over the malar surface. Other manifestations of this disease include pleurisy, pericarditis, renal or neurologic signs, anemia, polyarthralgia, arthritis, and fever.

The disease may present as a mild process or be extremely rapid in its destructiveness. Remission and exacerbation may become the norm for the patient. This unpredictable course may manifest itself as a vascular lesion of the kidney, which has a very poor prognosis. More frequently, arthritides that closely resemble rheumatoid arthritis will be seen. The accompanying arthralgias and joint swelling will be a part of the presenting picture in 90% of the cases. Lower extremity manifestations include avascular necrosis of the femoral head, peripheral neuropathy, and Raynaud's symptoms.

Polyarteritis Nodosa

Polyarteritis nodosa, also called *necrotizing vasculitis,* is a segmental inflammatory disorder of blood vessels, specifically medium- and small-caliber arteries. This disease occurs in middle-age men and has both acute and insidious presentations. There seems to be no typical picture, however. Commonly the patient may manifest a fever of unknown origin. Presentations such as this are extremely challenging to diagnose.

The patient may present initially with acute, severe abdominal pain or frequently with hepatic infarct, bronchopneumonia, cardiac failure, renal failure, or hypertension. Other associated illnesses are Kawasaki's disease in infants and children, Churg-Strauss syndrome, and Cogan's syndrome.

The lower-extremity manifestations are associated with either unilateral or bilateral peripheral neuropathy and arthralgias, edema, and subcutaneus nodules. Subcutaneous nod-

ules may be able to be palpated along the course of the affected artery. In the presence of this very confusing clinical picture, varying from acute gallbladder disease to coronary artery disease, only selective arteriography and biopsy can make the diagnosis. The gastrocnemius muscle should not be used for the biopsy unless it is the only muscle involved, because the risk for creation of a deep vein thrombosis is high. Laboratory tests other than a biopsy are necessary to exclude other diagnoses.

INHERITED DISORDERS

Marfan's Syndrome

Marfan's syndrome is an autosomal dominant inherited disorder that affects connective tissue. It presents most notably as arachnodactyly, and the severity of the disease varies from person to person. Patients will be taller than others in their family and for their age.

This disease can be debilitating. Ocular manifestations result in subluxations of the lens and sometimes in retinal detachment. There can be associated cardiac disease that is primarily the result of aortic abnormalities.

Lower-extremity and pedal manifestations of Marfan's syndrome are unusual joint and ligamentous laxity, genu recurvatum, kyphoscoliosis, and pes planus. Many other skeletal and developmental abnormalities may be seen. The extent of the disease determines treatment, but few treatments are successful.

Ehlers-Danlos Syndrome

Ehlers-Danlos syndrome is a poorly understood autosomal dominant disease with at least ten different forms. It is believed that there is a defect in the cross-linking of collagen fibrils that produces the common manifestations. As in Marfan's syndrome, excessive joint laxity may be present. The skin is often fragile and bruises easily. Minor trauma causes wide wounds that tend not to bleed much. Wound margins are very fragile and difficult to suture.

In the lower extremity, varicosities and other vascular problems may arise. Joint effusions (accumulations of fluid in the joint) frequently develop. This leads to a loss of function. Ankle sprains and joint dislocations are the most frequent presentations in the primary care setting.

ARTHRITIS

Rheumatoid Arthritis

Adult rheumatoid arthritis is a chronic non-suppurative inflammation of diarthrodal joints. Women are affected two to three more times as often as men. The onset is insidious. Aching and stiffness occur initially, with gradual increasing articular pain. Morning stiffness is a prominent complaint. Symptoms usually begin in the hands and feet at the proximal interphalangeal joints and metatarsophalangeal joints. Tenosynovitis of the flexor and extensor tendon sheaths is also seen in a bilateral and symmetric pattern.

There are many late changes seen in rheumatoid arthritis. Intra-articular effusions with swollen boggy joint, periarticular edema, and ulnar/fibular drift may be seen. Classically mentioned are the boutonniere deformity at the proximal interphalangeal joint (hyperextension at the distal interphalangeal joint) and the swan neck deformity (hyperextension at the proximal interphalangeal joints).

Lower-extremity manifestations include hallux valgus, osteoporotic changes, joint space narrowing at the proximal interphalangeal joint and metatarsophalangeal joints, and subchondral erosions. Aseptic necrosis, a very grave finding, is reported to be spontaneous or associated with the use of corticosteroids.

Juvenile Rheumatoid Arthritis

Juvenile rheumatoid arthritis occurs in persons before their 16th birthday. The onset is not uniformly distributed throughout all ages younger than 16, having bimodal peaks at ages 2 through 5 and 9 through 12. It is found more often in females. Juvenile rheumatoid arthritis is characterized by high spiking fevers in about 20% of the patients. The child is often profoundly sick and may also have hepatosplenomegaly, lymphadenopathy, and polyarthritis. Sexual maturation may be delayed in these children, yet early closure of the epiphys-

eal plates may occur. Fifty percent have growth abnormalities that are readily noted on physical examination. Surprisingly, 70% of these patients regain nearly normal joint function by adulthood.

Ankylosing Spondylitis

Ankylosing spondylitis is a chronic progressive form of arthritis affecting the sacroiliac joints, spinal epiphyseal joints, and paravertebral soft tissues. The vertebral disks may ossify. Also known as Marie-Strumpell disease, it affects men three times more frequently than women. The onset is insidious and begins with low back pain. Ten percent show sciatica-type pain and morning stiffness. Back motion becomes increasingly limited. Radiographically, "bamboo" spine is seen, with its characteristic appearance of thickening segments in the vertebral column. The patient may present to the podiatrist with gait abnormalities because of the restriction in the lower back. Pain is diminished by assuming a forward leaning position, increasing gait abnormalities.

Psoriatic Arthritis

Psoriatic arthritis, as the name suggests, is associated with psoriasis. Although only about 7% of all psoriatic patients are affected, overtly it is very important to recognize the manifestations of this process.

The variations in this disease range from very mildly debilitating asymmetric arthritides in the distal interphalangeal joints to involvement of large joints such as the sacroiliac. Resorption of the terminal phalanx and a "sausage toe" appearance are the classic hallmarks. Eighty percent of these patients will have nail pitting or psoriatic nail changes. This can be a severely crippling form of arthritis. Often skin and joint manifestations may appear simultaneously and remit at the same time.

Treatment is similar to the treatment of rheumatoid arthritis; however, antimalarial agents are added to the regimen with some, albeit limited, success. Other medications and modalities used in treatment are photochemotherapy, with psoralen and ultraviolet light (PUVA) and the chemotherapeutic agent etretinate. This very highly toxic drug is used in severe cases and only when there is no risk of pregnancy. Gold and other antirheumatoid treatments may also be used.

Reiter's Syndrome

Reiter's syndrome is a reactive arthritis. There are two recognized forms: sexually transmitted and dysenteric. It is a disease of young men, usually those in the 20- to 40-year age group. Women and children do not usually present with Reiter's syndrome. This syndrome is usually associated with *Chlamydia trachomatis* infection, but the enteric forms may be due to *Shigella, Salmonella, Yersinia,* or *Campylobacter.* More than half (63% to 96%) of those affected have the HLA-B27 tissue antigen.

The characteristic presentation is of urethritis, arthritis, conjunctivitis, circinate balanitis, and possible buccal ulcerations. The arthritis may be severe and asymmetric, involving multiple joints both large and small.

The pedal findings include enthesopathy with Achilles tendonitis or plantar fasciitis and keratoderma blennorrhagicum seen on the soles and palms. These hyperkeratotic lesions may also involve the nails.

Diagnosis is made following a 1- to 2-month period of arthritis and urethritis. Gonococcal cultures will be negative in Reiter's syndrome.

This is a self-limiting disorder lasting from 6 weeks to 6 months. However, recurrence is common. Treatment consists of anti-inflammatory agents, corticosteroid injections at the site of enthesopathy if necessary, and oral administration of either tetracycline or erythromycin, 500 mg, four times a day for 10 days if it is chlamydial. Both the patient and sexual partner(s) must be treated.

Degenerative Joint Disease

Degenerative joint disease (osteoarthritis) is a common noninflammatory disorder of the joints. Investigations in the United Kingdom suggest that there is, in fact, an inherited predisposition as well as a link in mechanisms to rheumatoid arthritis. This disease is seen in movable weight-bearing joints with a deterio-

ration of the articular cartilage. Formation of new bone is seen in subchondral areas and at the margins of joints.

This disease is always associated with the aging process by the general public and viewed as a normal part of aging. Although it is more prevalent in the elderly, the "wear and tear" phenomenon is seen also in morbid obesity, from acquired or developmental abnormalities, and in competitive athletes.

Joint pain after periods of rest, aching in inclement weather, crepitus, and spasms are common symptoms in osteoarthritis. Limitation of motion and malalignment are frequent signs noted by the clinician. In the foot, one may see fusifom swelling of the digits, hallux valgus, and atrophy of surrounding muscles.

Septic Arthritis

Septic arthritis is an invasion of the synovial membrane by living microorganisms. The factors that determine the occurrence of this are bacteremia, predisposition of certain organisms to invade the joint, and unusual host susceptibility, such as from trauma, surgery, and injection.

Any joint can be affected by microorganisms. All that is required is entry to the space. The joint becomes red, hot, and swollen. It may or may not drain, but constitutional signs and symptoms will most likely follow unless the responses are masked by drugs. Lymphangitis is a strong indication that action must be taken promptly.

Gout

Gout is one of the most commonly reported complaints historically. Once thought to be the disease of the rich, because of the association with meat consumption, this entity occurs today across all socioeconomic levels. The extremely painful acute attack is the result of the deposition of monosodium urate crystals in the synovial fluid and is usually monoarticular. Eventually these crystals can form a tophus in joints, kidney, and subcutaneous sites. The cause is a hyperuricemia either from overproduction or from decreased clearance or uric acid. Although an acute attack will likely be associated with a serum uric acid level greater than 7 mg/dL in men (1 mg less in women until menopause), the uric acid level may be within normal limits at the time of presentation to the office.

Primary gout is an inherited inborn disorder of metabolism. Eighty-five to 90% of these patients are male. The initial onset can be at any age but generally occurs about the fifth decade of life. The initial attack may be after a traumatic incident such as surgery, alcohol ingestion, or emotional depression. Gouty attacks may also be precipitated by drugs, the most common of which are the thiazide diuretics, insulin, and penicillin.

Onset of symptoms in the lower extremity is rapid. There is a predilection for the first metatarsophalangeal joint, where gout is called podagra. The joints of the tarsus, ankles, and knees can also be affected. Maximal pain occurs within hours of the initial onset of symptoms. Periarticular swelling, erythema, and severe pain are hallmarks of an acute gouty attack. Low-grade fever and leukocytosis may also be present. Diagnosis is definitive with aspiration of joint fluid containing urate crystals.

When the diagnosis is in doubt, colchicine is the preferred drug unless the patient is intolerant to colchicine. In established gout the nonsteroidal anti-inflammatory drugs are preferred. They include indomethacin, tolmetin, ibuprofen, or any of the other new nonsteroidal anti-inflammatory agents. Corticosteroids are seldom used but are a reasonable alternative when other therapies are unsuccessful. Following the acute attack, referral should be made to initiate therapies to prevent recurrence.

Chondrocalcinosis

Chondrocalcinosis is the presence of calcium salts in the fibrocartilage and hyaline cartilage in one or more joints. These salts include calcium pyrophosphate, calcium hydroxyapatite, and calcium orthophosphate.

Pseudogout is the appearance of acute or chronic inflammatory synovitis associated with the presence of calcium pyrophosphate dihydrate crystals in the joint fluid. There is also a cartilagenous calcification. This crystal-induced gout is associated with the elderly. It is seen in other medical conditions, including primary gout and such conditions as hyperparathyroidism, alkaptonuria, hemochromatosis, Wilson's disease, acromegaly, and diabetes mellitus. The onset is sudden, and the symptoms are usually of a 2-week duration. This disease affects the knees, large peripheral joints, hands, and feet. The diagnosis is conclusive with the presence of calcium pyrophosphate dihydrate in the joint fluid.

The treatment is with colchicine, 1 mg, intravenously, followed in 12 hours with a repeat dose if the symptoms and pain persist. Any synovial effusions should be drained. The prognosis is generally good.

CARDIOVASCULAR DISEASE
Congestive Heart Disease

Congestive heart disease is the failure of the heart to maintain an adequate output. This results in decreased blood flow to the tissues and congestion in the pulmonary and systemic circulation. The onset may be insidious or sudden. A gradual loss of energy, exertional dyspnea, and ankle edema may be seen in left ventricular failure. Dyspnea is generally the chief presenting complaint. In right ventricular failure there is ankle swelling that will be relieved at night. In late disease the swelling will become recalcitrant.

The lower-extremity manifestations will most certainly involve edema with concomitant irritation by shoes. This edema may be pitting or nonpitting. The application of compression stockings may be helpful.

Stasis dermatitis and stasis ulcers may manifest themselves in the lower extremities and the foot. Stasis dermatitis may be treated with compresses or colloid dressings. Later, as the skin integrity improves, a corticosteroid might be applied. Ulcers most certainly represent a threat to the patient and must be treated promptly. The application of an Unna boot (a zinc gelatin dressing) may be necessary. A colloid dressing might also be effective.

Pulmonary Hypertension

Pulmonary hypertension (cor pulmonale) occurs when there is an increase in pulmonary arterial pressure. This increased pulmonary arterial pressure may be the result of mechanically induced diminution of ventilation, or it can be the result of decreased respiratory drive. Occasionally there is idiopathic pulmonary hypertension, but by far the most frequent underlying cause is emphysema. Trauma, surgical removal, emboli, and many other pulmonary pathologic processes can induce cor pulmonale.

As in congestive heart failure, peripheral edema, especially at the ankle, is found. Clubbing at the finger may also be present.

Cerebrovascular Accident

Cerebrovascular accident, or stroke, is the destruction of brain substance secondary to an embolic event, thrombosis, hemorrhage, or vascular insufficiency. A space-occupying lesion may precipitate such an event, or it may be secondary to processes in or out of the brain itself.

The results of a cataclysmic cerebral event may be devastating. If sufficient tissue is lost or if damage is to primary centers of autonomic function, death can ensue. Frequently the patient will develop hemiplegia, gait abnormalities, and motor or sensory loss. This may impair any or all motor, proprioceptive, or sensory abilities.

An inability to recognize written words or symbols can occur, or there may be a loss of understanding of the spoken word. This becomes increasingly frustrating for the patient and caregivers because effective communication is nearly impossible.

Other significant deficits may occur as a result of stroke. Especially dangerous are changes in the ability to swallow, which can lead to aspiration and pneumonia. There may be complete failure to acknowledge the affected side of the body, which will distort the patient's view of the world and create a hazard to safety.

Lower-extremity manifestations of stroke may include edema, paralysis, and contractures. Neurologic manifestations may include both motor and sensory deficits, depending on the location and severity of the stoke. On examination, increased deep tendon reflexes,

spasticity, and a positive Babinski sign are common findings.

Subacute Bacterial Endocarditis

Bacterial infection of the endocardium is characterized by symptoms of infectious disease, such as chills, malaise, and fever. Also associated with subacute bacterial endocarditis is embolic pneumonia and the presence of vegetations in the endocardium.

The pedal signs of subacute bacterial endocarditis consist of clubbing in digits (most commonly the hands), Osler's nodes, Janeway lesions, splinter hemorrhages, and petechiae.

Janeway's lesions are hemorrhagic macular areas on the palms and soles. They are painless, although they may cause concern to the patient because of their appearance. Osler's nodes are small, raised, red-purple lesions that may or may not have a white center. They are found at the ends of the fingers and the toes. Splinter hemorrhages and petechiae may be found under the nails of the hand and feet.

The prognosis depends on the exact manifestations of the infection and on the location of emboli as well as on the extent of vegetations in the heart. Renal infarction may occur, adding yet another complication.

Treatment and prevention revolve around antibiosis. Penicillin in nonsensitive patients is often the drug of choice. Additional antibiotics may be required for resistant infections.

RENAL DISEASE

Renal failure is the acute and severe reduction of renal function leading to uremia. When the kidney is unable to successfully filter nitrogenous waste, pedal manifestations can ensue. Prerenal disease is secondary to a loss of perfusion to the kidney. Intrinsic kidney disease can be the result of a toxin or many other forms of renal tissue damage. Postrenal disease is associated with problems such as prostatism, calculi, or other forms of blockade to urinary flow.

There will be increases in serum creatinine, blood urea nitrogen, and potassium values. Sodium levels in the serum will fall. Other laboratory values that should be closely monitored include urinalysis and urine sodium and urine osmolarity tests.

Pedal signs include coarse muscular twitching, peripheral neuropathy, and muscle cramps. Changes in the skin include yellow-brown discoloration, uremic frost (crystalization of urea on the skin), and intense pruritus.

Treatment depends on the cause of the disease. Dialysis may be necessary, but there are other tools to management in the proper circumstances.

CARCINOMA OF THE PANCREAS

Patients with carcinoma of the pancreas present with some unusual manifestations in the lower extremity: a polyarthritis that does not respond to either nonsteroidal anti-inflammatory agents or corticosteroidal treatments, and subcutaneous nodules and fat necrosis that mimic those of erythema nodosum. Treatment will be focused on the carcinoma and not specifically aimed at these manifestations.

HEMATOLOGIC DISORDERS

Anemias are frequently associated with pedal symptoms. The anemia can be secondary to chronic blood loss, to the inability to produce red blood cells, or to exaggerated destruction of the red blood cells.

Pedal symptoms include vasomotor disturbances, neuralgic pain, numbness, and tingling. The nails may become spoon shaped, flat, or concave and excessively brittle.

The treatment is based on the laboratory findings. Simply giving ferrous compounds or other nonspecific treatment is never indicated. Prognosis once again depends on making the proper diagnosis.

Pernicious anemia is a chronic microcytic anemia seen in whites older than the age of 50. It is due to a vitamin B_{12} deficiency.

The pedal manifestations are similar to other anemias. Numbness of the hands and feet is often the precipitating cause for the appointment with the physician. A yellow tint to the skin very different from the jaundice of liver disease is also possible; it is sometimes referred to as a lemon tint. Forty percent of the patients will have a central nervous system

component to the disease, causing difficulty in walking. This difficulty will be aggravated by the darkness. There is also a loss of vibratory sense in the legs, hyperreflexia, and a positive Babinski sign if the lateral tract is affected. Hypotonia and hyporeflexia will be displayed if the posterior column is affected.

Sickle cell anemia is a chronic hemolytic anemia occurring most frequently in blacks. It is characterized by the sickle shape of the red blood cell as the result of a homozygous inherited hemoglobin (HbS). Valine is substituted for glutamic acid in the sixth amino acid of the β chain, causing the red blood cell to sickle at the site of low partial pressure of oxygen.

Pedal manifestations include arthralgia, a very painful symptom that may plague the patient throughout life. There may be punched-out ulcerations around the ankles. There are also neurologic disturbances, which may be due to cerebral thrombosis.

Hand-foot syndrome is a painful swelling of the dorsa of the hands and feet in infancy. This can be most distressing to the parents. Prevention is only possible through genetic counseling. Treatment is symptomatic and must include the control of pain as well as the treatment of any causes of diminished partial pressure of oxygen.

DIABETES MELLITUS

The inherited disease of diabetes mellitus is a disorder of carbohydrate metabolism. There is an intolerance to carbohydrates owing to a relative or absolute insufficiency of insulin. This may occur at any age. The disease may be aggravated by poor dietary management as well as obesity, infection, and other stressors. There are two general types of diabetes mellitus. Type I is insulin dependent, and type II is non–insulin dependent.

Although there remains some controversy over the effects of tight control, it is believed by most that maintenance of serum glucose levels to close to normal values will improve the long-term outlook for the diabetic.

There are many common and notable problems that arise from diabetes, including visual disturbances, neuropathy, nephropathy, and other systemic effects. The pedal manifestations occur within a triad of pathways: ischemia, neuropathy, and infection. Ischemic changes are often seen in the lower extremity as a loss of hair, thickened nails, shiny tight skin, and atrophy of subcutaneous fat. The examiner may then note temperature differences, specifically cold feet, the absence of pulses, and blanching on elevation. The dependent rubor that can be seen at the end of the examination also represents this small to medium-sized vessel disease that is so often a part of diabetes.

Neuropathy is an especially frustrating part of this disease. It may be painful but is usually anesthetizing. This sets the stage for a multitude of battles to defend the legs and feet from injury and loss. Ulcerations from pressure seem to develop instantaneously. There may be large ulcers that go unnoticed until there is drainage onto socks or bedclothes. Neurotrophic ulcers characteristically are painless and often have a white halo surrounding the margins. The treatment for these pedal manifestations includes thorough physical examination, nonvascular studies when indicated, close contact and frequent communication with other members of the health care team (especially the diabetologist), and close monitoring of serum glucose levels.

THYROID DISEASE

Graves' disease is the result of hyperplasia of the thyroid parenchyma. This results in excessive secretion of thyroid hormones. The metabolic rate is greatly increased when this occurs. Exophthalamos is the most frequently noted outward sign of the disease, causing much distress for the patient.

The pedal manifestations are related to the increase in the thyroid hormones and include increased perspiration of the feet, erythema, pruritus, increased hair growth, pretibial myxedema, and nail changes. The nails may show the appearance of Beau's lines, may be unusually small (onychtrophia) but of normal color and thickness, and may also be embedded in the ungualabia. Oddly, another manifestation may be large dystrophic nails with a characteristic gray-yellow powdery appearance.

Treatment of this disease consists of radioactive sodium iodine if the patient is older than 40, surgical removal of parenchyma, or propylthiouracil and methimazole. The concomitant use of beta-blockers may be included to relieve symptoms of adrenergic stimulation.

Hypothyroidism/myxedema is the body's reaction to the lack of thyroid hormones. It may result from the treatment of hyperthyroidism as primary hypothyroidism or as a secondary manifestation of pituitary hypofunction. Personality changes, an enlarged tongue, and a deepening voice herald the onset. The pedal manifestations include slowing Achilles tendon reflexes, dry skin, and pretibial myxedema.

LIVER DISEASE

The liver is responsible for many complex degradative, detoxifying, and biotransforming processes. Because of this vast array of functions the manifestations of disease in the liver can be quite pervasive as well as nonspecific. It is therefore important for the clinician to perform a very accurate review of systems as well as an astute interrogation for historical findings.

In the early stages of liver disease a patient may complain of malaise or fatigue. Other symptoms can be changes in sleep patterns, nausea, vomiting, or diarrhea. Men may complain of increased breast size, which is the result of circulating estrogens not inactivated by the diseased liver. Other tumors locally in the breast as well as distant sites will need to be ruled out.

In the lower extremity concurrent with the rest of the body, jaundice may be noted. Jaundice is a yellow-orange or yellow-green appearance to the skin that is a result of an aberration in the production of bile from senescent red blood cells.

Normally the heme ring of a red blood cell is cleaved by heme oxygenase. This converts the heme to biliverdin. The process continues with biliverdin reductase to yield bilirubin. Bilirubin is tightly bound to albumin and goes on to glucuronidation to make it a nontoxic water-soluble product. If there is a failure to release bilirubin from albumin, it will be trapped in tissues. This will be seen as bilirubin serum levels reach approximately 2 mg/dL.

Jaundice may be unobservable in the lower

extremities of darkly pigmented patients. In this instance the sclera may be icteric. The patient may have reported a concurrent lightening of the color of stools with a darkening of the urine. Another significant complaint will be that of pruritus. Intense itching may result in excoriations noted on the legs and feet and elsewhere on the body.

Because of alterations in cholesterol and lipid metabolism, a xanthoma may appear. A xanthoma presenting on the lower extremity, as in other parts of the body, will be one of five types. In its nodular form it is a tumorous lesion on the Achilles, patellar, or digital extensor tendons. Historical information is important since associated familial coronary artery disease is often acknowledged. Xanthomas may be seen as papular lesions on the thigh or buttocks or as linear lesions of the skin creases on the foot or leg. Other forms also exist but are seen more extensively outside the region of the lower extremities. Any form of recurring Achilles tendonitis, especially in females, with an associated xanthoma may be a warning that liver disease exists.

HUMAN IMMUNODEFICIENCY VIRUS INFECTION AND ACQUIRED IMMUNODEFICIENCY SYNDROME

Our understanding of the acquired immunodeficiency syndrome (AIDS) is continually expanding and changing. As this knowledge base evolves, better treatment for those affected and preventive measures will also take form.

The disease is caused by the human immunodeficiency virus (HIV), which is a retrovirus with the unique ability to attack the very core of the human immune system—the T4 helper cell. T-helper lymphocytes direct the other cells in the immune system to function. Ironically the virus uses the host's own genetic apparatus to reproduce itself. It does so using reverse transcriptase. This reproduces DNA from RNA correctly but backward. Thus the infected cell dies and along with it, albeit slowly at first, the immune system of the host.

The virus is transmitted through the exchange or contact with body fluids, especially blood. This makes shared needles among drug users one of the most dangerous practices.

One motivation for this behavior is the potential for injecting any drug left behind in the needle or syringe from previous use. Thus the contaminants also left behind are introduced directly into the circulatory system. Transmission can occur through other contacts with body fluids as in intimate sexual acts, from mother to infant, or from direct inoculation by sharp instruments or needles used in health care.

After infection the person may not test positive for the antibodies to the virus for weeks or months. The patient may experience flulike symptoms that subside quickly as the immune system attacks the virus. The symptoms may be so slight or of such a transient nature that the patient will hardly suspect any problem exists.

In general, there is a latent period when no outward signs of disease exist. This period often lasts 5 years or more, although it can be much shorter.

The first alarm may be a rare form of pneumonia caused by *Pneumocystis carinii*. This type of pneumonia is frequently the cause of death. Other opportunistic infections may appear, such as thrush, herpes zoster, or leukoplakia, which are often accompanied by night sweats, fatigue, weight loss, and diarrhea.

In the lower extremity the patient with AIDS presents with an especially rare form of onychomycosis known as proximal subungual onychomycosis. This lesion appears as a whitebrown area on the nail plate that eventually spreads across the entire nail.

Another common lower-extremity manifestation is Kaposi's sarcoma. This neoplasm is otherwise rare, especially outside certain African areas, and is not found in children. The population most often afflicted are renal transplant patients, elderly men of Mediterranean ancestry, and Jewish men. This malignancy begins as a dark purple or blue nodule on the feet or ankles. Occasionally it will be plaquelike instead of nodular. The lesions orient along cleavage lines to make oval papules and may insinuate themselves along any organ pathway including the gastrointestinal tract, respiratory tract, and lymphatics. Homosexual men with HIV appear to have a 20-fold higher incidence of Kaposi's sarcoma as compared with other HIV-infected persons.

HIV-infected persons may also develop peripheral neuropathy. In the lower extremity this is usually a distal symmetric polyneuropathy. It is strikingly similar to the diabetic polyneuropathy, presenting with a stocking-glove distribution of numbness, tingling, or other dysesthesias. Patients may also present with a Guillain-Barré–like motor neuropathy. This syndrome is short term, usually occurring while the patient is fighting some other opportunistic infection. There will be a generalized paralysis that gradually subsides. Supportive measures such as respiratory ventilation may be needed during this critical time.

Other forms of neurologic disturbance may also present in the lower extremity. Spinal cord dysfunction, although much less common, is alarming to the patient. The lower extremity will be hyperreflexive and spastic. The abdominal reflexes may be absent. Stroking of the plantar surface of the foot will cause a plantarward contraction of the foot (Babinski's sign).

Any other disease processes of the lower extremity will be magnified by the immunodepression associated with AIDS. Verrucae may manifest as massive warty protuberances or multiple mosaic warts. Treatment is extremely difficult. It is suggested that the CO_2 laser may be the best choice in the treatment of verrucae in the patient with AIDS.

Psoriasis may present for the first time in the person's history. Folliculitis may erupt with organisms resistant to penicillin. In short, any disease affecting the lower extremity may become a problem for the patient with AIDS and may be resistant to treatment.

SMOKING OF TOBACCO PRODUCTS

The use of tobacco in any of its many forms has long been associated with disease. In general, once a person has begun using tobacco products there are psychological and physiological imperatives to continue. The power of this addiction is often substantiated anecdotally by the familiar recounting of patients who have had a laryngectomy but continue to smoke through a tracheostomy.

The effects of long-term use of tobacco are only now being fully appreciated. Many years of research on animal models were rejected by the industry and the public at first. However, the repeated efforts of science and the office of the Surgeon General have finally sparked the awareness of the dangers of smoking.

Inhaled smoke from a cigarette contains many different chemicals. Most of these are by themselves considered dangerous. Carbon monoxide, formaldehyde, cyanide, and nicotine are the most notorious chemicals associated with tobacco smoke. When a person inhales smoke from the cigarette, the lung quickly absorbs the nicotine into the bloodstream to satisfy the smoker's addiction. The heart rate increases, the blood pressure rises, and the oxygen saturation of the blood drops precipitously. The extremities are immediately cooled because blood flow to the hands and feet is decreased.

The gases inhaled in cigarette smoking cause an increase in turbulent blood flow that allows for intimal damage and aids in plaque formation. It is also suggested that cigarette smoking keeps levels of triglycerides as well as low-density lipoproteins elevated. This adds to vessel occlusion and further increases in turbulent flow. This will be seen in the lower extremity as the diminution of pedal pulses, an increase in capillary filling time, and temperature changes. The patient may report periods of intermittant claudication.

Another devastating disease found in smokers is thromboangiitis obliterans. Also known as Buerger's disease, this disease is most often found in men aged 20 to 40 years who smoke cigarettes; it is rare to see this disease in women. The disease has been suggested to have a genetic link, since there is a prevalence of HLA-A9 and HLA-B5 phenotypes in these persons.

The small and medium-sized arteries, and in some instances the superficial veins, are damaged in the extremities. The first complaints are usually minor but soon progress to gangrene at the most distal tips of the extremities.

Pathologically, lymphocytes invade the intimal layer of the vessel. Endothelial cells proliferate, and a thrombus is formed. The patient may confide that there is a past history of phlebitis of the foot and/or leg veins. There may also be persistent coldness, tingling, or other kinds of dysesthesia. As the ischemia increases, the pain worsens and ulcerations appear. Pulses in one or more of the pedal arteries will probably be absent. The color of the foot will be pale on elevation and ruborous when returned to a dependent state.

Noninvasive vascular examination in the office setting is extremely useful in determining the extent of the impairment and to provide a baseline for further treatment and referral to a vascular surgeon when indicated. Arterial examinations most often employed are bidirectional Doppler studies, ankle-arm indexes, pulse volume recordings, and photoplethysmography.

The ankle-arm, or ankle-brachial, index is the systolic pressure taken at the ankle over the systolic pressure taken at the arm as one would measure any blood pressure. This fraction then indicates the severity of the disease. There are slight differences in the several scales used to interpret the ankle-arm index because of the variables involved in performing the test. It is a screening test and is used to determine the need for further arterial studies. It is not meant to render a definitive diagnosis. The following scale is recommended:

Normal: 1.0 or greater
Mild arterial disease: .76–.99
Moderate arterial disease: .51–.75
Severe arterial disease: below .50

The patient with thromboangiitis obliterans must be aided in the effort to completely stop smoking before any treatment is hoped to be of value. The patient should begin a walking program. A properly fitted shoe should be worn, and walking should be indoors whenever weather is inclement since cold exposure would be extremely detrimental. The patient should walk at least 25 minutes a day or 15 minutes twice a day to begin.

At night it may be helpful to use a semi-Fowler's position or to elevate the head end of the bed. This positioning may aid in arterial filling and prevent symptoms.

Regularly scheduled continous podiatric care must be given to prevent potentially devastating pedal injury. Frequent examinations, instruction in self-examination to be done daily by the patient, as well as proper padding can be immensely useful.

Most medications used in the past are ineffective in treating this problem. Some relatively new drugs may, however, be beneficial, such as pentoxifyline, some calcium channel blockers, and some of the thromboxane inhibitors.

BIBLIOGRAPHY

Arterial Doppler. IMEX 9000 systems manual, 1990.

Bodman M: Dermatology Lecture Notes. OCPM, 1992.

Cotran RS, Kumar V, Robbins SL (eds): Robbins Pathologic Basis of Disease, ed 4. Philadelphia, WB Saunders, 1989.

Fitzpatrick TB: Color Atlas and Synopsis of Clinical Dermatology. NY, McGraw-Hill Information Service Co, 1991.

Guyton AC: Textbook of Medical Physiology, ed 8. Philadelphia, WB Saunders, 1991.

Kompus D: Pedal Manifestations of HIV. Unpublished manuscript. OCPM, 1992.

Levy L, Hetherington VJ: Principles and Practice of Podiatric Medicine. New York, Churchill Livingston, 1990.

Merck Manual. Merck, Sharpe & Dohme Research Laboratory, Rahway, NJ, 1987.

Rakel RE: Textbook of Family Practice, ed 4. Philadelphia, WB Saunders, 1990.

CHAPTER 15

THE DIABETIC FOOT

William F. Todd
Todd Laughner
Brad G. Samojla

Diabetes mellitus is a multifaceted disease characterized by hyperglycemia and glucose intolerance caused by inadequate insulin utilization or faulty insulin production. Unfortunately, there are many other diseases associated with diabetes mellitus, including hypertension, peripheral vascular disease, coronary heart disease, and hypercholesterolemia. This results in retinopathies, nephropathy, and neuropathy. Despite the increased morbidity associated with diabetes, many persons can, with proper medical and personal care, go on living an enjoyable and productive life. Therefore, it is the purpose of this chapter to discuss the disease and treatments of its manifestations, so that primary care physicians may help their patients live as normal a life as possible.

The disease of diabetes mellitus can be described as a large circle. A point on the circle represents the beginning of the disease. As one moves around the circle, in the untreated patient, manifestations of the disease can represent points or parts of that circle. The circle ends with the death of the patient, usually as a complication of diabetes. As physicians our goal is to determine where the patient is on that circle and then to intervene and care for that patient. We must realize that to achieve this goal, podiatrists cannot and should not do this alone. To effectively manage a diabetic patient, the podiatrist must have a thorough understanding of the disease and be willing to be part of a diabetic management team. Besides a podiatrist, the team must include a diabetologist and vascular surgeon and may include pedorthists and social workers.

DISEASE TYPES

Historically, *diabetes mellitus* was a descriptive term used to characterize a collection of symptoms that followed a predictable and catastrophic course; however, over the past 30 years a more rigorous definition of diabetes has emerged. What follows is a brief description of the classification of diabetes mellitus as set forth by the National Diabetes Data Group (NDDG) and the World Health Organization (WHO).[1-3]

During the late 1970s and through the mid 1980s the NDDG and WHO established a classification system for diabetes mellitus.[1, 3] Furthermore, data they collected throughout this time clearly showed that diabetes mellitus is an etiologically and clinically heterogeneous group of disorders that share glucose intolerance in common. In general, their classification system has three groups of patients: (1) those with overt disease who have either fasting hyperglycemia or elevated plasma glucose levels after an oral glucose tolerance test; (2) an at-risk group, which is defined only by an oral glucose tolerance test in which there is an elevated plasma glucose level but not one that is elevated enough to be considered overt disease; and (3) an at-risk group with currently normal plasma glucose levels after an oral glucose tolerance test.

Insulin-Dependent Diabetes Mellitus

Type I, or insulin-dependent, diabetes mellitus (IDDM; formerly called juvenile-onset diabetes) has an abrupt onset in persons typically younger than 30 years old. Although the peak age at diagnosis is between 11 and 13 years of age, 32% of patients are diagnosed with IDDM after the age of 30.[4]

At the time of diagnosis, patients present with a sudden onset of severe symptoms that have been present from only a few days to a few weeks. The classic description of the presentation of IDDM is that of polyuria, polyphagia, polydipsia, and weight loss. However, it is much more likely that these patients present with only one or a few of the classic "polys." Because persons with IDDM are prone to diabetic ketoacidosis, this potential life-threatening problem may be the initial presentation. Most often, patients with IDDM are not obese; however, when they are, assignment into this group can be difficult.

IDDM is characterized by little, if any, circulating insulin (insulinopenia), and exogenous insulin is required for maintenance of life. After the beginning of treatment, some patients with IDDM may go into a period of remission that requires little if any exogenous insulin. This "honeymoon" period may last for weeks or even months but always results in an absolute requirement for insulin. After the honeymoon period, the patient often requires greater amounts of insulin than what was required before the remission. In a few persons resistance to exogenous insulin may occur.

Non–Insulin-Dependent Diabetes Mellitus

Type II, or non–insulin-dependent diabetes mellitus (NIDDM; formerly referred to as adult-onset diabetes), occurs in persons usually older than 30 years of age (average age at diagnosis is between 61 and 64 years).[4-6] Typically, the onset of symptoms in NIDDM is so gradual that the patient may not even be aware that a medical problem exists. In a study by Harris and coworkers,[6] it was estimated that diabetic retinopathy is present from 4 to 7 years before the diagnosis of NIDDM. Also, it is estimated that retinopathy occurs approximately 5 years after the onset of NIDDM.[7] Therefore, Harris and coworkers concluded that NIDDM may have an onset 9 to 12 years before diagnosis of the disease.[6]

Typically, patients with NIDDM present to their physician with a history of polyuria, polydipsia, polyphagia, fatigue, weight loss, dizziness, headaches, and blurred vision. Occasionally, they may present with more advanced complications of NIDDM, such as blindness, renal failure, cardiovascular disease, peripheral vascular disease, and neuropathy. Although some of these patients may have an initial weight loss, it is important to note that 50% to 90% of all patients with NIDDM are obese (>20% ideal body weight); therefore, NIDDM is further subclassified into obese and nonobese NIDDM.[8]

Non–insulin-dependent diabetics are resistant to their own insulin, and as a result they may have normal circulating insulin levels or mild insulinopenia or may even exhibit hyperinsulinemia. These patients are not dependent on exogenous insulin and may be treated with various sulfonylureas, diet, and exercise. Between 3% and 5% of persons in this group will eventually develop complete insulin deficiency.[8, 9] These persons are referred to as having insulin-requiring NIDDM and will require exogenous insulin to control hyperglycemia. Ketoacidosis may occur in NIDDM during periods of extreme stress.

Gestational Diabetes Mellitus

Gestational diabetes mellitus is an uncommon disorder that affects approximately 3% of all pregnancies.[6] This disease appears only in pregnancy and is usually a mild form and not life threatening to the woman. However, if this disease does occur, there is an increased risk for the woman to develop NIDDM later in life. According to the NDDG and WHO criteria, women with gestational diabetes mellitus, after parturition, should be reclassified as diabetic, as having impaired glucose intolerance, or simply as having a previous abnormality of glucose intolerance (most women are reclassified into this group).[6]

Impaired Glucose Tolerance

Persons whose fasting blood glucose levels are not high enough to qualify as a diabetic (i.e., less than 140 mg/dL) and whose oral glucose tolerance test (75 g of carbohydrate administered after a 12-hour fast, then plasma glucose measured 2 hours postprandially) results in a measured glucose level between normal and diabetic are classified as being impaired glucose tolerant. These patients have been previously known as "borderline," "subclinical," and "asymptomatic." This class is not defined by any clinical manifestation, only by plasma glucose criteria, and an oral glucose tolerance test is mandatory to place a patient into this category. The prognostic significance of impaired glucose tolerance is not fully understood; however, about one third of patients go on to develop diabetes in 5 to 10 years. The remaining two thirds revert back to normal glucose tolerance levels or remain with impaired glucose tolerance. Because persons with impaired glucose tolerance are at a greater risk of developing diabetes than the general population, this disorder should not be taken lightly.

High-Risk Classes

There appear to be at least several different groups that are at an increased risk of developing diabetes. The NDDG and WHO have classified these patients into two general at-risk groups.[3, 6] Both of these groups are characterized by normal fasting and oral glucose tolerance test glucose levels. The first group at risk for the development of diabetes includes those persons who have a history of diabetic hyperglycemia or impaired glucose tolerance but currently have normal glucose tolerance. These persons are known as having a previous abnormality of glucose tolerance and have spontaneously, or in response to a specific stimulus, reverted back to normal glucose tolerance. Persons within this group include gestational diabetics, obese diabetics who after losing weight are now normoglycemic, diabetics (or hyperglycemia) secondary to acute metabolic stress, and those who have been previously classified as having impaired glucose tolerance. Although there are few data to suggest otherwise, it is generally believed that if these persons are subjected to the same stress, they will again become diabetic or have impaired glucose tolerance.

The second group, known as having potential abnormality of glucose intolerance, is simply a statistical risk group of persons who have never exhibited abnormal glucose tolerance. These persons are at a higher risk than the general population for the development of diabetes. Persons who are at a higher risk for developing NIDDM include (in decreasing order of risk) the monozygotic twin of a patient with NIDDM; sibling, parent, or child of a patient with NIDDM; obese persons; mothers of neonates weighing more than 4 kg; and members of racial or ethnic groups with a high prevalence of diabetes, including Native Americans, South Pacific populations, and, to a lesser extent, Hispanic, blacks, and Maltese. Those persons at an increased risk for development of IDDM include persons with islet cell antibodies; the monozygotic twin of a patient with IDDM (HLA identical, HLA haploid, HLA nonidentical); and a child of a patient with IDDM. Although these persons have an increased chance of developing diabetes, the degree of risk is not well established. Furthermore, it needs to be stressed that the previous or potential abnormality of glucose tolerance is not a diagnosis. Persons should be placed into one of these two groups for epidemiologic purposes only.

INCIDENCE AND PREVALENCE

In 1987, 6.82 million persons in the United States were known to have diabetes, with an estimated equal number remaining undiagnosed.[10, 11] Between 1980 and 1987, diabetes increased by nearly 10% from 25.4 to 27.6 per 1000 residents.[11] During this 7-year period, diabetes was more prevalent in black than white males and almost twice as prevalent in black than white females.[11] Also, the age-standardized prevalence in blacks was higher by 33%.[11]

Complications from diabetes mellitus (i.e., infection) account for roughly 45% of all nontraumatic amputations in the United States and roughly 85% of all lower-extremity amputations from nonischemic causes.[12, 13]

IDDM. Worldwide incidence of diabetes varies greatly, with Finland having the highest incidence and Japan having the lowest.[14] Interestingly, worldwide, especially in rural United States, there is a dramatic seasonal variation in the clinical onset of IDDM, with the lowest incidence during the spring and summer and the highest incidence in the autumn and winter.[14]

NIDDM. NIDDM accounts for nearly 90% of all diabetics, and in some populations it is the only form of diabetes.[6] The main problem with studying NIDDM in the past has been inconsistent criteria used worldwide. The highest prevalence of NIDDM in the world can be found in the Pima Indians of Arizona (30% of adults).[14] Furthermore, it has been proposed that this high prevalence is a relatively new phenomenon, being present only since after World War II.[14] The next highest rate has been found in the Micronesian populations, which approaches the Pima Indian rate. High rates have been shown in migrant populations in South Africa, Trinidad, Singapore, and the United Kingdom and in Mexican Americans and Japanese.

In 1987, Harris and colleagues[10] studied the prevalence of diabetes and impaired glucose tolerance in the United States in persons between the ages of 20 and 74 years. These researchers did not characterize diabetic patients (as IDDM or NIDDM); therefore, based solely on the age of their study population, the results were more likely skewed toward NIDDM. What they found was that almost an equal number of persons, when randomly studied, had diabetes but were not previously diagnosed and were unaware of the fact they had diabetes. Furthermore, they clearly showed that diabetes was more prevalent in the elderly. For instance, 2.0% of the US population between the ages of 20 and 44 are diabetic, as compared with 17.7% between the ages of 65 and 74. Also this study showed that black Americans are at an increased risk of developing diabetes (3.1% in ages 20 to 44; 25.9% in ages 65 to 74). Finally, 4.6% of the population in the United States exhibit impaired glucose tolerance, which is more common in the elderly.

MORBIDITY

Wetterhall and coworkers studied the trends in diabetes along with specific complications.[11] Their data reveal that age-standardized mortality rates (for diabetes) have declined between 1980 and 1986 (2350 to 2066 per 100,000, respectively) and morbidity associated with diabetes has increased. For example, statistically of 1000 diabetic persons 133 are hospitalized for cardiovascular disease, 58.4 for ischemic heart disease, and 18.8 for stroke. In 1980, approximately 36,000 persons with diabetes had lower-extremity amputations, while in 1987 this figure rose to 56,000. The age-standardized rate, for this time period, rose from 6.3 to 8.1 per 1000 persons with males (8.8/1000) being more likely to undergo an amputation than females (8.1/1000). Race comparisons reveal that black diabetics (9.0/1000) are more likely to have an amputation as compared with white diabetics (6.3/1000).

DIABETES AND AGING

Approximately 40% of persons older than the age of 65 to 74 years have impaired glucose tolerance or diabetes. By the time a person reaches 80 years of age, the prevalence rises to 50%.[15] The number of elderly persons is increasing dramatically in the United States, where it is estimated that one fifth of the US population will be older than 65 by the year 2020.[15] Treatment of diabetes mellitus and management of its complications are made more complex by the fact that aging is associated with the development of chronic illness. In many instances, an elderly person will suffer from several chronic illness that requires a variety of medications, taken at several times throughout the day. Finally, social, economic, and psychological problems can result in a very difficult situation to adequately manage an elderly diabetic patient. Despite these seemingly insurmountable problems, with proper planning and a team approach, some of these problems can be minimized.

DIABETIC PATHOLOGY

Diabetes mellitus is a disease with interrelated metabolic, vascular, and neuropathic components. The metabolic derangements are characterized by one common feature—hyperglycemia. Hyperglycemia is a result of abnormal metabolism of carbohydrate, fat, and protein, secondary to irregularities of insulin secretion or use.

A process called hyperglycemic memory may contribute to many of the complications in both persons with IDDM and those with NIDDM. Hyperglycemic memory is a concept that refers to persistence or progression of hyperglycemia-induced pathology during periods of normoglycemia.[16] This memory may be an advanced glycation end-product that permanently alters tissue macromolecules.[16]

Dermatologic Disease

Lower-extremity cutaneous manifestations of diabetes are numerous and vary from trivial to life threatening. A few of the cutaneous manifestations may aid in the early diagnosis of diabetes, while others occur as a secondary finding to the disease.

Approximately 30% of diabetic patients demonstrate cutaneous signs during the course of the disease.[17, 18] Certain cutaneous disorders are noted to commonly occur in the diabetic patient. Diabetic dermopathy and necrobiosis lipoidica diabeticorum were thought to be pathognomonic for diabetes; however, these skin conditions were found to be present in nondiabetic subjects as well.[13, 19–21]

Diabetic dermopathy (shin spots) is a common cutaneous finding in diabetic patients.[19] These lesions are usually found on the anterior tibial region and may disappear after 1 or 2 years. These lesions are oval, flat-topped, dull, red, hyperpigmented papules that may be single or grouped. The risk of ulceration of this lesion is very small.

Necrobiosis lipoidica diabeticorum was once thought to be a skin lesion unique to the diabetic that occurs in approximately 0.3% of diabetics.[20–22] Since this disorder may precede the diagnosis of diabetes, its presence warrants further examination. Necrobiosis lipoidica diabeticorum occurs on the lower extremities and is often bilateral. The lesions are initially well-circumscribed red papules that present as a fine scale. These lesions extend radially and have hard, depressed, waxy, atrophic centers. The periphery of these lesions is raised and may be red-blue. A complication of this lesion is a superficial ulceration.[17, 19]

Vascular Disease

Vascular disease in the diabetic person is the major cause of morbidity and mortality.[23] Not only is vascular disease responsible for death from myocardial infarction and stroke, but it is also a major cause of limb loss.[23] Persons with NIDDM are two to four times more likely to develop coronary heart disease and suffer from its complications than the general population.[23, 24] In men with NIDDM, peripheral vascular disease occurs in between 27 and 47 per 1000 persons; in women with NIDDM, the occurrence is between 19 and 29 per 1000 persons.[25] Others have estimated that peripheral vascular disease occurs in approximately 3.2% of the diabetic population.[26] Comparatively, insulin-dependent diabetics have a cardiovascular mortality rate that is 11 times higher than the general population.[27] Although many studies have shown increased risk factor profiles for the diabetic patient, these studies have failed to show that diabetes itself is a risk factor.[24] Furthermore, the pathogenic process appears to be quite different between persons with IDDM and NIDDM.

IDDM AND VASCULAR DISEASE

Location

In general, diabetes causes an increased risk of developing atherosclerotic disease; however, the reasons for this increased risk are not well understood. Epidemiologic studies have attempted to explain the increased incidence of cardiovascular disease seen in diabetes.[24] What has emerged is a relationship between the development of vascular disease and the presence of renal disease.[24]

Although little data exist that reveal the incidence or prevalence of lower-extremity artery disease in IDDM populations, it does appear that lower-extremity arterial disease is rare before the age of 25.[24] After 25 years, a threefold increase is seen as measured by the ankle-brachial index (ABI); persons with an ABI of 0.80 or less were considered to have arterial disease. In another study, all persons with an ABI of less than 0.8 did not complain of intermittent claudication (as measured by the Rose questionnaire).[27] The fact that these persons did not feel intermittent claudication is most likely because of peripheral neuropathy. If macrovascular disease was purely a result of the diabetic process, then all locations of the vascular system would be affected equally. These findings suggest that there are some common manifestations of macrovascular disease and that different pathologic processes are probably responsible for the disease appearing in the various locations.[24]

Pathogenesis

According to Donahue and Orchard,[24] IDDM may be involved in contributing to cardiovascular disease in one of four ways: (1) it may initiate the atherosclerotic process earlier; (2) it may accelerate the process once it has started; (3) it may cause a greater severity in the disease; or (4) a combination of these factors may occur. Evidence from other studies indicates that IDDM accelerates the athero-

sclerotic process rather than initiating the process.[28]

Very little data are available to determine predictors of atherosclerotic disease in IDDM. Although glycosylated hemoglobin and blood glucose levels indicate the level of diabetes, they are not good markers for arterial disease.[24] Some markers have been identified for lower-extremity arterial disease and include low-density and high-density lipoprotein cholesterol levels and triglyceride/apoprotein A1 ratios.[24]

Nephropathy is more common in IDDM than NIDDM: it is present in about 25% of persons with IDDM and 8% of those with NIDDM.[23] Data show that cardiovascular mortality associated with IDDM is related to the presence of proteinuria.[29] This relationship led to the formation of the Steno (Clinic) hypothesis, which states that there is a subgroup of persons with IDDM who have a genetic predisposition to renal disease and that this predisposition causes an increased risk of cardiovascular disease and other complications.[30] This process leads to microalbuminuria, which ultimately results in vascular damage. Central to this theory is enzyme malfunction involved in heparan sulfate metabolism, which leads to altered connective tissue damage, resulting in renal and vascular disease. Lipoprotein lipase activity is altered; thus, characteristic lipoprotein disturbances occur, leading to cardiovascular disease. The usual cardiovascular disease risk factors (high blood pressure, increased lipid levels, and smoking) are still operative, but other defects (glycosylation and oxidation of lipoproteins, lipoprotein compositional changes, platelet aggregation, and clotting factors) also contribute in varying degrees to vascular disease.[16] Although the Steno hypothesis nicely explains a relationship between renal disease and macrovascular disease, parts of it are being challenged.[24]

NIDDM AND VASCULAR DISEASE

Location

In persons with NIDDM, studies indicate that elevated glucose levels significantly increase the risk for coronary heart disease. These patients tend to be older, weigh more, have higher systolic blood pressure, and have triglyceride concentrations with lower HDL concentrations. Central obesity, a predictor of congestive heart disease in men and women, is also seen in persons with NIDDM. Hyperinsulinemia is a concomitant finding of central obesity. It has been postulated that insulin resistance may be the common feature that associates atherosclerosis, coronary heart disease, and NIDDM.[24] Elevated insulin levels have been shown to predict the development of coronary heart disease in men with NIDDM.[24] Since insulin levels are difficult to measure, the relationship of C-peptide to coronary heart disease has been studied. The C-peptide value is in fact elevated in men with NIDDM with coronary heart disease as compared with men with NIDDM without heart disease. Therefore, interventions, such as exercise and weight loss, that reduce insulin levels or increase insulin sensitivity should reduce the risk of developing coronary heart disease.

Pathogenesis

Macroangiopathy, according to Campbell,[23] is no different in persons with NIDDM than in the general population. A major difference between the general population and diabetic groups is the anatomic locations at which plaques develop. In NIDDM, microvascular disease (retinopathy, basement membrane thickening) and metabolic derangements are less frequent, with macrovascular disease being more frequent and not responsive to the control of glycemia. In IDDM, neuropathy and metabolic disorders are more prominent, followed by rapid progression of disease.

The risk factors for the development and progression of arterial disease in the person with NIDDM include genetics, age, hypertension, cigarette smoking, hypercholesterolemia, and diabetes.[23, 24, 31-33] Eight percent of adult patients with diabetes have arterial disease when their diabetes is diagnosed, and this increases to 45% after 20 years.[34] Some authors believe that ischemic changes in the diabetic are caused by autonomic neuropathy, which results in abnormal arteriovenous shunting.[23, 35] The blood flow then bypasses the capillary beds, resulting in tissue ischemia. This tissue ischemia can lead to skin changes, ulceration, infection, and eventual amputation. The prac-

titioner should perform a vascular examination of each diabetic patient; however, it should not be assumed that each diabetic patient has peripheral vascular disease. In diabetics with lower-extremity arterial disease there is a greater tendency toward tibial and peroneal artery disease.[36] Also, medial calcinosis, which is calcification within the tunica media of small to large arteries, is commonly seen in diabetics.

The development of the atherosclerotic plaque is believed to be accelerated in diabetic populations.[24, 28, 37] Initiation of an atherosclerotic plaque occurs in regions of the arterial system, where hemodynamic forces provide shearing stresses against the wall of the artery.[28] This usually occurs where there is a reversing blood flow and stagnation of the blood. There is an aggregation of platelet and monocytes, with release of platelet-derived factors. This, in turn, stimulates smooth muscle growth and deposition of lipoproteins. Release of free radicals results in modification of these deposited molecules, which ultimately continues the deposition of more lipoproteins. Diabetes will alter many aspects of this process. Some of the processes that lead to an accelerated deposition of plaques include defective phagocytosis, impaired leukocyte function, increased platelet adhesion, and glycosylated proteins, which contribute to the formation of abnormally rigid proteins.[28]

Neurologic Disease

ETIOLOGY

Although many investigators have attempted to classify diabetic neuropathy based on clinical, pathologic, etiologic, or topographic categories, it is perhaps best described as a complex of syndromes with peripheral and autonomic nerve degeneration.[38-44] The etiology and pathogenesis of diabetic neuropathy is a subject of active research and debate. There are two prominent theories that have been proposed to cause diabetic neuropathy: the vascular theory and the metabolic theory.[41, 43] Both theories assume hyperglycemia as the foundation of causing neuropathy. In the metabolic theory, hyperglycemia directly results in nerve pathology; while in the vascular hypothesis, hyperglycemia results in vascular damage that eventually results in ischemic nerve damage. Although researchers from both groups continue to argue over which is more correct, other etiologic factors are being identified that may be as crucial to the pathogenesis of diabetic neuropathy.[16, 43] Therefore, it appears that no single mechanism is responsible for the development of diabetic neuropathy (Fig. 15–1).

Vascular Hypothesis

The vascular theory in the pathogenesis of diabetic neuropathy states that there is a decreased blood supply to nerves, which leads to nerve hypoxia and subsequent multifocal nerve degeneration.[43, 45] This theory is based on studies showing microvascular damage to the vasa nervorum in diabetics.[43, 46] Early studies showed hyperplasia in the walls of the small neural blood vessels in diabetic neuropathy.[46] Other studies confirmed these data and reported a thickening in the basal laminae of the small neural blood vessels.[47, 48] This basal lamina hyperplasia was found to be common

in chronic neuropathies but was statistically greater in diabetic subjects.[47, 48] Although some studies found intraluminal deposits of fibrin with occlusion of the neural blood vessels, others theorized that the distribution of axonal degeneration was indicative of embolization.[39, 40, 49] More recently, Yasuda and Dyck[50] showed not only that blood vessel basement membrane was thicker in diabetics but also that there was a positive association with the severity of the disease. Also, endothelial hyperplasia was found, which corresponded to the severity of disease.[50] Vascular disease is a likely mechanism for the development of a diabetic mononeuropathy but is a controversial mechanism for the development of other types of diabetic neuropathy.[39, 41, 42, 45, 51] Critics of the vascular hypothesis cite problems with many of the studies and question if the changes seen within vessels are reactive or primary to the disease.[36]

Metabolic Hypothesis

The metabolic hypothesis states that chronic hyperglycemia activates the sorbitol (polyol) pathway, leading to increased accumulation of

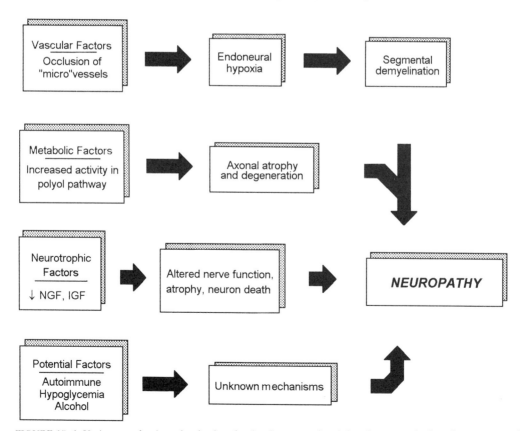

FIGURE 15–1. Various mechanisms that lead to the development of peripheral neuropathy have been proposed.

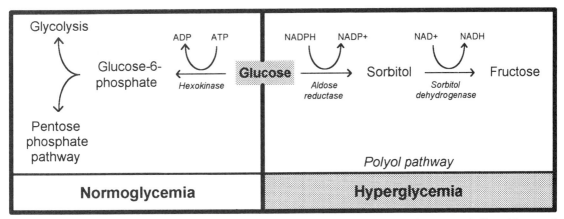

FIGURE 15–2. The polyol pathway. The left side of the diagram is the primary route for glucose metabolism with normal blood glucose levels. In states of hyperglycemia, glucose metabolism is shifted into an alternative pathway—the polyol pathway. In the polyol pathway, the rate-limiting step is the conversion of glucose to sorbitol by aldose reductase.

sorbitol with an associated depletion of myoinositol and reduced sodium–potassium adenosine triphosphatase (Na^+–K^+ ATPase) activity in the peripheral nerves.[41, 43] The polyol pathway is an alternative pathway for the utilization of glucose that consists of two enzymatic reactions that convert nonphosphorylated glucose to sorbitol and then to fructose and the reduced form of nicotinamide adenine dinucleotide (Fig. 15–2). The enzymes of this pathway are believed to be located within the cell protoplasm and are present in many mammalian tissue types, including peripheral nerves. The two enzymes involved in the pathway are aldose reductase and sorbitol dehydrogenase (see Fig. 15–2).[52] Aldose reductase is the limiting enzyme in this pathway.[53]

The activity of polyol pathway appears to be regulated by the intracellular concentrations of glucose. Brain, peripheral nerves, and other tissues that do not require insulin for glucose uptake are dependent solely on the plasma concentration of glucose. When plasma glucose levels are normal there is little need for the polyol pathway, and the concentration of the products from this pathway are low. However, during periods of hyperglycemia, glucose concentration within peripheral nerve increases, which, in turn, increases aldose reductase activity, thus increasing the intracellular concentration of sorbitol and fructose. Little evidence suggests that the accumulation of sorbital is responsible for nerve pathology.[52, 53]

Another molecule related in structure to glucose is myoinositol. Myoinositol is a water-soluble cyclic hexanol that is found throughout the body and in high concentrations. It is either obtained from our diet or synthesized. Myoinositol is used mainly for the synthesis of membrane phospholipids, specifically phosphoinositides. It usually circulates within plasma as a free molecule; then it is filtered and reabsorbed by the kidneys. Oxidation of myoinositol to glucuronic acid takes place within the kidneys. Myoinositol is actively transported into peripheral nerves by a sodium-dependent gradient generated by another transport system—Na^+–K^+ ATPase. The peripheral nerve concentration of myoinositol is usually 90 to 100 times the amount of myoinositol found in the plasma.[54]

In diabetic patients there is an increased amount of myoinositol found within urine, and significantly reduced concentrations occur within peripheral nerves.[54] It has been postulated that during states of hyperglycemia glucose competively binds to the sodium-dependent transport system, thus diminishing the amount of myoinositol transported into the nerve. Also, depletion of intracellular myoinositol appears to be associated with decreased Na^+–K^+ ATPase activity. Diminished Na^+–K^+ ATPase activity results in decreased transport of intracellular Na^+, resulting in high intracellular concentrations of sodium. The high intracellular concentrations of sodium block nodal depolarization and slow nerve conduction velocity.[55] In animal models, rapid normalization of glucose, in short-term diabetes, results in return to normal sodium gradient and function.[55] Similar results have been obtained in patients when normalization of glucose improves nerve conduction velocity and vibratory sense.[56]

How are the polyol pathway and decreased levels of myoinositol related to diabetic neuropathy? This relationship, at best, is poorly understood. Sorbitol, a byproduct of the polyol pathway, does not readily diffuse out of cells. Also, in animal studies, administration of aldose reductase inhibitors has been found to completely prevent diminished intracellular concentrations of myoinositol and diminished $Na^+–K^+$ ATPase activity. Thus, by a mechanism not fully understood, hyperglycemia results in increased polyol pathway activity, which results in myoinositol and $Na^+–K^+$ ATPase derangements.

Another cause of diabetic neuropathy is hypoglycemia. The development of a neuropathy has been reported with insulinoma-related hypoglycemia.[57] The role of hypoglycemia or the mechanism by which hypoglycemia leads to nerve damage is unclear.[43] The possibility of neuropathy induced by an autoimmune response has become increasingly more important. The presence of circulating antibodies may have a role in the pathogenesis of neuropathies associated with amyloidosis and of certain hematologic diseases. Antibodies against various nerves have been isolated, but again their role in the pathogenesis of neuropathy is unclear and is based on circumstantial evidence.[43] These antibodies may play a primary role in the development of neuropathy, or they may be reactive against products of nerve damage.[43]

Within the nervous system there are a number of cells that are dependent on growth factors for development, survival, and possibly regeneration.[58, 59] The neural crest–derived cells, dorsal root neurons, and sympathetic neurons are dependent on nerve growth factor.[60] Interestingly, decreased circulating levels of nerve growth factor have been reported in diabetic patients.[61] Nerve growth factors are also involved in the regulation of substance P synthesis in adult dorsal root ganglions.[62, 63] A variety of animal studies have shown nerve growth factors and insulin-like growth factors responsible for regeneration of nerve tissue.[43, 64] Although the mechanism of action is unknown, nerve growth factors are most likely involved in the pathogenesis of diabetic neuropathy. It is possible that a reduction in the nerve growth factors and insulin-like growth factors results in altered neuron function, atrophy, and possibly cell death, ultimately leading to a neuropathy.[43] Early treatment of neuropathies can be prevented by the administration of nerve growth factor.[65] Clearly, much additional work needs to be done to determine the role of these factors in diabetic neuropathy.

TYPES OF DIABETIC NEUROPATHY

The clinical picture of diabetic neuropathy varies from a painful to a painless form of neuropathy. The type of neuropathy depends on the type of nerve fiber involved. It is therefore useful to review the clinical manifestations of nerve degeneration and the affected nerve components (Table 15–1).

Sensory neuropathy is often an early finding of generalized diabetic neuropathy and has

---

TABLE 15–1. **Types of Diabetic Neuropathy**

Subclinical Neuropathy
Abnormal electrodiagnostic tests: decreased nerve conduction; decreased amplitude of evoked muscle or nerve action potential
Abnormal quantitative sensory testing: vibratory/tactile; thermal warming/cooling
Abnormal autonomic function tests: abnormal/altered cardiovascular reflex; abnormal biochemical response to hypoglycemia

Clinical Neuropathy
Autonomic neuropathy
    Cardiovascular autonomic neuropathy
    Abnormal pupillary function
    Gastrointestinal autonomic neuropathy: gastroparesis; constipation; diabetic diarrhea; anorectal incontinence
    Genitourinary autonomic neuropathy: bladder dysfunction; sexual dysfunction
    Hypoglycemic unawareness/unresponsiveness
    Sudomotor dysfunction
Focal mononeuropathy
    Mononeuropathy
    Mononeuropathy multiplex
    Amyotrophy
Diffuse somatic neuropathy
    Distal symmetric sensorimotor polyneuropathy
        Primary small fiber neuropathy
        Primary large fiber neuropathy
        Mixed fiber neuropathy

been described as the most critical factor in the formation of pedal ulcers.[66, 67] The ability of sensory input to protect the limb deteriorates to a point that mechanical stress, possibly in combination with ischemia, leads to tissue breakdown. This derangement paves the way for severe ulceration and potential infection. The critical point at which the sensory system fails to protect the soft tissue is termed the *protective threshold*.[20, 68] Once the sensory protective threshold is lost, the affected region is at high risk for the mechanical, chemical, and thermal insults.[20] Initially, patients are unaware of any sensory loss, even though they may have already lost over 50% of the nerve endings to the skin.[69]

The protective threshold level cannot be determined by subjective complaints of paresthesias, because patients complaining of paresthesia often have an adequate protective threshold. The use of Semmes-Weinstein monofilament wire probes offers an excellent reproducible means of assessing the protective threshold status and is described in detail later.

Diabetic neuropathy encompasses a wide range of abnormalities affecting both peripheral and autonomic nerve function. There has been much controversy in the literature as to the prevalence of diabetic neuropathy, with an incidence ranging from 5% to 60% in published studies.[41, 43] This wide variation in the reported incidence of this disorder is due largely to difficulty in defining diabetic neuropathy and establishing appropriate guidelines to measure its presence. It is often difficult to ascertain the extent of diabetic neuropathy since the manifestations of this disorder may go unrecognized by the patient and may only be detected by the physician through careful examination. The subtle nonspecific presentation of diabetic neuropathy in many patients is probably the cause of the discrepancy in the incidence reported in the literature. Neuropathy is not confined to a single type of diabetes, but it can occur in both IDDM and NIDDM and various forms of acquired diabetes.[41, 43] Most authors agree that neuropathy is the most common complication affecting persons with diabetes. The effects of this common disorder on the diabetic lower extremity are explored throughout this chapter.

Although many investigators have attempted to classify diabetic neuropathy based on clinical and pathologic, or etiologic, or topographic categories, it is perhaps best described as a "complex of syndromes" with peripheral and autonomic nerve degeneration. Established diabetic neuropathies can be grouped into three broad categories: (1) symmetric polyneuropathy, (2) focal and multifocal neuropathy, and (3) autonomic neuropathy.

Symmetric Distal Sensory Polyneuropathy

A somatic sensory polyneuropathy of insidious onset is by far the most frequent form of peripheral neuropathy presenting in diabetic patients. The onset is usually insidious; however, acute-onset presentations have been reported following stress on initiation of insulin therapy (insulin neuritis).[41] The deficit is predominantly sensory, with lesser involvement in the motor fibers. Brown and coworkers suggested that causes of diabetic sensory neuropathy constitute a spectrum: at one end are the patients with painless distal sensory loss (predominantly loss of position sense and depression of deep tendon reflexes); at the other end of the spectrum are patients with painful neuropathy and autonomic dysfunction with intact tendon reflexes and large fiber sensory modalities.[70]

In the majority of persons (those with sensory polyneuropathy), the symptoms are relative mild. Initially, the patient may be unaware of the sensory loss, although they may have degeneration of over 50% of the nerve endings supplying the skin.[41] The involvement of the peripheral sensorimotor nerves produces the "stocking-glove" distribution of sensory involvement, with the distal legs affected more commonly than the distal arms.[41] A single "glove" covering the distal extremity does not accurately reflect the neuropathy.[41, 43] It is best described as multiple "gloves" covering the limb: one "glove" for each modality and each with its own end point. The larger nerve fibers are affected first and have the most proximal neuropathic end point, whereas smaller nerve fibers have a more distal neuropathic end point.[41, 43] The sensory modalities affected depend on the involved nerve fiber type. The large nerve fibers are associated with a loss of deep tendon reflexes, proprioception, and vibratory sense. The small nerve fibers are associated with a loss of pain sensation and detection of temperature. Patients may experience symptoms of numbness or may be completely unaware of the disruption of sensation owing to the extreme insidious onset of the disorder.

In marked contrast to the patient who develops sensation of numbness from the symmetric sensory polyneuropathy are those who develop painful polyneuropathy. These patients develop predominantly small fiber neuropathy, which is manifested by a burning or sharp boring pain and paresthesia.

Mononeuropathy

Mononeuropathies are frequently encountered in diabetic patients. These neuropathies may affect any cranial or peripheral nerves. Nerves that are at a high risk for compression appear to be more susceptible to develop a mononeuropathy. The most commonly affected peripheral nerves are the ulnar, median, radial, femoral, lateral femoral cutaneous, and peroneal nerves. Thus it is possible for a diabetic patient to present with an isolated sensory, motor, or sensorimotor neuropathy. Although focal lesions may be seen in nondiabetic patients, they occur most frequently in diabetics.[41, 43] For example, isolated femoral nerve neuropathy is almost always associated with diabetes. Other examples include median nerve compression, which may result in a carpal tunnel syndrome, which is quite common in diabetics, and common peroneal nerve damage, which may develop into a dropfoot deformity.

Mononeuropathy multiplex represents multiple focal nerve involvement. Mononeuropathy multiplex may be difficult to differentiate from distal symmetric neuropathies. The onset of these mononeuropathies is usually abrupt, but it may be insidious. There is a poor correlation between systemic control and duration of diabetes with the development of these neuropathies.

Proximal Motor Neuropathy

Asymmetric muscle weakness and wasting may occur in the proximal lower extremity. The condition primarily affects the hip flexors and may involve the anterolateral muscle groups in the lower leg. This group of neuropathies can be further classified depending on their clinical presentations.

EVALUATION OF THE DIABETIC FOOT

A careful systematic history and physical examination is a critical component in treating a patient with diabetes. Through careful questioning alone, the practitioner can often develop an understanding of the effect the disease process has had on each particular patient. It is important to determine the length of time since diagnosis as well as overall glucose control. It is also important to elicit a thorough family history because of the genetic disposition for development of diabetes and its complications. Attention should be given to previous hospitalizations, surgery, amputations, ulceration, and, most importantly, the response of the patient to past treatment. The podiatrist should have a full grasp of the patient's medical status. Recent blood glucose values, diet, medication used, and length of time the patient has been under care are important factors to elicit to evaluate the patient's potential response to care. It is also important to question the patient as to the names of other specialists who are involved in the treatment of the patient's disease. Physical examination of the diabetic foot should include a systematic examination of the dermatologic, vascular, neurologic, and musculoskeletal systems.

Dermatologic Evaluation

HISTORY

Does the patient have a history of pruritus, chronic fungal infections, or ulcerations? Does the patient notice any area or areas of irritation from shoes? If there is a history of ulceration, the location of the ulcer and how it was treated should provide important clues to any current problems. If an ulcer is the presenting complaint, then it is extremely important to ascertain the onset, duration, and course of the ulcer. In addition, the specific methods by which the patient has been treating the ulcer should be obtained. If appropriate, does the patient have any systemic symptoms such as fevers or chills? Finally, it is important to obtain a list of any "salve," "ointment," or "lotion" the patient applies. Antibacterial ointments, "corn removers," and homemade remedies may cause or promote serious infections in diabetic patients.

PHYSICAL EXAMINATION

Good lighting and a thorough inspection of upper and lower extremities are essential to an adequate dermatologic examination. The texture and turgor of the skin are noted with special attention to variations in pigmentation and color. The presence of scars or of any break in the integument is also noted. Special attention is directed to the web spaces, and each interdigital space is inspected for the presence of maceration or ulceration. Interdigital areas are prone to maceration, with subsequent bacterial and fungal colonization. The importance of maintaining an intact integument, which serves as a barrier to invading organisms, must be stressed to each diabetic patient.

Corns, calluses, and onychomycotic nails must be debrided on a regular basis to prevent tissue breakdown. Discoloration in a nail or the presence of a central hemorrhagic spot within a hyperkeratotic lesion may indicate increased pressure and underlying tissue destruction (Fig. 15–3). Debridement may reveal subungual or subdermal ulceration.

Vascular Examination

HISTORY

A thorough history will often identify those diabetic patients who have developed peripheral vascular disease; therefore, it is important to ascertain their current activity level and identify any risk factors. Known risk factors such as tobacco smoking and high blood pres-

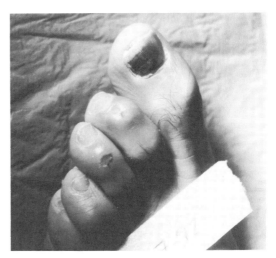

FIGURE 15–3. Subungual hematoma secondary to shoe pressure on a contracted hallux. Note the contractures of the lesser digits with subsequent superficial ulceration on the dorsal aspect.

sure predispose the patient to development of peripheral vascular disease.[24, 31, 32] Questions regarding ischemia-related problems must be included. Does the patient experience extreme pain in the foot, calf, thigh, or buttocks following periods of exercise that is relieved by rest? Does this pain recur in a reproducible and predictable fashion; for example, does the pain occur after every 50 steps? Diabetic patients may not present with classic ischemia symptoms, like intermittent claudication; therefore, it may be difficult for a patient to locate and characterize the pain. This vagueness of symptoms may be due to the presence of diabetic neuropathy. If this is the case, then ischemic problems are more advanced than the symptoms would indicate. Patients who complain of a severe burning pain in their legs that is present even during rest might have severe ischemic changes. These patients must be differentiated from those persons with radiculopathy, neuropathy, or phlebitis in whom the arterial examination will be normal or show mild disease. Does the patient have a history of coronary heart disease or bypass surgery of the lower extremity? Does the current list of medications include vasodilators, pentoxifylline, or other medications prescribed for peripheral vascular disease? Has the patient undergone previous noninvasive or invasive vascular tests? A thorough and complete history can aid the practitioner in identifying and treating the diabetic patient with vascular compromise.

PHYSICAL EXAMINATION

The examination begins with determining the vascularity of the patient's lower limb. The integument of both lower extremities is examined for hair growth, skin texture, and color. The ischemic foot often exhibits dry shiny skin, atrophy of soft tissue, absence of hair growth, and fissuring of the skin (Fig. 15–4).

All pulses should be palpated and graded, from the femoral to the dorsalis pedal artery. Furthermore, digital vascularity should be determined by measuring the time it takes for color to return to the tuft of the toe after digital pressure is used to blanch the toe (subpapillary venous return time). This test is most accurate when performed on the foot after a period of elevation, which measures the arterial capillary filling time. Lower limb elevation and dependency tests should be performed to determine arteriovascular disease. Last, the presence of edema and relative temperature gradient of both feet should be noted.

In the patient with vascular disease, pedal pulses are seldom easily palpable. In the diabetic patient there is a propensity toward anterior tibial and peroneal artery disease. The ischemic limb will reveal sluggish arterial capillary filling times and may demonstrate pallor with elevation and rubor on dependency.

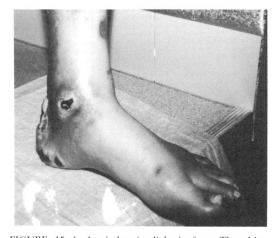

FIGURE 15–4. An ischemic diabetic foot. The shiny, atrophic skin and lack of hair growth should be noted, as well as the presence of several ischemic ulcers about the ankle.

Noninvasive Vascular Tests

Several noninvasive tests can be used to evaluate the avascular foot. An ABI should always be obtained. Although this index is automatically determined on most vascular analyzers, one does not need expensive equipment to accurately perform this test. A hand-held Doppler device and blood pressure cuff are sufficient. The ABI is determined by simply dividing the ankle systolic pressure by the brachial systolic pressure on the same side of the body. Normally the two systolic pressures are identical. If arterial disease is present in the lower limb, then the ankle systolic pressure is lower, resulting in an ABI less than 1. Care should be exercised when interpreting the results of an ABI greater than 1. Arteries that are calcified are difficult to compress and result in an unusually high ABI (Fig. 15–5). Furthermore, calcified arteries are not normal and may have a significant degree of occlusion, resulting in avascular signs and a high ABI.

Segmental examinations with digital pressures and waveforms should be obtained at the same time as the ABI. The pitch and waveforms of the pulses should correlate with the ABI. If they do not correlate, they should be considered inaccurate. If it is determined that arterial supply to the extremity is inadequate, then vascular reconstruction should be considered.

Angiography

The definitive method for determining if an arterial occlusion exists is to perform an angiogram. Considering the potential complications and adverse effects on the kidneys, this invasive test should be reserved for those patients who are potential candidates for arterial reconstruction.

Neurologic Examination

HISTORY

The history is aimed at trying to ascertain if neuropathy or myopathy exists. Does the patient have a history of burning sensations, numbness, or tingling in his or her hands, feet, or face? Does the patient see his or her limbs move but feel dissociated from them? Are

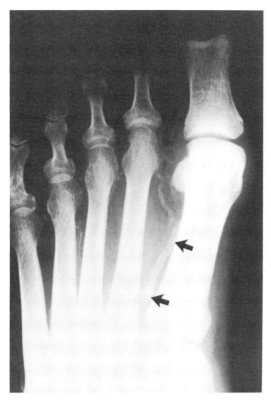

FIGURE 15–5. Calcification of the metatarsal *(tips of the arrows)* and digital arteries is apparent in this patient with NIDDM. The ABI was 1.58 secondary to calcification of the dorsalis pedis and posterior tibial arteries. This patient has subsequently had multiple amputations of the hallux and metatarsal secondary to gangrene.

symptoms bilateral or unilateral and well localized? Has the patient experienced any muscle weakness or loss of muscle strength? Neuropathy may have such a gradual onset that it may go unnoticed.

PHYSICAL EXAMINATION

A careful systematic neurologic examination is a critical component of the physical examination. Sensory, autonomic, and motor neuropathy often combine to initiate tissue breakdown, infection, arthropathy, and amputation. The early recognition of peripheral neuropathy will allow the practitioner to educate the patient and prevent complications.

It is clear that diabetic neuropathy affects many body systems. The presence of autonomic neuropathy affecting the cardiovascular system carries a poor prognosis.[41, 43] As such, the physical examination of the neurologic sys-

tem should not be confined to the lower extremity.

Sensory neuropathy (vibration, proprioception, pain, temperature, and touch) is often an early finding of generalized diabetic neuropathy and has been described as the most critical factor in ulcerogenesis.[66, 67] The ability of sensory input to protect the limb deteriorates to a point that both mechanical stress and tissue ischemia may go undetected. Sensory testing should enable the practitioner to assess the degree of degeneration of the various sensory components. All sensory testing should be performed bilaterally on the forefoot, midfoot, ankle, knee, and hip. Because neuropathy is not confined to the lower limb, a similar type of examination should be performed on the upper extremity as well. If a sensory deficit is detected, then the level at which that deficit ends should be noted.

Although special instrumentation has been designed to assist with the evaluation of some sensory functions, these instruments are not readily available to most practitioners. Vibratory sense is easily evaluated with a 128-cps tuning fork placed on bony prominences in the extremity (Fig. 15–6). The patient is considered to have impaired vibratory sensation if he or she perceives the vibratory end point before the examiner's end point (usually 10 seconds or more).[71] Proprioception and sensory ataxia are evaluated by gait examination and the Romberg test. Small-fiber sensation,

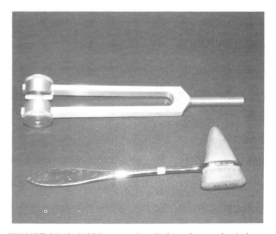

FIGURE 15–6. A 128-cps tuning fork and neurologic hammer used to assess neurologic status. These instruments are readily available and amenable to use in the office setting.

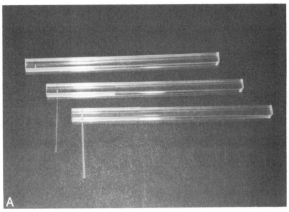
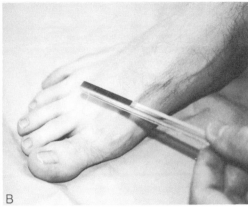

FIGURE 15–7. *(A)* Semmes-Weinstein monofilament aesthesiometers. These probes are easy to use and offer reproducible gradation of sensation in the diabetic patient. The three most commonly used wires are the 4.17 (finest), the 5.07, and the 6.10 (coarsest). The 5.07 and 6.10 are the most commonly used to test sensation in the foot. *(B)* Demonstration of the correct method in using the monofilament wires. Pressure is exerted on a 5.07 probe until buckling of the wire is noted.

light touch, and temperature can be tested in a variety of ways. A cotton wisp stroked lightly against the skin tests light touch. Tubes filled with ice and warm water evaluate temperature sensation. Superficial pain sense is performed by using a broken cotton-tipped applicator. When this examination is performed on the diabetic patient, care must be taken to protect the integument from injury. The ability to detect deep pain is tested by firmly squeezing the Achilles tendon just proximal to its insertion. Deep tendon reflexes and muscle testing are also important areas that require investigation to complete the routine neurologic examination.

The protective threshold is evaluated using the Semmes-Weinstein monofilament wires (Fig. 15–7). Various authors have provided a thorough description of these devices and have demonstrated reproducibility and specificity for assessing the protective threshold.[68]

Musculoskeletal Examination

HISTORY

Subjective complaints of decreased muscle strength or of changes in joint range of motion should be noted. For example, increased digital motion or subluxation or the description of a "collapsing arch" along with a warm foot may indicate an acute Charcot process. Other subjective complaints of "tripping, falling, or stubbing toes" may be manifestations

of loss of proprioception or focal peroneal nerve degeneration (a focal mononeuropathy). The patient should be questioned as to the rate and progression of such findings.

PHYSICAL EXAMINATION

The musculoskeletal examination should begin with a general visual examination of each lower extremity, noting muscle atrophy, structural alignment, and any frank dislocation of joints. The presence of digital deformities, such as hallux abductovalgus and hammer toes, should be noted. In the diabetic neuropathic foot, these structural deformities may predispose the patient to ulceration at the tip of the digits, on the dorsal aspect of the interphalangeal joints, or plantar to the metatarsophalangeal joint (see Fig. 15–3; Fig. 15–8).

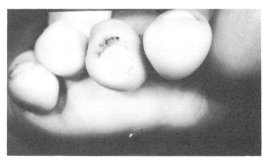

FIGURE 15–8. Mallet-toe deformity with superficial ulceration at the distal aspect of the third digit. This patient is neuropathic and was unable to detect the stress that initiated the ulcer.

Range of motion should be evaluated for all joints in the lower extremity. The presence of limited joint motion, crepitation, or osseous subluxation warrants further investigation with radiographs. Structural or functional limb length discrepancies and suprastructural deformities should be documented. A biomechanical examination is routinely performed to assess function of the forefoot and rearfoot.

Muscle strength testing should be performed both statically and during gait. Each muscle group should be isolated and tested by having the patient actively contract the muscle against applied force. A standardized grading system of muscle strength should be used for documentation purposes and to assess progression. Patients are asked to perform heel and toe walking to assess relative strength of ankle plantarflexors and dorsiflexors. The presence of equinus should be noted since it may place a great deal of stress on the forefoot. This increased stress combined with sensory neuropathy may predispose the patient to plantar ulceration or development of Charcot deformity.[72]

A computerized gait analysis can provide further clues to proprioceptive disturbances, muscle weakness, selective muscle substitution or stabilization, and a variety of biomechanical faults that may provide the dynamic forces responsible for joint destruction or ulceration.

DIABETIC COMPLICATIONS

Diabetic Ulcerations

EPIDEMIOLOGY

It has been estimated that 15% of the diabetic population will develop a foot ulcer during their lifetime.[73] Statistically, 20% of all diabetics who enter the hospital are admitted for foot problems.[73] In the majority of these cases, the admitting diagnosis is diabetic foot ulceration and infection. Approximately two thirds of the 50,000 nontraumatic amputations performed in the United States are those of the diabetic patient.[74, 75] Once the diabetic patient has had a major lower-extremity amputation, the contralateral limb and the life expectancy of the patient are at risk. Following the first major amputation, there is between a 32% to 68% incidence of amputation of the contralateral limb within 5 years.[76, 77] The life expectancy of the diabetic amputee approximates 50% in 3-year survival rates.[78] Considering the morbidity and mortality associated with lower-extremity amputation in the diabetic patient, the goal of treating the diabetic ulceration is limb preservation.

PATHOGENESIS

Diabetic foot ulcerations are the result of many intrinsic and extrinsic factors.[20] Intrinsic factors that initiate tissue breakdown include pathologic changes in the vascular, neurologic, and immunologic systems. Extrinsic factors that must be considered include social, occupational, physical, and environmental factors. The majority of diabetic foot ulcerations are the result of painless trauma incurred by the patient with peripheral neuropathy and the resulting insensitive foot. The presence of vascular disease compounds the problem, making healing a difficult process. Other important considerations are the level of each patient's knowledge of diabetic foot care and family support. It is of vital importance to identify and recognize the causative factors (intrinsic and extrinsic) that have combined to initiate the diabetic ulceration. Failure will certainly result if one attempts to treat a diabetic ulceration without identifying and addressing all factors that have initiated its occurrence.

Neuropathic Ulceration

Brand[79] defined the protective threshold as "the retention of enough nerve function to prevent injury by feeling a threat and adequate sensation to prevent the use of an injured part." Neuropathic ulcerations are primarily caused by repeated pressure, which results in inflammation and autolytic breakdown of the skin in the insensate diabetic foot.[66, 67, 80] In addition to the loss of protective threshold (sensory deficit), many of these patients have varying degrees of damage in the autonomic and motor innervation to the lower extremity. The resultant dysfunction in these systems often contributes directly to the pathogenesis of the diabetic ulceration. Autonomic neuropathy in the lower extremity often manifests itself as anhidrosis. The resultant dry, inelastic, cracked skin may pave the way for ulceration.

Damage to the motor innervation of the lower extremity can result in atrophy of the intrinsic and extrinsic musculature. Atrophy and weakness of the extrinsic leg muscles can result in equinus deformity and severe alteration of foot biomechanics. With weakness of the intrinsic muscles of the foot (intrinsic minus foot), the stability of the digits is lost; the direct result is that of digital contracture (hammer toe and claw toe deformity).[81] Those prominent contracted digits in the neuropathic patient are then prone to ulceration. The digital contractures also incur a retrograde buckling force on the metatarsal heads, causing osseous prominence and increased susceptibility to plantar ulceration (Fig. 15–9).

Coleman and Brand[69] described three separate groups of causative events that lead to ulceration in the diabetic neuropathic foot. The result of damage from one of these three initiating events is a wound or ulceration.

The first group of initiating events includes those events that impact directly on the exposed skin surface and initiate breakdown in those areas. Most commonly, the injury is induced by stepping on a sharp object. This type of injury may also be induced by thermal or chemical insult. Human skin is extremely resilient and can tolerate high pressures without breaking or tearing. The foot will generally accept the whole body weight with each step, except when this weight is transferred to a narrow or sharp object. In this case, the area of contact is small and the resultant stress exceeds the capacity of the skin. This results in tissue destruction. An example of this type of injury would be that of a neurotrophic patient stepping on a tack that had become lodged in carpet. The resulting wound is then susceptible to infection and possibly gangrene.

Thermal and chemical insults are also examples of direct damage. Accompanying the loss of cutaneous sensation is that of loss of thermal discriminatory sense. As a result, these patients are at high risk for thermal injury (burns and cold exposure). A thermal injury can easily be incurred by stepping into a hot bath or warming the feet by a fire or heater (Fig. 15–10). The neuropathic foot is also susceptible to damage from chemical agents. Most commonly, these chemical injuries occur as a result of application of caustic chemicals to the skin. An example of this type of injury is the application of commercially available chemical "corn removers" to the insensate diabetic foot. These agents may induce a chemical burn with resultant tissue destruction.

The second group of events includes injuries induced by the application of low-level stresses for prolonged periods of time. The result of this type of stress is decreased local tissue perfusion, ischemia, and subsequent ulceration. In a sensate patient, the local tissue ischemia would result in pain followed by patient recognition and removal of the offending stress. In the neuropathic patient, ulceration of tissues may result as the sensory warning system fails to alert the patient and initiate a response. A common cause of pressure sores in the diabetic patient is from ill-fitting, tight shoes.

The third group of initiating events is the most common cause of ulceration[69]—moderate repetitive stress applied to the body part. The amount of pressure that is involved is found to be between that of direct trauma and ischemia. The pathologic process that underlies this mechanism (repetitive stress) is that of inflammation, edema, and migration of inflammatory cells. The results of inflammation

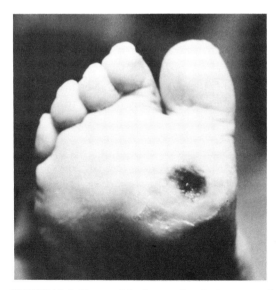

FIGURE 15–9. Neuropathic ulcer on the plantar aspect of the first metatarsal head. The patient has severe dorsal contracture at the first metatarsophalangeal joint, and the retrograde forces resulted in this plantar ulcer.

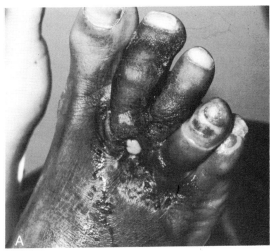 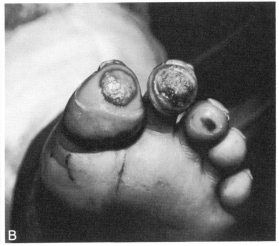

FIGURE 15–10. This neuropathic patient fell asleep in front of a fireplace. The patient was not aware of the second- and third-degree burns on his feet. *(A)* Right foot. *(B)* Left foot.

are decreased tissue compliancy and suscepti-bility to autolytic tissue destruction. This type of stress is experienced by nondiabetic patients as well; however, the pain associated with the inflammation prompts the person to rest the affected parts.

Various authors have recognized that areas on the foot (the plantar aspects of the heel and metatarsophalangeal joints, especially the first, are most common) that are subjected to repetitive stress and subsequent ulceration also exhibit an increase in skin temperature.[75, 81–84] This increase in skin temperature is most likely due to the underlying inflammatory process.[82] This observation is of vital importance to the clinician caring for diabetic patients, since this increased local skin temperature can serve as an indicator of ensuing ulceration.[82] Routine skin temperature screening of all diabetic pa-tients, noting any areas of increased tempera-ture, can be a valuable diagnostic tool in pre-venting ulcerations (Fig. 15–11). With proper education, the patient can include assessment of skin temperature as part of daily foot in-spection.

Diabetic Ischemic Ulceration

Since diabetic patients are at an increased risk of developing macrovascular disease, they are also subsequently at risk for development of ischemic ulcerations and ulcers that are both ischemic and neuropathic. It is important to differentiate between ischemic and neuro-pathic ulcerations since their treatment will vary. Typically, an ischemic ulceration is very painful and debilitating. Along with the ulcer-ation the patient may also complain of other symptoms indicative of peripheral vascular dis-ease, such as pain in the calf, leg, or buttocks.

When diabetic neuropathy is present, the patient may develop ischemic ulcerations with minimal or no discomfort. These lesions are the result of painless trauma to the vascular compromised lower limb. A common ulcera-tion exhibiting this phenomenon is the decu-

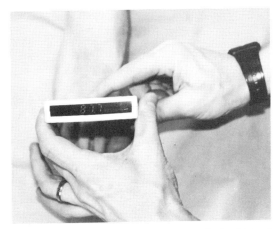

FIGURE 15–11. Skin temperatures are routinely obtained from all diabetic patients using a sensitive infrared skin temperature device. Routine screening may indicate po-tential sites of ulceration or the beginning of a Charcot foot deformity.

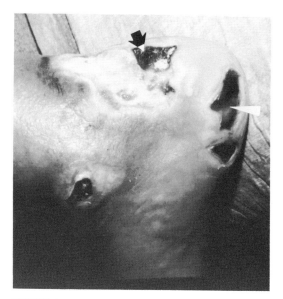

FIGURE 15-12. Ischemic heel ulcers occurred in this diabetic patient after prolonged hospitalization. Note the black necrotic base *(tips of the arrows)* of these ulcers.

bitus heel ulceration (Fig. 15-12). These ulcerations can be commonly found in neuropathic patients who have been confined to prolonged bed rest. The patient develops this ulceration as a result of prolonged pressure on the posterior aspect of the heel, which leads to local tissue ischemia and eventual ulceration. The presence of neuropathy prevents the activation of the sensory warning system and removal of the stress. The resultant ulceration combined with poor peripheral circulation affords a tenuous prognosis.

PHYSICAL EXAMINATION

The ulceration should be carefully examined and the location, diameter, depth, odor, and presence of infection determined. The ulcer should be probed with a metal nasal probe or other suitable device to determine the extent of the ulceration (Fig. 15-13). The presence of sinus tracts or involvement of deeper structures must be determined. Radiographs are essential to rule out gas formation or osteomyelitis in cases of infected ulcerations. A thorough clinical examination of the vascular, neurologic, and musculoskeletal systems is of vital importance to identify the factors that have led to the breakdown of the skin.

The quality of the ulcer base may provide

clues as to the vascularity and should be noted. A red, granular bed is likely well vascularized, while a firm, fibrotic, "rubbery" bed is likely poorly vascularized.

The neuropathic ulceration typically occurs in areas of osseous prominence and repetitive stress. The ulceration is typically well circumscribed and surrounded by thick callous tissue (Fig. 15-14). The ulceration may develop under an area of thick callous buildup, such as corns and plantar tyloma. Ulcerations that develop under areas of callous tissue are termed *mal perforans ulcerations.* Often these ulcerations are discovered clinically by debridement of the hyperkeratotic tissue. The patient may also identify the problem and present to the clinic complaining of drainage from these sites. Any calloused tissue that contains a hemorrhagic appearance is suspect for underlying ulceration. Hemorrhage present under a hyperkeratotic lesion usually indicates dermal bleeding and should be debrided thoroughly.

The ischemic ulceration typically occurs on the digits or areas of bony prominence. The

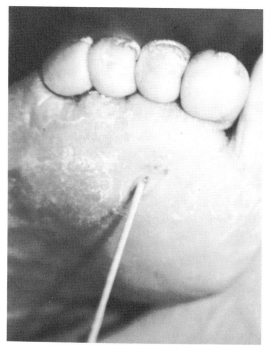

FIGURE 15-13. Blunt probing used to determine depth and presence of sinus tracts in diabetic ulcers. The ulcer was probed to the underlying metatarsal heads. Radiographs revealed osseous destruction typical of osteomyelitis. The patient subsequently underwent surgical debridement.

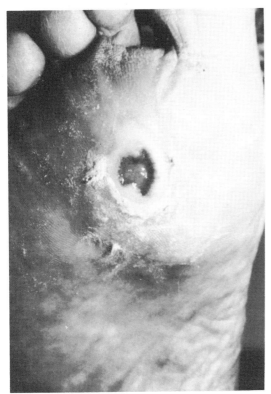

FIGURE 15–14. Example of a typical diabetic neuropathic ulcer. Note the irregular border and hypertrophic rim. Usually after debridement a red granulation tissue base that readily bleeds is noted.

ulcerations may also be found on any part of the foot, including the dorsum, that has been subject to a stress that exceeds the circulation in that area. The ischemic ulcer typically has a well-defined border, with little if any hyperkeratotic tissue surrounding the site. The characteristic "beefy red" granular tissue typical of a neurotrophic ulceration is replaced with that of a necrotic, pale, fibrotic-appearing tissue.[85] The ulcerations often appear as if they were punched out of the skin with a cookie cutter. They may also be covered with a leathery, tough eschar.

CLASSIFICATION OF ULCERS

The rationale for developing a grading system is to provide assistance for the practitioner who must decide on a treatment plan that is appropriate for the pathology. The most commonly used grading system for diabetic ulcerations is the one proposed by Wagner.[86, 87] Keep in mind that at times it may be difficult

to assign an ulcer to one grade or another. The fact is that ulceration of tissue occurs as a continuum. These grades are not absolute but rather serve as a means to assess treatment and provide prognosis.

Grade 0 or Preulcerative or Healed Ulceration. Treatment is aimed at prevention and education. Areas of potential breakdown should be accommodated with appropriate shoe modifications, or, if appropriate, surgical management should be considered.

Grade 1 or Superficial Ulceration. This ulcer penetrates the superficial structures only. Typically it seems as though the skin has been worn through. The ulcer usually does not extend to the level of the deep fascia. The treatment plan for the ulcer is to convert it to a grade 0 through appropriate local wound care (Fig. 15–15).

Grade 2 or Deep Ulcerations. This ulcer penetrates the deeper tissues of the body, usually to the level of the tendon or joint capsule. This ulcer is localized, rarely penetrating into the deep compartments of the foot. In general, this ulcer is not infected; however, because of the amount of tissue loss, a patient is susceptible to a serious infection. Treatment of these ulcers is best accomplished by surgical debridement. After debridement, appropriate braces or non–weight bearing of the ulcer is necessary for healing.

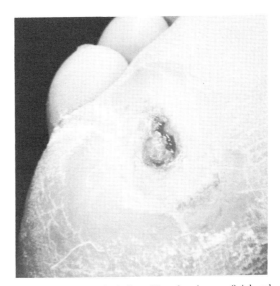

FIGURE 15–15. Grade 1 ulcer. The ulcer is superficial and does not involve deeper structures. There is a loss of the skin only.

On occasion it is difficult to distinguish a grade 2 ulcer from a more serious ulcer (see Fig. 15–13). Ulcers that probe to bone yet that are clinically or radiographically not infected are especially problematic, especially for those practitioners who do not regularly treat serious ulcers. In these situations it is best to consider the ulcer the more serious grade 3. It is better to have surgically debrided an ulcer and obtained deep cultures that yielded "no growth" than to let an occult infection fester in a diabetic foot for months.

Grade 3 or Deep Abscess. This is the progression of the grade 2 ulcer to a deep abscess, often with obvious signs of osteomyelitis (Fig. 15–16). Because of the depth of the ulcer and the involvement of bony tissue, radical surgical debridement is often necessary. It is essential that all necrotic tissue be removed in these patients. Of special concern are those patients with underlying vascular compromise who may need revascularization or partial amputation to promote healing.

Grade 4 or Partial Gangrene. In this patient an ulcer is the focal point for the beginning of a serious infection and resultant necrosis. In these patients the ulcer may not be evident; however, gangrenous changes are noted on parts of the foot (Fig. 15–17). Usually only the digits or part of the forefoot are involved and local amputation is the treatment of choice.

Grade 5 or Total Pedal Gangrene. This represents the most disastrous end stage of an ulcer. It is characterized by total gangrene of the foot and no local procedures can be con-

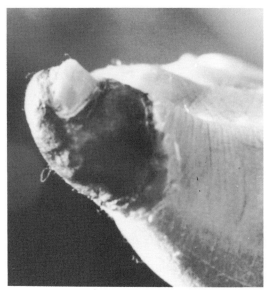

FIGURE 15–17. Grade 4 ulcer. Dry gangrene of the hallux secondary to infection and peripheral vascular disease. This diabetic patient subsequently underwent amputation of the necrotic hallux and healed uneventfully.

sidered. The treatments of choice are proximal amputations at the level of tissue viability.

TREATMENT

Neuropathic Ulcers

Treatment of the neuropathic ulceration is aimed at removal of all initiating factors, local wound care, and patient education. For the superficial ulceration with no clinical signs of infection, appropriate debridement of all hyperkeratotic and fibrotic tissue is necessary to promote healing. Saline wet to dry dressings are instituted, and the patient is instructed to change the dressing once or twice daily.

Other topical therapy and dressings, such as povidone iodine, hydrogen peroxide, and topical enzymes, have been found to be inhibitory to healing.[88–90] Currently, research has emphasized the development of tissue growth factors that may be applied to wounds and ulcer sites to promote healing.[91] Pending clinical trials, approval by the Food and Drug Administration, and continued research, these topical growth factors may prove invaluable to the successful treatment of diabetic ulcerations in the future.[91] Therapeutic soaks and whirlpool therapy are not currently indicated for treatment

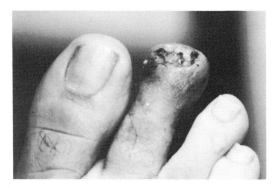

FIGURE 15–16. Grade 3 ulcer. The ulcer at the dorsal aspect of the second digit probes to bone, and radiographs revealed complete dissolution of the phalanx. Note the edema of this digit.

of diabetic ulcerations. Soaking can cause a drying effect on the skin and can actually seed an infection. Culturing of an ulceration that is not clinically infected is not recommended. Often, positive culture results are obtained that reflect the presence of skin contaminates and normal skin flora. Cultures should be routinely performed only in the presence of infection. Dispensing antibiotics for a noninfected ulceration may predispose the patient to development of a superinfection with resistant organisms.

If the ulceration probes to bone or the ulcer is deeper than it is wide, surgical debridement is indicated to remove all necrotic tissue. If the ulceration appears infected, additional steps should be taken. Antibiotic therapy and surgical intervention are often required. Treatment of diabetic infections is discussed later in the chapter. Although local wound care is the priority in treating diabetic ulcerations, one must also identify the source of the stress that initiated the ulceration. Therefore, a crucial portion of the treatment relies on identification of the intrinsic and extrinsic factors that have initiated tissue breakdown. If the ulceration developed secondary to ill-fitting shoes or a structural deformity, one must address these problems. Proper-fitting shoes are essential for the neuropathic foot. The ulcer site must be relieved of extrinsic force to promote healing. Often fabrication of a custom-molded healing sandal, a healing brace, or accommodative orthotics is necessary to promote healing (Fig. 15–18).[92]

Although the contact casting technique is perhaps the best method of treating these ulcers, felted foam has also been used successfully.[93–97] It is important that the ulcer be thoroughly evaluated before the application of a contact cast. Contact casts are contraindicated in patients with infected ulcers or severe edema. Although not specifically contraindicated, contact casts should be used judiciously on patients with severe equinus and psychological disorders.

Once these ulcerations have healed, the practitioner must take steps to prevent recurrence. Patient education is an essential part of treatment and prevention of the diabetic ul-

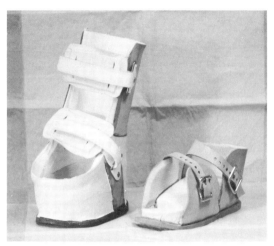

FIGURE 15–18. Custom-molded healing sandal and healing brace fabricated to relieve pressure on the ulcer site. (Courtesy of Leighton & Son Foot Lab, Ypsilanti, Michigan.)

ceration. Structural deformities must be surgically corrected or accommodative shoes constructed to prevent recurrence. Elective surgical intervention is not contraindicated in diabetic patients with adequate peripheral circulation and metabolic control.

Ischemic Ulcers

The mainstay of treatment for ischemic ulcers is to ensure adequate blood supply to the tissue. A thorough vascular examination is of paramount importance. In most cases it is necessary to consult a vascular specialist. Often these patients may require invasive revascularization of the lower extremity to promote healing and prevent further breakdown of tissue.

Ischemic ulcers are not debrided as aggressively as neurotrophic ulcers because of the poor vascular supply to the tissues. Treatment is aimed at removing necrotic debris, off-weighting the ulcer, and ensuring an adequate blood supply to the tissue. Appropriate drug therapy may be helpful in those cases in which surgical intervention is not indicated or when underlying medical problems prevent surgical intervention.

In those cases in which surgical intervention is not indicated or when underlying medical problems prohibit such measures, local wound care can be instituted. Debridement of these ulcerations is very conservative, so as not to inflict further tissue damage. The noninfected wound can be covered with several commercially available occlusive dressings.

Diabetic Neuropathic Osteoarthropathy

Charcot, in 1868, was the first to describe joint changes in the neuropathic foot of tertiary syphilis.[98] However, many other diseases are known to produce the deformity, including leprosy, tabes dorsalis, syringomyelia, spina bifida, meningomyelocele, alcoholic neuropathy, and spinal cord and peripheral nerve injuries.[72, 99] Since then, the same changes have been shown to occur in diabetes mellitus.[100] Today diabetes is the leading disease associated with Charcot deformity.[101] Charcot joint disease or neuropathic osteoarthropathy is a process characterized by bony destruction followed by excessive bony repair. Diabetic neuropathic osteoarthropathy (DNOAP) is the form of neuropathic arthropathy associated with diabetes mellitus.

EPIDEMIOLOGY

DNOAP is an uncommon but severe complication of diabetes mellitus. Unfortunately this complication of diabetes is not tracked by the NDDG and WHO; therefore, the incidence will vary according to the study and the geographic location.[34] The incidence of DNOAP ranges from 0.08% to 0.5% among all diabetics.[101] The average age at onset for this deformity is 57 years.[101]

Although somewhat controversial, it is generally believed that the most important etiologic factors are peripheral neuropathy with loss of protective sensation, trauma, and increased osseous blood flow secondary to autonomic "autosympathectomy."[43, 101]

What puts a patient at risk for developing DNOAP? Unfortunately there is no straightforward answer to this question. Although some factors or complications of diabetes clearly put patients at risk, other factors are not so apparent. The presence of peripheral sensory and autonomic neuropathies has been previously documented to be the main risk factor in the development of DNOAP. In patients with peripheral neuropathy, the incidence of DNOAP increases to 29%.[102] The extent of the neuropathy can be quite variable and still the patient may develop DNOAP. In fact, in one study it was reported that 32% of those patients studied had joint pain with no known neuropathy.[103, 104] The duration of disease also appears to be a risk factor. The range of time from the diagnosis of diabetes mellitus to the development of DNOAP is 12 to 18 years.[101] Eighty percent of patients with DNOAP have been diabetic for more than 10 years, while only 60% have been diabetic for more than 15 years.[101] Apparently minor trauma is a factor as well. There is an 80% unilateral occurrence (20% bilateral), but neglect of the contralateral limb during treatment often induces a bilateral Charcot deformity.[101, 105] Treatment of other diabetic complications can also induce DNOAP. For example, renal transplantation associated with corticosteroids has been associated with DNOAP.[105]

PATHOGENESIS

Many theories have emerged over the years to explain the destructive changes seen in DNOAP.[97] Banks and McGlammery[72] have combined the two previous theories (neurotraumatic and hypervascular) into a "unified theory" that, they hypothesize, describes the development of DNOAP. After an autonomic neuropathy develops, there is an increase in the flow of blood to the lower extremity. Because of the increased blood flow, osteopenia results and the skeletal structures weaken. Secondarily, a motor neuropathy develops that results in muscle imbalances, which ultimately results in pathologic forces being placed on the foot without the ability to react. Coupled to this is a sensory neuropathy that may be so significant that the patient may not be able to detect a problem within his or her foot. Ultimately, even mild normal weight-bearing forces may be of sufficient strength to result in failure of skeletal structures, ultimately resulting in the classic Charcot foot.

PHYSICAL EXAMINATION

Vascular examination may reveal a warm, edematous, erythematous area often associated with recent trauma. Skin temperature provides clues for early diagnosis as well as progression and should be routinely measured. Bounding pulses are almost always noted, except in the cases of medial calcification of pedal arteries.

Dermatologic examination may reveal the presence of neurotrophic ulcerations with or without associated infection. Hyperkeratosis, anhidrosis, redness, erythema, and taut skin may also be seen (Fig. 15–19).

Neurologic examination will reveal sensory neuropathy including absent or diminished vibratory and light touch sense, with a loss of the protective threshold (inability to detect a 5.07 Semmes-Weinstein monofilament). Deep tendon reflexes may be diminished or, most likely, absent. The patient may complain of an

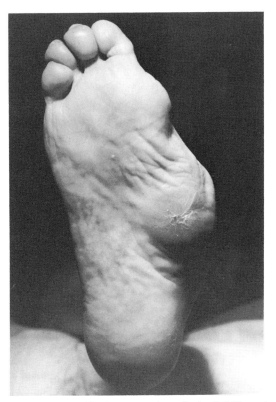

FIGURE 15–20. Classic presentation of a healed Charcot deformity. The patient has had a partial resection of the first ray, and there is a large osseous prominence at the talonavicular joint.

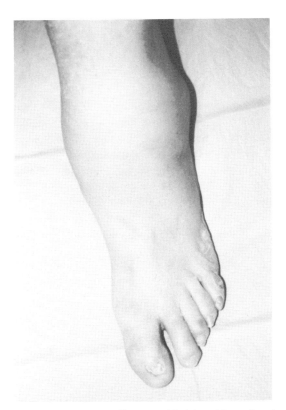

FIGURE 15–19. Acute Charcot ankle joint with profound dermatologic changes. Note the extreme edema, tautness of the skin, and erythema (discoloration) about the ankle joint. Skin temperatures were found to be 10°F higher than on the contralateral foot.

aching or shooting pain in a previously insensate foot. This presentation is common and warrants prompt attention.

Musculoskeletal examination may reveal a rocker-bottom foot deformation, Lisfranc's dislocation, equinus, and crepitation. Hypermobility due to ligamentous laxity and joint capsule expansion from abnormal joint stresses allows subluxation or dislocation to occur (Fig. 15–20).

Classification and Radiographic Appearance

Radiographic changes associated with DNOAP are classified into two main categories: atrophic and hypertrophic. Atrophic changes include bony resorption, osteolysis, juxta-articular cortical erosion, tapering of the metatarsal shafts, pencil-in-cup deformity of the metatarsophalangeal joints, joint effusions, subluxation, and dislocation (Fig. 15–21). The atrophic phase may be thought of as a destruc-

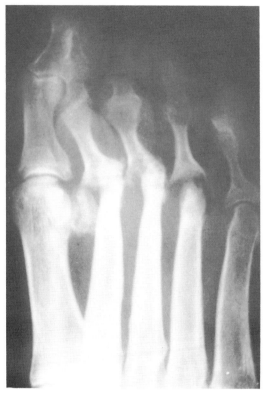

FIGURE 15–21. Atrophic Charcot deformity. Note the juxta-articular erosions of the central metatarsals and the pencil-in-cup deformity of the fourth metatarsophalangeal joint.

tive phase, with hyperemia predominating and leading to resorption and softening of the bone.

Hypertrophic changes range from osteochondral fragmentation to periosteal new bone formation, subchondral sclerosis, and bony fusion (Fig. 15–22). The hypertrophic phase can be thought of as a repair phase in which absorption of fine debris and fusion of large bony fragments with hypertrophic bone formation occurs. Stabilization is increased in this phase owing to the osseous bridging of bony fragments.

Eichenholz[106] further divided the disease process into three useful stages with various radiographic findings. These stages are developmental, coalescent, and reconstructive. The developmental stage represents the destructive or acute phase of a neuropathic osteoarthropathy. Joint effusion, soft tissue swelling, subluxation, osteochondral fractures, and fragmentation ("joint mice") are characteristic of this

phase (see Fig. 15–22). Both atrophic and hypertrophic changes are seen. The coalescent phase is a stage of initial repair with increased edema, absorption of fine debris, and coalescence of larger fracture fragments. Periosteal new bone formation and subchondral sclerosis are also seen in this phase. The reconstructive phase is the final stage of bone healing. Ankylosis and hypertrophic proliferative bone changes occur in this stage. Exostosis, osteophytes, and ligaments and cartilage calcification may occur. Rounding of bone ends with decreased sclerosis occurs in areas that are not ankylosed.

Locations

Although neuropathic osteoarthropathy may be found at multiple sites throughout the body, including the hip, knee, spine, shoulders, and elbow, DNOAP is confined to the bones and joints of the foot and ankle, with few exceptions. The reported distribution of bone and joint involvement varies depending on the source. A review of the literature reveals an increased affinity for the tarsometatarsal joint and the metatarsophalangeal joints, followed by the tarsal and interphalangeal joints.[72, 99, 100]

Previous researchers have found it beneficial to describe Charcot foot according to different patterns of disintegration. Steindler[97] distinguished between only different patterns of bony destruction, that occurring within the axis of the leg and one occurring in the forefoot. Harris and Brand[81] described disintegration occurring in one of two ways: by either

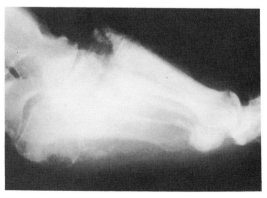

FIGURE 15–22. Subluxation and dorsal osteochondral fragmentation of the tarsometatarsal joint.

(1) a process of slow erosion and shortening of the foot, which is associated with ulcerations plantar to the metatarsophalangeal joints, or (2) proximal disintegration of the tarsus in which mechanical processes often determine the onset and progress of the condition.[81] They describe five patterns of disintegration of the foot: (1) posterior pillar, (2) central, (3) anterior pillar–medial arch, (4) anterior pillar–lateral arch; and (5) cuneiform-metatarsal base.

Sanders and Mrdjenovich[129] have more recently characterized five different patterns of DNOAP. Their system is more useful in attempting to characterize a patient with DNOAP because it incorporates the entire skeletal structure of the foot, not just the tarsus.[81, 97, 101] Pattern I of DNOAP is located in the forefoot of the affected extremity. In all reported cases of DNOAP the forefoot has been involved 26% to 67% of the time.[101] Furthermore, in 91% of all patients with this pattern of involvement an ulceration is noted. This ulceration may be a marker for the pres-

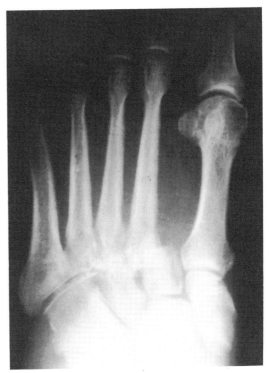

FIGURE 15–24. Pattern 2 of DNOAP affecting the tarsometatarsal joint.

ence of DNOAP (Fig. 15–23).[101] This pattern affects the distal metatarsal, the phalanges, and their joints. Usually the changes are atrophic and destructive. Osteopenia, osteolysis, juxta-articular cortical erosions, and subluxation are often noted. Since this pattern is so frequently associated with an ulcer, a clinician's first impression is often that of acute osteomyelitis.

Pattern II pedal DNOAP affects the distal aspect of the midfoot, especially the tarsometatarsal articulations (Fig. 15–24). In all cases of pedal DNOAP, this pattern is present 15% to 43% of the time. In this pattern, early changes are very subtle, often indicated only by a local increase in skin temperature and swelling. Late changes include joint destruction and ulceration plantar to the apex of the deformity.

Pattern III of pedal DNOAP affects the bones and joints of the lesser tarsus. Specifically, the naviculocuneiform, intercuneiform, talonavicular, and calcaneocuboid articulations are involved in 32% of those with pedal DNOAP. Classic radiographic findings are dorsal osteolysis with sharply defined borders at

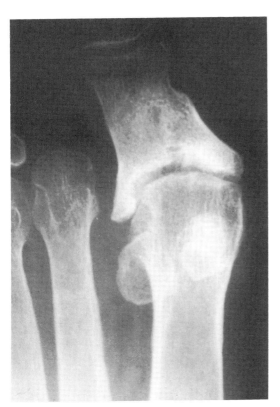

FIGURE 15–23. Pattern 1 of DNOAP affecting the metatarsophalangeal joint. Note the atrophic destruction of the joint.

the talonavicular joint on a lateral film. Without treatment, this pattern will progress to a rocker-bottom deformity.

Pattern IV is the most severe form of DNOAP that affects the ankle joint and is seen in only 3% to 10% of reported cases (Fig. 15–25). Harris and Brand state that mechanical forces determine the onset and progress of the condition.[81] They hypothesize that in an abnormal foot, weight-bearing forces do not follow normal trabecular patterns that are designed to accommodate those forces.[81] Instead, weight-bearing forces act obliquely to the trabecular patterns, thus weakening them and eventually causing "minor fractures." Thus in the insensitive foot, continued weight bearing results in additional fractures and eventual destruction of the bone and associated joints. The most trivial of trauma may result in significant joint destruction and collapse.

Pattern V involves the calcaneus (Brand's posterior pillar) and is the least common pattern seen with DNOAP (Fig. 15–26).[81] The patterns of involvement that have been described seldom occur by themselves; usually several patterns occur together in the affected foot.

TREATMENT

Once osseous disintegration has begun, treatment of DNOAP can be extremely difficult and frustrating. The most effective means of preventing severe foot destruction is by *prevention*. The patient must understand diabetes

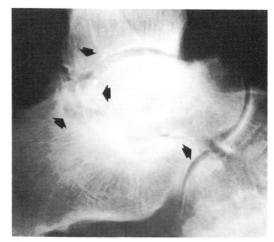

FIGURE 15–26. Pattern 5 of DNOAP affecting the calcaneus. Note the bony destruction of the calcaneus near the posterior aspect of the talus. Also note the anterior process fracture of the calcaneus.

and its complications. For those patients most at risk, daily checks for local increased temperature are essential. Early aggressive treatment is the most effective way to increase the chances of preventing the severe destructive changes that occur from continued ambulation on the acute stages. However, early treatment would require screening examinations on every known or suspected diabetic patient. The undiagnosed, noncompliant, or improperly treated patient will continually alternate between the developmental and coalescent stages of the disease with prolonged atrophic destruction. The net result is often joint collapse and subluxation with abnormal osseous prominence, leading to chronic ulceration, infection, and amputation.

It is occasionally difficult to determine if the changes seen on radiographic examination are due to DNOAP, osteomyelitis, or both. Although the clinical appearance may be similar, laboratory values may provide important information leading to a diagnosis. For example, in osteomyelitis the white blood cell count is often elevated, with a shift in the differential count toward increased polymorphonuclear leukocytes. Technetium and gallium bone scans are usually positive for both DNOAP and osteomyelitis and are therefore of little value.[107] An indium-111 scan has been shown to have a 67% to 89% specificity and a 100% sensitivity for osteomyelitis,[108–110] although, re-

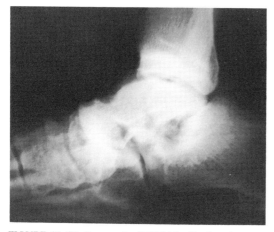

FIGURE 15–25. Pattern 4 of DNOAP affecting the ankle joint. Range of motion was restricted with crepitation. This is the same patient as in Figure 15–19.

cently, rare false-positive results of indium-111 scanning have been reported.[107] Even with these false-positive scans, however, indium-111 scanning is indicated to differentiate between DNOAP and osteomyelitis. If an indium-111 scan is reported as being positive, then a follow-up bone biopsy is indicated.

Once the diagnosis of Charcot foot has been made, early and aggressive treatment must be instituted. If ulcers are present, local aggressive debridement and wound care should begin. Complete bed rest may be the ideal treatment for this condition, but this is usually impractical and may lead to noncompliance. Total contact casting has been successfully employed for the resolution of neurotrophic ulceration and promotion of Charcot coalescence. If a total contact cast is employed, then the patient is instructed in not putting weight on the affected limb. Initially the cast is checked at 3- to 5-day intervals until edema subsides. The patient gradually changes to full weight bearing of the extremity along with an increased interval between cast changes. Total contact casts are contraindicated in the presence of an infection or excessive edema.

Surgical procedures should be contemplated only after resolution of the acute developmental stages. Surgery is prophylactic, and such procedures are aimed at removing bony prominences, digital stabilization, and triceps surae lengthening. Panmetatarsal head resection is occasionally a viable and successful alternative to submetatarsal head ulceration, particularly owing to prior metatarsal head or ray resection and DNOAP in the metatarsophalangeal joint. Although complications are frequent in these procedures, Banks and McGlamry[72] have reported "good" results with such procedures as Lisfranc's, triple, and pantalar arthrodeses. Proper osseous alignment and fixation is often difficult but absolutely essential with these procedures. Strict avoidance of weight bearing is essential after such procedures to guard against reinitiation of the Charcot process. In addition, the contralateral limb must be routinely assessed during this period to prevent development of Charcot deformity.

Regardless of the location or severity of the Charcot process, the goal is the gradual return to full weight bearing and as normal a gait pattern as possible. Initially, crutches or a walker are employed to keep the patient from putting weight on the affected limb. These aids are then used to provide stability during partial and gradual return to weight bearing of the extremity. Custom "tridensity" inlays, custom shoes, modified shoes, healing braces, and healing sandals may all be necessary during the course of treatment of a Charcot deformity.

Diabetic Infections

Infections in patients with long-standing diabetes mellitus are common and must be treated more aggressively than in patients without diabetes.[111–114] Infection is a commonly encountered and serious complication of the disease. Diabetic foot infections are associated with prolonged and costly hospital stays, disability, and mortality.[111, 114, 115] Nearly one half of lower-extremity amputations in diabetic patients occur as a result of uncontrolled infection even in the presence of an adequate blood supply.[114, 116] The etiology of the diabetic foot infection is multifactorial, and often a team approach is required for successful management.[117–120]

PATHOGENESIS

There are three major factors that predispose the diabetic foot to the development of infection.[111, 112, 119–122] The pathologic alteration in the vascular, neurologic, and immunologic systems increases these patients' susceptibility to infection. The presence of peripheral neuropathy increases the susceptibility of the diabetic patient by allowing injuries of the foot to go undetected. As a result of the loss of protective sensation, breakdown of the skin may remain unnoticed. Once the protective barrier (skin) has been violated, there is a portal of entry for microbes. Accompanying the sensory loss in many of the diabetic patients is motor and autonomic neuropathy. Motor neuropathy is responsible for muscle atrophy, altered biomechanics, and subsequent structural deformities, all of which increase the potential for breakdown of the integument.[116] Anhidrosis is a result of autonomic neuropathy and is seen as dry, inelastic, and cracked skin; there-

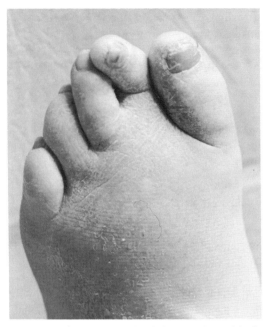

FIGURE 15–27. The foot of a diabetic patient with dry scaly skin on its dorsal aspect. The digital subluxation and deformity of the second digit represents an atrophic Charcot deformity affecting the proximal interphalangeal joint. Note the thickened, mycotic toenails.

fore, the bacteriostatic action of the sweat is lost (Fig. 15–27).[21]

The presence of diabetic immunopathy and its role in the pathogenesis of infections is a subject of controversy and debate.[123, 124] Most investigators agree that there is an alteration in the immune mechanism of diabetic patients. The disagreements are centered around whether the immunopathy is a result of humoral or cellular functions.[122, 124–126] Humoral immunity in patients with diabetes mellitus appears to be normal, and often the patient will actually have elevated levels of circulating immunoglobulins.[124–126] However, cellular immune function has been shown to be impaired with hyperglycemia, and hyperglycemia has been shown to impair leukocyte function and intracellular killing.[124–126]

Infections of the diabetic foot can be divided into four general categories: (1) skin and skin structure infections, (2) necrotizing skin and soft tissue infections, (3) dermatophytosis, and (4) osteomyelitis.[127]

Skin and Skin Structure Infections. Infections of the skin or of the underlying soft tissue structures are generally the most common of all infections in the diabetic foot.[123, 124, 127] Quite frequently, these infections precede a breach in the integument that allows for ingress of microbes. Corn and coworkers[128] distinguished three subsets of soft tissue infection according to the initiating event. In this series, more than two thirds were associated with tissue ulceration, paronychial involvement accounted for 21%, while trauma-induced infections were found in 11%. The common event preceding the infections was breakdown in the integument. Because of a possible sensory neuropathy in diabetic patients, this breach in the integument may go unnoticed until a complication develops. There are varying degrees of these soft tissue infections, ranging from the infected ingrown toenail to the plantar space infection. Treatment of these soft tissue infections must always be individualized according to the severity and extent of involvement.

Necrotizing Skin and Soft Tissue Infections. These severe and often life-threatening infections are frequently caused by synergistic interaction of multiple bacteria, including both aerobes and anaerobes.[115, 129] These infections are distinguished from others by how quickly these infections spread and by the massive tissue destruction that is involved. Within this group of infections are synergistic necrotizing fascitis and nonclostridial anaerobic myonecrosis.[115, 127] Patients typically present with pronounced systemic involvement, including septicemia, high white blood cell count, and fever.[130] The extremity may show local signs of cellulitis, foul odor, or gangrene (Fig. 15–28). These types of infections are associated with high mortality rates (20% to 50%) and are considered surgical emergencies.[115, 130, 131]

Dermatophytosis. Fungal infections of the diabetic foot are common and involve the toenails (onychomycosis) or the pedal skin (tinea pedis).[132] The infection and organisms involved do not appear to be any different than that encountered in nondiabetic patients.[21, 76] Whether fungal infection is more common in the diabetic population compared with that of the nondiabetic population is a source of debate.[132–134] However, the potential sequela of these infections is more significant in the diabetic patient. The presence of a fungal infection of the skin may provide an opportunity for ingress of opportunistic bacteria. As an ex-

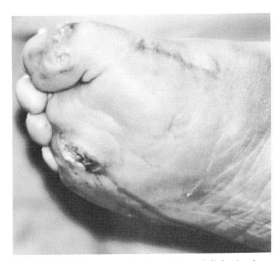

FIGURE 15–28. An example of an infected diabetic ulceration with edema, cellulitis, and a purulent discharge. The patient is a 62-year-old black female and had undiagnosed diabetes. The ulcer had a foul odor and purulent discharge, and probing showed that the ulcer extended to the dorsal aspect of the foot. This diabetic infection required radical surgical debridement of soft tissue and bone. Intraoperative cultures were positive for anaerobic as well as aerobic organisms.

ample, intertriginous fungal infection presents as maceration of the web spaces, which may fissure and ultimately ulcerate. This then provides a portal of entry for bacterial invasion.

Osteomyelitis. Infection of bone is a commonly encountered complication of the infected diabetic foot. In one study, approximately one third of 247 patients with osteomyelitis were diabetic.[135] In diabetics, most cases of pedal osteomyelitis develop as a sequela of chronic ulceration.[109, 136] Several studies have shown that pedal osteomyelitis was found to underlie chronic ulceration in between 68% and 94% of patients.[124-126]

It is often difficult to make a clinical diagnosis of osteomyelitis based on physical examination alone. The patient may present with an overlying soft tissue infection, cellulitis, or edema. In some persons there may be minimal clinical signs that indicate osteomyelitis. If there is an overlying ulceration that probes to bone or if the bone is visible in the wound, then one should consider the bone infected.[110]

Gram's stain and aerobic and anaerobic cultures should be obtained on all infected lesions. Deep tissue cultures or bone biopsy are essential for accurate bacteriologic diagnosis.[137] Laboratory testing should include complete blood cell count with differential count, erythrocyte sedimentation rate, and renal profile. Although standard radiographs may provide the diagnosis of osteomyelitis, radiographic signs are not evident until 10 to 14 days after the destructive process has proceeded and 30% to 50% of the involved bone has been destroyed.[107, 138, 139] Since the radiographic changes seen in Charcot joint are often similar to those of osteomyelitis, bone scans are often necessary to differentiate between DNOAP and osteomyelitis. Since technetium scans, including triphasic scans, have been found to be positive in both osteomyelitis and DNOAP, indium-111–labeled leukocyte scans should be used to differentiate osteomyelitis from neuroarthropathy.[107] Indium-111 leukocyte imaging has been shown to be close to 100% specific for acute osseous or soft tissue infection.[108-110, 140-142]

Bacteriology

The microbiology of the diabetic foot infection is quite complex. These infections are often polymicrobial, containing a combination of organisms, including gram-positive cocci, gram-negative rods, and anaerobes. Many investigators have confirmed the polymicrobial flora of the diabetic foot infection.[126, 143-148] Sapico and colleagues,[147, 149] in a quantitative study of deep tissue microbiology of amputated diabetic feet, found an average of 4.8 microorganisms per specimen. The majority of these specimens were noted to have a mixture of aerobic and anaerobic bacteria. These studies emphasize the importance of appropriate culture techniques in determining the identity of the pathologic organisms.

MANAGEMENT

The management of diabetic foot infections must be individualized. Individual considerations include presence of neuropathy and peripheral vascular disease and the overall metabolic control of the patient. Local considerations include location of the infection, extent and severity of the soft tissue and bony involvement, and the response to the infection. The presence of sepsis and a marked elevation of the blood glucose level warrants prompt and aggressive control.[150] Examination of the infected foot should be complete and include all aspects of the history and physical examination. The practitioner should elicit all previous treatment, antibiotics taken for the infection, presence of fever or night sweats, and initiating causative events. The location, depth, and presence of drainage are noted on examination. The infected site may be probed with a sterile nasal probe to determine the depth and presence of sinus tracts. Presence of cellulitis and its proximal extension are noted as well as enlargement of the popliteal or inguinal lymph nodes.

Bacteriologic identification is of paramount importance in treating these diabetic foot infections. Gram stain as well as aerobic and anaerobic cultures should be taken from deep tissue if possible to obtain an accurate representation of pathogens. Sharp and coworkers[151, 152] compared the results of 58 superficial and deep cultures in diabetic infections and found only 10 instances of comparative results. Therefore, deep tissue cultures are encouraged while superficial swabs and aspirates of wound sites are not recommended.

Standard laboratory tests that should always be done to evaluate an infection include complete blood cell count with differential count, erythrocyte sedimentation rate, and determination of the serum creatinine and blood urea nitrogen values. It is important to order kidney function studies in these patients (renal profile) to evaluate the presence and severity of diabetic nephropathy. Because most antibiotics are excreted by the kidneys, their functional capacity is of paramount importance to antibiotic selection. Standard radiographs should be taken to determine if any soft tissue abnormalities, such as gas, are present and if any osseous changes indicative of osteomyelitis are seen.

Although each case is unique, certain general guidelines can be used to identify those patients who require inpatient treatment. Patients who must be hospitalized include those with systemic signs of infection, such as fever, increased white blood cell count, ascending cellulitis, and, most importantly, the need for surgical debridement. The decision to hospitalize a patient rather than use aggressive outpatient therapy is frequently encountered. As a general rule, if this decision is debatable, the patient should be admitted to the hospital. Surgical debridement should always be performed if an abscess is present or if osteomyelitis is noted on radiographs. The presence of a rapidly spreading infection such as necrotizing fasciitis or the presence of tissue gas warrants prompt surgical debridement. Appropriate consultations with the vascular surgeon, infectious disease specialist, and internist should be made if the patient is admitted to the hospital.

Fungal Infections

Topical antifungal agents are used first for most cases of tinea pedis. Antifungal lotions are used for interdigital involvement while creams are used for noninterdigital areas. Regular changes of socks, improvement in pedal hygiene, and patient education are all essential parts of a successful treatment plan. Oral antifungal agents should be instituted in cases of secondary bacterial involvement.

Thickened, dystrophic, mycotic nails are frequently encountered in the diabetic patient. This nail deformity may initiate subungual ulceration in the neuropathic patient, owing to retrograde pressure applied by shoes. It is important to prevent ingrowth of these nails as well as to reduce the bulk of the nail plate with debridement. Periodic debridement of nails and ensuring proper fitting of shoes help to reduce the possibility of subungual ulcerations.

Antibiotic Therapy

Empiric antibiotic therapy for the diabetic should be based on clinical presentation, Gram stain results, and a knowledge of the most frequently isolated organisms in a particular infection. Joseph[122] describes three general clinical degrees of diabetic infections and recommends appropriate empiric antibiotic therapy for them. For a mild infection with minimal cellulitis and no systemic involvement, amoxicillin/clavulanic acid or clindamycin, both given orally, is recommended. For moderate soft tissue infections, such as an early plantar space infection, with cellulitis localized to the foot and minimal or no systemic involvement, parenteral therapy with ticarcillin/clavulanic acid or ampicillin/sulbactam is preferred. These two agents can be combined with aztreonam to cover gram-negative bacteria, and clindamycin may be used for the patient who is allergic to penicillin. Severe limb-threatening infections should be treated with imipenem/cilastatin as an adjunct to surgical intervention.

Surgical Intervention

Surgical intervention is often indicated in the infected diabetic foot to arrest tissue destruction and promote healing. Proximal progression of an infection, presence of soft tissue gas, or abscess formation as well as osteomyelitis are just a few examples that warrant surgical debridement. Antibiotic therapy alone is not sufficient to eradicate the infection in these cases, and delay in surgical intervention may result in lower limb amputation, sepsis, or even death. Debridement of all necrotic tissue and bone will reduce the inoculum size and will enable the host defense system to function. The presence of peripheral vascular disease in the infected diabetic foot is not an absolute contraindication to surgical intervention. The vascular status should not prevent the clinician from debriding the infection when it is warranted. Once the septic process has been controlled, revascularization can be attempted to promote closure of the wound. In these cases, a vascular consultation is essential.

Osteomyelitis

Osteomyelitis in the diabetic foot is difficult to eradicate with medical management alone. In the past, a 6-week course of intravenous antibiotics directed at the pathogens identified on bone culture was advised. This 6-week course of intravenous antibiotics was followed with a prolonged course of oral antibiotics.[153, 154] However, relapses and other complications were noted with this regimen.[153, 154]

Currently, combination antibiotic therapy, surgical debridement, and local wound care are paramount for successful management. Necrotic bone is removed along with any devitalized tissue. The wound is then left open to heal by secondary intention; or if adequate skin coverage is possible, primary or delayed primary closure may be performed. A 6-week course of intravenous antibiotic therapy, local wound care, and medical management is still utilized. The patient is monitored with serial plain film radiography. Once the wound appears noninfected, a followup indium-111 scan is performed.

PATIENT EDUCATION AND ROUTINE CARE

Primary care podiatrists can have a significant role in establishing the diagnosis of diabetes. The American Diabetes Association has proposed guidelines for screening for diabetes.[155] The primary purpose of this screening program is to identify those persons who are likely to meet the criteria for diabetes. If these persons can be identified and referred to a diabetologist for appropriate treatment of hyperglycemia, then some of the complications of diabetes may be delayed or even prevented. Screening for diabetes should be limited to persons with one or more risk factors, pregnant women, and persons presenting with possible complications of diabetes.[155]

When a patient presents to the office or clinic for the first time, a detailed podiatric history must be obtained and physical examination must be performed. If the person is unaware of any diabetes, then a family history must be obtained and, if appropriate, blood glucose testing should be ordered. If the patient is a known diabetic, then a detailed history of the course of the disease must be obtained. At the end of each visit the patient should be counseled on the disease. This is best performed by a nurse educator. As a part of each visit the feet must be examined for any breaks in the skin and any signs of breakdown. Hyperkeratotic tissue should be appropriately debrided to prevent ulceration, and digital nails should be trimmed. A previous misconception is that aggressive debridement of diabetic nails is necessary. This is not necessarily the case; in fact, trimming the nails to ensure an even edge without sharp medial and lateral borders and reducing the bulk found in severely mycotic nails is all that is necessary.

Furthermore, educating the patient as to the proper type of shoe to wear or providing the patient with an appropriate orthotic device to prevent tissue breakdown is important. If the patient has Charcot deformity or a history of ulcerations, the patient should routinely check skin temperatures and return to the office if any increase of greater than 3°F is noted. Often patients are willing to purchase a skin thermometer to prevent a recurrent ulceration or exacerbation of Charcot deformity.

Appropriate home care instructions for the diabetic are essential. These instructions must include daily foot examinations, examination of shoes before wear, and avoidance of foot soaks. If for medical reasons it is necessary to use "soaks," application of gauze pads saturated in saline solution and changed at regular intervals is recommended.

Diabetic patients without diabetic neuropathy will have a different tolerance to activities than a patient without any sensation. Patients with Charcot foot deformity or with a previous history of ulceration may need to limit the amount of walking. Some of these persons have led a full and active life up to the point of developing an ulcer or Charcot foot. These patients must understand that if they continue to be as active after developing any of the these complications, then their condition may worsen. In young patients who have been recently diagnosed with diabetes, this could be very difficult for them to understand. Compassion and understanding of their circumstances may lead to better patient compliance. For example, with appropriate monitoring these patients may be able to continue to have a healthy lifestyle. Active patients may want to monitor the distance they walk with a pedometer and look for signs of inflammation with skin temperature readings. In those patients who are recovering from Charcot foot or an ulceration, it is important that there is a gradual return to normal function, otherwise there may be a worsening or delay in the healing process. As primary care podiatrists, we often are the first to recognize a medical problem and may find ourselves in the role of organizing the health care of the patient.

REFERENCES

1. Harris MI, Hadden WC, Knowler WC, Bennet PH: International criteria for the diagnosis of diabetes and impaired glucose tolerance. Diabetes Care 8:562, 1985.
2. Modan M, Harris MI, Halkin H: Comparative evaluation of World Health Organization and National Diabetes Data Group criteria for impaired glucose: Results from two national samples. Diabetes 38:1630, 1989.
3. National Diabetes Data Group: Classification and diagnosis of diabetes mellitus and other categories of glucose tolerance. Diabetes 28:1039, 1979.
4. Melton LJ, Palumbo PJ, Chu CP: Incidence of diabetes mellitus by clinical type. Diabetes Care 6:75, 1983.
5. Bennet PH, Bogardus C, Tuomilehto J, Zimmet P: Epidemiology and natural history of NIDDM: Nonobese and obese. In Alberti KGMM, DeFronzo RA, Keen H, Zimmet P (eds): International Textbook of Diabetes Mellitus, p 147. New York, John Wiley & Sons, 1992.
6. Harris MI, Klein R, Weborn TA, Knuiman MW: Onset of NIDDM occurs at least 4–7 years before clinical diagnosis. Diabetes Care 15:815, 1992.
7. Jarrett RJ: Duration of non-insulin diabetes and development of retinopathy: Analysis of possible risk factors. Diabetic Med 3:261, 1986.
8. Harris MI, Zimmet P: Classification of diabetes mellitus and other categories of glucose intolerance. In Alberti KGMM, DeFronzo RA, Keen H, Zimmet P (eds): International Textbook of Diabetes Mellitus, p 3. New York, John Wiley & Sons, 1992.
9. Holman RR, Turner RC: Oral agents and the treatment of non-insulin dependent diabetes mellitus. In Pickup JC, Williams, GP (eds): Textbook of Diabetes, p 462. Oxford, Blackwell Scientific, 1991.
10. Harris MI, Hadden WC, Knowler WC, Bennett PH: Prevalence of diabetes and impaired glucose tolerance and plasma glucose levels in US population aged 20–74 years. Diabetes 36:523, 1987.
11. Wetterhall SF, Olson PR, DeStefano F, et al: Trends in diabetes and diabetic complications, 1980–1987. Diabetes Care 15:960, 1992.
12. Most RS, Sinnock P: The epidemiology of lower extremity amputations in diabetic individuals. Diabetes Care 6:87, 1983.
13. Nelson RG, Gohdes DM, Everhart JE, et al: Lower-extremity amputations in NIDDM: 12 years of follow-up study in Pima Indians. Diabetes Care 11:8, 1988.
14. Jarrett RJ: The epidemiology of diabetes mellitus. In Pickup JC, Williams, GP (eds): Textbook of Diabetes, p 47. Oxford, Blackwell Scientific, 1991.
15. Peters AL, Davidson MB: Aging and diabetes. In Alberti KGMM, DeFronzo RA, Keen H, Zimmet P (eds): International Textbook of Diabetes Mellitus. New York, John Wiley & Sons, 1992, p 1103.
16. Brownlee M: Glycation products and the pathogenesis of diabetic complications. Diabetes Care 15:1835, 1992.
17. Bauer M, Levan NE: Diabetic dermangiopathy: A spectrum including pigmented pretibial patches and necrobiosis lipoidica diabeticorum. Br J Dermatol 83:528, 1970.
18. Gilgor RS, Lazarus GS: Skin manifestations of diabetes mellitus. In Rifkin H, Raskin P (eds): Diabetes Mellitus, p 313. Bowie, MD, Brady, 1981.
19. Binkley GW: Dermopathy in the diabetic syndrome. Arch Dermatol 92:625, 1965.
20. Jenkin WM, Palladino SJ: Environmental stress and tissue breakdown. In Frykberg RG (ed): The High-Risk Foot in Diabetes Mellitus, p 103. New York, Churchill Livingstone, 1991.
21. Samitz MH: Metabolic disorders. In Samitz MH (ed): Cutaneous disorders of the lower extremities, ed 2, p 101. Philadelphia, JB Lippincott, 1981.

22. Nell SE, Sibbold GR: The skin in diabetes mellitus. In Pickup JC, Williams, GP (eds): Textbook of Diabetes, p 753. Oxford, Blackwell Scientific, 1991.

23. Campbell DR: Diabetic vascular disease. In Frykberg RG (ed): The High-Risk Foot in Diabetes Mellitus, p 33. New York, Churchill Livingstone, 1991.

24. Donahue RP, Orchard TJ: Diabetes mellitus and macrovascular complications: An epidemiological perspective. Diabetes Care 15:1141, 1992.

25. Kreines K, Johnson E, Albrink M, et al: The course of peripheral vascular disease in non-insulin dependent diabetes. Diabetes Care 8:235, 1985.

26. Janka HU, Standl E, Mehnert H: Peripheral vascular disease in diabetes mellitus and its relation to cardiovascular risk factors: Screening with Doppler ultrasonic techniques. Diabetes Care 3:207, 1980.

27. Dorman JS, Laporte RE, Kuller LH, et al: The Pittsburgh insulin-dependent diabetes mellitus (IDDM) morbidity and mortality study: Mortality results. Diabetes 33:271, 1984.

28. Schwartz CJ, Valente AJ, Sprague EA, et al: Pathogenesis of the atherosclerotic lesion. Diabetes Care 15:1156, 1992.

29. Borch-Johnsen K, Kreiner S: Proteinemia: Value as a predictor of cardiovascular mortality in insulin-dependent diabetes mellitus. Br Med J 294:1651, 1987.

30. Deckert T, Feldt-Rasmussen B, Borch-Johnsen K, et al: Albuminuria reflects widespread vascular damage: The Steno hypothesis. Diabetologia 32:219, 1989.

31. Ford ES, Newman J: Smoking and diabetes mellitus: Findings from 1988 behavioral risk factor surveillance system. Diabetes Care 14:871, 1991.

32. Jarrett RJ: Risk factors for coronary heart disease in diabetes mellitus. Diabetes 41(Suppl 2):1, 1992.

33. Taskinen MR: Quantitative and qualitative lipoprotein abnormalities in diabetes mellitus. Diabetes 41(Suppl 2):12, 1992.

34. National Diabetes Data Group: Diabetes in America: Diabetes Data Compiled 1984. Publication No. 80-1468, p 1. Bethesda, MD, National Institutes of Health, 1984.

35. Boulton AJM, Scarpello JHB, Ward JD: Venous oxygenation in the diabetic neuropathic foot: Evidence of arteriovenous shunting. Diabetologia 22:6, 1982.

36. LoGerfo FW, Coffman JD: Vascular and microvascular diseases of the foot in diabetes: Implication for foot care. N Engl J Med 311:1615, 1984.

37. Colwell JA: Peripheral vascular disease in diabetes mellitus. In Davidson JK (ed): Clinical Diabetes Mellitus: A Problem-Oriented Approach, p 486. New York, Thieme Medical Publishers, 1991.

38. Dyck PJ: Clinical and neuropathological criteria for the diagnosis and staging of diabetic polyneuropathy. Brain 108:861, 1985.

39. Dyck PJ, Karnes JL, O'Brien PO, et al: The spatial distribution of fiber loss in diabetic polyneuropathy suggests ischemia. Ann Neurol 19:440, 1986.

40. Dyck PJ: Pathology. In Dyck PJ, Thomas PK, Asbury AK, et al (eds): Diabetic Neuropathy, p 223. Philadelphia, WB Saunders, 1987.

41. Thomas PK, Eliasson SG: Diabetic neuropathy. In Dyck PJ, Thomas PK, Lambert EH, Burge R (eds): Peripheral Neuropathies, ed 2, p 1173. Philadelphia, WB Saunders, 1984.

42. Vinik A, Mitchell B: Clinical aspect of diabetic neuropathies. Diabetes Metab Rev 4:223, 1988.

43. Vinik AI, Holland MT, Le Beau JM, et al: Diabetic neuropathies. Diabetes Care 15:1926, 1992.

44. Weinberg CR, Pfeiger MA: Development of a productive model for symptomatic neuropathy in diabetes. Diabetes 35:873, 1986.

45. Boulton AJM: Diabetic neuropathy. In Frykberg RG (ed): The High-Risk Foot in Diabetes Mellitus, p 44. New York, Churchill Livingstone, 1991.

46. Fagerberg SE: Diabetic neuropathy: A clinical and histological study on the significance of vascular affections. Acta Med Scand 164(suppl 345):1, 1959.

47. Powell HC, Rosoff J, Myers RR: Microangiopathy in human diabetic neuropathy. Acta Neuropathol 68:295, 1985.

48. Vital C, LeBlanc M, Vallel JM, et al: Etude ultrastructurale du nerf periipheriques et 16 neuropathies non diabetiques. Acta Neuropathol (Berl) 30:63, 1974.

49. Timperly WR, Ward JD, Preston FE, et al: Clinical and histological studies in diabetic neuropathy: A reassessment of vascular factors in relation to intravascular coagulation. Diabetologia 12:237, 1976.

50. Yasuda H, Dyck PJ: Abnormalities of endoneurial microvessels and sural nerve pathology in diabetic neuropathy. Neurology 37:20, 1987.

51. Raff MC, Sangalang J, Asbury AK: Ischemic mononeuropathy multiplex associated with diabetes mellitus. Arch Neurol 18:487, 1968.

52. Clements RS: Diabetic neuropathy: New concepts of its etiology. Diabetes 28:604, 1979.

53. Sherman WR, Sterwart MA: Identification of sorbitol in mammalian nerve. Biochem Biophys Res Comm 22:492, 1966.

54. Greene DA, Lattimer SA: Altered myoinositol metabolism in diabetic nerve. In Dyck PJ, Thomas PK, Asbury AK, et al (eds): Diabetic Neuropathy, p 289. Philadelphia, WB Saunders, 1987.

55. Brismar T, Sima AAF, Greene DA: Reversible and irreversible nodal dysfunction in diabetic neuropathy. Ann Neurol 21:504, 1987.

56. Service FJ, Rizza RA, Daube JR, et al: Near normoglycemia improved nerve conduction velocity and vibratory sensation in diabetic neuropathy. Diabetologia 28:722, 1985.

57. Jaspan JB, Wollman RL, Bernstein L, Rubenstein AH: Hypoglycemic peripheral neuropathy in association with insulinoma: Implication of glucopenia rather than hyperinsulinism: Case report and literature review. Medicine (Baltimore) 61:33, 1982.

58. Rich KM, Luszczynski JR, Osborne PA, Johnson EM: Nerve growth factor protects adult sensory neurons from cell death and atrophy caused by nerve injury. J Neurocytol 16:261, 1987.

59. Sidenius P, Jakobsen J: Axonal transport in human and experimental diabetes. In Dyck PJ, Thomas PK, Asbury AK, et al (eds): Diabetic neuropathy, p 260. Philadelphia, WB Saunders, 1987.

60. Levi-Montalcini R, Calissano P: The nerve growth factor. Sci Am 240:68, 1979.

61. Faradji V, Sotelo J: Low serum levels of nerve growth factor in diabetic neuropathy. Acta Neurol Scand 81:402, 1990.

62. Lindsay RM, Harmer AJ: Nerve growth factor regulates expression of neuropeptide genes in adult sensory neurons. Nature 337:362, 1989.

63. Schwartz JP, Pearson J, Johnson EM: Effect of exposure to anti-NGF on sensory neurons of adult rats and guinea pigs. Brain Res 244:378, 1982.

64. Jacobsen J, Brimijoin S, Skau K, et al: Retrograde axonal transport of transmitter enzymes, fructose-labeled protein, and nerve growth factor in streptozotocin-diabetic rats. Diabetes 30:797, 1981.

65. Apfel SC, Lipton RB, Arezzo JC, Kessler JA: Nerve

growth factor prevents toxic neuropathy in mice. Ann Neurol 29:87, 1991.

66. Harrison MJG, Faris IB: The neuropathic factor in the aetiology of diabetic foot ulcers. J Neurol Sci 28:217, 1976.

67. Lang-Stevenson AI, Sharrard WJW, Betts RP, Duckworth T: Neurotrophic ulcers of the foot. J Bone Joint Surg [Br] 67:438, 1985.

68. Birke JA, Sims DS: Plantar sensory threshold in the ulcerative foot. Lepr Rev 57:261, 1986.

69. Coleman W, Brand PW: The diabetic foot. In Davidson JK (ed): Clinical Diabetes Mellitus: A Problem-Oriented Approach, p 494. New York, Thieme Medical Publishers, 1991.

70. Brown MJ, Asbury AK: Diabetic neuropathy. Am Neurol 15:2, 1984.

71. Dyck PJ, Karnes J, O'Brien PC: Detection thresholds of cutaneous sensation. In Dyck PJ, Thomas PK, Asbury AK, et al (eds): Diabetic Neuropathy, p 107. Philadelphia, WB Saunders, 1987.

72. Banks AS, McGlamry ED: Charcot foot. J Am Podiatr Med Assoc 79:213, 1989.

73. Levin ME: Pathophysiology of diabetic foot lesions. In Davidson JK (ed): Clinical Diabetes Mellitus: A Problem-Oriented Approach, p 504. New York, Thieme Medical, 1991.

74. Bild DE, Selby JV, Sinnock P, et al: Lower extremity amputation in people with diabetes: Epidemiology and prevalence. Diabetes Care 12:24, 1989.

75. Frykberg RG: Diabetic foot ulceration. In Frykberg RG (ed): The High-Risk Foot in Diabetes Mellitus, p 151. New York, Churchill Livingstone, 1991.

76. Goldner MG: The fate of the second leg in the diabetic amputee. Diabetes 9:100, 1960.

77. Roon AJ, Moore WS, Goldstone J: Below-knee amputation: A modern approach. Am J Surg 134:153, 1977.

78. Knighton DR, Fiegel UD, Doucett M, et al: Treating diabetic foot ulcers. Diabetes Spectrum 3:51, 1990.

79. Brand PW: The insensitive foot (including leprosy). In Jahss MH (ed): Disorders of the Foot, p 1266. Philadelphia, WB Saunders, 1982.

80. Delbridge L, Ctereteko G, Fowler C, et al: The aetiology of diabetic neuropathic ulceration of the foot. Br J Surg 72:1, 1975.

81. Harris JR, Brand PW: Patterns of disintegration of the tarsus in the anaesthetic foot. J Bone Joint Surg [Br] 40:4, 1966.

82. Bergtholdt HT, Brand PW: Temperature assessment and plantar inflammation. Lepr Rev 47:211, 1976.

83. Chan AW, MacFarlane FA, Bowsher DR: Contact thermography of painful diabetic neuropathic foot. Diabetes Care 14:918, 1991.

84. Fernando DJS, Masson EA, Veves A, Boulton AJM: Relationship of limited joint abnormality to abnormal foot pressures and diabetic foot ulceration. Diabetes Care 41:8, 1991.

85. Roenigk HH: Diabetic leg ulcers. In Roenigk HH, Young JR (eds): Leg Ulcers: Medical and Surgical Management, p 177. New York, Harper & Row, 1975.

86. Wagner FW Jr: A classification and treatment program for diabetic, neuropathic and dysfunctional foot problems. In: AAOA Instructional Course Lectures, vol 28, p 143. St. Louis, CV Mosby, 1979.

87. Wagner FW Jr: The dysvascular foot: A system for diagnosis and treatment. Foot Ankle 2:64, 1981.

88. Branemark PI, Ekholm R, Albrektson B, et al: Tissue injury caused by wound disinfectants. J Bone Joint Surg [Am] 49:48, 1967.

89. Oberg MS, Lindsey D: Do not put hydrogen peroxide or povidone iodine into wounds! Am J Dis Child 141:27, 1987.

90. Rodeheaver G, Bellamy W, Kody M, et al: Bactericidal activity and toxicity of iodine-containing solutions in wounds. Arch Surg 117:181, 1982.

91. Ondrick K, Samojla BG: Angiogenesis. Clin Podiatr Med Surg 9:185, 1992.

92. Diamond JE, Sinacore DR, Mueller MJ: Molded double-rocker plaster shoe for healing a diabetic plantar ulcer. Phys Ther 67:1550, 1987.

93. Coleman WC, Brand PW, Birke JA: The total contact cast: A therapy for plantar ulceration on insensitive feet. J Am Podiatr Med Assoc 74:548, 1984.

94. Kominsky SJ: The ambulatory total contact cast. In Frykberg RG (ed): The High-Risk Foot in Diabetes Mellitus, p 449. New York, Churchill Livingstone, 1991.

95. Laing PW, Cogley DI, Klenerman L: Neurotrophic foot ulceration treated by total contact casts. J Bone Joint Surg [Br] 74:133, 1991.

96. Ritz G, Kushner D, Friedman S: A successful technique for the treatment of diabetic neurotrophic ulcers. J Am Podiatr Med Assoc 82:479, 1992.

97. Steindler A: The tabetic arthropathies. JAMA 96:250, 1931.

98. Hoche G, Sanders LJ: On some arthropathies apparently related to a lesion of the brain or spinal cord, by Dr. J.M. Charcot, January 1868. J Hist Neurosci 1:75, 1992.

99. Johnson JTH: Neuropathic fractures and joint injuries: Pathogenesis and rationale of prevention and treatment. J Bone Joint Surg [Am] 49:1, 1967.

100. Jacobs JE: Observations of neuropathic (Charcot) joints occurring in diabetes mellitus. J Bone Joint Surg [Am] 40:1043, 1958.

101. Sanders LJ, Frykberg RG: Diabetic neuropathic osteoarthropathy: The Charcot foot. In Frykberg RG (ed): The High-Risk Foot in Diabetes Mellitus, p 297. New York, Churchill Livingstone, 1991.

102. Cofield RH, Morrison MJ, Beabout JW: Diabetic neuroarthropathy in the foot: Patient characteristics and patterns of radiographic change. Foot Ankle 4:15, 1983.

103. Brower AC, Allman RM: Pathogenesis of neurotrophic joints: Neurotraumatic versus neurovascular. Radiology 139:349, 1981.

104. Brower AC, Allman RM: Neuropathic osteoarthropathy. Orthop Rev 14:295, 1985.

105. Clohisy DR, Thompson RC: Fractures associated with neuropathic arthropathy in adults who have juvenile-onset diabetes. J Bone Joint Surg [Am] 70:1192, 1988.

106. Eichenholz SN: Charcot Joints. Springfield, IL, Charles C Thomas, 1966.

107. Kerr R, Sartoris DJ, Fix CF, Resnick D: Imaging of the diabetic foot. In Frykberg RG (ed): The High-Risk Foot in Diabetes Mellitus, p 79. New York, Churchill Livingstone, 1991.

108. Maurer AH, Millmond SH, Knight LC, et al: Infection in diabetic osteoarthropathy: Use of indium-labeled leukocytes for diagnosis. Radiology 161:221, 1986.

109. Newman LG, Waller J, Palestro CJ, et al: Unsuspected osteomyelitis in diabetic foot ulcers: Diagnosis and monitoring by leukocyte scanning with indium in 111 oxyquinoline. JAMA 266:1246, 1991.

110. Newman LG, Waller J, Palestro CJ, et al: Leukocyte scanning with ^{111}In is superior to magnetic resonance imaging in diagnosis of clinically unsuspected osteomyelitis in diabetic foot ulcers. Diabetes Care 15:1527, 1992.

111. Joseph WS, LeFrock JL: The pathogenesis of diabetic foot infections: Immunopathy, angiopathy and neuropathy. J Foot Surg 26:S7, 1987.

112. Leichter SB, Schaefer JC, O'Brien JT: New concepts in managing diabetic foot infections. Geriatrics 46(5):24, 1991.

113. Sapico F, Bessman AN: Diabetic foot infections. In Frykberg RG (ed): The High-Risk Foot in Diabetes Mellitus, p 197. New York, Churchill Livingstone, 1991.

114. Whitehouse FW: Infections that hospitalize the diabetic. Geriatrics 28:97, 1973.

115. Sapico FL: Foot infections in patients with diabetes mellitus. J Am Podiatr Med Assoc 79:482, 1989.

116. Lippman HI: Must loss of limb be a consequence of diabetes mellitus? Diabetes Care 2:432, 1979.

117. Goldberg D, Neu HC: Infectious disease of the diabetic foot. In Brenner M (ed): Management of the Diabetic Foot, p 98. Baltimore, Williams & Wilkins, 1987.

118. Joseph R, Cavuoto JW: The latest theories and treatment of diabetic foot complications. Clin Podiatr Med Surg 8:249, 1991.

119. Joseph WS, Axler DA: Microbiology and antimicrobial therapy of diabetic foot infections. Clin Podiatr Med Surg 7:467, 1990.

120. Tan JS, Flanagan PJ, File TM: Team approach in the management of diabetic foot infections. J Foot Surg 26:S12, 1987.

121. Bernhard LM, Bakst M, Coleman W, Nickamin A: Plantar space abscesses in the diabetic foot: Diagnosis and treatment. J Foot Surg 23:283, 1984.

122. Joseph WS: Handbook of Lower Extremity Infections, p 85. New York, Churchill Livingstone, 1990.

123. Larkin JG, Frier BM, Ireland JT: Diabetes mellitus and infection. Postgrad Med 61:233, 1985.

124. Rayfield EJ, Ault MJ, Keusch GT, et al: Infection and diabetes: The case for glucose control. Am J Med 72:439, 1982.

125. Bagdade JD, Root RK, Bulger RJ: Impaired leukocyte function in patients with poorly controlled diabetes. Diabetes 23:9, 1974.

126. Mowat AG, Baum J: Chemotaxis of polymorphonuclear leukocytes from patients with diabetes mellitus. N Engl J Med 284:621, 1971.

127. Axler DA: Microbiology of diabetic foot infections. J Foot Surg 26:S3, 1987.

128. Corn DB, O'Keefe RG, McCarthy DJ: Soft tissue infections of the foot and ankle. J Am Podiatr Assoc 67:508, 1977.

129. Bessman AN, Sapico FL, Tabatabai MF, Montgomerie JZ: Persistence of polymicrobial abscesses in the poorly controlled diabetic host. Diabetes 36:448, 1986.

130. Carlow SB, Jacobs RL, Vedder DK: Limb salvage in a diabetic with necrotizing fasciitis: A case report and literature review. Foot Ankle 16:199, 1986.

131. Jelinek JE: Cutaneous markers of diabetes mellitus and the role of microangiopathy. In Jelinek JE (ed): The Skin in Diabetes, p 37. Philadelphia, Lea & Febiger, 1986.

132. Alteras I, Saryt E: Prevalence of pathogenic fungi in toe webs and toenails of diabetic patients. Mycopathologica 67:157, 1979.

133. Jolly HW, Carpenter CL: Oral glucose tolerance studies in recurrent *Trichophyton rubrum* infections. Arch Dermatol 100:26, 1969.

134. Rothman S: Systemic disturbances in recalcitrant *T. rubrum* infections. Arch Dermatol 67:239, 1953.

135. Waldvogel FA, Medoff G, Swartz MN: Osteomyelitis: A review of clinical features: Therapeutic considerations and unusual aspects. N Engl J Med 282:198, 260, 316, 1970.

136. Bamberger DM, Daus GP, Gerding DN: Osteomyelitis in the feet of diabetic patients: Long-term results, prognostic factors, and the role of antimicrobial and surgical therapy. Am J Med 83:653, 1987.

137. Caprioli R, Testa R, Counoyer RW, Esposito FJ: Prompt diagnosis of suspected osteomyelitis by utilizing percutaneous bone culture. J Foot Surg 25:263, 1986.

138. Butt WP: The radiology of infection. Clin Orthop 96:20, 1973.

139. Sachs W, Kanat IO: Radionucleotide scanning in osteomyelitis. J Foot Surg 125(4):311, 1986.

140. Forstrom L, Hoogland D, Gomez L, et al: Indium-111 oxine labeled leukocytes in the diagnosis of occult inflammation or abscess. J Nucl Med 20:659, 1979.

141. Merkel KD, Brown ML, Dewanjee M, et al: Comparison of indium-labeled leukocyte imaging with sequential technetium scanning in the diagnosis of low-grade musculoskeletal sepsis: A prospective study. J Bone Joint Surg [Am] 67:465, 1985.

142. Schauwecker DS, Park HM, Mock BH, et al: Evaluation of complications of osteomyelitis with Tc99m, MDP In 111 granulocytes and Ga-67 citrate. J Nucl Med 25:849, 1984.

143. Fierer J, Daniel D, Davis C: The fetid foot: Lower extremity infections in patients with diabetes mellitus. Rev Infect Dis 1:210, 1979.

144. LeFrock JL, Blais F, Schell RF, et al: Cefoxitin in the treatment of diabetic patients with lower extremity infections. Infect Surg 2:361, 1983.

145. Leichter SB, Allweiss P, Harley J: Clinical characteristics of diabetic patients with serious pedal infections. Metabolism 37(Suppl 1):22, 1988.

146. Louie TJ, Bartlett JG, Tulley FP, Gorbach SL: Aerobic and anaerobic bacteria in diabetic foot ulcers. Ann Intern Med 85:461, 1976.

147. Sapico FL, Witte JL, Canawati HN, et al: The infected foot of the diabetic patient, quantitative microbiology and analysis of clinical features. Rev Infect Dis 6(Suppl 1):S171, 1984.

148. Wheat LJ, Allen SD, Henry M, et al: Diabetic foot infections: Bacteriological analysis. Arch Intern Med 146:1935, 1986.

149. Sapico FL, Canawati HN, Witte JL, et al: Quantitative aerobic and anaerobic bacteriology of infected diabetic feet. J Clin Microbiol 12:413, 1980.

150. Schoenbaum SC: How to minimize infectious complications of diabetes. Geriatrics 34:51, 1979.

151. Sharp CS, Bessman AN, Wagner FW Jr, et al: Microbiology of deep tissue in diabetic gangrene. Diabetes Care 1:289, 1978.

152. Sharp CS, Bessman AN, Wagner FW Jr, et al: Microbiology of superficial and deep tissues in infected diabetic gangrene. Surg Gynecol Obstet 149:217, 1979.

153. Ingerman M, Abrutyn E: Osteomyelitis, a conceptual approach. J Am Podiatr Med Assoc 76:487, 1986.

154. Little JR, Kobayaski GS, Sonnenwirth AC: Infection of the diabetic foot. In Levin ME (ed): The Diabetic Foot, ed 4, p 133. St. Louis, CV Mosby, 1988.

155. American Diabetes Association: Screening for diabetes: Position statement. Diabetes Care 15(suppl 2):7, 1992.

CHAPTER 16

FOOT INFECTIONS

Warren Joseph

If a primary care provider is one who serves as the patient's entry point into the medical system, then the practitioner who diagnoses and treats lower-extremity infections truly fits this criterion. One excellent example is the patient with a diabetic foot infection. Often this patient presents with no previous history of diabetes mellitus. He or she may have not sought medical care for years and relates that he or she has been as "healthy as a horse" until this foot infection caused him or her to see a doctor. Careful questioning, however, unveils a medical, social, and family history consistent with diabetes, and simple testing reveals that, indeed, this patient has diabetes. This patient is then referred to an internist or diabetologist and may need hospitalization for surgical intervention or parenteral administration of antibiotics. Generally there are consultations with numerous other specialists, including vascular surgeons and ophthalmologists. Indeed, this patient has now entered into the system, and it is hoped that after the acute event the patient will remain with the initial practitioner for prevention and coordination of services.

The purpose of this chapter is to discuss approaches to diagnosis and treatment of lower-extremity infections. The focus is directed toward diagnostic and therapeutic procedures that are usually performed in the practitioner's office or clinic and not toward the more technical aspects of infectious diseases, such as sophisticated laboratory testing and parenteral administration of antibiotics.

DEFINITION OF INFECTION

Too many textbooks and papers are written on the topic of infectious diseases with the assumption, sometimes incorrect, that the actual definition of the term *infection* is understood. This failure to actually explain what an infection really is can lead to misunderstanding and inappropriate treatment. For purposes of this chapter, an infection can be defined as the *pathologic* presence of bacteria in a tissue as evidenced by inflammation, purulence, or both. This definition stresses the point that the mere presence of bacteria on a wound or in a tissue is *not* diagnostic of an infection! Infection is a clinical diagnosis made on clinical grounds, not by laboratory identification of organisms.

DIAGNOSIS OF INFECTION

The diagnosis of a lower-extremity infection should be made by using data obtained from three sources of information:

1. Clinical history and examination
2. Laboratory data including bacteriology
3. Radiographic studies

Clinical History and Examination

PATIENT HISTORY

Use of the usual preprinted "Welcome to our Office" type of history form does not provide sufficient information to determine the source and type of an infection. Even usually mundane questions of medical history, allergies, social history, and current medications take on special importance in the presence of an infection.

Medical History. The obvious question to pose to any patient presenting with a lower-extremity infection is whether he or she has diabetes mellitus. Reports of an increased prevalence of infections in patients with diabetes can be debated. However, when a patient presents with a foot infection more severe than expected given a reportedly minimal insult, the first suspicion that comes to mind is that the patient has diabetes. To this end, questioning should include whether the patient has ever been diagnosed with the disease. A surprising number of cases of previously undiagnosed diabetes have been uncovered because of a foot infection. If occult diabetes is suspected, questioning should determine the presence of polyuria, polydipsia, polyphagia, sudden weight gain or loss, and family history of the disease. If the patient is being treated for diabetes, then the patient's last blood glucose test result, his or her method of control

and self-monitoring, and the date of the last visit to the patient's physician should be documented. The practitioner should not accept the seemingly universal answer of "fine" when querying the patient as to the quality of his or her control but should ask specifically for a numerical value for the latest glucose test result. Devices to test the serum glucose level through a simple finger stick are readily available and are invaluable for checking on a patient's reported control or even for making a presumptive diagnosis.

Another condition of importance that should be determined in the patient's medical history is immune compromise. This may include the acquired immunodeficiency syndrome, cancer chemotherapy, or prolonged use of corticosteroids. The presentation of the actual infection may be altered in the presence of one of these conditions. Furthermore, the efficacy of various antibiotics may be changed.

Hypertension or cardiac history should also be determined. There is little direct relationship between blood pressure and the prevalence or presentation of infection (other than possible hypotension in septicemia). The importance is more in antibiotic selection. Patients on diuretic agents may present with an electrolyte imbalance that may be exacerbated by the use of certain antibiotics. This is more evident in some of the parenteral preparations that may have significant sodium loads. The specter of fluid retention, fluid overload, and congestive heart failure is always looming but infrequently reported.

Finally, it is important to determine whether the patient has renal or hepatic disease. All antibiotics are going to be metabolized or excreted through one or both of these systems. The vast majority of commonly used drugs are cleared through the kidneys, so renal disease will have a potentially significant effect on drug selection and dosage. Techniques for monitoring renal excretion of drugs are covered in the section on laboratory testing.

Allergies. When presented with the question of drug allergy, many patients will relate being "allergic" to penicillin. If taken at face value, this response may have important consequences when selecting an antibiotic. Many of these patients have had an adverse reaction to a drug and have been incorrectly advised that they were allergic. By definition, an allergy is an immune-mediated side effect that is, in fact, fairly uncommon. Questioning of a patient who reports an allergic reaction should include the type of reaction—gastrointestinal, urticarial, or immediate hypersensitivity. The surprisingly large number of patients reporting gastrointestinal upset as an allergy will immediately alleviate the doctor's concern for an actual allergic response in a majority of the patients. Those patients relating a "rash or itch" should be questioned further as to which specific agent caused the reaction. Also, the practitioner needs to ask what other drugs the patient has taken without any problem. Frequently, a patient relating an allergic rash to penicillin has been subsequently treated with a cephalosporin without any problem. This same question should be asked of patients reporting anaphylactic-type reactions to drugs. Cross-reactivity between cephalosporins and penicillins is probably more a perceived than a real threat.

Social History. Probably the most difficult and uncomfortable area in which to delve is the patient's social history. Unfortunately, diagnosis of many infectious diseases that affect the lower extremity may require questioning in this area. Of course the most obvious is infection with human immunodeficiency virus. The lowered CD4 counts in patients with full-blown acquired immunodeficiency syndrome may predispose to lower-extremity infections. Tinea pedis and onychomycosis may be more common. Neuropathy, either from the disease process or from drugs used in its therapy, could predispose to mal perforans ulcerations. New outbreaks of multiresistant tuberculosis are being accompanied by increasing reports of skeletal tuberculosis, including cases affecting the foot. Universal precautions recommended by the Centers for Disease Control and Prevention are to be followed in every office for every patient.

Sexual practices and parenteral drug use can lead to other lower-extremity infections. Gonococcal septic arthritis should be considered in any patient who is sexually active and presents with an inflamed joint or transient arthritis. Syphilis was one of the first reported causes of lower-extremity neuropathy (tabes dorsalis), and the number of cases is increas-ing. Intravenous drug abusers appear to have a predisposition to infection with multiresistant organisms, including *Pseudomonas aeruginosa,* anaerobes, and methicillin-resistant staphylococci. By injecting these organisms directly into their blood they might allow a hematogenously spread infection to settle into the foot. Furthermore, "skin popping" into the lower extremities may lead to necrotic ulcerations that are difficult to heal.

Beyond these usual queries that are a routine part of a patient history, other specific questions directly related to the onset and progress of the infection should be asked:

1. How long has the patient been experiencing signs and symptoms of infection? This is important because certain organisms may present more aggressively while others are of lower virulence and may not be evident for long periods of time. The classic example of this is a prosthetic implant infection frequently caused by *Staphylococcus epidermidis.* It is well accepted that clinical signs and symptoms of infection may not present for 5 to 10 years following implantation. Likewise, fever and pain experienced by a patient the evening following surgery under general anesthesia would most likely be a normal postoperative consequence and not an infection. An infection following clean elective surgery usually does not become evident for at least 48 hours. There are, of course, exceptions to all of these patterns.

2. How does the patient feel on this initial visit? A patient with a localized, mild to moderate infection may only be experiencing symptoms localized to the part in question. If the patient reports he or she is "not feeling well" or classically mentions something like "I would have come in sooner but I think I had the flu for the past few days," then a more systemic involvement needs to be considered.

3. Has the patient noticed any pain or lumps behind the knee or in the groin? Are there any red streaks traveling up the foot (patients may know this as "blood poisoning")? Lymphadenitis and lymphangitis are frequently noticed by the patient without their understanding what the relation is to the infection. Furthermore, popliteal and,

to a lesser extent, inguinal lymph nodes may be difficult to palpate on examination, yet the patient can readily point to a newly identified "mass."

4. What has the patient done to make the area feel better or worse? The patient may describe having had unbearable pain in an area with massive edema and erythema. The patient either "lanced it" or noticed a spontaneous rupture with frank drainage. The site now feels significantly improved. If the pain in an "infected toe" is greater when the leg is elevated and relieved by dependency, the possibility of an ischemic rest pain, rather than pain secondary to infection, may be considered.

5. Has the patient taken any antibiotic that was either prescribed or found in the medicine cabinet? If the patient has been taking antibiotics with no improvement in the condition, then this may be helpful in directing empiric therapy because another class of agent may be warranted. Conversely, if the drug has been providing relief and improvement, then there is no need for change.

PHYSICAL EXAMINATION

After a complete history is obtained, the physical examination should be performed. This examination can be broken down into two parts: a local examination and a systemic examination.

Local Examination

The local examination is used to inspect the infected area to determine the etiology and severity of the infection.

Cellulitis. As defined earlier, for an area to be considered infected, the body must be defending against the invading organisms. The primary defense mechanism is inflammation of the tissues, which is known as cellulitis. Through this process the vessels dilate, perfusion to the area increases, capillary leaks develop that allow migration of the leukocytes, and the bacteria can be phagocytized. This is evidenced clinically in the five usual clinical signs of infection:

1. Rubor (erythema)
2. Tumor (edema)
3. Dolor (pain)
4. Calor (heat)
5. Functio laesa (loss of function)

All five of these signs do not necessarily have to be present to make the diagnosis of infection; however, in the majority of cases they are. Likewise, the presence of any or all of these five signs is not pathognomonic for infection. Other conditions such as trauma, venous disease, and arthritides can also present in a similar manner.

Lymphadenitis and Lymphangitis. These two processes represent the body's attempt to clear infectious products away from the actual site of the infection. Any area proximal to the infected site should be examined for lymphangitis. This will appear as one or two erythematous streaks following a tortuous course along lymphatic channels. These channels end in lymph nodes that act as reservoirs and filters along the vessels. The most commonly involved nodes in the lower extremity include the popliteal and inguinal groups. The popliteal nodes are more difficult to palpate. Just because these cannot be found to be enlarged does not mean that the inguinal nodes are not involved. They, too, should be palpated and are generally easier to find.

Drainage. Pus is generally composed of leukocytes, bacteria, and other skin cells. Not all pus is infectious, because any inflammatory process can develop a sterile form consisting mostly of leukocytes. When pus is associated with an infectious process, however, there may be characteristic colors and odors that may aid in the identification of the involved organism. Some general statements describing pathologic organisms are listed below:

Staphylococcus aureus: golden yellow color with no odor

Staphylococcus epidermidis: white color with no odor

Pseudomonas aeruginosa: green color, characteristic "fruity" odor

Anaerobes: watery brown/red color and fetid or foul odor

Streptococci: watery clear to white color and minimal odor

Systemic Examination

Systemic signs of infection are generally noted when the process has broken through the local defenses and toxins have been released throughout the rest of the body. This process is also known as septicemia or sepsis. *Sepsis* can be defined as the physiologic response of the body to microorganisms and their byproducts. Bacteria do not have to be isolated from the blood (bacteremia) for this to occur. In fact, asymptomatic bacteremia is a frequent event of little concern to an otherwise healthy patient. Commonly the patient with systemic involvement will appear lethargic, be diaphoretic, and have a fever.

Fever. The most important systemic manifestation of infection is the presence of fever. Fever represents the body's response to both endogenous and exogenous pyrogens formed by the bacteria (exogenous) or the monocytes (endogenous). In a localized infection of the toe or foot, the chances are that the patient will not have a fever. Monitoring the temperature in these conditions is not mandatory. If, however, there are any signs that the infection may have spread systemically, the fever should be monitored and recorded. Fevers tend to have a normal diurnal pattern with spikes in the late afternoon and early evening hours. Fever is also useful to determine the adequacy of therapy. If a patient continues to spike fevers despite antibiotics and drainage, then the possibility of antibiotic resistance or residual abscess should be considered.

Laboratory Testing

For the purpose of simplicity, laboratory testing in the diagnosis of lower-extremity infections can be broken into two sections: hematology and bacteriology.

HEMATOLOGY

Blood is drawn from the infected patient for both direct examination of the blood specimen and performance of various tests that reflect the operation of other body systems.

Complete Blood Cell Count. Probably the most direct indicator of the body's response to infection is the complete blood cell count with differential count. As the severity of an infection increases the body will produce and release more leukocytes into the peripheral circulation. For this reason, monitoring the specific leukocyte count will give a good idea as to the severity of the infection. As with fever, in the patient with a common localized lower-extremity infection, the leukocyte count will rarely be elevated. Once the marrow's ability to form mature leukocytes is overwhelmed by a significant infection, immature cells, known as "band forms" or "bands," will be released. This increase in bands is known as a *left shift.*

Erythrocyte Sedimentation Rate. An infection or inflammation may cause the erythrocytes to lose their natural tendency to repel one another. When this occurs, the cells will clump together and form rouleaux, which are heavier than a single cell. For this reason, when placed in a narrow column these clumps of cells will tend to sink faster than individual cells. This sink rate is measured by the erythrocyte sedimentation rate (ESR or sed rate). The problem with this test is that it is too nonspecific for infection and will be positive with any inflammatory process. Thus its use is limited to the ancillary role of tracking the progress of more chronic infections, such as osteomyelitis. When the ESR decreases, the infection is improving. In diagnosis of an infection, however, the use of the ESR is limited.

C-Reactive Protein. A more sensitive, although no more specific, test of inflammation is the C-reactive protein (CRP). The CRP tends to increase more rapidly than the ESR and return to normal earlier. However, its use in the actual diagnosis of infection is limited.

Blood Chemistries. The battery of blood chemistry tests exists to determine the level of function of various organ systems. Although not really related to the diagnosis of infection, these tests become important in its therapy. Probably the most important blood chemistry test is evaluation of the serum creatinine level. Although this is an indirect test of renal function, it provides enough information to allow a general idea of the patient's status. It should be ordered for any patient who is receiving parenteral antibiotics that are cleared through the kidney.

Other chemistries that may be considered are liver function studies (in patients receiving antibiotics metabolized by the liver), electrolyte studies, and serum glucose determination. A hemoglobin A1c test can be useful in determining a patient's long-term diabetes control.

This may be important given the debatable data pointing to an immune compromise in poorly controlled diabetes.

BACTERIOLOGY

Once it is suspected through history and physical examination that the patient is infected, the causative organism should be identified. In the vast majority of lower-extremity infections, this can be empirically accomplished without any testing at all. The most common pathogen in the lower extremity is *Staphylococcus aureus*. This is followed by *S. epidermidis* and the streptococci. Many commonly used oral antibiotics will easily eradicate these organisms, so that by the time the culture report is returned, the infection has cleared. In those patients in whom an unusual pathogen is suspected or in whom the infection fails to clear with standard empiric selections, the two most commonly performed bacteriologic tests are the Gram's stain and the culture and sensitivity. Remember, the diagnosis of infection is a clinical judgment. The mere presence of bacteria does not constitute an infectious diagnosis.

Gram's Stain. An easy to perform, inexpensive, underutilized, in-office technique is the Gram's stain. With a readily available set of four compounds and a microscope with oil immersion, a wealth of information can be determined in less than 5 minutes. The Gram's stain will show the presence of leukocytes, and leukocytes plus bacteria indicates pus, which should signal infection. A Gram's stain will also give a hint as to the organism present by revealing the morphology and staining characteristics of the bacteria. For example, *Staphylococcus* will stain as gram-positive (blue-purple) cocci (spheres) in clusters. This is in contrast to streptococci, which present as gram-positive cocci in chains.

Culture and Sensitivity. By far the most important aspect of performing a culture and sensitivity test, and the one under the most control by the physician, is the harvesting of the sample. The most sophisticated bacteriologic testing technologies cannot compensate for a poor specimen.

1. Does the site need to be cultured at all? Superficial ulcerations and wound dehiscence that show no clinical evidence of infection will surely grow superficial contaminants that may lead to inappropriate therapy. If the patient has been taking antibiotics and the infection is improving, then culture and sensitivity determination is probably not indicated.

2. Was a proper specimen taken? Pus may contain dead bacteria. Sinus tracts may be contaminated with multiple organisms that have no bearing on the infection. Bone should be harvested through a clean site to avoid contamination. Deep tissue is the best specimen. Use of superficial swabs should be avoided. Proper decontamination of surrounding tissues should be performed before taking a deep culture.

3. What tests should be ordered? The standard aerobic culture and sensitivity study is all that is needed in most primary care settings. Some laboratories will automatically perform an anaerobic study if the specimen is sent in the proper medium. Anaerobic studies are required only in special cases, such as deep diabetic abscesses, animal bites, puncture wounds, necrotizing infections, or when possible anaerobic infection is suggested from findings of the history or physical examination. Special studies such as those for fungi and acid-fast bacilli should be considered if infection is present but cultures are negative. Transport of the specimen to the laboratory should be expeditious.

Radiographic Diagnosis of Infection

With new technologies in the area of radiology, clinical imaging, and nuclear medicine emerging rapidly, one might be lulled into a false sense of security that these modalities can diagnose infection. Despite all of these advances the bottom line remains the same: diagnosis of infection is a clinical judgment! Despite claims to the contrary, the problem of sensitivity versus specificity remains. In the field of infectious disease diagnosis, radiology is only confirmatory.

RADIOGRAPHY

The traditional plain film remains the technique of choice. Radiographs are relatively inexpensive, and most outpatient facilities are equipped to obtain them. Their use in the diagnosis of soft tissue infections is severely limited. In fact, all that can be seen is either nondescript soft tissue swelling or, in very rare cases, tissue gas. Probably the most valuable use for radiographs in soft tissue pathology is as a gauge to monitor the depth of ulcerations and sinus tracts. They remain useful for the diagnosis of osteomyelitis. If any of the classic changes of osteomyelitis, periosteal elevation, bone destruction, sequestra, and so on are seen when an infection is clinically suspected, then there is little need to go forward with other studies.

BONE SCINTIGRAPHY

Despite promotional claims to the contrary, whether one is using technetium-99m, gallium citrate, HMPAO, indium-111, or any other new isotope, the same problem remains: these are all nonspecific for infection. Acute arthritides, trauma, Charcot foot, and postoperative changes may all be reported as false-positive results. Bone scans may be useful to make an early diagnosis of osteomyelitis before changes are seen on plain films. A good example would be in a puncture wound of the foot. However, if radiographic changes are definitive, bone scintigraphy is a costly redundancy.

IMAGING

Magnetic resonance imaging has been shown to be very useful in the diagnosis of osteomyelitis and soft tissue infections. Although bone itself does not image well, the changes seen in the magnetic resonance image can be characteristic for infection. Soft tissue abscesses can also be visualized and therefore aid in the planning of surgical intervention and drainage. Despite wide use and acceptance, the modality is not perfect. The technology is expensive. Again, if plain films show an infectious process, then the spending of extra money is unnecessary. Furthermore, false-positive results can be found, especially in patients with acute gouty arthritis. The differentiation between a Charcot foot and osteomyelitis is still not definitive.

Hospitalization of the Infected Patient

Most lower-extremity infections can be treated on an outpatient basis. Even the moderately severe diabetic foot infection can be treated in the primary care setting with aggressive treatment and appropriate follow-through. There will be cases, however, when the primary care provider will have to admit the patient to a hospital for more intensive workup and therapy. Instead of listing these instances by infectious condition (e.g., a diabetic foot infection), it is more appropriate to give guidelines pertaining to the severity of the infectious process[1]:

1. Severe infection identified by
   a. High fever (above 101°F)
   b. Elevated leukocyte count (above 13,000/mm^3)
   c. Systemic involvement as evidenced by signs of sepsis
2. Failure to respond to previously attempted outpatient therapy
3. Need for parenteral antibiotics
4. Need for surgical debridement requiring general anesthesia
5. Underlying systemic disease

COMMON LOWER-EXTREMITY INFECTIONS

The most common lower-extremity infections seen by the primary care practitioner are the superficial skin and soft tissue types. Deep abscesses, severe widespread osteomyelitis, and necrotizing infections tend to be handled in the tertiary care setting.

Cellulitis. Although *cellulitis* is a term frequently used to describe any inflammation of skin and connective tissues, it is also the proper name for a specific acute spreading infection of the skin. The disease cellulitis is most often described as being caused by streptococci, although staphylococci may also be found. There is an ill-defined border and acute spreading inflammation (Fig. 16–1). Rarely is there an open sinus or drainage. For this reason actual culturing of the lesion is difficult. Aspiration of the leading edge of cel-

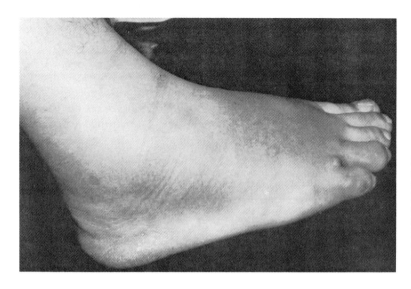

FIGURE 16–1. Cellulitis of the foot secondary to an abscess in the fourth interdigital space. Note the loss of normal topography as a result of massive edema. (From Joseph WS: Infections. In Levy LA, Hetherington VJ (eds): Principles and Practice of Podiatric Medicine, p 277. New York, Churchill Livingstone, 1990.)

lulitis results in a low success rate and may implant organisms more deeply into the tissues. Empiric antibiotic therapy is begun on the assumption of a gram-positive infection. Culturing, possibly through biopsy, becomes necessary only if remission is not noted on therapy.

Paronychia. More questions can be raised about the treatment of paronychia (Fig. 16–2) than about any simple infection. Is it necessary to culture? Is it necessary to obtain radiographs? When should a biopsy be performed on the granulation tissue? Are antibiotics necessary? These questions are mentioned because of the number of medicolegal actions that have arisen over this condition. The common presenting scenario is remarkably consistent. The patient, who is frequently a young healthy adult or older child, has been to his or her "family doctor." He or she is placed on an oral antibiotic with little attention given to the invading nail spicule other than vague instructions to "soak your foot." The patient continues to have pain and drainage. The lesion becomes chronic, and the pain may diminish. On presentation there is generally acute inflammation of one or both nail borders. Simple digital anesthesia followed by excision of the involved borders and a light dressing will resolve the problem in the majority of cases. In the rare instance when drainage persists, the patient may seek another medical opinion. Radiographs are ordered and show erosions on the distal phalanx. The patient is

referred to a surgeon, and the toe is amputated.

This scenario has occurred on more than one occasion, and the physician performing the original avulsion has been sued for malpractice. The claims are usually the failure to diagnose an osteomyelitis and the failure to culture the wound and give "appropriate antibiotics." The fact is that the patient probably never had an osteomyelitis. Radiographs showed erosion common to any chronic inflammatory process. No cultures or pathologic studies are ever performed on the amputated toe, so this procedure is difficult to defend. Furthermore, culturing of the wound would

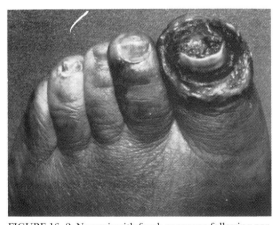

FIGURE 16–2. Necrosis with frank gangrene following paronychia in a patient with diabetes. (From Joseph WS: Infections. In Levy LA, Hetherington VJ (eds): Principles and Practice of Podiatric Medicine, p 291. New York, Churchill Livingstone, 1990.)

have shown staphylococci and streptococci, by far the most common organisms isolated in these cases. Since the inflammation is probably secondary to irritation from the ingrown nail spicule, there may not even be an infection. If there is no infection, no antibiotics are necessary. The question of biopsy of granulation tissue is raised because of the outside chance of an amelanotic melanoma. If the paronychia is recurrent or presents in an unusual fashion, it may be advantageous to send the tissue sample for pathologic analysis.

Bacterial Interspace Infections. These wet, macerated, foul-smelling infections are often mistaken for fungal infections and termed *athlete's foot*. In fact, a fungal element usually is involved. Leyden[2] has shown that dermatophytic fungi may initially be present in an interspace. These fungi may cause some initial tissue damage to the area and set up a true interdigital tinea pedis (dermatophytosis simplex). Given the proper local conditions of occlusion commonly seen in interspaces, a secondary bacterial infection may arise in the previously damaged area. These infections are frequently caused by gram-positive organisms but may also become colonized by gram-negative organisms (dermatophytosis complex). The number of fungal isolates actually decreases as the severity of the infection worsens, and it is postulated that this is caused by fungal inhibitory factors produced by the bacteria. Treatment usually consists of reversing the local factors that potentiated the infection in the first place. Antibiotics may be used, but the bacteria, through contact with an antibiotic-like substance produced by the fungi, may be resistant to many drugs. Topical or short-term systemic antifungal agents may also be useful.

Infected Diabetic Ulcerations. The emphasis here is on the word "infected." Many patients will present with diabetic mal perforans ulcerations that appear clean with no surrounding inflammation, no drainage, and a healthy granulating bed. Treatment of these ulcers consists of strict adherence to local care principles, in particular, removal of pressure. Culturing of these lesions is counterproductive because a superficial swab is bound to grow organisms. These tend to be harmless commensals and not infecting pathogens. Placing the patient on an antibiotic based on these results may lead to colonization with resistant organisms and will surely not heal the ulcer. If, however, the ulceration has surrounding cellulitis, purulent drainage, or a necrotic base, then infection should be considered. Cultures should be performed only after the surface has been prepared to ensure minimizing the isolation of contaminants. Deep tissue samples are the best specimen, although swabs of deep tissue may be useful. Careful probing of the wound should be performed to ensure no tracking to bone. Empiric antibiotic selection should be based on the assumption that the infecting organisms are either staphylococci or streptococci (usually group B). The threat of anaerobic pathogens, which is often written about in articles on the diabetic foot, is minimal in these infected ulcerations.

Impetigo. Although most common on the face of children, this superficial skin disease may also occur on the foot. These foot infections are most common in the young and the elderly. The clinical presentation is similar to the facial variety with "honey gold" crusts and purulent drainage (Fig. 16–3). The disease is highly contagious. The common organism is group A streptococci, although staphylococci may also be isolated. Treatment, traditionally through oral antibiotics, is now handled effectively with the topical agent mupirocin.

Folliculitis. Infection of the hair follicle most commonly presents on the dorsum of the foot or toes (there are no hair follicles on the plantar aspect). The initial presentation is of a painful red papule. If the papule is not treated, the area of inflammation spreads and may "come to a head." If more than one follicle is involved, the lesion may be termed a *carbuncle*. Treatment consists of warm compresses and topical antibiotics. Surgical drainage may be necessary in more severe or unresponsive cases.

ANTIBIOTIC SELECTION

The choice of an antibiotic agent before the return of the culture results, or in cases in which cultures are deemed unnecessary, is referred to as *empiric selection*. To determine the drug of choice, three rules should be followed:

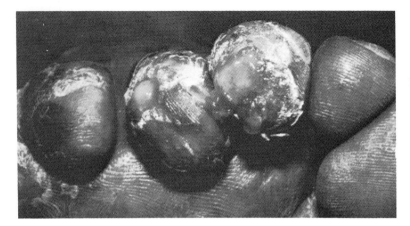

FIGURE 16–3. Impetigo of the toes previously misdiagnosed, and treated unsuccessfully, as tinea pedis. Classic honey-colored crusts and Gram's stain showing gram-positive cocci are useful in making the diagnosis. (From Joseph WS: Infections. In Levy LA, Hetherington VJ (eds): Principles and Practice of Podiatric Medicine, p 283. New York, Churchill Livingstone, 1990.)

1. *The antibiotic selected should have activity against those organisms suspected to be the cause of the infection.* This is the most important of the three rules. An antibiotic must be effective against the causative organism for the patient to improve. To make the proper selection really amounts to an educated guess of the identity of the infecting bacteria. Fortunately, when dealing with community-acquired lower-extremity infections, the possibilities are relatively limited. The vast majority of the organisms found in these infections are the gram-positive organisms. Specifically, *S. aureus* is, by far, the most common. This is followed by *S. epidermidis,* which for years was considered merely a contaminant and is now known to cause infection. Various species of the streptococci round out the list. Despite this preponderance of gram-positive organisms there will occasionally be infections caused by the gram-negative organisms. These community-acquired gram-negative organisms include *Proteus mirablis* and *Escherichia coli.* All of the above-mentioned organisms are relatively susceptible to most of the oral antibiotics, such as the first-generation cephalosporins, which are commonly prescribed in the outpatient setting.

There are rare special cases that may present to the primary care provider in which other, more resistant organisms may be suspected. In a patient presenting a history consistent with the following situations, antibiotic selection may not be as clear-cut as above:

a. Puncture wounds. Although staphylococci and streptococci remain the most frequent causes of soft tissue infection following a puncture wound, *Pseudomonas aeruginosa* has been most frequently isolated in cases of osteomyelitis. The reasons for this prevalence are theorized but poorly documented.

b. Bite wounds. Infections of both animal and human bite wounds are caused by organisms different than the usual community-acquired pathogens. Although staphylococci and streptococci may be found, it is the normal bacterial flora of the mouth that becomes a problem in these wounds (Fig. 16–4). The mouths of humans and animals contain large numbers of organisms, including anaerobic bacteria, various unique species of streptococci, and unusual organisms such as *Eikenella corrodens, Pasteurella multocida,* and the unnamed alpha-numer-

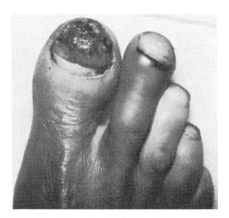

FIGURE 16–4. Wound to the right hallux and the right second digit. (From Myers RA, Littel ML, Joseph WS: Bite wound infections of the lower extremity. Clin Podiatr Med Surg 7(3):501–508, 1990.)

ics. Some of these tend to be resistant to the first-generation cephalosporins that may otherwise be selected.

c. Aquatic injuries. Infections of wounds sustained while the patient is swimming or walking in water may be caused by unusual bacteria that are only found in the aquatic environment. These include *Aeromonas hydrophilia* and *Vibrio* species. Again, these organisms tend to be resistant to commonly prescribed oral agents.

d. Lyme borreliosis. A patient may present with a cellulitis of the lower extremity that does not improve with the usual antibiotics. There may be a history of living in or visiting an endemic region of Lyme disease. The cellulitis may in fact be a case of erythema chronicum migrans, which is the initial presenting symptom of Lyme disease. Treatment with doxycycline should rapidly clear the lesion.

2. *The antibiotic selected should be the least expensive choice if a number of agents fit rule 1.* Once a particular organism is suspected, a number of equally efficacious antibiotics may be available. Given everything else as equal, then the most inexpensive drug should be prescribed. Usually the less expensive choice is a generic product. Some physicians and patients have a bias against the use of generic drugs, feeling, correctly or incorrectly, that they may not be as effective. Some of the older, less-expensive drugs may have to be given more frequently than newer agents, which tests a patient's compliance. It is well known that as the number of times per day a drug must be taken increases, the actual amount taken by the patient decreases. How cost-effective is a drug if it is forgotten and not taken? The cost of the whole prescription should be determined, not just the cost of each pill. A drug taken once a day can be *four times* the cost (per pill) of a drug taken four times a day and still be the same cost per prescription. These factors all have to be considered when discussing the relative expense of an antibiotic selection.

3. *The antibiotic selected should be the safest and best tolerated of those that fit the first two rules.* Most of the currently available oral agents are relatively safe and well tolerated. There-

fore, this rule becomes less of a concern in the primary care setting then it would in the hospital. However, there are still slight differences in tolerance on an individual patient basis.

To clarify the above three principles it may be helpful to present an illustrative case:

A male patient presents with a draining pustule on the foot. Cellulitis extends for 4 cm around the area. The drainage is creamy yellow and odorless. Gram's stain reveals gram-positive cocci in clusters. The assumption is made that the patient has an uncomplicated *S. aureus* infection. There is no history of allergy to penicillin, and the patient seems reliable and compliant. What antibiotic should be prescribed?

The following five antibiotics may be considered:

Dicloxacillin, 500 mg four times a day
Cephalexin, 500 mg three times a day
Cefadroxil, 500 mg twice daily
Erythromycin, 500 mg four times a day
Ciprofloxacin, 500 mg twice daily

In following rule 1, ciprofloxacin can be immediately removed from the list. This drug has excellent activity against resistant gram-negative organisms but has had significant resistance develop to *Staphylococcus* while patients have been on therapy. The other four drugs perform consistently better and all would have excellent activity, thereby passing rule 1.

Applying rule 2 would eliminate cefadroxil. When compared with cephalexin, which is given three times a day, this drug, although only given twice a day, is two to three times more expensive. The activity of the two drugs is identical. Rule 2 would also eliminate dicloxacillin. Although its per pill cost is similar to cephalexin, dicloxacillin should be given four times per day. Cephalexin can be effectively dosed three times a day, making it less expensive on a daily basis. This leaves only cephalexin and erythromycin on the list.

Erythromycin is significantly less expensive than cephalexin, but rule 3 would eliminate it from consideration. A majority of patients who take erythromycin develop significant gastrointestinal distress, so much so that this drug is not often considered a viable alternative for skin and soft tissue infections in adults. Therefore, by applying the above principles, cephalexin would be considered the drug of choice in this clinical scenario.

ANTIBIOTIC AGENTS

Because the focus of this book is on primary care, this chapter has concentrated on infections and antibiotic usage in that setting. In this section only the orally available antibiotics are discussed because these are the drugs used most commonly by the primary care provider. With the popularity of home infusion it is true that some cases can be treated with parenteral agents, but in relative numbers this is still rare.

The oral antibiotics discussed here are listed by class of compound. Each entry includes generic name, trade name (if applicable), spectrum of activity, and dosing. Any important adverse effects specific to an agent are also listed. This listing is not meant to be all-inclusive. There are probably close to 50 different oral antibiotics available on the market. Of these, only a percentage have any real application to lower-extremity skin and skin structure infections, and these are discussed here.

Penicillins

There are a variety of classes of penicillins: the natural penicillins, aminopenicillins, penicillinase-resistant penicillins, and penicillin/β-lactamase inhibitor combinations. Of these the natural penicillins have such a limited spectrum of activity as to be useless unless the infection is caused solely by streptococci. Since this is a rare occurrence and there are other agents that work equally as well against these organisms, the natural penicillins are not included in the list. Likewise, aminopenicillins such as amoxicillin are also too limited in their spectrum. With no activity against the staphylococci and increasing resistance against gram-negative organisms, these, too, are not individually listed.

Dicloxacillin. This is the prototypical penicillinase-resistant penicillin. It is similar in most respects to the other orally available agent, oxacillin. The use of one over the other depends on personal preference. Because they are relatively older, less frequently prescribed drugs, some pharmacies may not carry one or the other.

Spectrum: Staphylococcus, Streptococcus
Dosing: 250 to 500 mg every 6 hours on an empty stomach

Amoxicillin/Clavulanic Acid (Augmentin). This is the first orally available β-lactamase inhibitor combination. The addition of clavulanic acid, by inhibiting the activity of the β-lactamases through binding with them, significantly increases the spectrum of the amoxicillin. This drug combination is an ideal empiric selection for mildly infected diabetic foot lesions and bite wounds.

Spectrum: Staphylococcus, Streptococcus, enterococcus, community-acquired gram-negatives, anaerobes
Dosing: 250 to 500 mg every 8 hours with food and a full glass of water. Because of a fixed amount of clavulanic acid in both forms, giving two 250-mg tablets does not equal one 500-mg pill.
Side effects: Significant incidence of diarrhea reduced with co-administration of food

Cephalosporins

Although the differences between them are more and more seemingly arbitrary, cephalosporins are still generally classified into three "generations." Although we have always been taught that the earlier generation agents have better gram-positive activity that decreases with later agents in inverse proportion to the activity against the gram-negative organisms, these distinctions have blurred. The one general statement that can still be made is that as the generations advance from first through third, the activity against certain gram-negative organisms increases. Date of release has nothing to do with the classification since some newer second-generation drugs were released after some third-generation agents.

Cephalexin (Keflex, Keftab). Although not the earliest first-generation drug, cephalexin has endured as the most commonly used. This is because of its excellent activity against most of the common skin pathogens and reliable safety profile. In the generic form its low price combines with the above features to make it the drug of choice for almost all community-acquired skin and skin structure infections of the lower extremity.

Spectrum: Staphylococci, streptococci, community-acquired gram-negative organisms
Dosage: 250 to 500 mg every 6 to 8 hours. Although its short half-life would suggest dosing of every 6 hours, it is as effective and easier for the patient to take at the less frequent interval.

Cefadroxil (Duricef). The addition of a hydroxy group to the cephalexin molecule yields cefadroxil. The sole advantage of this chemical manipulation is a longer serum half-life, which allows less frequent dosing. The problem is that without a generic form its price is incredibly high (three times that of generic cephalexin for 500 mg) with minimal appreciable benefits.

Spectrum: Identical to cephalexin
Dosage: 500 to 1000 mg every 12 to 24 hours

Cefuroxime Axetil (Ceftin). This second-generation cephalosporin has the advantage of actually having better in vitro activity against staphylococci and streptococci than either of the two previously mentioned first-generation agents. Along with this advantage against the gram-positive organisms it also has a broader spectrum against some common gram-negative organisms. Its twice-daily dosing, broader spectrum, and, in some locations, lower price may make this a preferable agent over cefadroxil.

Spectrum: staphylococci, streptococci, community-acquired gram-negative organisms, *Proteus vulgaris,* and some first-generation resistant *Klebsiella* and *Haemophilus*
Dosage: 250 mg every 12 hours

Cefprozil (Cefzil). A newer second-generation agent, cefprozil is very similar in activity and dosing to cefuroxime axetil. Less is known about its action against skin and skin structure infections, and it is primarily marketed for respiratory tract infections.

Spectrum: same as cefuroxime axetil
Dosing: same as cefuroxime axetil

Cefaclor (Ceclor). Probably the first second-generation oral cephalosporin, cefaclor's activity is similar to the first-generation agents with the exception of slightly better *Haemophilus* activity. The similar activity, along with thrice daily dosing and relatively high price, does not give it any advantage over the first-generation products. It remains more popular for respiratory tract infections.

Spectrum: similar to cephalexin, *Haemophilus*
Dosage: 250 to 500 mg every 8 hours

Loracarbef (Lorabid). This drug is very similar to cefaclor in most respects. The major difference is that it can be dosed every 12 hours as opposed to the every-8-hour regimen for cefaclor. This drug can be thought of as "b.i.d. Ceclor." It is mostly marketed for respiratory tract infections.

Spectrum: Same as cefaclor
Dosage: 200 to 400 mg every 12 hours

Cefpodoxime Proxetil (Vantin). This is the only third-generation oral cephalosporin that may have usefulness in skin infections. An earlier third-generation product, cefixime (Suprax), had the disadvantage of no gram-positive coverage. Cefpodoxime, although not a drug of choice for *Staphylococcus,* does have some activity against this organism. Both of these drugs have gram-negative activity that is similar to that of the parenteral third-generation agents. They are not effective against *Pseudomonas aeruginosa.*

Spectrum: Moderate activity against *Staphylococcus* and *Streptococcus;* typical third-generation activity against the Enterobacteriaceae. Resistance may develop to these organisms through the production of inducible β-lactamase.
Dosage: 200 mg every 12 hours. (Package insert states 400 mg for skin infections, but there is no evidence that this higher dose is more effective than the 200 mg.)

Macrolides

The prototype agent for the macrolide (large molecule) class of antibiotics is erythromycin. Although the spectrum of this drug is conducive to use in lower-extremity infections, the side-effect profile renders erythromycin mostly useless. Although throughout the years there have been manipulations of the original molecule's base, really significant changes have been recent.

Azithromycin (Zithromax). This newer macrolide has a few advantages that may make it very interesting for the treatment of lower-extremity infections, especially in those patients allergic to penicillins and cephalosporins. Probably the most unusual aspect is the extremely long tissue half-life of the drug. This makes once-daily dosing possible. Furthermore, the drug only has to be given for 5 days to obtain tissue levels comparable to 10 days of therapy with traditional agents. This dosing regimen, although convenient to the patient, comes at a high per pill cost. This is a prime example of the importance of cost of therapy, not just cost of each pill. Five days of therapy with azithromycin is equivalent to 10 days of therapy with other drugs and costs about the same.

Spectrum: Staphylococcus, Streptococcus; probably will work against community-acquired skin gram-negative organisms but the data are lacking. (Most of the attention on the gram-negative organisms has been directed toward the respiratory pathogens.)
Dosage: 250 mg, two the first day followed by one per day the next 4 days for a total of 5 days of therapy

Clarithromycin (Biaxin). Released a few months earlier than azithromycin, this drug got a bit of a head start on the market. This may account for its popularity, especially among the family physicians who use it extensively to treat upper respiratory tract infections. It may also have an advantage against some mycobacterial infections common in patients with the acquired immunodeficiency syndrome. For the lower extremity there is little advantage to this drug over any other

agent. It does not have the more convenient dosing of azithromycin.

Spectrum: Similar to azithromycin; possibly some in vitro differences that are probably not clinically significant
Dosage: 250 to 500 mg every 12 hours

Quinolones

One of the most misunderstood, overpromoted, and overprescribed class of antibiotics, the quinolones are not the panacea that marketing may lead one to believe. There has been significant development of resistance, especially against *Staphylococcus.* This has led some researchers in the infectious disease community to state that the quinolones are not drugs of choice for the treatment of these infections. When used in the proper situation, however, these drugs are excellent, effective antibiotics that can be life and limb saving. The greatest advantage of these agents is their activity against the gram-negative pathogens. These include organisms that may have become resistant to later-generation cephalosporins. Infections caused by such bacteria as *P. aeruginosa* and *Serratia* may be treated with quinolones as oral single agents. Although development of resistance has been reported for some gram-negative organisms, especially *Pseudomonas,* this remains fairly isolated, mostly found in intensive care units and tertiary care hospitals. All quinolones should be avoided in children because of the possibility of cartilage damage. This has been shown in animals but not substantiated in humans. Interactions with theophylline and caffeine occur to a debatable extent with most quinolones, although these interactions seem to be the most common with ciprofloxacin.

Ciprofloxacin (Cipro). The first quinolone marketed that is effective for skin and skin structure infections, ciprofloxacin has gained a lion's share of the market. As with other quinolones, the drug is expensive and should not be routinely used for empiric therapy of lower-extremity infections. As stated many times previously, the bulk of these infections are caused by *Staphylococcus* and *Streptococcus,* two organisms against which ciprofloxacin is not the most effective. When a culture report is returned demonstrating infection caused by a gram-negative organism, ciprofloxacin may be considered as an appropriate selection. Another potential use is the combination of ciprofloxacin with amoxicillin/clavulanic acid or clindamycin for oral therapy in patients with moderately severe diabetic foot infections.

Spectrum: Excellent broad-spectrum against most gram-negative pathogens, including *Pseudomonas.* It may be ineffective against some *Acinetobacter* species. Resistance develops rapidly in the gram-positives organisms, and it is generally ineffective against anaerobes.
Dosage: 500 to 750 mg every 12 hours

Ofloxacin (Floxin). The second quinolone released for the treatment of skin infections was ofloxacin. The main difference between this agent and ciprofloxacin is in vitro susceptibility. Ciprofloxacin seems to be more effective against the gram-negative organisms while ofloxacin is more effective against the gram-positive organisms. The clinical significance of this difference is not known. Another difference is cost. At the 500-mg dose, ciprofloxacin is less expensive than 400 mg of ofloxacin. However, some may argue that a more appropriate comparison would be 750 mg of ciprofloxacin to 400 mg of ofloxacin. At this dosing, the ofloxacin has the price advantage.

Spectrum: Similar to ciprofloxacin with the above-discussed differences
Dosage: 400 mg every 12 hours

Lomefloxacin (Maxaquin). Currently only approved for urinary tract infections and respiratory infections, lomefloxacin has been marketed to some physicians for skin infections. The only advantage that this agent seems to possess is once-daily dosing.

Miscellaneous Antibiotics

There are a number of classes of drugs that have useful agents for lower-extremity infections. Because most of these have only one or two compounds, they are grouped together.

Clindamycin (Cleocin). A very good selection for skin and skin structure infections of the lower extremity, clindamycin was the recipient of bad press early in its existence. Cases of serious colitis were associated with the drug, and the warning was quickly spread. Fortunately, the truth is that the incidence is exaggerated and the drug is relatively safe. It is also a very effective, convenient antibiotic. It is especially useful in patients allergic to penicillin and cephalosporins who have mild to moderate diabetic foot infections.

Spectrum: Staphylococcus, Streptococcus, anaerobes
Dosage: 300 mg every 8 to 12 hours
Side effects: Although the incidence of true pseudomembranous colitis is overstated, the antibiotic can still cause diarrhea. The patient should be made aware of this and advised to discontinue the drug and notify the physician if diarrhea occurs. The diarrhea is usually self-limiting.

Trimethoprim-Sulfamethoxazole (Bactrim, Septra). Traditionally thought of as a urinary tract agent, this compound is very well absorbed from the gastrointestinal tract (so much so that levels with oral dosing are comparable to those of parenteral dosing). It is very effective in skin and soft tissue infections. It has a broad spectrum that attacks not only common pathogens but also some unusual organisms. It is a relatively safe drug in doses used for these infections, as long as the patient does not have a sulfa allergy. This broad-spectrum and efficacy also comes at an inexpensive price. The generic product can be found for less than 10 cents per pill (double strength).

Spectrum: Staphylococcus (including methicillin-resistant variety), *Streptococcus,* broad spectrum of gram-negative organisms *except P. aeruginosa* but effective against other *Pseudomonas* species, and unusual pathogens, including *Xanthomonas.*
Dosage: 1 double-strength (160/800 mg) tablet every 8 to 12 hours
Side effects: Take with plenty of water to avoid crystalluria. Hemolysis may occur in patients with glucose-6-phosphate dehydrogenase deficiency. Allergy including Stevens-Johnson

reaction is possible. Interactions occur with some oral hypoglycemic agents.

Tetracyclines. Although the original tetracycline compound now has limited uses secondary to multiple side effects, there are two newer agents that may prove useful. Minocycline (Minocin) has the best antistaphylococcal activity and may be considered as alternative oral therapy in patients infected with methicillin-resistant *Staphylococcus.* Dosage is 100 mg every 12 to 24 hours. A loading dose of 200 mg is frequently given. The second agent is doxycycline (Vibramycin). The primary use for this drug is in patients with Lyme borreliosis. The dosing is the same as with minocycline.

Metronidazole (Flagyl). Usually considered for infections of the urinary tract caused by *Trichomonas vaginalis* and amebae, this drug has excellent activity against the anaerobic bacteria that may be found in more severe diabetic foot infections. It may also prove useful as the drug of choice for the treatment of pseudomembranous colitis caused by *Clostridium difficile.*

Spectrum: Anaerobes including *Bacteroides*
Dosage: 500 mg every 8 hours

REFERENCES

1. Joseph WS: Handbook of Lower Extremity Infection. New York, Churchill Livingstone, 1990.
2. Leyden JL: Progression of interdigital infections from simplex to complex. J Am Acad Dermatol 28:S7–S11, 1993.

CHAPTER 17

PODIATRIC BIOMECHANICS AND ORTHOPEDICS

Allan M. Spencer

With regard to orthopedic evaluation and diagnostic methods in primary care podiatric medicine, practitioners must obtain the maximum amount of information with the most effective use of their time. If the patient has a complaint with a mechanical etiology, it is clear that a biomechanical evaluation and gait analysis will be primary in the establishing of a diagnosis and the development of an effective treatment program. On the other hand, orthopedic problems seen by podiatrists are often caused by local or systemic medical disorders. It is, therefore, important to obtain as much information as possible from the patient's history and chief complaint. This chapter discusses problems that have a mechanical cause.

GAIT ANALYSIS

When a gait analysis is done it is important that it be performed in sequence and then followed by the biomechanical examination. This is to ensure that subjective gait observations can be objectively evaluated in the biomechanical examination.

The objective is to visualize malalignment and imbalances that occur during gait on the frontal, sagittal, and transverse body planes. The patient should be observed while wearing a swimming suit or similar outfit so that body landmarks can be clearly seen. It is important to have an area where the patient can walk in his or her normal gait pattern for a distance of 15 to 20 feet. The practitioner should have the patient walk two or three times back and forth before recording any observations. Use of a portable tape recorder that can be carried in the pocket or held in the hand will allow the podiatrist to document his or her comments on the gait analysis and biomechanical examination expeditiously. This information is transcribed at a later time. In this manner, the practitioner can record conversation with the patient during the gait analysis and biomechanical examination that includes comments and questions that may offer additional insight into the patient's symptoms.

Developing a routine method of examination will facilitate observation and documentation. It is recommended that the analysis begin proximal at the head and move distally. The majority of time will be spent examining the lower extremities; however, the influence of the upper body and arms is equally important.

Segmenting the Body During Gait Analysis

Frontal Plane (Inversion—Eversion)
   Head tilt
   Shoulder level
   Spinal curves (Scoliosis)
   Hip level
   Femoral angulations
   Tibial-fibular angulations
   Rearfoot
   Forefoot
Sagittal Plane (Dorsiflexion—Plantarflexion)
   Head tilt (front—back)
   Shoulders
   Spinal curves (lordosis)
   Hip level (anterior–posterior tilt)
   Femoral angulations
   Tibial-fibular angulations
   Rearfoot
   Forefoot
Transverse Plane (Adduction—Abduction)
   Head position
   Shoulder position
   Hip position
   Femoral angulations
   Patella position
   Tibial-fibular angulation
   Foot position

Most of the information obtained in the gait analysis will be evaluated and authenticated in the biomechanical examination.

As the patient walks toward the examiner the most effective observations are made on the frontal and transverse planes. On the frontal plane one can observe any head tilting, shoulder tilting, and hip levels. Lateral spinal curves are also evident. The relationships of the femurs (femoral varum or valgum) and the tibias (tibial varum or valgum) are visually evaluated. At the foot level the examiner should look for any inrolling (inversion) or rolling out (eversion) of the entire foot. Any move-

ment between the forefoot and rearfoot at midstance should be noted. This is a "quiver" type movement that may be an attempt by the foot to get into a locked position to move into a propulsive phase of gait. This motion is observed in the excessively pronated foot. Where the foot "locks" should be documented. Some feet lock in, or close to, a normal, neutral functional position. Others lock in a maximally pronated or a relatively apropulsive position. All feet lock at the midtarsal joint at some point in space and time. I propose that this "quiver" motion is the forefoot's moving into this maximally pronated position (eversion, abduction, and dorsiflexion) to ensure locking of the foot.

On the transverse plane two basic observations are very important. The first is the location of the patella during the swing phase of gait. If it is directed medially or laterally, one should consider a femoral problem, either positional or torsional, that occurs on the transverse plane. If the patella faces directly forward but the foot is directed outward, one must consider excessive tibial torsion. The second observation is foot placement. At the foot level the abduction component of pronation may contribute to an externally directed gait. The examiner should try to estimate the number of degrees of external or internal position by referring to the face of a clock. External position of 30° would appear as 1 o'clock. As the patient moves away, the examiner should be aware of how quickly the heel is lifted, which can suggest an equinus problem. At midstance, the examiner should observe tilting of the calcaneus (inversion—eversion) and how much of the lateral side of the foot can be seen. In an excessively pronated foot it will be noted that more of the foot can be seen owing to the abduction component of pronation.

It is helpful to use specific lines to aid in demonstrating abnormal movements during the gait analysis. This can be done by drawing lines as illustrated in Figure 17–1.

BIOMECHANICAL EXAMINATION
Non–Weight-Bearing Rearfoot Evaluation

The patient is placed prone on an examination table with the foot extending over the end

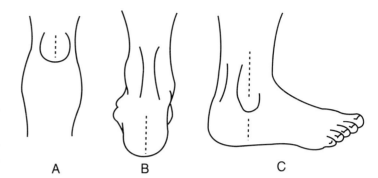

FIGURE 17–1. The observer should draw lines to observe abnormal movements. *(A)* Line bisecting the patella. *(B)* Line bisecting the calcaneus. *(C)* Lines serving as a visual check for alignment between the foot and leg.

of the table and the posterior surface of the heel directly vertical. The heel is bisected into equal halves with a marking pen. The leg is bisected at the level of the popliteal fossa, and the lower leg is bisected between the medial and lateral malleoli. Next the points between the popliteal fossa and the posterior ankle area are connected. The calcaneus is inverted and everted at the subtalar joint, and the point of rotation is noted (Fig. 17–2). With the aid of a protractor, the amount of inversion and eversion in relationship to the leg line is determined (Fig. 17–3). The point of rotation is used as the reference point to determine the angular relationship (see Figs. 17–2 and 17–3). The total number of degrees obtained is added to determine the total range of motion. According to Root's rule of neutral subtalar position, neutral position is determined to be a point that on measurement is one third in the direction of inversion from the most everted position. For example, if the measurement is 23° inversion and 7° eversion, then the total range of motion is one third or 30°, which equals 10° back from 7° eversion, giving a value of 3° inverted (varus) as the neutral subtalar position.

Non–Weight-Bearing Forefoot Evaluation

The relationship between the forefoot and the rearfoot in the frontal plane is the major focus of the non–weight-bearing evaluation. Is it inverted (varus) or everted (valgus) in its relationship with the rearfoot when the subtalar joint is in neutral subtalar position? It is therefore necessary to know the neutral subtalar joint position before finding the forefoot measurement. The patient is maintained in the prone position with the leg extended over the edge of the table. The foot is placed with the subtalar joint neutral, and the forefoot is loaded or pushed in dorsiflexion for only as long as the subtalar joint can be maintained in neutral (Fig. 17–4). Most importantly, as the subtalar joint moves in an everted (pronation) direction, more forefoot to rearfoot motion becomes available and the locking mechanism is impaired. In this case it can be stated that motion begets motion. After loading the foot correctly, the examiner notes the position of the forefoot by placing a tongue blade on the plantar surface of the metatarsal head with double-sided adherent tape to determine the

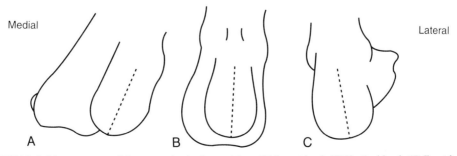

FIGURE 17–2. Measurement of the neutral subtalar position. *(A)* Invert heel. *(B)* Vertical heel. *(C)* Evert heel.

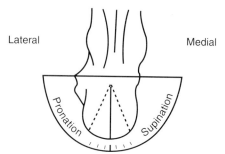

FIGURE 17–3. Direct measurement of the neutral subtalar position with a protractor.

frontal plane relationship to the neutral rearfoot. This measurement may be less accurate in non–weight-bearing owing to many factors, such as plantarflexed first ray; hence, more value is placed on the weight-bearing determination of this relationship.

Non–Weight-Bearing Foot to Leg Relationships

SAGITTAL PLANE

Equinus is a very powerful pronating influence on the foot because foot pronation is one of the most common compensations for equinus. The evaluation for equinus is performed by first maintaining the subtalar joint in neutral and then dorsiflexing the entire foot on the leg and measuring the lateral column of the foot in relationship to the lower leg. It is commonly reported that 10° of motion at the ankle joint with the subtalar joint neutral is required to function normally and not exert a deforming pronating influence on the foot.

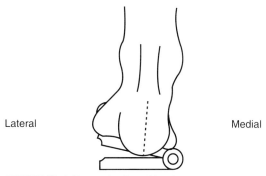

FIGURE 17–4. Determination of forefoot varus with a tractograph.

FRONTAL PLANE: TIBIAL VARUM

Measurement of tibial varum is obtained by having the patient standing with the subtalar joint neutral and by observing the frontal plane angulation of the lower leg with the foot. The best device for obtaining this value is a gravity goniometer, which is placed on the anterior border of the tibia. This has traditionally been considered to be a lower leg relationship that should be added to the neutral subtalar joint position to obtain the neutral rearfoot position. I believe that a small amount (2° or 3°) of tibial varum can be added to the subtalar joint neutral position to determine the neutral rearfoot position. It has been suggested that this tibial varum influence has a pronating effect on the rearfoot; however, when these amounts are in the 3° to 5° range, I do not add them, and, indeed, when they are above the 5° range, I suggest that they might better be subtracted from 5° when considered in the rearfoot position. The rationale is based on the rotation point within the subtalar joint on the frontal plane. If the line of gravity from the tibia above falls medial to this point, a pronating influence would be present. If the line of gravity falls directly over it, no frontal plane influence would occur; however, if the line of gravity from the tibial influence falls lateral to the frontal plane rotation point, it would have a supinating effect on the rearfoot. If one notes the number of excellent athletes who have very high tibial varum values and have extremely effective propulsive foot function, one has to question whether tibial varum is a positive or a negative influence on rearfoot position and foot stability and function.

Weight-Bearing Biomechanical Examination

There are times in an office practice when it is important to gain preliminary information about a patient's biomechanical values. In these situations a brief weight-bearing assessment is required.

This evaluation is based on the ability of the examiner to determine neutral subtalar position by palpation and talocalcaneal congruency. If one palpates the foot just in front of the medial and lateral malleoli, a concavity is noted. When the foot is in subtalar neutral position, the concavity is of equal depth on both sides of the talus; however, when the foot is inverted or everted, this congruence will not be present and the subtalar joint is not in its neutral position.

Another method that has been presented by Root and coworkers is that when the foot is observed from behind, a concavity is seen above and below the lateral malleolus. When these two curves are identical, this is the neutral subtalar position (Fig. 17–5).

To determine the neutral position, a vertical line is drawn on the back of the calcaneus, bisecting the heel into two halves while the patient kneels with his or her knee on a chair. Now the patient is asked to stand and is observed from behind. The examiner observes the line and notes any deviation of the line in relationship to the floor. If the line deviates laterally (everts), this is the Helbing sign, which is an indicator of flexible flatfoot or excessive midstance pronation. This is considered to be the relaxed calcaneal stance position and is directly related to the motion that occurs between the forefoot and the rearfoot as a compensation so that the forefoot may contact the weight-bearing surface. If one assumes that this foot motion is fully compensated, it follows that this angular relationship of the calcaneal line to the weight-bearing surface is the amount of forefoot varus. The patient is now asked to actively invert and evert the root, and the examiner palpates for congruency in front of the ankle joint, as previously described. The patient is placed in neutral subtalar position, and the line on the posterior surface of the calcaneus is observed and measured with a protractor to determine the relationship of the line to the ground. This angulation is a representation of the neutral subtalar position. This test can be carried out with a simple protractor and a small ruler. It takes little time and gives a great deal of information as to subtalar joint neutral position and the amount of forefoot to rearfoot motion that occurs on weight bearing. When the calcaneal bisection line inverts (deviates medially) on weight bearing, one should consider a forefoot valgus or plantarflexed first metatarsal ray.

The proper utilization of the information obtained during the gait analysis and biomechanical examination is to accurately assess the biomechanics of the foot as it functions within the environment. The ultimate objective of therapy is to make foot function as mechanically efficient as possible in both static position and dynamic motion. This implies limiting abnormal motion and promoting normal motion.

Through the work of Root and colleagues we now have a much better understanding of foot function. It is now generally accepted that the foot must function as both a flexible adaptor and a rigid lever during the stance phase of gait, between the time period of heel contact to toe off. The mechanics involve the subtalar joint, which consists of the calcaneus and talus. Since the talus also articulates with the tibia and fibula, it can be considered as a torque converter that converts movements from both the proximal leg and the distal foot. It is important to recognize that the subtalar joint is the key to the proper locking and unlocking of the foot. The midtarsal joint, which is dependent on the subtalar joint, is made up of articulations between the talus and navicular and the calcaneus and cuboid. When the axes of motion between these articulations are parallel, motion is available; and when these axes intersect, a decrease of available motion is noted and the foot becomes locked or rigid. When more motion is available, a condition

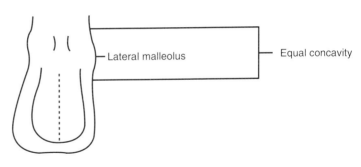

FIGURE 17–5. Observation of the neutral subtalar position.

that is described as pronation occurs; and when less motion is present, a condition of supination is present.

During the period of closed kinetic chain weight bearing, pronation consists of the motions of eversion, abduction, and dorsiflexion and supination consists of inversion, adduction, and plantarflexion. This is a relationship between the forefoot and rearfoot and also the leg. Stance phase is divided into three periods: contact period, which makes up 27% of the stance phase; midstance period, which makes up 40% of stance phase; and propulsive period, which makes up the remaining 33% of stance. It is important to remember that the foot should be in a flexible adaptive mode on initial heel contact and then progressively move into a rigid propulsive arm to permit normal propulsion to occur. This occurs by means of subtalar joint position and the resultant effect distally through the midtarsal joint and the first metatarsal ray segment.

In a treatment program directed toward proper foot function it must be recognized that initial pronation at heel strike is normal. Indeed, it is needed to absorb shock so that it not be excessive proximally in the knees, hips, and back. The most important fact to consider with pronation is that it not occur for a prolonged period during the stance phase. The subtalar joint should be in neutral position at two points during stance phase. The first is at initial heel contact, and the second is at the middle (50%) of the stance phase. As noted earlier, if pronation occurs for a prolonged period, the foot remains flexible and skeletal malalignments occur not only in the foot but also in the leg, knee, hip, and back. This relationship has been described by Jones in his book *The Postural Complex,* in which the relationship of posture to neuralgic pain in various parts of the body is discussed. It is therefore extremely important that the primary podiatric practitioner recognize the impact of abnormal foot function on the entire skeletal system.

TREATMENT METHODS

Taping

Flexible casting is a type of adhesive taping that was developed by Dye. Dye developed various taping methods, but the two that are commonly used by podiatrists are the high Dye and low Dye tapings. Taping is an excellent method to assess the reduction in symptoms in the podiatric patient with abnormal foot function due to faulty biomechanics of the foot. The decision as to which taping method to use involves the biomechanical findings, specifically the range of motion of the subtalar joint and neutral subtalar position. If the patient has a rearfoot varus of over 4°, the high Dye taping is used to control the foot adequately. If, on the other hand, the rearfoot neutral is less than 4° and the primary biomechanical abnormality is between the forefoot and the rearfoot, a low Dye taping is used. The rationale for this is that the high Dye taping has a much greater vector of force on the frontal plane to position the foot in neutral subtalar position. The low Dye taping is of benefit in that it keeps the flexible, unstable forefoot varus in a close packed position with the rearfoot at the midtarsal joint. I suggest using the tapings only until it can be determined that correct positioning of the foot is benefiting the patient and his or her orthopedic symptoms.

Foot Orthotic Devices

Most podiatrists use the services of a professional orthotic laboratory when choosing the most effective orthotic device. This choice involves many factors, such as type of material, amount of control, length of the device, and amount of posting on forefoot or rearfoot. One method that addresses the requirements of the podiatric orthopedic patient involves considering the requirements in terms of quality and quantity of control. Quality involves the material of the shell of the orthotic and is frequently described in four categories: rigid, semirigid, semiflexible, and flexible.

Rigid orthotics have classically been made of Rohadur (Rohm and Haas, Philadelphia, PA), an acrylic polymer which is of limited availability; however, other materials such as graphite laminates are being promoted. The advantage of graphite is that the same rigidity as with Rohadur can be obtained but with less thickness, which takes up less space in shoes.

The original idea of posting with rigid devices was a rigid post on the rearfoot of dental acrylic to position the foot in neutral subtalar position. This was fabricated with a 4° grind off on the medial side to permit shock absorption. This posting was also used on the forefoot to create the proper angulation of the forefoot for weight transfer, which was determined during the biomechanical examination. There are several points that should be evaluated when considering why these devices are so effective when used correctly.

The rearfoot post creates the angular relationship of the foot in the shoe of neutral subtalar position, which is important in the proper locking of the distal joints of the foot. A secondary benefit is that of the heel lift effect, which acts to neutralize the effect of equinus that is seen very often in the patient with pronated feet. The main compensation is excessive pronation with equinus; and when a rearfoot posted orthotic is used, this compensation of pronation is no longer required owing to the heel lift effect of the angulated rearfoot post.

The second effect relates to the application of the extrinsic forefoot post, which is added to the front of the orthotic on the plantar surface. In many cases of plantar keratoses it is noted that the lesions improve or in some cases disappear after extrinsic posted orthotics are worn. There is no doubt that proper control or locking of the foot decreases the shearing force on the transverse plane, which plays a major role in the etiology of the hyperkeratosis; however, there is the additional effect of a metatarsal bar that changes the weight transfer on the metatarsal heads and creates a new fulcrum for propulsion on the sagittal and frontal planes. This effect may be a reason for using the extrinsic post rather than the intrinsic post, which depends on cast modification for any angular imbalance such as forefoot varus or valgus; however, it does not change the fulcrum in propulsion to as great an extent as the extrinsic post.

Semirigid devices offer more flexibility than rigid devices. Materials utilized are the various polymer composites. With the limited availability of Rohadur, these materials appear to be more popular, especially in athletes. A major benefit of these materials is the spring effect of the shell. During walking when weight stresses increase to 125% of body weight and in running when the increase is three to four times body weight and the orthotic shell is depressed at midstance, as the foot moves into propulsion a springing back effect directs a supinatory effect on the foot, making this type of device very effective in athletes. This type of patient needs both control and shock absorption.

Semiflexible devices might be thought of as giving more flexibility and less control. Such materials as cork or latex and wood-flour materials that can be molded on a cast are commonly used. These materials provide control by bulk, which creates a problem in the proper fit of shoes. This type of device is indicated in the patient who cannot tolerate a more rigid device or who requires more shock absorption and less control.

Flexible devices can be used most effectively when very little control is required but shock absorption is the major consideration. Examples of this could be the patient with the rheumatoid foot with prominent metatarsal heads or the diabetic patient with a poor weight transfer pattern that results in excessive loading on specific metatarsal heads and potential ulceration. Materials may vary, but a foamed polyethylene of closed cell construction or open cell foams that do not bottom out are very effective.

Quantity of Control

An important factor that is frequently overlooked is the time of control or effect of the foot orthotic device. This depends on the length of the device.

If one considers a rigid or semirigid device, which by the nature of the material requires that its forward edge be proximal to the metatarsal heads, one has a high quality of control but a low quantity or time of control. This is an important factor because when an individual moves into propulsion the foot is past the major controlling influence of the device. On the other side of this situation is the patient who has a semiflexible device that ends distal to the metatarsal heads or is full length. Although the quality of control might be low, the quantity of control is high. These two considerations of quantity and quality of control can be very helpful in orthotic selection for the podiatric patient.

BIBLIOGRAPHY

Dye RW: Dye Technique of Foot Correction. Sandy Lake, Pennsylvania, 1969 (unpublished monograph).

Root ML, Orien WP, Weed JH, et al: Biomechanical Examination of the Foot, vol I. Los Angeles, Clinical Biomechanics Corporation, 1971.

Root ML, Orien WP, Weed JH: Normal and abnormal function of the foot. In Clinical Biomechanics, vol II. Los Angeles, Clinical Biomechanics Corporation, 1977.

Spencer A, Shadle JH, Watkins CA, et al: Practical Podiatric Orthopedic Procedures. Ohio College of Podiatric Medicine, 1978.

CHAPTER 18

SPORTS MEDICINE

James E. Lichniak

Sports medicine, as a subspecialty of orthopedics, emerged in the 1920s concurrent with the increased interest and participation in various forms of sports. Growth of the field continued as additional peaks of interest followed World War II, with the medical community eventually recognizing the need for further development of sports medicine as a specialized branch of medicine. Further increased interest in physical fitness, particularly during the early 1960s, emphasized the need for specialized training and research relative to the athletic patient, and sports medicine as a recognized field was officially born. Today, sports medicine, as a specialty, continues to grow as interest in athletics and fitness continues to expand.

Recognizing the predominance of lower extremity conditions associated with athletic and fitness activities, podiatry has expanded into the sports medicine field. Sports medicine has become a part of the curriculum at each of the colleges of podiatric medicine. Additionally, the American Academy of Podiatric Sports Medicine (AAPSM) was founded in 1976 to foster dissemination of information, interest, and research in podiatric aspects of sports medicine. By 1991, the AAPSM had about 1000 active members. Sports medicine education moves forward through this organization at its annual meeting held each May in addition to other sponsored continuing education programs. Fellowship status in the AAPSM is granted by examination.

Sports medicine basically involves five areas of concern:

1. *Preparticipation preparation.* This area is concerned with helping a participant begin an athletic or fitness program and advising the participant on safe ways to proceed with his or her program. This may involve recommendation of the type of activity, restrictions to activity, and ways to begin activity. All too often, athletic and fitness programs are prematurely discontinued owing to injury or loss of interest because the participant was either ill-informed or not in-

formed at all as to how to begin and progress through the program safely. This area may also involve the identification of conditions that may disqualify an athlete from particular types of activity.

2. *Injury prevention and conditioning.* This area includes the recommendation of proper training and conditioning methods and activities as well as the identification of improper training or conditioning activities and their subsequent correction. Also included are identification of mechanical abnormalities that may lead to injury and correction of such abnormalities to prevent injuries. This may involve the identification and correction of muscular tightness or weakness and of biomechanical foot faults or gait abnormalities that frequently predispose the participant to injury.

3. *Diagnosis and treatment of injury.* This area is concerned with the physical detection and clinical diagnosis of athletic-related injury by the use of physical and laboratory tests and the subsequent treatment recommendations appropriate for specific conditions. This involves not only acute and symptomatic care but also, more importantly, the identification of predisposing conditions that may promote injury and their correction.

4. *Rehabilitation following injury.* The proper rehabilitation and reconditioning of the athletic patient is necessary to resolve injury, correct mechanical problems, and allow the athlete to return to activity at the highest safe level of participation at the earliest time. This is based on the recognition that structure and function must be returned or restored to as close to normal as possible before the athlete is allowed to return to full and unrestricted participation in an attempt to prevent reinjury or aggravation of the existing injury.

5. *Recommendation for equipment and rules.* This area includes the recommendation for the use of proper equipment by the individual athlete as well as making recommendation for general equipment improvement. This has been evident with the significant improvement noted in the manufacture of running shoes prompted by recommendations from the sports medicine physician.

Knowledge of athletic participation also stimulates the creation or modification of rules of play to allow the athlete to participate with less chance of injury.

THE ATHLETIC HISTORY

Although many practitioners may label athletic patients difficult to work with and demanding (desiring to be better yesterday) and frequently noncompliant, those practitioners who routinely deal with the athletic patient find this to be a misconception. Athletic patients tend to be knowledgeable, rational, and able to become actively involved in a treatment program when they are provided with truthful, informative, and reasonable advice. Athletic patients are generally ''goal oriented,'' whether that goal is toward specific athletic accomplishment or toward general physical benefits of fitness. Therefore, when dealing with the athletic patient, the practitioner must rely on a strong base of information, provide reasonable plans for treatment of injury and correction of mechanical problems, and provide alternatives for activity during the rehabilitation period without placing undue restrictions or demands on the athletic patient's lifestyle.

Although the history of the athletic patient is essentially quite similar to that of most other podiatric patients, in some ways it is vastly different. Chief complaints may be similar, but the manner in which they are produced tend to be different. In the athletic patient, injury can result from activity that produces high stresses, which are frequently associated with improper training techniques, improper use or selection of equipment or footgear, and mechanical faults or flaws. It thus becomes essential to investigate, by history, the many factors that may be responsible for injury production, such as the training history and footgear, in addition to simply characterizing and quantifying the chief complaint.

The athletic patient generally presents with a chief complaint relating to discomfort, dysfunction, or deformity. This may be similar to the presentation of the nonathletic patient and should be investigated in a similar fashion by obtaining information concerning the onset, location, intensity, radiation, duration, timing, and character or quality of the complaint; precipitating or aggravating factors; and relieving factors. Other areas that should be investigated include any prior treatment for the same or similar conditions, how the condition was managed, how long ago the similar condition occurred, how long was treatment continued, and what was the success of the prior treatment.

It is also helpful to look at the course of the current or prior injury. In athletes experiencing a *persistent* problem, the cause is generally an uncorrected mechanical problem, inadequate prior treatment or treatment of an insufficient duration without adequate healing time, or resulting loss in strength or flexibility. In athletes experiencing *intermittent* problems, some training "variable" or occasional training error may be responsible for the condition. When an athlete presents with a *recurrent* problem, an uncorrected biomechanical flaw may have been adequately treated in the past but has returned because of wear and tear of orthotic devices, footgear, or body tissues as a result of increasing stresses and loads.

By far, discomfort is the most frequent complaint related by the athletic patient. When discomfort is present, the first consideration is whether it is significant. It is not unusual for an athlete to relate occasional discomfort for various reasons that may not be considered significant. A problem should be considered when discomfort

- Has been present 2 or more consecutive days
- Interferes with normal function or activity
- Worsens rather than improves
- Occurs following acute trauma
- Is associated with a feeling of instability
- Is associated with edema
- Is significant to alter the level of physical activity
- Increases with continued activity and persists at rest

STAGING OF INJURIES

If the timing of the discomfort is noted, it may also be possible to stage the injury according to its severity. This can be particularly helpful in patients with chronic, overuse injuries in which no definite acute event precipitating the injury can be identified, but the insult to tissues is produced by chronic overuse and stress.

Stage I injuries present as pain, frequently described as a tightness or stiffness before activity but no pain, stiffness, or tightness during activity. As this stage progresses, complaints of pain, stiffness, or tightness may return after activity has been completed. The duration of the postactivity complaint frequently reflects the increasing severity of the condition. Injuries in this stage tend to worsen with time without proper training, conditioning, or functional control and, if left unchecked, tend to progress to stage II injuries. However, if the injuries are correctly treated during this stage, the best prognosis results.

Stage II injuries may cause pain, stiffness, and/or tightness before and after activity, but their particular characteristic is that pain or other dysfunctional complaints now occur during activity as well. During this stage, however, the athlete is still generally able to continue activity at some level. The more severe the discomfort or dysfunction during the activity period, the more consequential the injury. This stage can also be subdivided into degrees. Early stage II injuries may have a pain-free period at the beginning of activity with pain occurring only later or toward the end of activity. The athlete may even be able to complete the intended workout. As the injury progresses, however, the athlete may experience pain at the beginning of activity, followed by a pain-free period, only to have the discomfort return later in the exercise session. As further progression occurs, pain or other dysfunctional complaints persist throughout the entire activity session to the point where activity must be prematurely discontinued. Unfortunately, most athletes seek advice only after the chronic, overuse injury has progressed to some degree of stage II. As a result, treatment tends to be longer and generally more involved and the injury develops some characteristics of chronicity.

In stage III injuries, the athlete can no longer participate in the activity of choice. The injury has become significant enough to prompt the athlete to discontinue the chosen activity and participate in some form of alternative activity, such as swimming or water running. The injury has become more chronic, and treatment generally tends to be prolonged with a later return to the chosen activity. In this stage, any activity, even of a low intensity, tends to produce pain. However, when at rest the athlete may experience little or no actual pain. A typical example of this may be the tibial or fibular stress fracture.

In stage IV injuries, pain tends to be present with or without activity. Obviously, prognosis of this stage is more guarded than in previous stages. Because of persistent complaints, the athlete may be severely restricted in activity or unable to participate in any activity at all.

Dysfunction and deformity are, as previously mentioned, frequent complaints of the athletic patient. Dysfunction can be related by the athlete in a variety of different forms. It may be perceived as tightness or stiffness, weakness, instability, clicking, popping, or grinding, or even abnormal shoe wear, and may be initially recognized by the athlete in the form of decreased productivity, such as diminishing mileage, speed, or quickness. Deformity may be *acute,* resulting from sudden injury, *progressive,* such as in the athlete with hallux abductovalgus deformity, or *static,* such as may be the case in genu varum.

THE TRAINING HISTORY

The "training history" sets the historical evaluation of the athlete in a different light. The training history is important for three reasons. First, it assists the practitioner in evaluating the athlete's overall level of fitness or conditioning. Second, by revealing the athlete's limitations due to symptoms, the practitioner may be able to recognize what the athlete may or may not be able to continue to do during the recovery period. Third, and possibly most important, with training errors being a common origin for many "overuse" injuries, by the uncovering of such errors, treatment, including the correction of these recognized errors, has a significantly greater chance of success. The trap of treating only the symptoms is avoided when the cause of mechanical injuries, as revealed in the training history, is treated.

In a study by Pagliano and colleagues of 3000 long distance runners, 40% of the prob-lems encountered involved a training error or training changes, most notably in either effort or running distance. Therefore, the investigation of activity attitudes, schedules, warm up and cool down activities, mileage, pace and speed, and environmental factors becomes an integral part of the athletic history.

Activity

It is important to determine the various activities in which an athlete is involved. Different activities seem to predispose the athletic patient to different problems. The athlete's "workout" should be evaluated for activity types and alternative activities, such as weight training, which may not be the primary activity.

Length of Program

The practitioner needs to determine how long an athlete has been participating in a particular activity program. In general, the longer an athlete has seriously participated in a particular activity, the better acclimated the tissues are to the stress of that particular activity. As the length of participation increases, the athlete's general knowledge of the activity also increases.

Schedule

The athlete's daily and weekly schedule is also of prime importance. How much of what activity is being done and when is it being done? Occasionally, simple aspects such as the time of day in which the activity takes place may have an effect on the development of an injury. For example, if an athlete has limited flexibility, it may be better for participation in the activity to occur later in the day when he or she is more flexible. On the other hand, if an athlete has a problem with weakness, participation earlier in the day is better when he or she tends to be stronger. The daily and weekly schedule should also denote specific variations from the typical, such as long runs, speed work, and swims, which are not regularly encountered.

Warm Up and Cool Down

The "warm up" helps the athlete get the body ready for activity. Investigation of warm up activities and of progression and duration of the warm up should be performed. The "cool down" after activity allows the body to return to normal resting levels as well as assists in muscle relaxation and removal of metabolic wastes. Although not all athletes approach warm up and cool down as diligently as they should, even those who are conscientious often make mistakes in sequences or techniques. They "ease into and out of" activity less effectively, and this detracts from the overall effect of warm up and cool down.

Mileage, Distance, and Duration

It is important not only to discover an athlete's immediate daily or weekly mileage but also to inquire into the mileage of the preceding 6 to 8 weeks, particularly that period before the onset of injury or symptoms. Frequently practitioners see the onset of musculotendinous and bony overuse syndromes as a result of excessive increases in mileage over too short a period of time. This is the typical "too much, too soon" phenomenon as an athlete drastically increases the workload applied to tissues more rapidly than the tissue's ability to respond and adapt to the increased levels of stress. This, in fact, may be the most typical training error seen in a sports medicine practice.

Runners should be advised not to increase their overall mileage by more than 10% to 15% per week. Increases over this level commonly produce injury. Novice runners, who run less than 10 miles per week, demonstrate tissues with only minimal adaptation to stresses, which are therefore more prone to injury with more radical changes in activity schedules. Low mileage runners, in general, possess less skill and knowledge and are more prone to training mistakes. Provided a runner has been exposed to gradually increasing levels of stress by slow and progressive mileage increases, distances of 10 to 30 miles per week tend to be a relatively safe level of activity with adequate tissue adaptation and cardiovascular conditioning. As distances past these levels are reached, there may again be an increase in the frequency of overuse injury owing to expanding levels of microtrauma and stress superimposed on biomechanical abnormalities and limitations.

Pace and Speed

As is similarly seen with mileage, the running pace should be gradually increased over time. Drastic increases in speed may precipitate injury by subjecting the athlete to levels of stress that cannot be handled well by the body tissues. Additionally, some conditions or symptoms may worsen with faster speeds or paces while other conditions or symptoms may worsen with slower speeds or paces. There should also be some correlation between "training" paces and "racing" paces. Ideally, the racing pace should be no more than 1 minute per mile faster than the training pace.

Activity Purpose

Persons become involved in athletic endeavors for different purposes. Some work toward fitness and are dedicated to improving cardiovascular and respiratory efficiency. To this person, activity becomes a significant part of one's lifestyle and daily routine in an effort to improve the overall quality of life. These individuals tend to be very driven, knowledgeable, and often skillful. This may differ from the recreational athlete, who simply enjoys participating in whatever athletic event is available with less concern for detail, skill, or intensity. On the low end of the scale is the "weekend" athlete, who has little concern for mechanical efficiency, conditioning, or skill and, therefore, is frequently prone to macrotraumatic as well as microtraumatic injury.

Environmental Factors

SURFACE

The surface on which one participates in an athletic endeavor is of concern in the training history. Although the hardness or softness of a playing surface may be a major consideration, how level the surface is and the traction coefficients also need to be investigated. Some surfaces for particular activities may be too hard, adding to shock absorption–related problems, and some surfaces may be too soft for other activities. An excessively soft surface may create undue levels of adaptations of the foot and excessive amounts of foot motion and require added muscular work. Unevenness of a surface leads to mechanical compensations similar to those seen in cases of limb-length discrepancies, creating an artificial or environmental problem of asymmetry. This may be seen as a runner runs on the side of a crested road where the limb farthest from the crest may function as a short limb and the limb closest to the crest may function as a long limb, producing a syndrome suggestive of asymmetry when, in fact, no structural difference in limb length exists. Furthermore, surface traction may predispose to injury. With the emergence of artificial turf, first metatarsophalangeal joint injuries (turf toe) and ankle and knee joint injuries have increased.

SHOES

Footgear technology has changed dramatically over the past few years, both to the advantage and disadvantage of the athlete. Although it can be stated that structurally and functionally today's athletic shoes are superior to those of 5 to 10 years ago, the athlete is now left with so many choices of styles and modifications that it has, in some ways, become difficult for the athlete to choose the right shoe. The first consideration is that the shoe match the activity. Running shoes are not appropriate for court sports and vice versa. Simply stated, each type of shoe has different functional requirements according to the demands of the respective activity. General trends, in regard to shoe attributes, involve improved shock absorption, improved stability, and improved fit. There has also been a desire for shoes to become lighter and more durable. Because of the wide variety of shoes now available, the question that is frequently asked is "What is the best shoe?" This becomes difficult to answer since what may be the best shoe for one athlete may be the worst shoe for another. It is important that the shoe, with all its multiple variations, match the needs and physical attributes of the athlete. The choice of shoes is also complicated

by the rapid change in available shoes dictated by the evolution in shoe manufacture.

Another factor that may be important when evaluating shoes is in regard to recent shoe changes. Changing the shoe may precipitate injury if the new shoe does not match what is required by the athlete. It is also important to investigate shoe wear. Abnormal wear patterns related by the athlete and verified by examination of the shoe may reflect various biomechanical and functional abnormalities, either in the location or in the rapidity of the wear.

PHYSICAL EXAMINATION OF THE ATHLETIC PATIENT

The physical examination of the athletic patient includes all of the aspects of a general podiatric physical examination but with special emphasis on the diagnosis of injury and on the investigation of predisposing and aggravating factors. The physical examination generally begins with inspection of the injured area, identifying visible findings such as deformity, edema, effusion, and erythema. Precise palpation aids to identify injured and involved structures by the presence of tenderness, warmth, masses, deformity, and so on. Specialized physical examination techniques, such as the drawer test in the ankle and the spring, McMurray, Apley, Lachman, and Clark tests in the knee, are employed according to the specific area of injury.

The evaluation of joint range of motion of muscular flexibility is of critical importance. Muscular tightness or limitations in joint range of motion may be either precipitating factors behind the development of injury or the sequelae of previous injury. Limited range of motion and limited flexibility are also significant detriments to rehabilitation following injury. Muscle strength must also be evaluated. This can be performed by manual muscle testing, grading muscle strength by resistance to motion provided by the examiner. Muscle strength can also be quantitatively measured by devices such as the Cybex or Biodex apparatus, which provide a "printout" of muscle parameters such as strength, power, and endurance. The biomechanical or arthrometric evaluation is vital to identify intrinsic structural and functional problems that may occur in midtarsal, subtalar, ankle, and superstructural joints that frequently are the source of injury. The biomechanical examination should always be coupled with a visual gait analysis, which should mirror abnormalities identified in the flexibility and range of motion, strength, and biomechanical examinations. Limb lengths should be measured. Asymmetry of limb lengths is a common cause of overuse injury. This is particularly true when unilateral complaints are encountered or, in the instance of paradoxic injuries, when one limb suggests pronatory complaints while the other suggests supinatory problems.

It is also important to perform an "extrinsic" examination to involve evaluation of footgear, orthotic devices (if applicable), and other miscellaneous equipment. First the athletic shoe type should be checked to see if it matches the athlete's activity. Next, does the shoe last shape match satisfactorily the shape of the foot? This can be checked by direct comparison of the foot or bare footprint to the shoe outsole and upper. Also, does the construction of the last match the athlete's particular structural needs? The shoe wear patterns to the outsole and midsole should be evaluated and the counter inspected. Any excessive torque in the shoe may indicate frontal plane abnormalities or compensations in the foot. It is not uncommon for excessive wear or the improper shoe to be the source of injury. If the athlete uses orthotic devices, it is also necessary to evaluate whether the devices match the athlete's particular biomechanical need in regard to orthotic type, materials, fit, and compatibility with the foot and shoe and posting. Finally, other equipment that may contribute to the development of injury, such as ski gear, skates, or even exercise equipment (e.g., the height of the bicycle seat), should be evaluated.

RUNNING BIOMECHANICS

With normal biomechanical function of the foot to guide or determine foot activity, most of the stresses and loads applied to the foot during gait can be satisfactorily dissipated or accommodated to prevent injury or structural damage to muscles, joints, and bones. However, in athletics, running activity is a frequent denominator between many sports. During running, the stresses and loads applied to the foot and leg can be significantly increased. Furthermore, biomechanical faults or flaws have a tendency to augment the effect of applied stresses and loads. As a result, the athlete involved in running activities is particularly vulnerable to the development of injury due to the added stresses applied to the less than perfect biomechanical function. The problems that may develop in the runner may be related to (1) the inability to sufficiently absorb shock; (2) abnormal motions or function that may force compensations to occur that in themselves cause injury; (3) abnormal function that forces other areas to work harder with larger resulting energy expenditure; (4) the loss of overall functional efficiency; and (5) adaptive soft tissue and bone changes over time.

As podiatrists, we tend to rely on the standard biomechanical examination to determine normal versus "abnormal" biomechanical function and compare our findings with the "normal," which may be defined by the typical Root criteria. Our standard biomechanical evaluation has limitations that may be particularly critical to evaluation of biomechanical function in runners. The typical biomechanical examination is basically a static examination, and we need to correlate our findings with that which we observe during an active gait evaluation. What we see with a patient statically prone on the table does not always coincide with what we see with the patient in active motion. Those values and functions considered normal for the average walking gait are not always appropriate for the running gait. The running gait should have a new set of standards owing to significant differences between running and walking. This prompts the discussion of the basic differences between the walking gait and the running gait, each of which has its own special requirements, adaptations, and principles.

Differences Between Walking and Running

To begin with, perhaps the simplest difference may be in terminology. In various texts, the contact phase may also be referred to as "foot strike," midstance referred to as "midsupport,'' and the propulsive phase referred to as the "take off" phase. Swing phase also takes on new terminology. Although in walking, the swing phase is rarely broken down into segments, in running, swing phase takes on added meaning. A good deal of momentum and inertia needs to be maintained in swing phase. Physical limitations in swing can significantly affect stance. Initially in the swing there is the "follow through" or "push off" phase followed by "forward swing" or "float/double float" phase. This float phase is significant in that it is a time when neither limb is in contact with the ground, which sets it apart from the walking gait, when at least one limb is in contact with the ground at all times. Swing terminates with the "foot descent" or "reach" phase as the foot begins to approach the ground to commence stance. Swing phase differences are discussed to a greater extent later in this chapter.

In considering overall stresses, as would be expected, as speed increases, body momentum also increases. Momentum is a function of body mass times the velocity of gait. The mass in running remains unchanged, but the velocity increases, thereby increasing momentum. As momentum increases, forces, stresses, and loads to the foot and leg also increase and may reach levels of three times or more body weight. Additionally, as stresses increase, they frequently become more localized, such as may be encountered in the forefoot of the sprinter when the fore part of the foot contacts the ground earlier in stance and remains in contact with the ground the longest. Larger stresses over smaller areas must contribute to the overall picture of injury development. Furthermore, as stresses increase, joints such as the subtalar joint and the midtarsal joint, among others, are stressed and forced to go through a greater range of motion, sometimes to their absolute limits, which also serves as a focus for injury.

Base of Gait

When a person walks, the normal walking base of gait, or the separation between the medial malleoli, is 2 to 4 inches. If a line is drawn down the center of a walkway and the subject asked to walk this line, the right foot

would normally hit just to the right of the line and the left foot would normally hit just to the left of the line, assuming the center of gravity is adequately maintained generally over the line down the runway. However, the running gait normally demonstrates what may easily be termed a *straight line progression*. Instead of the right foot hitting on the right side of the line and the left foot hitting on the left side of the line, the right foot hits directly on the line, sometimes even crossing over to the left side of the line, and the left foot also hits directly on the line or with occasional crossover. Because the feet now strike more directly under the center or midline of the body, the legs must therefore assume a more inverted or varus attitude from the hips to the heels. This creates what may be termed a *runner's* or *functional varus*, an excessively inverted position of the heel at heel contact compared with the typical walking gait. Therefore, to get to vertical position of the heel and to absorb the increased varus, more motion is forced at the subtalar and midtarsal joints in the direction of eversion. The subtalar and midtarsal joints are forced to go through more of their range of motion in a pronatory direction, placing added stress on the subtalar and midtarsal joints. This also frequently adds increased compensation and stress at the ankle, knee, hip, and lower back, particularly if the subtalar and midtarsal joints cannot accommodate the increased need for more motion.

Angle of Gait

In the normal walking gait, the feet are usually mildly abducted to 10° to 15°. However, as a runner increases speed, this abducted foot angle of gait diminishes. Therefore, as speed increases, the angle of gait conversely decreases. This may be explained by the fact that as running speed increases, more time is spent on the forefoot and less time on the rearfoot. The forefoot hits directly ahead and occasionally is mildly adducted. Coupled with the functional varus as previously described, the angle of gait decreases.

Contact Progression

With walking, in the normal gait, the heel contacts the ground first. During the first 15%

of stance, the forefoot approaches the ground until a flat foot position is achieved. The forefoot then loads during late contact and through midstance as the leg now begins to move forward and over the foot. The propulsive phase begins at the time of heel off, the point at which the heel leaves the supporting surface. The end of stance is when the toes leave the supporting surface at toe off. Therefore, the contact progression of the foot on the ground in the normal walking gait is heel contact—foot flat—heel off—toe off. With running, this contact progression changes as the runner increases speed. At slower running speeds, the contact progression may be similar to that of the walker, as described earlier. However, as speed increases, the heel and forefoot may begin to strike the supporting surface simultaneously, thereby eliminating the brief period of time between heel contact and flat foot periods. As speed continues to increase, the forefoot may, in fact, contact the supporting surface *before* the heel, with the foot rocking back on the heel, producing a contact progression of forefoot contact—heel contact—heel off—toe off. As would be expected, the overall time of heel contact with the supporting surface is also decreased. With significantly faster speeds, such as in sprinting, the foot tends to strike excessively on the forefoot and the heel may descend toward the ground, briefly touching or, in some cases, never touching the supporting surface. This may have a significant implication in the use of orthotic devices in that rearfoot control would seem to have a diminishing effect in the faster runner if, in fact, there is not significant heel contact or well-defined midstance phase around which the success of many typical orthotic devices depends. Forefoot control would, on the other hand, increase in significance and be most appropriate. Additionally, with excessive forefoot contact with increased speed, various injuries may be seen to rise in incidence, such as Achilles tendonitis and propulsive plantar fasciitis.

Swing vs. Stance Proportion

In the normal walking gait, the proportion of the typical gait cycle can be divided into about 65% of the time constituting stance phase and 35% of the time constituting swing phase. However, with running, during swing, there is a period of time when no limb is in contact with the supporting surface, which significantly influences the proportion of the swing phase time to stance phase time. As running speed increases, stance phase time decreases as the runner tries to contact the ground for the shortest possible time. The longer the foot is on the ground, the slower is the speed. Additionally, with the development of the float phase of swing, swing phase time increases in proportion to stance, thus changing the ratio of stance to swing phase durations. Running speed can be increased either by increasing the number of strides per minute or by increasing the stride length.

In the slower runner there is a very short float phase and the foot stays fixed to the ground only slightly shorter than with walking. The float phase develops most likely due to a mild increase in stride length. Stance phase is still longer than swing in total duration, but the ratio of stance to swing decreases. As speed increases, swing phase continues to increase as the stride length continues to lengthen, but stance is still longer than swing, probably because added speed results from an increase in the number of strides per minute and not because of the effect of the increased stride length. The stance versus swing ratio is becoming closer to 50:50. As speed continues to increase, swing phase time eventually equals stance phase time, and eventually swing surpasses stance as the take off becomes more explosive; increased momentum continues into the follow-through phase, increasing the overall float or airborne time. In sprinters, stance becomes very short in duration and swing phase time now overwhelms stance phase time as the sprinter spends stance phase time primarily on the forefoot, significantly decreasing contact time with the ground and increasing float time owing to the forcefulness of take off and follow through.

Swing Phase Changes

The swing phase takes on new meaning and importance in the running gait. Swing phase becomes a period of time when, for maximal running efficiency to occur, inertia and momentum developed in stance must be maintained and carried over into the next stance period. Swing phase can be divided into separate phases each with their own characteristics, requirements, and limitations.

PUSH OFF OR FOLLOW-THROUGH PHASE

This phase of swing occurs immediately after toe off. At this point the leg is behind the body mass and the foot is leaving the ground and beginning to move forward in space. At the beginning of push off/follow through, the hip is hyperextended, the knee is extended, and the ankle is plantarflexed. The subtalar and oblique midtarsal joints are supinated, and the longitudinal midtarsal joint is pronated. Physical limitations that may restrict and limit the effectiveness of push off/follow through may include tight hip flexors or weakness of the foot plantarflexors. With hip flexor tightness, extension and hyperextension of the hip is limited, which would decrease the push off angle of the leg and thereby diminish speed. With weak plantarflexors, push off strength would be diminished, lessening momentum and forward thrust.

FLOAT OR DOUBLE-FLOAT PHASE

This phase may also be called the forward swing phase. During this intermediate period in swing, the leg is most actively moving forward with its greatest overall horizontal velocity. This phase in the running gait is unique in that during this portion of the stride neither leg is in contact with the ground, which typifies the running gait. The runner is actually "floating" through air. The time and length of the float depend on push off force and the angle of the push off. Any restriction diminishing the push off force will subsequently decrease the float and thereby decrease the speed. Since the push off force determines the time and momentum in float, conditions decreasing the force of push off will decrease the force or momentum and time in swing. Such limitations may be weakness of the hamstrings or weakness of the plantarflexors. Conditions that decrease the momentum in moving the leg forward will also limit float, such as may be seen with weak hip flexors limiting the force of the leg being pulled forward. A second important factor is the angle of push off. Factors that alter the push off angle will therefore also limit the length of the float. If the push off angle is too vertical, the force may also be too vertical, possibly creating a higher but shorter length of float. Also, body mass may alter float in that increased mass tends to decrease float. In summary, any factor decreasing float time will decrease momentum and thereby decrease speed.

REACH OR FOOT DESCENT PHASE

In this phase, the foot is descending toward the ground with the leg a distance in front of the body before contacting the ground. During this phase, the horizontal velocity of the foot is decreasing so that at the time of foot contact the horizontal velocity will be near 0 to limit the amount of longitudinal shear stresses on the foot in early stance. Ideally, when the foot contacts the ground the tibia should be just short of perpendicular. In cases of overstriding, the tibia is far short of perpendicular, leading to posterior impingement problems as well as shock-related complexes. When a runner understrides, the tibia is past perpendicular, creating excessive sagittal plane stress and anterior impingement problems. In this latter case, the knee is also excessively flexed at foot contact, creating excessive stress on the patellar tendon and producing patellar tendonitis. During the reach or foot descent phase, the hip should ideally be in 30° to 40° of flexion at the time of heel contact. With degrees greater than this (excessive flexion), significant strain is placed on the knee and patellar tendon as well as possibly increasing patellofemoral contact pressures, which are a source for patellofemoral pain syndromes. If the hip is flexed less than 30°, speed is usually diminished. Factors that decrease the effectiveness of the reach phase tend to decrease speed. Such physical limitations include weak hip flexors or tight hamstrings or hip extensors, both of which may limit the forward progression of the leg.

Stance Phase Changes

FOOT STRIKE PHASE

At the instant of foot strike or heel contact, the horizontal velocity of the foot should be close to 0, which allows the foot to remain stable on the ground without excessive shear. In other words, despite the increased momentum in running, there comes that point when, while body momentum and velocity must be maintained, the foot achieves a period of 0 velocity when it becomes fixed to the ground, thus going from a time of rapid movement in swing to a time of essentially no forward movement relative to the supporting surface. The heel generally hits in an inverted position, usually somewhat more inverted as compared with walking because of the possible "functional" or "runner's" varus. Therefore, it would not be unusual to see more lateral heel wear on a person's running shoe than on the person's casual walking shoe. Because of the increased varus attitude of the running heel at the time of ground contact, the foot may need to pronate more to adapt to the surface and absorb shock. If only limited motion is available in the subtalar and midtarsal joints, other joints of the superstructure of the body may need to absorb more shock, which may produce injury in more proximal structures. A common area of compensation is in the knee, which is frequently visualized as excessive knee flexion after contact, placing excessive amounts of stress on the anterior knee structures. As the foot contacts the supporting surface, vertical ground reactive forces experience their first rise, with eventual peak forces being two and one-half to three times or more body weight. In some reports, ankle stresses have been even higher, estimated in some cases to be up to eight to ten times body weight. Initially, these forces are not dissipated by muscle decelerating contractions. This occurs slightly later, with initial forces tending to be taken up by bone and joint structures. Although the previously described events describe slower running gaits, as running speed increases, the heel contact phase diminishes. This may occur simultaneously with forefoot contact or after forefoot contact, or eventually it may not occur at all in some sprinters. Therefore, as the heel contact phase diminishes, less importance on rearfoot mechanics is required and the midtarsal joint becomes the dominant joint in biomechanical control as well as the major area of shock dissipation and ground adaptation in the foot.

MIDSUPPORT PHASE

In the slower runner, the midsupport phase probably remains the most critical period of stance. The pedal conversion from a pronated foot to a supinated foot occurs and, as in the walking gait, identifies the subtalar joint neutral position. As would be similarly seen in the walking gait, excessive subtalar joint pronation occurs if there is a delay in reaching this neutral position, with the foot remaining pronated far into midstance. In this slower runner or jogger, the intent of biomechanical control still revolves around maintaining the proper time for conversion from pronation to supination. Orthotics are, therefore, still created as a midstance controlling device. In the faster runner, as would be expected, midsupport bears little resemblance to walking midstance by a proportionally shorter or even absent midsupport phase, which may be seen in some sprinters. Posterior leg muscle tightness tends to be particularly destructive in the late midsupport phase in joggers and slower runners. In the late midsupport phase the body needs to move "over" the foot. If there is limited posterior muscle group flexibility (i.e., gastrocnemius or gastrocnemius–soleus equinus or even ankle joint or bony equinus), the foot may compensate by any of a number of factors. These compensations include excessive subtalar joint pronation, excessive knee flexion in the midsupport phase, or an early heel off. All of these may produce overuse symptoms. If the foot continues to move forward during the midsupport phase, frictional problems in the foot, such as the "runner's toenail" or blisters, may occur.

TAKE OFF PHASE

In early take off or propulsion phase, ground reactive forces peak again as the heel leaves the ground and the body passes over the fixed forefoot, concentrating forces in the fore part of the foot. Again, forces peak at two to three times body weight. Foot strike and midsupport phase, as previously described, may be significantly altered or even essentially absent in some sprinters. This highlights the importance of forefoot control in sprinters because of the proportionally long take off phase with the significantly shortened preceding phases.

In summary, although it would be nice to apply our biomechanical guidelines and concepts of what we think as "normal," regardless of how arbitrary and even artificial they may be to all aspects of gait, running has biomechanical characteristics all its own. Running activities and body requirements may be significantly different from the "normal" walking gait. Therefore, the biomechanics and gait analysis of walking do not necessarily correspond to the biomechanics and gait analysis of running. As a result, with orthotic prescription and intervention, these differences in biomechanical characteristics must be considered.

ATHLETIC FOOTGEAR

Over the past decade, there has been a tremendous evolution in the design of athletic shoes. As podiatrists have become more knowledgeable about the needs of particular athletes regarding footgear, athletic shoe technology has attempted to coincide with our recognition of those particular needs. As a result, the market has become flooded with new athletic shoe technology, so much so that it is difficult to keep up with the multitude of newer changes. This is compounded by the not too uncommon disappearance of styles we finally get to know and understand. There is no "universal" shoe that is appropriate for all athletes and all sports. All too frequently, athletic injuries, particularly running injuries, may be secondary to the use of the wrong shoe or a shoe that is excessively worn. Shoe evaluation, therefore, becomes a critical component in the physical podiatric examination of the athletic patient.

Although different athletic activities require different attributes in respective footgear, each athlete also has different functional and structural attributes that must be addressed in his or her shoe prescription. These needs are reflected in an athlete's running style, activity, body build, and biomechanical needs determined by his or her individual biomechanical function or flaws.

When recommending the appropriate athletic shoe to athletic patients two major factors must be considered. First, podiatrists need to understand the particular activity and biomechanical requirements of the athlete in regard to his or her footgear. Second, podiatrists need to be able to match as closely as possible particular mechanical aspects and innovations of athletic shoes to the particular needs of the patient. Most of those particular aspects revolve around motion control and stability, shock absorption characteristics, fit and sizing, and overall shoe durability. Therefore, the selection of the "right" shoe depends on first understanding the needs of the athletic patient and then trying to match a patient with the shoes that satisfy his or her needs. It is, therefore, important that podiatrists become not only proficient in evaluation of the needs of the patient but also knowledgeable in the composition of athletic shoes.

Anatomy of the Athletic Shoe

It is important to understand the basic anatomy of the athletic shoe to lay a foundation for further understanding of the many modifications that are possible to meet the athlete's needs. The athletic shoe comprises the upper, the insole, the midsole, and the outsole, each with its own component parts (Figs. 18–1 through 18–4).

THE UPPER

The *upper* is the portion of the shoe that covers the top and sides of the foot, attached in various manners to the midsole below. Ideally, the upper should be lightweight, durable, and stable. In running shoes, nylon or nylon mesh is a common material from which the upper is made. Nylon is lightweight, relatively durable, breathable, and generally soft and nonabrasive. However, nylon or nylon mesh is not sufficiently rigid to maintain shape well. Therefore, the upper is commonly reinforced by strips of leather or suede, called foxing, particularly to the toe box, sides, and counter region to add needed support and stability. In athletic shoes requiring more inherent stability of the upper, such as in court shoes, aerobic shoes, cross-trainers, and cleated shoes, the upper may be made entirely of leather. Leather provides more support than nylon but also adds weight to the shoe, tends to crack and

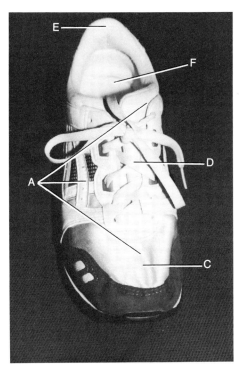

FIGURE 18–1. Front/top view of a running shoe. (A, upper; C, toe box; D, laces/eyelets; E, pull tab/Achilles pad; F, insole/sock liner)

deform with time, and is generally more abrasive. An advantage to leather is that it can be shaped to areas of pressure or irregular contour for fit. The upper of most athletic shoes is covered on the inside with a soft, nonabrasive lining.

The Counter

The *counter* is, perhaps, one of the most important individual parts of the athletic shoe. The counter is the rigid internal heel cup surrounding the heel medially, laterally, and posteriorly within the upper of the shoe. The counter is intended to provide stability and limit rearfoot motion of the heel in the shoe. Ideally, the counter should be largely inflexible and firmly attached to the midsole. The counter should snugly fit the heel without allowing excessive motion of the heel on the frontal plane as well as on the transverse plane. Early counters were frequently made from a thin fiberboard material. In recognition of the need for counter stability, the trend is now toward plastic counters. In addition to increasing the effectiveness of the counter by increasing its rigidity, the counter can be lengthened longitudinally or heightened to add to efficiency. For example, for a runner with excessive pronation, an extended medial counter will provide more medial support and stability to the shoe. The counter effectiveness can also be increased by reinforcement by additional materials and foxing. Even with a rigid counter, a firm attachment of the counter to the midsole is vital. This attachment can also be reinforced by a plastic or rubber strip, an external heel stabilizer that covers and strengthens the junction between the counter and midsole. Finally, a firmer midsole provides a more stable foundation on which the counter rests. Softer materials under the heel, while initially providing added shock absorption, allow more counter instability. Therefore, this fact must be considered in determining the relative needs of shock absorption and stability in the same shoe for the needs of a particular athlete.

The Toe Box

The *toe box* is the area of the upper that covers and encases the toes. This area tends to

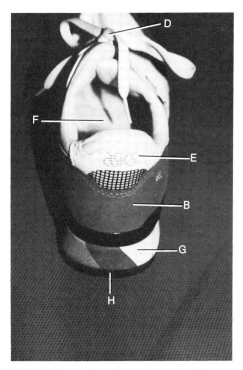

FIGURE 18–2. Rear view of a running shoe. (B, counter; D, laces/eyelets; E, pull tab/Achilles pad; F, insole/sock liner; G, midsole; H, outsole)

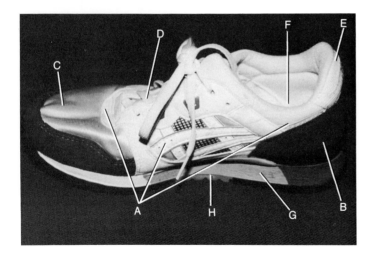

FIGURE 18–3. Medial view of a running shoe. (A, upper; B, counter; C, toe box; D, laces/eyelets; E, pull tab/Achilles pad; F, insole/sock liner; G, midsole; H, outsole)

be reinforced with foxing to provide stability of the toe box and lift and hold the upper off the toes. There should be enough room in the toe box area for the toes to comfortably rest, allowing a slight amount of free motion of the toes without dorsal friction. The toe box should be slightly longer than the "longest" toe and slightly higher. Toe boxes that are too short or too low tend to produce jamming problems of the nails, such as in the "runner's toe," producing subungual hematomas and eventual nail irregularities in addition to producing excessive wear of the toe box from pressure from the digits against the inside of the toe box.

Lacing and Eyelets

The *lacing* and *eyelet* system is intended to hold the shoe snugly on the foot to prevent excessive motion within the shoe. The eyelets may be "in line" or may be staggered (variable width laces), allowing for variable lacing patterns and tensions, and can be helpful in accommodating various foot deformities. Speed lace systems employ plastic eyelets, which, when the laces are run though the eyelets, provide a more even tension along the lacing. Rearfoot laces are used in some shoes, with laces or straps coursing behind the heel.

The Pull Tab or Achilles Pad

The *pull tab* or *Achilles pad* is the variable shaped and sized extension on the back of the shoe above the counter in the region of the Achilles tendon. This tab can be grasped to assist in putting on the shoe and may mildly cushion around the tendon itself. This minor cushioning generally extends around the open

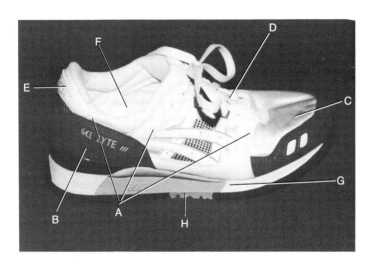

FIGURE 18–4. Lateral view of a running shoe. (A, upper; B, counter; C, toe box; D, laces/eyelets; E, pull tab/Achilles pad; F, insole/sock liner; G, midsole; H, outsole)

part of the shoe medially and laterally, forward to the laces as the *collar*.

THE INSOLE

The *insole* or *sock liner* is the inner portion of the shoe on which the plantar aspect of the foot contacts and rests. The purpose of the insole is to provide a smooth, conformed inner liner to help in shock dissipation, increase cushion, decrease shear and friction plantarly, and, to some degree, absorb sweat. Most running shoes have a removable insole that can be modified further by added cushioning or pad placement (e.g., metatarsal pads, arch "cookies," heel pads, buttress pads) and wedges (e.g., lifts, forefoot and rearfoot frontal plane wedges). Insoles are most frequently composed of plastazote or similar closed cell foams that may improve the contour and fit by gradually conforming mildly according to pressure. Other materials commonly seen in the insole may include open cell foams for improvement of shock absorption or neoprene rubber (e.g., Spenco [Spenco Medical Corporation, Waco, TX]) to decrease shear and friction.

THE MIDSOLE

The *midsole* is the portion of the shoe between the upper and the outsole. The midsole is an area of the athletic shoe that has received a great deal of attention over the past few years as a large number of modifications have been made in an attempt to improve shock-absorbing capabilities of a shoe as well as increasing inherent stability. The midsole is a plate of material extending the full length of the shoe; it is generally thicker in the rearfoot and thinner toward the forefoot. The function of the midsole is to provide cushion and shock absorption, add stability to the shoe, protect the rearfoot and forefoot, and provide a stable base on which the upper can rest.

The midsole is composed of a foamy material, commonly either ethylvinyl acetate, which provides a comfortable, softer feel, or polyurethane, which tends to be more durable than ethylvinyl acetate but less cushioning. These materials can, however, be manipulated in regard to their density or firmness. The firmness of the material is measured in durometers. High durometer materials (i.e., 45) are firmer,

are more stable, compress less, and provide a more stable base for the counter and upper. They are also less shock absorbing. Low durometer materials (i.e., 25) are softer, more shock absorbing, and more compressible. Although lower durometer materials may provide more shock absorption and cushioning, they also tend to "bottom out" faster and actually, with time, impart a firm feeling. It is not unusual to see a variable density midsole in which the midsole durometer may be manipulated within the shoe to place higher durometer material in areas where more stability is needed and lower durometer materials in other areas where shock absorption or cushioning is required.

The quest for shock absorption has been a major focus in the midsole evolution. Simple methods of increasing shock absorption, in addition to using softer materials, may include the addition of perforations or transverse holes under areas requiring more cushioning to "soften" the midsole in that area. This is commonly seen in the forefoot under the metatarsal heads and in the lateral rearfoot. A variety of additional modifications have been added to include gas or air encapsulation systems, silicone gel or fluid systems, flexible plastic beds of varying designs over open air chambers, open tubes, or "honeycomb" systems in an effort to improve shock absorption.

The midsole has also been subject to the placement of various wedges, lifts, and flares according to the varying needs of different athletes. A medial flare on the rearfoot midsole, particularly of a more dense material, may provide additional antipronatory stability, but if it is too large it may actually "clip" the opposite ankle as the leg swings through. A lateral flare of a higher density material may provide more lateral stability, which may be helpful in individuals with a tendency for inversion ankle sprains. However, this lateral flare may increase pronatory forces as the flare forces a rapid pronatory motion after contacting the ground, placing added stress on the posterior tibial muscle and tendon, possibly resulting in tendonitis or posterior shin splints. Similarly, a posterior flare forces a rapid plantarflexion of the ankle after heel contact, placing added stress on the tibialis anterior, possibly resulting in tendonitis or anterior shin splints. The "biased heel" or "shin splint cut off" is a rounded or beveled modification of the posterior portion of the midsole allowing a more gradual "rolling" transition from posterior heel contact at foot strike to a flat foot position. This may be helpful in anterior shin splints because of the diminished work now required of the anterior compartment muscles in decelerating plantarflexion following heel strike, but it may place added stress on the Achilles tendon and aggravate Achilles tendonitis.

More shoes are also adopting a contoured or anatomical midsole or last in which the midsole is contoured to the plantar surface. This is intended to provide a better overall fit of the shoe by allowing the foot to sit deeper in the shoe for better stability. It also may help in reducing the weight of the shoe by reducing some of the midsole material. This shoe would provide a more "natural" feel of the midsole, compatible with the foot. By its lack of a flat footbed, however, the contoured last may cause difficulty in orthotic device compatibility with the shoe, should such a device be prescribed.

THE OUTSOLE

The *outsole* is the contact surface of the shoe to the ground that requires a durability sufficient to resist friction and abrasion but must be flexible enough to allow normal foot-bending motions. The outsole is intended to protect the rest of the shoe from friction and, to a degree, compression, as well as to improve traction of the shoe on the athletic surface.

The outsole is a rubberized sheet from heel to toe plantarly, which can be of varying consistency. Blown rubber has a tendency to be somewhat softer and thus is concentrated in areas where shock absorption and softness may be an attribute. Carbon rubber, on the other hand, has a tendency to be harder and more durable and thus is placed in areas where durability would be an asset. The tread pattern of the outsole is also important. "Waffle" patterns with multiple nubs function similarly to a cleat, which allows improved traction on softer surfaces and increased flexibility but may irritate tender areas lying directly in line with a stud. Waffle pattern outsoles also tend to be less durable, with excessive wearing of the waffle studs. Herringbone-type outsole patterns with multiple ripples tend to be stiffer and more durable on harder surfaces but with generally lower adherent properties. Many of the current outsole patterns are hybrids with modifications of each of the above patterns, and it is unusual to see a purely waffle or herringbone pattern. Furthermore, a more recent trend is to decrease some of the bulk of the central outsole longitudinally while mildly raising the peripheral outsole tread in the "center of pressure" design. This may decrease the overall weight of the shoe as well as increase central shock absorption as the foot depresses over the lessened outsole centrally.

THE LAST

The *last,* or form, of the shoe can be described according to both its construction and its shape. The last is the mold or shape around which each shoe is made. Each shoe company has its own last or shape, which can be different for each style of shoe. Therefore, not only will the last vary between different shoe companies, but it will also vary between styles within the same shoe company. The last is important because by its construction type it can provide either stability or flexibility to the shoe depending on the needs of the runner and because by its shape it can be used to fit different foot types.

The athletic shoe last can be constructed in a variety of different forms (Fig. 18–5). In the conventional (also called board, machine, cement) last, the upper opens plantarly, attached by glueing or stitching to the midsole with a cardboard or fiberboard plate and then glued over the plantar opening of the upper to the midsole. When the inside of the running shoe is examined, this is demonstrated by a full-length piece of cardboard or fiberboard under the insole, covering the midsole. This type of last provides a stiffer, more stable, rigid shoe, which may assist in limiting excessive foot motion. The slip or moccasin last consists of an upper that is sewn together plantarly, creating a "moccasin"-like effect. The upper is then attached to the midsole. A seam is visible extending the length of the shoe plantarly within the upper, and the midsole is not seen when the insole is removed. This type of last creates a more flexible upper, which may also

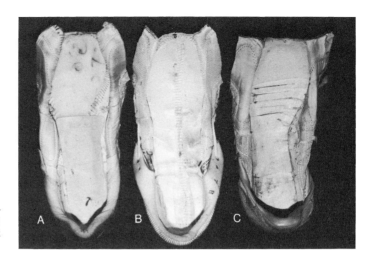

FIGURE 18–5. Last construction. (*A*) Combination last. (*B*) Slip or moccasin last. (*C*) Conventional, board, machine, or cement last.

produce a better, snugger fit. A combination last in a shoe combines the attributes of both the conventional and the slip lasts: the rearfoot portion of the shoe demonstrates a conventional type last for increased rearfoot stability, while the forefoot portion demonstrates a more flexible, snug-fitting effect by slip lasting. In combination, a shoe is formed imparting rearfoot stability with forefoot flexibility.

The last shape is critical in matching the shape of an athlete's foot with the shape of the shoe. Foot to shoe incompatibility in regard to shape can produce abnormal wear of the shoe or induce injury as the shoe becomes incompatible with structural and functional attributes of the foot. The last shape can be determined by bisecting the plantar surface of the shoe. In a straight last shoe, the bisection creates roughly equal mass on each side of the bisection, which courses directly up the middle of the outsole. Although the straight-lasted shoe best fits a rectus foot structure, some suggest that this shape may be appropriate for many runners, providing additional medial support and therefore producing an antipronatory effect. However, there are few truly straight-lasted shoes available and they may create fitting problems in athletes with a more rigid, adductus foot type. The curved or inflare last shoe demonstrates an inward curve forward of the midfoot. The outsole bisection, therefore, reveals more shoe medial to the bisection than lateral. This type of last is appropriate in a forefoot adductus foot type and in many cavus feet but is not appropriate for most runners. If the inflare is too excessive,

the runner exhibits lateral cramping of the foot in the shoe, frequently giving the appearance of the lateral border of the foot and upper extending over the lateral midsole and lateral digits wearing through the toe box. As a compromise, a semi-curved or semi-inflare last is available. In fact, most shoes are made around a semi-curved last, which appears to satisfactorily fit most athletes. A shoe with this type of last is somewhere between a straight-lasted shoe and a curve-lasted shoe. Again, the shape of the last curve should roughly match the shape of the foot. The foot should fit comfortably within the shoe without medial or lateral crowding. Besides simple visual matching of the last shape to the foot, in a shoe that has been sufficiently worn, the impression of the foot should be roughly centered on the sock liner in an appropriately matched last.

Recommendations

In recommending or selecting athletic shoes, a number of factors must be taken into consideration:

1. *Purpose.* The type of shoe selected should match the activity. For example, a running shoe is appropriate for running, primarily a forward progression activity, around which requirements the running shoe is made. It is, however, inappropriate for court sports requiring multidirectional movements; the running shoe is not designed with sufficient lateral directional

stability. On the other hand, court shoes are made for court activities and generally do not provide the proper attributes for running longer distances. A hybrid may be the cross-trainer, which has attributes of both running and court-type activities. Nonetheless, athletic shoes created for specific activities should be used for those activities alone.

2. *Fit and sizing.* It is important that the shoe should fit in width as well as length. The podiatrist should advise athletes to make sure to try on both shoes with the proper socks and firmly laced before purchasing. If the shoe does not feel comfortable, he or she should not assume that it will with time as it "breaks in." All too frequently, when the shoe becomes "broken in," it has become excessively worn and needs to be replaced. The suggestion should be made to the athlete to have the shoes fit later in the day when the foot may be slightly larger, which may, to some degree, simulate mild foot expansion that may occur with athletic activity. This may prevent the shoe from feeling too snug during times of activity.

3. *Last.* The shoe should be selected according to the most appropriate last construction for the athlete. Athletes requiring added stability may require a board-type last, whereas athletes requiring more flexibility may benefit from a slip-type last. Combination-lasted shoes tend to provide more rearfoot stability with forefoot flexibility. The last shape should also be matched to the shape of the foot. More rectus type feet should be in a straighter or less curved last, whereas more adductus type feet may require a more curved last.

4. *Stability and motion control.* The question should be asked concerning what may be a particular athlete's need for stability and control of motion followed by the question asking which shoes meet those particular stability needs. A number of stability modifications may be sought in a shoe. These may include the rigidity and the size or extension of the counter, the stability of the midsole, and the counter–midsole junction reinforcement, among others. Conversely, what are the shoe flexibility requirements of a particular athlete and does the shoe flex adequately in the appropriate area according to need?

5. *Shock absorption and cushion.* Some athletes may have a problem with shock absorption and require a shoe that better helps to dissipate shock. For other athletes, this may not be as much of a problem. Some injuries appear to be shock related and may be improved or prevented with a more shock-absorbing shoe. In the past, shock-absorbing shoes tended to be softer and therefore less durable. As time has progressed, there has been more of a merging of shock absorption and durability with both cushioning systems and motion control devices within the same shoe. There are a number of shock-absorbing type shoe modifications available in athletic shoes through a number of different manufacturers.

6. *Weight.* A desirable attribute in an athletic shoe would be low weight. In the past, racing flats tended to weigh less than training shoes but overall offered less protection and were generally inappropriate for daily training. However, while more devices have been added to shoes, the overall weight is decreasing; in many cases, the lighter weight shoe is seen as a goal for many shoe manufacturers. This has largely been accomplished by reduction of midsole and outsole material, which are major contributors to the weight of the shoe. Most likely, the weight of the shoe will continue to decrease.

Evaluating Footgear During the Physical Examination

It is important to be able to evaluate shoes as part of the physical examination of the athlete. A number of factors need to be considered.

1. *The upper.* The upper should be searched for areas of excessive wear. Uppers that appear to be excessively extending over the lateral midsole in the forefoot tend to represent a shoe that is too small or a last that is too curved. Excessive wear in the toe box area from the digits may be due to a shoe

that is too short or a toe box that is too low. This may also reflect a last shape that does not match the foot shape or the presence of underlying digital pathology, such as a hallux extensus at the interphalangeal joint in hallux limitus.

2. *The counter.* The shoe is placed on a table. The counter should be vertical. A counter that is tipped medially may represent excessive pronatory forces, whereas a counter that is tipped laterally may represent a supinatory force. The firmness and stability of the counter are evaluated, and any cracks or defects that may be due to excessive counter stress are sought. Also, the counter–midsole junction should be inspected. If excessive motion is available at this junction, the effectiveness of the counter is markedly diminished.

3. *Inside shoe.* By running a hand inside the liner of the shoe, areas of excessive wear can be noted that may not yet be noticeable in the external portion of the upper. Also, the insole and foot bed should be inspected for areas of depression, which may reflect points of excessive plantar pressure secondary to structural or functional foot deformities.

4. *Midsole.* The midsole is evaluated for areas of excessive compression. In most cases, the height of the medial and lateral midsole in the rearfoot should be roughly equal. A disparity between the medial and lateral sides may reflect excessive pronatory or supinatory forces that have been uncontrolled, forcing the respective side to "bottom out." Defects or wear at the counter–midsole junction should be sought as well as at the midsole–outsole junction. Also, the overall flexibility of the shoe should be examined. Normal flexible shoes may bend mildly in the midfoot–forefoot region with finger pressure. The shoe should be evaluated for excessive flexibility or excessive stiffness, each of which may be detrimental in the susceptible athlete.

5. *Outsole.* The outsole is inspected for areas of excessive wear. Normal wear is indicated by a small triangular "wear spot" on the posterolateral heel, mild and even midfoot wear, mild wear under the central metatarsal heads, and mild wear under the hallux.

In excessive pronatory conditions there may be excessive wear along the medial heel extending toward the medial forefoot, whereas in supinatory conditions there may be excessive lateral wear of the heel extending toward the lateral forefoot. In equinus conditions there may be a pronatory wear if compensatory pronation is dominant or there may be excessive distal forefoot wear in uncompensated situations. Limb-length discrepancies may be reflected by grossly asymmetric outsole wear patterns.

6. *Torque.* The shoe is held upside down and examined for longitudinal torque. Apparent forefoot to rearfoot twisting may reflect uncontrolled frontal plane abnormalities of the foot that have produced a torque effect on the midsole. For example, a varus torque (forefoot inverted to the rearfoot) noted in the shoe may represent a varus imbalance of the forefoot.

OVERUSE INJURY TO SOFT TISSUE

Although many soft tissue injuries have an acute, violent, macrotraumatic etiology, such as podiatrists see with ankle sprains, soft tissue is also vulnerable to repetitive, cyclic stresses and loads that over a period of time may produce injury. These chronic, microtraumatic injuries are also known as overuse injuries. As soft tissues are overloaded, they are subject to repetitive microtrauma. With time, owing to excessive cyclic strain, the soft tissue demonstrates a diminished ability to withstand repetitive loading and begins to break down. This results in overuse injury.

Soft tissue, like bone, has the ability to remodel and adapt, to a degree, in response to stresses and loads. However, also as in the case of bone, soft tissue remodels slowly. With low levels of mechanical stress and strain, soft tissue can usually withstand the load. However, in situations demonstrating rapidly increasing levels of stress and strain, soft tissue becomes unable to keep up with the added load and will eventually fail. This is particularly so if the imposed stresses and strains are superimposed on structural or functional abnormalities, such as those seen with biomechanical foot faults, muscle imbalances, or limb-length discrepancies. These excessive, repetitive, cyclic stresses eventually promote the breakdown in collagen cross linkages, which functionally weakens connective tissue structures. As stresses continue, shearing between collagen fibers occurs and microinjury results. The injury then stimulates an inflammatory response, resulting in pain and diminished function and performance.

Soft tissue stresses can be of a variety of different forms. Frictional stress can produce injury, as can be demonstrated in the microtraumatic, inflammatory changes of the retropatellar surface seen in patellofemoral pain syndrome or chondromalacia patellae. Traction stresses can produce overuse injury at particularly vulnerable locations, such as the calcaneal apophysis (Sever's disease) or tibial tubercle (Osgood-Schlatter disease) in the adolescent athlete. However, by far the most significant stress is tension stress, which can be applied to musculotendinous, ligamentous, and capsular structures. This form of stress tends to be responsible for the overuse tendonitis, such as is commonly seen in the Achilles, posterior tibial, anterior tibial, and peroneal tendons. It is also the form of stress identified in chronic capsulitis, shin splint syndrome, and a variety of other conditions.

Most studies seem to suggest the incidence of soft tissue overuse injury at greater than 50% of all encountered athletic injuries. The overall incidence may be even higher than estimated, in that many overuse injuries go unreported. Overuse injuries are often overlooked by the athlete because he or she is unable to recognize any particular inciting incident. As the discomfort and decreased productivity build, the athlete may self-prescribe a lowered activity level with subsequent reduction in symptoms. When activity is resumed, if at a lower and more gradually increasing level, problems may not redevelop. If, however, activity is resumed at high, intense levels, the problem returns and the athlete seeks assistance.

Historically, most athletes will relate a sudden or dramatic increase in the intensity or duration of athletic activity. This is the "too much, too soon" phenomenon. Improper training techniques, training errors, and poor conditioning are also frequently encountered. The participation surface and equipment,

such as inadequate footgear, are commonly contributing factors. When these errors are superimposed on particular physical limitations, overuse injuries occur.

There is generally no preexisting defect in the tissue or any chemical abnormality in the blood before the onset of injury. Most frequently there is some structural or functional defect that may predispose the tissue to injury. Biomechanical abnormalities, particularly excessive subtalar joint pronation, are common accomplices to excessive stresses. Muscle imbalances, such as those encountered with abnormal agonist to antagonist muscle strength ratios or limited flexibility, as well as limb-length discrepancies and malalignment syndromes, are also seen in association with overuse soft tissue injuries. Frequently, these structural or function limitations may produce no significant problems when they occur in conjunction with low stress levels. However, with excessive stress levels, these faults may accentuate the stress and strain imposed on soft tissue.

For example, in overuse posterior tibial tendonitis, the posterior tibial muscle apparatus functions early in stance as a decelerator to subtalar joint pronation and later to assist in resupination of the foot. If the athlete pronates excessively, particularly with high stress levels such as may be seen in running activities, the posterior tibial muscle and tendon must work harder to decelerate subtalar joint pronation and assist in supination. The stresses become larger than the tendon's ability to withstand them and, owing to the delay in functional adaptation to the added stress, the tissue becomes overloaded and overuse injury results. Additionally, less conditioned muscles and tendons demonstrate a decreased ability to absorb and withstand increased stresses and loads, further adding to the potential for injury.

When overuse injury occurs in muscle, the focus of stress and injury tends to be at the weakest point in the musculotendinous unit. In younger persons, this may be at the point of attachment around an epiphyseal or apophyseal plate. In older persons, the tendon itself appears to be more vulnerable, possibly owing to its relatively lower vascularity and limited ability to repair itself. Muscle fiber itself is very fragile. However, the strength of the muscle fiber is supplied by the extensive network of connective tissue surrounding each fiber, bundle, and muscle. Muscle, therefore, has the ability to stretch somewhat, which may be mildly protective. Tendon, on the other hand, has a notably higher tensile strength than muscle, being composed largely of collagen. Although tendon has characteristically more strength than muscle, it also has a lower elasticity. Tendinous collagen fibers are wavy and, when stretched, appear straighter. However, when tendon is stretched beyond approximately 8%, cross linkages in the collagen break and structural weakness and breakdown occur.

When overuse injury to soft tissue occurs and inflammation ensues, healing must take place in an attempt to return the tissue to normalcy. Healing occurs through the inflammatory phase, followed by a proliferative stage when collagen regeneration occurs. It is desirable for soft tissue to heal with normal tissue and remodel accordingly to tension and stress. Unfortunately, tenocytes have only a limited potential for regeneration. Therefore, healing may frequently occur with scarring and fibrosis. This, when coupled with muscle deconditioning, joint and muscle stiffness, and defective proprioception following injury, promotes chronic tissue deficits, making the athlete prone to further injury. Thorough and complete rehabilitation and identification and correction of structural and functional abnormalities must be accomplished in a maximal effort to prevent reinjury.

Treatment

Initial treatment of overuse soft tissue injury revolves around relief of pain, control of inflammation, and limitation of stress and loading to the injured part. Inflammation, while essential in healing, if excessive can actually be a detriment by promoting local tissue hypoxia and elevated proteolytic activity at the injury site. The use of nonsteroidal anti-inflammatory agents may assist in controlling inflammation and discomfort. Treatment should be supported by appropriate physical therapy modalities and activity modification. Later stages of treatment rely on the correction of underlying

mechanical imbalances as predisposing causes. This can take the form of orthotic devices, lift therapy, stretching, strengthening, and correction of malalignments. Attention must also be given to recommendation of appropriate footgear and rectifying improper training and conditioning techniques. When activity is resumed, the load should be significantly lowered and the stress levels gradually and safely increased over time.

OVERUSE INJURY TO BONE (STRESS FRACTURE)

Although the overall incidence of stress fractures of the lower extremities differs in many studies, it can be roughly estimated that approximately 10% of all sports-related overuse injuries in the lower extremities may involve stress fracture. The actual incidence of stress fracture has been noted to increase. With the increased interest and involvement in physical activity and physical fitness, activity levels of a larger portion of the general population have increased, thus increasing the potential for stress-related injury to bone. Additionally, with the increased use of technetium bone scanning and its ready availability, suspicion of possible stress injury to bone with associated negative radiographs has led to the diagnosis of stress fracture on the basis of positive bone scans.

Bones of the lower extremity that appear to be most commonly involved with stress fracture include the tibia, fibula, metatarsals, and calcaneus. Other bones in which stress fracture is not as common but occasionally occurs include the tarsal navicular, the pelvis, and the femur. Although theoretically no bone of the foot is "immune" from stress fracture development, stress fractures of the cuneiforms, cuboid, and talus are only rarely seen.

With activity, bone is subjected to repetitive, cyclic stresses that produce tension and compression loads within the bone. This stress to bone is generally neutralized by the external or cortical and internal structure or trabeculation of the respective bone. Furthermore, bone exhibits "plastic" characteristics, meaning that bone will yield by bending when stress is applied. This is also protective, allowing bone to "give" when subjected to various loads. Bone, however, appears to be more subject to fatigue in the areas of plastic deformation or "fatigue zones." Also, according to Wolff's law, bone will change in architecture in response to prolonged stresses; however, this change occurs only over extended periods of time.

Etiology

The proposed etiology of lower extremity stress fracture has been frequently debated within the literature. With excessive stress applied to a bone, such as may be seen with increased activity levels or drastic activity changes, bone attempts to remodel in response to that stress. The stresses most commonly implicated involve actual bending stresses, in most cases applied to the bone particularly in a bone's bending or "plastic" region. This bending stress is most likely produced by excessive muscular activity applied to the bone near the region of muscle attachment. Compression or longitudinal loading-type stresses are less frequently the cause of stress fracture, particularly that which occurs in long tubular bones. As the bone is caused to bend, the convex side undergoes a tension stress, while the concave side of the bone undergoes a compression stress. This bending, producing a tension side versus compression side of the bone, stimulates the production of a piezoelectric current effect. The tension side of the bone assumes a relative electropositivity, while the compression side of the bone becomes more electronegative. A current flow is thereby induced from the electropositive to the electronegative side of bone. On the convex, tension, electropositive side, osteoclastic activity predominates and bone is resorbed. On the concave, compression, electronegative side, osteoblastic activity predominates and bone is laid down. The bone thus undergoes remodeling. As long as the rate of remodeling can keep up with the rate of stress, no problem occurs. It is when the amount of applied cyclic stress over a period of time is of a sufficient level that actual remodeling lags behind the amount of required remodeling to withstand stress that stress injury to bone occurs.

History

During history taking, it is very typical to find a change in activity intensity or other related contributing factors such as changes in shoes, the surface on which the athlete is participating, or alterations in training patterns. The athlete frequently relates an initial vague discomfort, present during activity in the early stages. With time, however, the discomfort intensifies and is present even during times of rest or inactivity. Although the site of maximal pain and tenderness may become localized, there is frequently a generalized surrounding discomfort. At this point, the athlete usually relates a significant decrease in his or her productivity and activity level, prompting him or her to seek assistance.

Evaluation

General physical findings are frequently nonspecific, involving well-localized tenderness over the involved bone. Overlying soft tissue erythema and edema are frequently present. Occasionally, placing a vibrating tuning fork or passing an ultrasonic wave over the suspected fracture site produces increased discomfort over the localized area. Biomechanical foot and leg faults, muscle imbalances concerning either strength or flexibility, and limb-length inequalities are frequently observed and may, in fact, be the precipitating factor behind the development of stress fracture when burdened by increased stress and load levels of activity. It is important to recognize that stress fractures generally occur in otherwise normal persons without abnormalities noted in serum calcium, phosphate, or protein levels and with no preexisting defect or intrinsic weakness in bony structure.

The diagnosis of stress fracture, therefore, requires a certain degree of clinical suspicion. It has been estimated that between 30% and 70% of all stress fractures, when initially radiographed, appear normal without overt radiographic evidence of stress fracture. The variation in time between the onset of symptoms and the appearance of changes on plain radiographs may be anywhere between 2 weeks to 3 months. Therefore, an initial negative radiograph does not rule out the presence of stress fracture. Tarsal bones are particularly notorious for negative radiographs in the presence of stress fracture. Therefore, the clinician may frequently initiate treatment for stress fracture without definite radiographic evidence of such if clinical suspicion is sufficient to warrant treatment.

Although the appearance of stress fractures may vary among different bones, when positive they tend to exhibit particular characteristics. When occurring in epiphyseal areas or in areas of large concentrations of cancellous bone (e.g., the calcaneus), the fracture line tends to appear more sclerotic and there may be minimal if any periosteal new bone formation. When occurring in diaphyseal areas or in regions predominantly composed of cortical bone, periosteal and endosteal new bone formation or lucent cortical breaks are generally seen. Periosteal new bone formation presents as cortical thickening or callus formation. Endosteal new bone formation is demonstrated as a narrowing of the endosteal canal in the region of the stress fracture and may also be seen as transverse sclerotic bands extending across the endosteal canal. Frequently radiographs must be obtained in multiple views and angles to demonstrate these changes. It is also helpful to place a radiopaque lesion marker adjacent to the area of suspected stress fracture before obtaining the radiograph to localize the site of interest on radiography.

Frequently the clinician may rely on other methods of evaluation to satisfy the suspicion of stress fracture such as thermography, computed tomography, magnetic resonance imaging, and technetium bone scanning.

Thermography, either infrared or liquid crystal, while being relatively sensitive, is often nonspecific, unable to distinguish between increased temperature from the stress fracture or soft tissue inflammation. Thermography, therefore, may be more helpful in the diagnosis of stress fracture in areas with scanty amounts of overlying soft tissue. However, in a study by Pagliano and Heaslet, when proper diagnostic criteria are employed, such as the size of the hot spot, the temperature gradient, and comparison to the opposite side when evaluating tibial stress fractures, thermography has a sufficient predictive value to make it useful in diagnosis.

Computerized tomography in many cases may be no more sensitive than plain radiography, but when positive it may be more specific. This may be particularly true in cases of stress fractures, which are typically difficult to image, such as those of the navicular and calcaneus in which the fracture characteristics and orientation may be better appreciated. The same could be said for plain tomography.

Magnetic resonance imaging, owing to physiologic inflammatory changes in the endosteal canal and in collections of trabecular bone, may show signal changes, with a decreased signal on T1-weighted images in the marrow cavity and an increased signal on T2-weighted images in the marrow cavity because of the presence of inflammatory edema.

Technetium-99m bone scanning still remains the most used ancillary modality of evaluation, next to plain radiography. Because of the lack of sensitivity of plain radiographs and the possible delay in diagnosis, in cases in which suspicion needs to be satisfied, bone scanning may be helpful. The bone scan may become positive within 6 to 72 hours after the onset of pain. However, it should be recognized that the bone scan is nonspecific, only indicating an area of osseous "turnover" that may be due to any process producing accelerated bone remodeling, such as neoplasm, infection, and other conditions, as well as stress fracture. When bone scans are supportive of stress fracture, there tends to be a focal increase of radionucleotide uptake or "hot spot" in the area of the stress fracture. Linear, nonfocal increases in uptake may be seen indicating excessive bone remodeling, as demonstrated in tibial stress syndrome, without evidence of stress fracture. Overall, the bone scan may be considered worthwhile, particularly in the evaluation of bones that tend to demonstrate significantly delayed findings of stress fracture, such as the pelvis, femur, calcaneus, and navicular.

Treatment

Treatment of stress fracture, in most cases, is conservative. The initial phase of treatment generally involves control of discomfort through physical therapy, nonsteroidal anti-inflammatory medications, and modified activity or rest of the involved area. Depending on the stress fracture site, weight bearing is usually allowed (with the navicular being a particular exception) with the offending stress eliminated. Frequently, alternative activities, such as swimming, cycling, or "water running" are preferable as long as they do not aggravate symptoms or add particular stress to the injured area. Rigid immobilization, in most stress fractures, is usually not required unless symptoms dictate that immobilization would provide more initial comfort. If required, however, this period of immobilization time is generally brief. Lesser forms of immobilization in the form of braces or rigid soled shoes may occasionally be used for comfort and protection.

Flexibility exercises may be allowed if they do not produce symptoms. Excessive muscular activity with strengthening is usually avoided during this period of time. It is also during this initial phase that any contributing or inciting factors responsible for the development of the stress fracture be identified and corrected. The key to overall success in treatment is the identification of the offending cause and risk factors and taking all measures to avoid their return once activity is again begun. When the athlete becomes pain free, gradual resumption of activity in a slow and planned fashion is generally allowed. Some stress fractures, however, require a more aggressive approach to treatment. Such is in the case of diaphyseal fifth metatarsal and tarsal navicular fractures. In these cases, more persistent immobilization or surgical intervention may be required.

BIBLIOGRAPHY

Clement DB, Taunton JE, Smart GE, et al: A survey of overuse running injuries. Phys Sports Med 9(5):47–58, 1981.

Goodman PH, Heaslet MW, Pagliano JW, Rubin BD: Stress fracture diagnosis by computer-assisted thermography. Phys Sports Med 13(4):114–132, 1985.

Herring SA, Nilson KL: Introduction to overuse injuries. Clin Sports Med 6(2):225–239, 1987.

Hershman E: The profile for prevention of musculoskeletal injury. Clin Sports Med 3(1):65–84, 1984.

James SL, Bates BT, Osternig LR: Injuries to runners. Am J Sports Med 6:40–50, 1978.

Janis LR: Results of the Ohio Runner sports medicine survey. J Am Podiatr Med Assoc 76:586–589, 1986.

Kerner JA, D'Amico JC: A statistical analysis of a group of runners. J Am Podiatr Assoc 73:160–164, 1983.

Koplan JP, Powell KE, Sikes RK, et al: An epidemiological study of the benefits and risks of running. JAMA 248:3118–3121, 1982.

Lysholm J, Wiklander J: Injuries in runners. Am J Sports Med 15:168–171, 1987.

McKeag DB: The concept of overuse: The primary care aspects of overuse syndromes in sports. Primary Care 11:43–59, 1984.

McKenzie DC, Clement DB, Taunton JE: Running shoes, orthotics and injuries. Sports Med 2:334–347, 1985.

Nicholas JA, Hershman EB: The Lower Extremity and Spine in Sports Medicine, vol 2. St. Louis, CV Mosby, 1986.

O'Donoghue DH: Treatment of Injuries to Athletes, ed 3. Philadelphia, WB Saunders, 1976.

Pagliano JW, Jackson DW: The ultimate study of running injuries. Runners World 15(November):42–50, 1980.

Pollock ML, Gettman LR, Milesis CA, et al: Effects of frequency and duration of training on attrition and incidence of injury. Med Sci Sports 9(Spring):31–36, 1977.

Powell KE, Kohl HW, Caspersen CJ, Blair SN: An epidemiological perspective on the causes of running injuries. Phys Sports Med 14(6):100–114, 1986.

Renstrom P, Johnson RJ: Overuse injuries in sports: A review. Sports Med 2:316–333, 1985.

Ross CF, Schuster RO: A preliminary report on predicting injuries in distance runners. J Am Podiatr Assoc 73(5):275–277, 1983.

Smith LS, Bunch R: Athletic footwear. Clin Podiatr Med Surg 3(4):637–647, 1986.

Solomonow M, D'Ambrosia RD: Biomechanics of muscle overuse injuries: A theoetical approach. Clin Sports Med 6(2):241–257, 1987.

Stanish WD: Overuse injuries in athletes: A perspective. Med Sci Sports Exercise 16:1–7, 1984.

Stanitski CL, McMaster JH, Scranton PE: On the nature of stress fractures. Am J Sports Med 6:391–396, 1978.

Subotnick SI: Lower extremity problems in athletes: A biomechanical approach. Arch Podiatr Med Foot Surg 5(2):23–29, 1978.

Walter SD, Sutton JR, McIntosh JM, et al: The aetiology of sports injuries: A review of methodologies. Sports Med 2:47–58, 1985.

Williams JCP: Wear and tear injuries in athletes: An overview. Br J Sports Med 12:211–214, 1979.

CHAPTER 19

PEDAL NAIL AND SKIN PROBLEMS

Myron A. Bodman

The clinical characteristics and management principles of many of the pedal nail and skin problems seen by podiatrists are described in this chapter. Some conditions are encountered many times each day, while others are rarely noted. Nearly every podiatric patient exhibits nail and/or skin pathology. Certainly, nail and skin problems are the most frequently treated conditions in primary podiatric practice.

Nail disorders are discussed first, followed by the superficial skin infections, eczemas, hyperkeratotic disorders, sweat disorders, and some manifestations of diabetes. Textbooks of dermatology and podiatric medicine are additional resources for the many other interesting dermatologic diseases that can be manifested by podiatric patients.

PEDAL NAIL DISORDERS

Structure of the Nail Unit

Dawber and Baran have described the clinically significant topographic features of the nail unit.[1] They include the nail plate, nail folds, lunula, cuticle, hyponychium, distal groove, and, less obviously, onychodermal band. The nail unit is firmly attached to the underlying distal phalanx and follows its contour and its shape.[2]

Normally the nail plate is characteristically transparent and clear while attached to the underlying nail bed. This allows the visualization of the rich vascular pink nail bed beneath it. It is actually composed of three layers: (1) the thin dorsal layer derived from the inferior surface of the proximal nail fold, (2) the thick intermediate layer formed by the proximal nail root, and (3) the ventral layer of the plate from the nail bed.[2]

The nail folds medially and laterally form grooves of varying depths. They may be angulated toward the center of the nail plate proximally, contributing to onychocryptosis. The proximal nail fold actually has a dorsal and a ventral epidermal surface. It covers the proximal fifth of the nail plate.

The lunula can be seen as a crescent-shaped white zone projecting from beneath the proximal nail fold. It represents the distalmost extension of the nail root. It is white because the nail matrix cells here are still nucleated. Clear nail plate is always composed of non-nucleated flattened layers of interlocked keratinocytes.

The hyponychium is the slightly thickened skin just below the free edge of the normal nail in the distal groove. It represents the accumulated keratinocytes streaming distally from the superficial surface of the nail bed.

The onychodermal band is clinically seen as a barely perceptible, pale, 1-mm-wide, transverse band, just proximal to the distal free-edge zone of the nail plate. The vascular supply to this band responds differently from the remainder of the nail bed. When the nail plate is repeatedly pressed, the onychodermal band turns brighter pink while the remainder of the nail bed remains unchanged. This color difference is enhanced in the leukonychia of cirrhosis and in acrocyanosis.[3]

Nail Unit Growth and Development

The development of the nail unit starts in the fetus at about 10 weeks of age. The entire nail unit is derived from ectoderm and the resulting epidermis. A wedge of matrix primordium starts as a dimple and grows proximally and deeper to follow the contour of the distal phalanx. The nail plate is often clinically seen to follow the form and function of its supporting bone throughout its lifetime.

The nail plate is formed continually by a process of flattening of the basal cells of the matrix or root. The maturing process continues with fragmentation of the nuclei and condensation of the cytoplasm to form flat horny cells that are strongly adherent to each other, just as in hair formation.

The matrix is the sole structure responsible for the formation of the nail plate. Thus, if one excises or destroys the entire nail matrix, then the nail plate will not regrow. The normal nail plate lies on and follows the shape of the distal phalanx. If the shape of the bone

changes with time or trauma, the nail plate shape and contour will also change.

The nail bed extends from the lunula to the hyponychium. It does not make nail plate nor does it move distally as the nail grows, but instead it allows the nail plate to move over the nail bed gradually while still being firmly attached to it. Once a nail bed is exposed, without an intact covering nail plate, it will thicken somewhat and become harder skin but will not grow true translucent plate. The nail bed can become pathologically affected, allowing deviation and distortion of the forward growth of the overlying nail plate. Intermittent shoe pressure may cause reactive subungual nail bed thickening and hyperkeratosis of the nail bed and hypertrophy and distortion of the nail matrix, resulting in onychogryphosis. Dermatophytic infection of the nail bed can also cause subungual separation (onycholysis) and hyperkeratosis, further distorting and lifting the nail plate.

The proximal nail fold anatomy is usually not well appreciated. It is actually composed of two opposed layers of epidermis like a fold of skin. The first layer of the proximal nail fold is the dorsal epidermal covering of the digit over the base of the distal phalanx. The second layer is the ventral portion of the proximal nail fold that covers the superior proximal portion of the nail plate over the nail matrix. The horny layer of the ventral portion of the proximal nail fold becomes adherent to the surface of the newly formed nail plate. These cells move distally with the nail plate for a short distance, becoming the horny portion of the ventral nail fold known as the cuticle.

The cuticle eventually and gradually falls off or desquamates from the nail plate while acting as a natural seal to protect the proximal fold from bacterial or fungal invasion. The cuticle should be left intact and undisturbed. Patients should be encouraged to refrain from cosmetically inspired orange stick manipulations because this invites chronic inflammation and possible paronychia. Paronychia means any inflammation of the proximal, medial, or lateral nail folds. Pedal paronychia can vary in intensity from early paronychia, presenting as just soreness about a curved nail edge to acute paronychia manifesting as redness, pain, and drainage with possible abscess formation. Paronychia can become chronic and recurrent with granuloma formation and nail lip hypertrophy.

Skin diseases that commonly affect the proximal nail fold, such as infection, eczema, and psoriasis, can also affect the nail plate surface, causing ripples, pits, or grooves.

The nail plate is composed of dead keratin (a protein) and does not grow itself. The nail plate is more porous to water than the epidermis. The brittleness and hardness of the nail is directly related to its water content. Water- or alcohol-based preparations penetrate the nail plate better than oil-based compounds. The calcium content of nail plate is only 0.2% and is not related to nail hardness, nor has gelatin ever been shown to specifically encourage nail growth or nail strength. The rate of nail growth is solely determined by the rate of cell division of the nail matrix. Fingernails grow faster than toenails, perhaps because of the relatively higher upper limb temperature and rate of blood flow as compared with the foot. Nails of individual digits grow at slightly different rates, with the thumb nail growing at about 0.1 mm per day and the hallux nail plate growing at about 1 mm per month. The rate of nail growth is greatest in the second decade and then declines slightly thereafter with increasing age. Increased growth is seen in the summer and in warmer climates, while slower rates are observed in the winter and in colder climates.

The thickness of nail plate is directly proportional to the number of germinal cells of the matrix. If the matrix is flattened and longer distally, the nail plate becomes thicker throughout its entire length.

Systemic diseases can cause slowing of nail growth and thinning or grooving of the nail plate. These nail changes are seen weeks after the systemic illness because of the slow rate of nail maturation. Acute viral illnesses such as mumps or measles are the most frequent cause of these changes.

Starvation, malignancy, and drugs such as oral corticosteroids, methotrexate, and cytotoxic chemotherapeutic agents all decrease nail growth. Increased nail growth may be seen in pregnancy, psoriasis, and nail biting and after trauma to the extremity.

Removal of the nail plate, either traumati-cally or surgically, seems to actually speed the regrowth of the new nail plate. In avulsion the nail bed is denuded and the hyponychium is lost. The epidermis of nail bed is restored by the migration of epidermal cells from the lateral nail folds. If the matrix stays tightly adhered to the bony phalanx and is not disturbed, then the nail plate has a good chance to be normal, smooth, and thin. If there is any damage to the nail matrix in the process of avulsion, then there is a good chance for later nail scarring and permanent deformity.

Patterns of Nail Unit Pathology

See Table 19–1 for a glossary of nail disorders.

Atrophy of the Nail Matrix. Atrophy of the nail matrix can occur for a few weeks, causing transverse grooves called Beau's lines, or for a continual or sustained period of time, in which the nail plate becomes thin and fragile or sometimes is completely absent.

Hypertrophy of the Nail Plate. Hypertrophy of the nail plate results from the chronic intermittent microtrauma to the nail unit from shoes or a supporting surface that stimulates the nail matrix to generate a thickened nail plate, resulting in clinical onychauxis. If this microtrauma continues, subungual hyperkeratosis, thickening of the nail bed, and elevation of the nail plate occurs. This can cause an upward distortion of growth, resulting in clinically quite thickened and deformed ram's horn–like nail termed *onychogryphosis*. Acute trauma can also scar the nail unit and cause onychogryphosis. Hereditary congenital overgrowth of all 20 nails can occur and is called pachyonychia congenita.

Abnormal Keratinization. Abnormal keratinization within the nail matrix can cause leukonychia, onychoschizia, or onychorrhexis.

Leukonychia occurs when there are localized accumulations of abnormally nucleated keratinocytes creating clinical white spots within the nail plate. These faulty cells may desquamate, leaving pits or grooves like potholes on the nail plate. Onychoschizia is lamellar dystrophy or layering of the free edge of the nail, as in brittle nails, and is associated with repeated episodes of wetting and drying

TABLE 19–1. **Nail Disorders**

Disorder	Description
Koilonychia	Spoon-shaped or thin concave nails
Onychatrophia	Atrophy of the nails
Onychauxis	Overgrowth or thickening of the nail caused by trauma
Onychectomy	Excision of a nail or nail bed
Onychia	Inflammation of the nail matrix resulting in the shedding of the nail plate (onychitis)
Onychoclasis	Breaking of the nail plate
Onychodystrophy	Malformation of the nail plate
Onychogryphosis	A deformed, thickened overgrowth of a permanently scarred nail producing a hooked or incurvated nail
Onycholysis	Loosening or separation of all or part of the nail plate from its nail bed
Onychomadesis	Complete shedding of the nails
Onychomalacia	Softening of the nail plate
Onychomycosis	Any fungal infection of the nail, by either dermatophyte, saprophyte, or yeast
Onychopathy	Disease of the nail
Onychophagia	The habit of biting the nails
Onychophosis	Calloused nail groove or nail lip
Onychorrhexis	Spontaneous longitudinal splitting or breaking of the nails
Onychotillomania	Neurotic picking at the nails
Onychotomy	Incision of the nail
Paronychia	Inflammation involving the folds of tissue surrounding the nail
Tinea unguium	Fungal infection of the nail caused by only dermatophytes

Definitions adapted from Dorland's Illustrated Medical Dictionary, 27th ed. Philadelphia, WB Saunders, 1988.

of the nails.[4] Alternating hydration and dehydration produces a deformity analogous to weathered plywood. Columbo and Gerber[5] used oral biotin, 2.5 mg/d, to resolve brittle fingernails.

Onychoschizia has been reported in chondrodysplasia, polycythemia vera, and lichen planus and in patients using oral retinoids.[1]

Abnormal keratinization can produce a series of narrow longitudinal parallel furrows that look like they have been scratched on the nail plate with an awl. These longitudinal striations may be physiologic in some persons, becoming more prominent with age, or may be associated with lichen planus, rheumatoid arthritis, peripheral vascular insufficiency, or Darier's disease. Wider furrows can be due to tumors, warts, or cysts of the proximal nail fold.[6]

Clubbing. Clubbing or hippocratic fingers

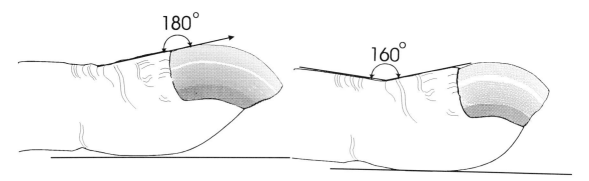

A

B

FIGURE 19–1. Signs of clubbing. (A) Lovibond's lateral profile sign in nail clubbing. This quantifies the relationship between the nail plate and the proximal nail fold. It is normally about 160°, while in clubbing it measures 180°. (B) Curth's modified profile sign. This sign measures the angular relationship between the distal phalanx and the middle phalanx at the interphalangeal joint. Normally it measures about 180°, while in clubbing it reduces to 140° to 160°. (Redrawn from Dawber RP, Baran R: Physical signs. In Baran R, Dawber RP (eds): Diseases of the Nails and Their Management, pp 26, 27. Boston, Blackwell Scientific Publications, 1984.)

were first described in patients suffering from thoracic empyema, which is a large abscess in the thoracic cavity. Two morphologic changes are seen in clubbing: (1) longitudinal and transverse overcurvature of the nail and (2) enlargement of the subungual and fingertip soft tissue structures. The increased curvature can affect all the nails but has a predilection for the radial three digits of the hands. Lovibond's lateral profile sign is used to measure the degree of clubbing (Fig. 19–1A). It measures the angle between the curved nail plate and the proximal nail fold. This angle is normally 160° but exceeds 180° in clubbing. Clinical clubbing can also be detected by Curth's modified profile sign (Fig. 19–1B). It measures the angle between the middle and distal phalanx at the interphalangeal joint. Normally the distal interphalangeal joint of the finger is straight (180°) when viewed laterally. In severe clubbing this angle may be reduced to 160° or even to 140° observed with the distal interphalangeal joint in neutral.

Koilonychia. Koilonychia is the converse of clubbing. The nail is concave with the edges everted, the so-called spoon-shaped nail. This nail dystrophy is more easily clinically appreciated when the nail plate is viewed laterally, just as in clubbing. Koilonychia more often affects several fingers, especially the thumb and less frequently the toes (Fig. 19–2). There are hereditary and congenital forms that occur with other developmental anomalies.[6] Koilonychia can be found more frequently in the toenails of unshod children living, for example, in a kibbutz (32%) than in urban children (17%).

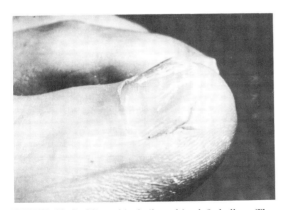

FIGURE 19–2. Idiopathic koilonychia, left hallux. The right hallux was also affected. The lesser toes have only minor involvement.

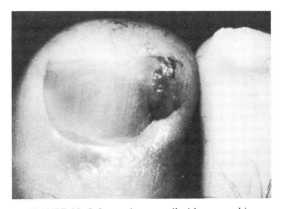

FIGURE 19–3. Ingrowing toenail with paronychia.

This form is temporary and seems to decrease with development. In infants there is a significant correlation with koilonychia and iron-deficiency anemia. The spooned-shaped nails may be noted before clinical or laboratory signs of anemia develop. Koilonychia can also be found in patients with hemochromatosis (a disorder of iron metabolism), lichen planus, and hypothyroidism. Pierre[8] lists many other associations with koilonychia.

Paronychia. Paronychia is inflammation involving the folds of tissue surrounding the nail unit. Clinically it can present in its early form as a sore nail lip caused by minor mechanical trauma or onychocryptosis. Later, secondary infection by bacteria, yeasts, or viruses can produce a severe chronic form with redness, pain, drainage, and nail fold edema that can extend all around the nail plate periphery. Paronychia is often associated with diabetes but can be found in 3% of nondiabetic female patients. Early paronychia on the toes is commonly found associated with incurvated nail edges, especially on the great toes. Simple excision of the adjacent offending nail plate allows the nail lip to drain (Fig. 19–3). Cleansing with hydrogen peroxide, followed by a topical antibiotic ointment for several days, is appropriate. Proximal nail fold inflammation is usually due to skin disease such as eczema, psoriasis, contact dermatitis, or Reiter's syndrome, rather than to infection. A surprisingly painful crack in the nail lip, usually extending from distal to proximal for 2 to 3 mm, is called a hangnail. It should be clipped flush with the skin at its triangular base with a tissue nipper or nail clipper rather than be torn back into intact skin.

Onycholysis. Onycholysis is the pathologic separation of the nail plate from the nail bed usually starting at the distal lateral attachments first. This may progress to produce spontaneous separation of the entire nail plate with its subsequent shedding, which is termed *onychomadesis*. Onycholysis is really a reaction pattern of the nail unit responding to many different potential etiologies. Pedal onycholysis is most commonly caused by microtrauma to the nail unit, while fingernails are continually chemically assaulted by a variety of agents, such as x-ray developer, cutting oils, solvents, and detergents. Fungi and bacteria can cause onycholysis. *Pseudomonas* bacteria apparently secrete keratolytic enzymes that allow more rapid spread. In addition to the customary pitting, onycholysis is a key clinical finding in psoriasis; however, psoriatic lysis is likely to be more yellow and irregular in its proximal extension. Both piroxicam and tetracycline have been associated with onycholysis occurring as a photosensitivity reaction. Onycholysis can also occur in lichen planus, in atopic dermatitis, and in hyperthyroidism, in which it has been designated Plummer's nails. Sculptured onycholysis can occur through overzealous self-cleaning of the underside of the nail plate with a sharp instrument.

Onycholysis of the toenails has two main causes: onychomycosis and trauma. Baran writes, ''in distal and subungual onychomycosis of the toenails, the horny thickening (caused by continuing microtrauma to the nail unit from foot gear) raises the free edge of the nail with disruption of the normal nail bed plate to nail plate attachment; thus giving rise to secondary onycholysis.''[6(p55)] Traumatic onycholysis occurs quite frequently from relatively minor digital malpositions, such as contracted toes, hammer toes, mallet toes, and toe length disproportions and even as a result of biomechanical compensation for hallux limitus. More severe forefoot deformities such as hallux valgus with digital overlap can cause microtraumatic onycholysis and onchodystrophy.

Subungual Hemorrhage. Another pattern of nail bed pathology is the accumulation of blood under the nail plate. Subungual hemorrhage can present as a total or partial subungual hematoma (Fig. 19–4). The common total subungual hematoma is traumatically

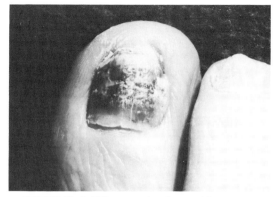

FIGURE 19–4. Old traumatic subungual hematoma.

induced and, if seen acutely before it coagulates, often needs to be anesthetized with hallux ring block and drained. The nail plate is often loose and may need to be avulsed totally. It is important to rule out a distal phalangeal comminuted fracture by radiography. (I have seen an elderly woman with a total subungual hematoma and fractured phalanx that failed to clot after drainage because of liver-induced coagulopathy of alcoholism.) Partial subungual hematomas are much smaller, are induced by microtrauma, and are localized to the proximal portion of the nail unit. The entire nail plate is still intact and not loose. Drainage of the coagulated blood is not necessary. Measuring the distance from the lesion to the cuticle and watching for distalward migration of 1 mm per month to exclude the possibility of an occult subungual melanoma is appropriate. Splinter hemorrhages are thrombosed linear capillaries occurring in the distal third of the nail bed. They can be associated with dozens of conditions, especially peripheral and systemic vascular diseases, but are diagnostic of none.

Longitudinal Melanonychia. Longitudinal melanonychia is a tan, brown, or black longitudinal streak within the nail plate (Fig. 19–5). Often it is clinically important to differentiate benign from malignant streaks. Single bands can be non-neoplastic and are caused by acute or chronic trauma, postinflammatory hyperpigmentation, a foreign body such as a splinter, or carpal tunnel syndrome. Neoplastic single bands can be due to melanocytic nevi, basal cell carcinoma, Bowen's disease, verruca vulgaris, or a histiocytoma. Multiple bands of

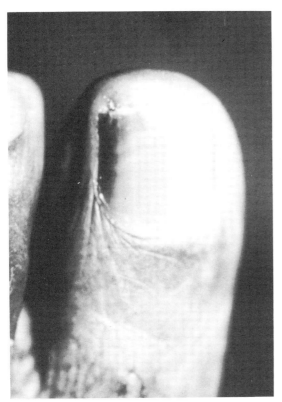

FIGURE 19–5. Common benign longitudinal melanonychia.

TABLE 19–2. **Mycobacterial Examinations in Pedal Onychomycosis**

Pathogen	Author	
	Baran*	Abramson†
Dermatophytes	12.8%	25%–30%
Saprophytic molds	69.4%	50%–60%
Yeasts	17.8%	10%–15%
Bacteria (Corynebacteria)	None reported	

*Data from Baran R: Onychia and paronychia of mycotic, microbial, and parasitic origin. In Pierre M [ed]: The Nail. New York, Churchill Livingstone, 1981.

†Data from Abramson C: Culture identification and therapy of fungal infections of foot and nails. Podiatric Pathology Prints 9:2, 1991. Baltimore, Podiatric Pathology Laboratories.

uli. Melanin can be differentiated from hemosiderin deposits by chemical staining of a biopsy specimen.

Onychomycosis

Onychomycosis is a general term for nail infections caused by a variety of nail pathogens (Table 19–2). *Tinea unguium* is the term correctly reserved for nail infections caused by only the dermatophytes. Regardless of the pathogen, individual mycotic nails clinically appear similar. They all exhibit, to various degrees, clinical onycholysis, discoloration (either white, yellow, brown, or green), thickening, hypertrophy, or subungual hyperkeratosis or crumbling. Not all of these signs are evident within each mycotic nail. Some nails present with only distal onycholysis yet are culture positive. Others exhibit only thickening and hypertrophy. Each nail can be at a different stage of onychomycosis (Fig. 19–6), depending on the primary cause of the mycosis and or the duration of the infection (Table 19–3). Most mycotic pedal nails are first initiated by repetitive microtrauma from the shoe or reactive forces during ambulation impacting on the nail unit.[10] Other causes include overt trauma or

longitudinal melanonychia are most commonly caused by variations in racial skin pigmentation with nearly all of black Americans older than the age of 50 demonstrating multiple nail streaks. Other causes include lichen planus, drugs, microbial infections, and systemic conditions such as hyperthyroidism, pregnancy, and porphyria.[9] Suspicions of subungual melanoma should be raised if the streak of longitudinal melanonychia clinically exhibits any of the following: failure to grow distalward at a rate of 1 mm per month, widing or blurring of the edges of the streak, change in color of the streak, leaking of pigment into the proximal nail fold or the surrounding nail bed (Hutchinson's sign), or any accompanying distortion of the overlying nail plate. Subungual melanoma occurs more frequently in lightly pigmented persons older than 50 years of age, on the thumb or index finger or great toe, within a traumatized digit, or in a patient with a history of malignant melanoma. The normal nail matrix does have usually quiescent melanocytes that can react to a variety of stim-

TABLE 19–3. **Stages of Onychomycosis**

Distal subungual onychomycosis
Superficial white onychomycosis
Proximal white subungual onychomycosis
Total secondary dystrophic onychomycosis
Total dystrophic primary onychomycosis

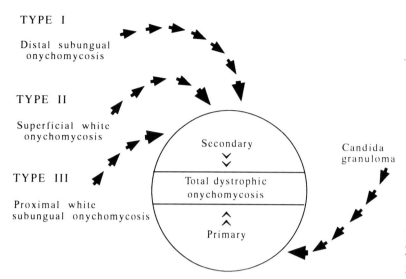

TYPE I

Distal subungual
onychomycosis

TYPE II

Superficial white
onychomycosis

TYPE III

Proximal white
subungual onychomycosis

Secondary

Total dystrophic
onychomycosis

Primary

Candida
granuloma

FIGURE 19–6. Clinical stages of onychomycosis. (From Pierre M: The Nail. Edinburgh, Churchill Livingstone, 1981.)

injury, systemic candidiasis, primary fungal infection, and even acquired immunodeficiency syndrome (AIDS)-related complex.

Proper media selection is necessary to culture the saprophytic molds that account for about half of the cases of onychomycosis. Dermatophyte test medium specifically suppresses saprophytes and should be used to screen for tinea pedis. Sabouraud agar without cyclohexamide or cyclohexamide should be used for nail fungal culturing. Species identification requires investigation in a mycology laboratory. Abramson reports that 25 different saprophytic genera can be found with 2 to 10 species per genera, many of which are resistant to the common antifungal agents.[11] The plant pathogens *Hendersonula toruloidea* and *Scopulariopsis brevicaulis* have been proven capable of primary invasion, while the others are probably secondary opportunistic organisms.[12]

Distal subungual onychomycosis starts as onycholysis that allows mycobacterial invasion of the hyponychium with proximal spread that, if not treated, often causes total nail dystrophy (Fig. 19–7). Linear yellow streaks are often seen in the nail bed. Management of this stage includes debridement of all dystrophic nail plate, application of an appropriate topical antifungal agent, and control of the initiating forces caused by ill-fitting shoes. It is the limiting of the digital impingement from shoes by the patient, wearing appropriately fitting shoes, rather than the potency of the antifungal agents, that most often determines improvement at this stage.

Superficial white onychomycosis is a far less common form of onychomycosis than distal subungual onychomycosis. It starts as small white patches on the surface of the toenail plate caused by direct invasion of dermatophytes, especially *Trichophyton mentagrophytes*, yeasts, or molds (Fig. 19–8). It seems to occur in the elderly with overlapping digits that cover the affected nail plate. This can progress to pits, grooves, and delamination of the nail plate and finally to total nail dystrophy. This form of onychomycosis can often be resolved on the first visit by careful superficial debridement of the diseased nail plate with a bur down to clean translucent nail plate. Topical antifungal agents can prevent recurrence.

Proximal subungual onychomycosis is usually a very rare form of onychomycosis that starts under the proximal nail fold above the lunula

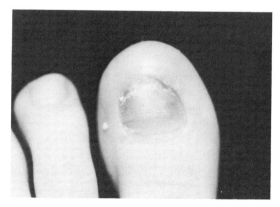

FIGURE 19–7. Distal subungual onychomycosis secondary to a long great toe impinging on the toebox of the shoe. The shorter second toenail is spared.

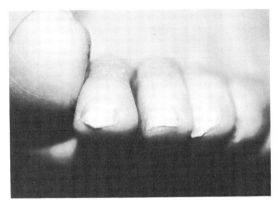

FIGURE 19–8. Superficial white onychomycosis in an elderly woman.

and spreads distally under the nail plate to produce total nail dystrophy (Fig. 19–9). Dermatophytes are cultured in the majority of cases. Proximal subungual onychomycosis is rarely found in human immunodeficiency virus (HIV)-negative patients but is the dominant type of onychomycosis (88%) in HIV-positive patients with a high frequency (83%) of pedal involvement.[13]

Total dystrophic onychomycosis is the most advanced stage of the previously discussed types. The nail matrix has become permanently scarred by chronic infection. The nail is thickened, elevated, and more dense or opaque. The nail bed is often hypertrophic and distorted with central humping. The axis of nail growth has become deviated dorsally and laterally from the long axis of the distal phalanx (Fig. 19–10). Total dystrophic onychomycosis does not resolve with oral or topical antifungal agents, regardless of the vehicle or the potency. Thorough periodic debridement with

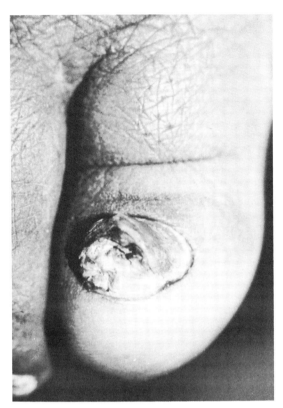

FIGURE 19–10. Total dystrophic onychomycosis.

thinning and rounding of the nail plate to a more normal contour often controls the patient's symptoms and prevents subungual pressure ulceration. Limiting the forces of impinging shoes and frequent use of simple emollients are useful. Surgical removal is seldom necessary. On rare occasions, total dystrophic onychomycosis occurs as a primary infection caused by *Candida*.

Nail Changes in Common Systemic Diseases

Psoriasis. Psoriasis is a papulosquamous skin and joint disease commonly seen in podiatric practice. Approximately one third of patients with psoriasis have a family history of the disease. Most podiatric patients relate their history of psoriasis, but some are first seen and diagnosed by the podiatrist. Psoriatic changes occur in the fingernails and toenails in about 50% of patients with psoriasis. If nail changes are watched for in an individual patient with psoriasis over his or her lifetime, 90% percent of the patients will have some psoriatic nail

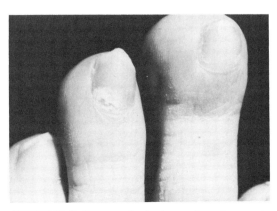

FIGURE 19–9. Rare, proximal subungual onychomycosis.

changes. The most classic psoriatic nail change is pit formation in the nail plate. These pits are the visible end products of punctate parakeratotic horn formation within the nail matrix. These immature keratinocytes fail to adhere properly to each other and desquamate prematurely, leaving superficial nail plate potholes or dents that grow out with the elongating nail plate.[2] The presence of more than 20 fingernail pits suggests psoriasis, and it is unlikely to find more than 60 nail pits in the absence of psoriatic nail changes. Other nail changes also occur commonly in psoriasis. These include yellow discoloration of the nail plate (''oil spot''), onycholysis, grooving, and subungual accumulations of crumbly hyperkeratotic debris (Fig. 19–11A).[14] These changes clinically appear similar to distal subungual onychomycosis and should be differentiated by fungal culture (Fig. 19–11B).

Lichen Planus. Lichen planus affects the nail unit in about 10% of patients with lichen planus. Many changes are possible, but characteristic of severe lichen planus is the pterygium formation or wing-shaped overgrowth and scarring of the proximal nail fold and cuticle. The nail bed is scarred, and the nail plate is quite dystrophic, with lateral wing-shaped nail plate spicules. In addition, longitudinal pigmented bands, fissuring, atrophy, and longitudinal ridging are all changes that may occur in the nails of patients with less severe lichen planus.[15]

Peripheral Vascular Disease. Peripheral vascular diseases are accompanied by a variety of nail changes. Arterial insufficiency often produces thin, brittle, or longitudinally split nail plates, presumably due to the overall loss of water and nutrients to the nail matrix. The subcutaneous structures supporting the nail plate and matrix can atrophy and increase the transverse overcurvature of the nail plate, contributing to onychocryptosis. Thin, vascular insufficient nail folds are predisposed to ulceration and paronychia. Onycholysis, onychomadesis, and subungual hemorrhage are common in vascular-insufficient lower extremities.

Lymphedema, if chronic, is associated with the so-called yellow nail syndrome in which the nail plate color changes from its normal white translucence to a pale yellow, varying to a slightly greenish color with the lateral edges being slightly darker. The nail plate appears thicker and more transversely overcurved with the distal one third to one half being more involved.[16] Perhaps the lymphedema decreases digital skin perfusion, resulting in a slowed nail growth rate.

Arthritis. Degenerative joint disease can also effect nail changes, such as excessive ridging and bending of the nail edges contributing to onychocryptosis. Osteoarthritis accompanying hallux valgus, mallet toes, and hammer toes commonly causes onychauxis, onycholysis, onychomycosis, and onychogryphosis. Psoriatic arthritis favors the distal interphalangeal joint, with nail plate changes ranging from simple pit formation to total dystrophy. The nail changes commonly precede the development of arthritis.[15]

The nail changes in Reiter's syndrome may be clinically and histologically indistinguisha-

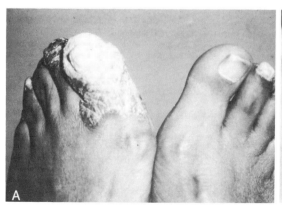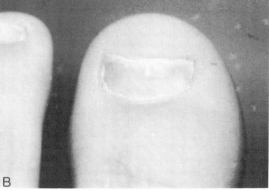

FIGURE 19–11. (A) Hallux with psoriatic nail and skin signs. (B) Hallux of 18-year-old man with brachyonychia, pits, grooves, onycholysis, and dactylitis of psoriasis. Previous treatment with griseofulvin was unsuccessful.

ble from the nail changes of psoriasis. These include paronychia, onycholysis, thickening, longitudinal ridging and splitting, subungual hyperkeratosis, and yellow or brownish red discoloration. Small, yellow to brown subungual pustules may develop and then dry up and resolve.

Subungual partial hematomas and onychauxis with atrophy of the adjacent skin are frequently seen in patients with rheumatoid arthritis. In severe generalized rheumatoid arthritis, nail growth may be reduced, producing Beau's transverse lines. Palmar flushing and erythema of the fingertips are more common in rheumatoid arthritis. In rheumatoid vasculitis, small infarcts around the nails can occur.[16]

Benign Tumors of the Nail Unit

Periungual verrucae are benign, weakly contagious, fibroepithelial growths with rough hyperkeratotic surfaces occurring around the nail unit. They are caused by a variety of human papillomavirus serotypes and specifically affect the proximal and lateral nail folds as well as the nail bed. They seem to be the most resistant of all clinical wart types, especially if the nail plate is not at least partially avulsed during treatment.

Pyogenic granuloma or "proud flesh" is a localized superficial ulcerated polypodal new growth of vascular tissue that results from irritation of the skin. It often accompanies ingrown toenails or pressure-induced subungual blisters and represents exuberant neovascularization (Fig. 19–12). It is not caused by pus or infection as its name seems to imply. It is easily and painlessly removed, and then a hemostatic agent such as silver nitrate is applied. If the irritating source, such as the offending nail spicule, is removed, the granuloma will spontaneously resorb within several days.

Periungual fibromas are rare benign tumors of the proximal nail fold that may be either acquired or associated with tuberous sclerosis.[17] Acquired periungual fibrokeratoma spontaneously develops, perhaps from previous trauma, and presents as painless proximal nail fold protrusions that may cause a longitudinal groove within the nail plate. The lesions have

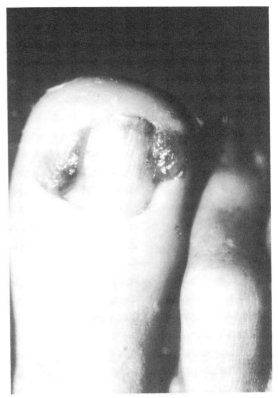

FIGURE 19–12. Pyogenic granulomas accompanying ingrown toenails.

a hyperkeratotic tip and a narrow base (Fig. 19–13). Thorough surgical excision with exploration beneath the nail plate and proximal nail fold may be required to prevent recurrence. *Koenen's tumors* are periungual fibromas that develop in 50% of the patients who have tuberous sclerosis. Tuberous sclerosis is a congenital disease in which a variety of lesions in the skin, nervous system, heart, kidney, and other organs develop because of a limited hyperplasia of ectodermal and mesodermal cells. The most frequent clinical manifestations constitute a triad of sebaceous adenoma, epilepsy, and mental retardation. Koenen's tumors appear between the ages of 12 and 14 years, increasing in size and number with time.[18]

Myxoid cysts are firm, tender nodules and tumors arising from the dorsolateral dermis between the distal interphalangeal joint and the proximal nail fold (Fig. 19–14). They are frequently seen in fingers of females with Heberden's nodes of osteoarthritis and may be a cause of nail dystrophy. They may spontaneously drain clear fluid that resembles syno-

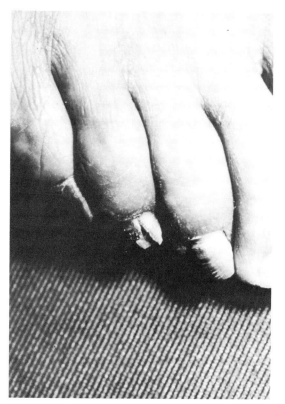

FIGURE 19–13. Traumatically acquired periungual fibro-keratoma.

plate can become elevated. It occurs between the ages of 10 and 25 and favors males in a ratio of 2:1.[12] Osteochondroma can be easily confused with a subungual wart. Radiographic examination demonstrates a well-defined, tra-beculated bone growth resembling a sesamoid bone arising from the phalanx. Histologic ex-amination reveals a hyaline cartilage cap cov-ering normal-appearing bone (Fig. 19–15).

Glomus tumors are small (several millimeters in diameter), painful, benign growths that are usually found subungually but can occur as a bluish red papule anywhere in the skin.[20] The glomus apparatus normally serves to regulate distal digital blood flow. The nail bed of the fingers and toes have between 93 and 501 glo-mus arteriovenous anastomoses per square centimeter. The pain is characteristically in-tense, is often pulsating, and can be triggered by changes in environmental temperature or the pressure of firm palpation. Sometimes the pain peaks nocturnally. Seventy-five percent of the cases occur in the hand, with an average age at onset of 30 to 50 years. The tumor can be seen through the nail plate as a bluish to

vial fluid but actually is mucoid degenerated collagen. These cysts have been managed by aspiration and injection of corticosteroids or by surgical excision.[19]

Osteochondroma is a painful subungual be-nign bone tumor. There may be a history of trauma to the digit. Impingement from shoes may cause subungual ulceration, and the nail

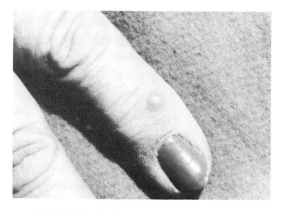

FIGURE 19–14. Myxoid cyst of the fifth finger.

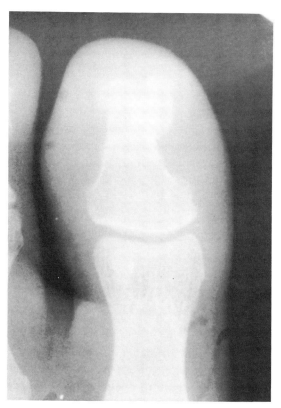

FIGURE 19–15. Osteochondroma in a 15-year-old girl.

reddish discoloration. Nail deformities are detected in 50% of the cases. Bony erosions or cysts can be seen in about half of the patients. Arteriography reveals a star-shaped, telangiectatic pattern.[18] Avulsion of the nail plate with careful complete excision of the lesion should resolve the problem.

Malignant Tumors of the Nail Unit

Although malignant transformation is unlikely within the nail unit, it should always be considered in any patient with a chronic nail infection or growth that fails to respond to treatment or fails to heal. Accurate diagnosis can be made only by biopsy. Squamous cell carcinoma, basal cell carcinoma, melanoma, and metastasis are discussed here, but other even rarer tumors are possible.

Squamous cell carcinoma in the nail unit is a slow-growing tumor that rarely involves the phalanx, and then only late in its progression. Most squamous cell carcinomas occur in the thumbs and index fingers, but hallucal involvement along with a longitudinal pigmented band has been reported.[21] Clinically, carcinoma can present with pain, swelling, inflammation, elevation of the nail plate, or ulceration; as a tumor mass; or even as an ingrowing toenail with an apparent pyogenic granuloma. Unfortunately, the duration of symptoms is more than 12 months in more than 50% of the cases before the correct diagnosis is made by biopsy.[18]

Subungual basal cell carcinoma of the toes has not been described, and fingernail involvement has been reported infrequently. Three cases of Kaposi's sarcoma of the toes have been reported (Fig. 19–16).[18]

Malignant melanoma of the nail unit can arise from the skin structures of the nail lips, the nail bed, and even the nail matrix, which normally has a few quiescent melanocytes. The incidence of malignant melanoma within the nail unit has been reported as 2.5% of all melanomas occurring in whites and 15% of all melanomas occurring in blacks. Subungual melanomas generally occur in older, lighter pigmented persons, with the mean age at onset being between 60 and 80 years.[9] They are often asymptomatic, and pain or discomfort is

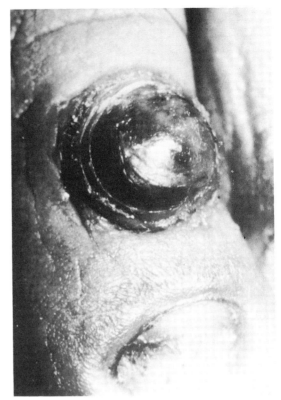

FIGURE 19–16. Kaposi's sarcoma of the great toe. (Courtesy of Donald Kushner, DPM, Ohio College of Podiatric Medicine.)

rarely noted until quite late. Twenty-five percent of melanomas are amelanotic. Suspicions should be raised and biopsy considered if a pigmented lesion in the nail bed widens or fails to grow distalward at the rate of 1 mm per month or if the pigment appears to leak into the proximal nail lip (Hutchinson's sign).[19] Subungual melanoma has a poor prognosis, with the reported 5-year survival rates being from 35% to 50%.[18]

Internal malignancies metastasize to the skin about 4% of the time, while metastasis to a lower extremity nail unit is even rarer. Recorded primary tumors with nail unit metastasis have included carcinoma of the larynx, squamous cell carcinoma of the lung, and medullary breast carcinoma.[22]

PEDAL SKIN DISORDERS
Superficial Bacterial Infections

Erythrasma. Interdigital erythrasma is a mild, localized, superficial, and often chronic skin infection caused by *Corynebacterium minutissimum* that is underdiagnosed.[23] Interdigital erythrasma is the most common bacterial infection of the foot, yet it is often not recognized. It most commonly manifests as an intertriginous web space infection that occurs more frequently in diabetics.[24] Erythrasma presents as chronic nonresolving maceration with fissuring or scaling of the toewebs. The diagnosis is confirmed by the presence of coral-red fluorescence on Wood's light examination. The fluorescent porphyrins are not easily washed away by bathing within the previous 20 hrs before examination. *C. minutissimum* is a fastidious organism and cannot be cultured routinely. Treatment requires drying of the web spaces and application of topical erythromycin in a gel base; erythromycin may also be administered orally. Erythrasma does not respond to griseofulvin or most other topical antifungal agents.[23] The newer imidazoles or naftifine may have sufficient antibacterial activity to be useful.

Pitted Keratolysis. The lesions of pitted keratolysis are conspicuous, superficial, discrete, circular, plantar erosions with a punched-out appearance. Hyperhidrosis, sometimes with a green or brown discoloration and a foul odor, can further help identify this superficial, often bilateral *Corynebacterium* infection. The superficial pits and erosions measure 1 to 4 mm in diameter but can become confluent and enlarge to several centimeters. They are characteristically not painful. The hyperhidrotic plantar skin is often quite macerated, with accentuated skin folds. The usual causative *Corynebacterium* organism is difficult to culture, and it is difficult even to find evidence of its filaments on a potassium hydroxide wet mount preparation. Some cases are caused by *Actinomyces keratolytica*, *Streptomyces*, or *Dermatophilus congolensis*.[25] It is interesting that pitted keratolysis can be experimentally induced in 5 of 10 normal persons by placing feet covered by socks in plastic bags that are left in place for 8 to 24 hours.[26] Treatment must be centered about the management of the underlying hyperhidrosis by first prescribing the daily use of antibacterial soaps such as povidone-iodine or chlorhexidine gluconate (Hibiclens) followed by naftifine topical cream. A topical antibacterial astringent such as 20% aluminum chloride

hexahydrate (Drysol) or erythromycin, either topical or oral, may be needed.

Superficial Interdigital Web Space Infections

If the dorsal surface of the foot is thought of as an arid plain and the plantar foot as a potential wetland with its poor drainage, then the lesser toe webs are an Amazon rain forest. This microbial ecologic niche is complicated and varies over time, with the dominant species often producing clinical infection at the expense of other floral competitors.

Toe web infections may present as a relatively asymptomatic, mild peeling condition (dermatophytosis simplex) or as a painful, exudative, macerated inflammatory process often accompanied by a foul odor (dermatophytosis complex).[27, 28] The normal microbial flora of the toe web space is composed of coagulase-negative staphylococci, aerobic diphtheroids, gram-negative bacteria, yeasts of the genus *Candida*, and dermatophytes.[27] As the web space becomes macerated, the dermatophyte population multiplies, actually producing antibiotics to suppress the competing susceptible bacterial flora and allowing the dominance of antibiotic-resistant populations.

In managing toe web infections the podiatrist should consider which fungus, bacteria, or yeast is the current dominant organism and focus therapy appropriately. This may require Wood's light examination, fungal culture, bacterial culture and sensitivity testing, and potassium hydroxide wet mount preparation. Whatever the antimicrobial agent selected, it is very important to dry out the web space with astringents, cotton, or lamb's wool spacers and control any underlying hyperhidrosis.

Tinea Pedis

In addition to athlete's foot, common synonymous terms for tinea pedis include *ringworm*, *jungle rot of the foot*, and *foot fungus*. Tinea pedis is a very common foot problem, accounting for one third of all pedal skin disease. The incidence of tinea pedis is about 38.7 cases per 1000 persons. To put this statistic into perspective, acne occurs in 68 of 1000 persons while verrucae of all types occur at a rate of 8.5 cases per 1000 persons.[29]

In general, tinea pedis is a disease of adult life. The stratum corneum of children is apparently too thin to readily support the growth of dermatophytes that only grow on dead keratin. Causative organisms can be cultured from fomites such as shoes, socks, flooring, and clothing, but simple contact with infected scales is not enough to cause infection. The real cause of tinea pedis involves the chronically moist, dark environment of the shoe, which favors the overgrowth of various fungal floral organisms. Chronic dry scaly tinea pedis is usually directly caused by the dermatophyte *Trichophyton rubrum;* however, on occasion it can be caused by *Epidermophyton floccosum.* Vesicular tinea pedis is usually caused by *T. mentagrophytes,* which has a granular appearance on culture. The interdigital form of tinea pedis is caused by the downy-appearing interdigital variety of *T. mentagrophytes.*[30] Fungi other than the dermatophytes on occasion can cause tinea pedis, such as the saprophyte *Hendersonula toruloidea,* which is resistant to commonly used antifungal agents.[31]

The clinical diagnosis of tinea pedis is all too often unconfirmed by appropriate culture or potassium hydroxide wet mount. Dermatophyte test medium, in addition to Sabouraud dextrose agar, contains cycloheximide, gentamicin, and chlortetracycline. These agents prevent bacterial growth and inhibit saprophytic fungi. In addition, a phenol red indicator is present that changes the color of the medium from yellow to red in the presence of dermatophytes. Mycosel or Myco-Biotic fungal cultures contain Sabouraud dextrose agar with chloramphenicol to inhibit bacterial growth and cycloheximide to inhibit many contaminants. Both of these media select for dermatophytes, the usual cause of tinea pedis, but can miss the saprophytes.[30] Potassium hydroxide wet mount preparations are easily performed but often difficult to interpret. Identification is made easier by the use of chlorozol and black E fungal stains in dimethylsulfoxide and potassium hydroxide (Dermatological Lab and Supply, Inc, Council Bluffs, IA), which colors the squamous cells light gray and the hyphae a refractile green.

Hyperkeratotic tinea pedis presents as widespread, fine scaling in a "moccasin" distribution. Careful inspection will reveal many clearly defined polycyclic lesions with scaly borders and superficial peeling. This dry chronic form of tinea pedis is often asymptomatic and unrecognized by the patient. Scraping of the peeling peripheral scales at the rim of the lesions produces the highest positive yield on potassium hydroxide and fungal culturing.

Vesicular tinea pedis presents as pruritic eczematous vesicles and even bullae or pustules on the dorsal or plantar skin. Culturing or examining the inferior surface of the roofs of the vesicles produces the highest fungal yield.

The most common clinical form of tinea pedis is the intertriginous variety (dermatophytosis simplex), which presents as mild to severe scaling, peeling, maceration, and fissures favoring the fourth and fifth toe webs bilaterally. It is seldom found in the first interdigital web space. Warm, dark, moist, basic pH zones favor fungal growth. Tight digital apposition due to plump toes and narrow shoes, slip-on shoes, and tight pantyhose all predispose to this infection. Intertriginous tinea pedis with secondary bacterial infection (dermatophytosis complex) is a subsequent form of the simplex variety heralded by malodor, proximal erythema, edema, or dorsal web tenderness (Fig. 19–17). At this stage the primary or initiating dermatophytes are difficult to detect because they have been suppressed by antifungal action of the bacteria, whose mean counts have now tripled.[32]

The differential diagnoses that should be considered in tinea pedis depend on the proper evaluation of the history, primary and secondary lesion characteristics, and distribution detected at the clinical examination. The hyperkeratosis of chronic tinea pedis suggests a different list of differential diagnoses than do the vesicles of acute inflammatory tinea pedis (Table 19–4). It is more efficient to consider the differential disorders and collect specimens for fungal culture and potassium hydroxide wet mount preparation at the time of initial evaluation than after a clinical trial of antifungal agents has failed to improve the condition.

Management. Management of all three types

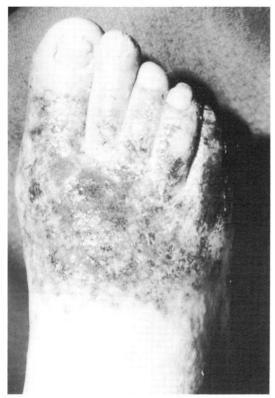

FIGURE 19–17. Dermatophytosis complex with cellulitis requiring hospital admission.

of tinea pedis can vary widely but in general should deal with acute care, long-term treatment, and prevention.

Prophylactic measures are aimed at controlling or altering the environmental factors of heat, moisture, and maceration. Patients should be instructed in proper daily washing with soap and water and thoroughly drying between the toes as a primary measure to remove hyperkeratotic debris. A useful adjunct is an absorbent powder such as Zeasorb, which contains 45% microporous cellulose that has a relative absorbency of water almost twice that of talc-based powders.[28] Talc-based powders such as baby powder should be used to reduce friction and lubricate the skin. Hyperhidrosis must be controlled because a tinea infection is unlikely to clear in the presence of soggy wet keratin. Clothing, socks, shoes, and towels should not be shared because infected keratinocytes can easily be spread from a site of infection to a susceptible spot. It is good advice to change socks once or twice daily and even to alternate pairs of shoes every other day. Patients should

avoid wearing nylon stockings, pantyhose, and occlusive vinyl shoes. Early detection can be accomplished by daily inspection of the toe webs before the fungus can spread. This is especially important in diabetics and in patients with arterial insufficiency but is often quite difficult to accomplish in the elderly patient with poor vision and limited flexion capabilities caused by osteoarthritis or obesity.

Local therapy for acute inflammatory lesions involves decompression of the larger blisters while leaving the roofs of the blisters intact. Cool soaks or wet to dry sterile dressings are anti-inflammatory and antipruritic and promote vasoconstriction. One Bluboro powder packet or tablet to 1 pint of water produces a 1:40 concentration that can be repeated four to six times a day for about 15 minutes in the acute inflammatory phase. A combination of antifungal and corticosteroid creams such as Lotrisone (clotrimazole and betamethasone) can be applied sparingly after the soak up to three times a day for several days until the lesions begin to dry up and the pruritus has subsided. This corticosteroid combination should not be used for longer than 2 weeks without a treatment rest period to avoid tachyphylaxis. Some of the imidazoles and naftifine have been identified as antifungal agents that

TABLE 19–4. **Differential Diagnoses of Tinea Pedis**

Chronic Hyperkeratotic Tinea Pedis
Pressure callus
Xerosis, common form
Psoriatic plantar keratoderma
Hereditary palmar plantar diffuse keratoderma
Chronic hyperkeratotic contact dermatitis
Ichthyosis, hereditary
Juvenile plantar dermatosis

Acute Vesicular Tinea Pedis
Dyshidrotic eczema (pompholyx)
Contact dermatitis due to shoes
Atopic eczema
Pustular psoriasis
Keratoderma blennorrhagicum of Reiter's syndrome
Poison ivy, *Rhus* allergy

Intertriginous Tinea Pedis
Hyperhidrosis or bromhidrosis
Heloma molle
Erythrasma
Candidiasis
Dermatophytosis complex
Psoriasis, macerated plaque

TABLE 19–5. **Principal Topical Antifungal Agents**

Topical Antifungal	AY	FC/FS	AB	AI	Freq	RX/OTC
Allymine class						
Naftifine (Naftin)	Yes	FC	No	Yes	qd	RX
Terbinafine (Lamisil)	Yes	FC	No	Yes	qd	RX
Olamine class						
Ciclopirox (Loprox)	Yes	FS	Yes	No	bid	OTC
Imidazole derivatives						
Clotrimazole (Lotrimin)	Yes	FS	Yes	Yes	bid	OTC
Econozole (Spectazole)	Yes	FS	Yes	Yes	qd	RX
Ketoconazole (Nizoral)	Yes	FS	Yes	Yes	qd	RX
Miconazole (Micatin)	Yes	FS	Yes	Yes	bid	OTC
Oxiconazole (Oxistat)	Yes	FS	Yes	Yes	qd	RX
Sulconazole (Exelderm)	Yes	FS	Yes	Yes	qd	RX
Tolnaftate (Tinactin)	No	FS	No	No	tid	OTC

AY, anti-yeast; FC, fungicidal at minimum inhibitory concentrations; FS, fungistatic at minimum inhibitory concentrations; AB, significant antibacterial action; AI, anti-inflammatory effect; Freq, recommended frequency of application; RX, prescription required; OTC, available over the counter.

have an intrinsic anti-inflammatory effect by inhibiting polymorphonuclear leukocytes (Table 19–5).[28]

Chronic hyperkeratotic tinea pedis is usually managed by topical antifungal agents but for longer duration of therapy (Fig. 19–18). The thick infected stratum corneum of plantar tinea is replaced about every 56 days, while the thinner dorsal skin turnover is every 28 days. Sufficient amounts of topical antifungal creams are required so the patient can continue to apply the cream throughout the entire plantar epidermal turnover period. About 1 gram for each application to both feet is required. Keratolytic agents such as Whitfield's ointment (6% benzoic acid, and 3% salicylic acid) may be used to soften and dissolve the thick keratin and enhance antifungal penetration. A gel vehicle combined with a potent antifungal agent such as naftifine is especially effective in penetrating plantar hyperkeratosis.[33]

The simple form of interdigital tinea pedis responds quickly to improved hygiene and miconazole cream, while the complex recurrent form requires fungal and bacterial culturing. An antifungal agent with antibacterial effects such as econazole nitrate 1% (Spectazole) has been shown to be especially effective.[34] A drying agent such as Drysol applied twice daily along with cotton between the toes may be required in persistent cases. Long-term prevention of recurrence can be accomplished with an absorbent powder combined with tolnaftate (Zeasorb AF powder).

Systemic oral antifungal agents, because of their potential for adverse side effects, are used infrequently in tinea pedis, although they have a role in recalcitrant infections.[28] It is essential to first identify the causative agent as a susceptible dermatophyte. Griseofulvin is the most often prescribed oral antifungal agent and is only fungistatic against dermatophytes. It is of no value against yeasts, bacteria, or tinea versicolor. Penicillin-sensitive patients may be allergic to the drug, and it may cause photosensitivity. Griseofulvin is contraindicated in patients with a history of porphyria. Most clinicians suggest pretreatment baseline blood studies with re-evaluation every 6 weeks. Oral ketoconazole is very effective in tinea pedis but has been associated with liver toxicity. Fluconazole (Diflucan) is highly effective but is very expensive and probably should be

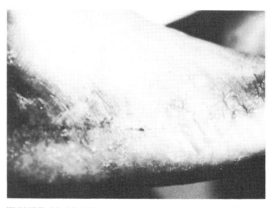

FIGURE 19–18. Chronic hyperkeratotic tinea pedis in a "moccasin" distribution.

reserved for severe widespread deep fungal infections.

Recalcitrant resistant tinea pedis may on rare occasion be actually a phaeohyphomycotic dermatomycosis. This is an opportunistic infection caused by dematiaceous fungi such as *Hendersonula toruloidea* and *Scytalidium hyalinum*.[35] Both organisms are resistant to griseofulvin and ketoconazole. The growth of *H. torluloidea* is also unaffected by miconazole, tolnaftate, haloprogin, and itraconazole. One case seemed to respond to ciclopirox olamine, and it has been suggested that topical amphotericin B (Fungizone) may be the agent of choice.[31]

A new member of the allylamine class, terbinafine (Lamisil), is available topically. It is primarily fungicidal with a minimum inhibitory concentration that is very low. It is the most potent antifungal agent to date, with demonstrated efficacy against a wide range of pathogenic fungi.[36]

Viral Infections

PEDAL VERRUCAE

Warts are a common nuisance that can plague both the podiatrist and the patient. They are a benign, usually self-regressing papilloma of the skin and adjacent mucous membranes caused by a specific human papillomavirus that multiplies within epidermal cell nuclei. Papillomaviruses are DNA viruses that have a variable incubation period that experimentally ranges from 1 to 20 months, with an average of 9 months. It apparently takes quite awhile for these viruses to successfully invade and take over epidermal nuclei. The chance for clinical infection to occur varies also with the age of the patient, the moisture content of the skin, and the host immune surveillance and response. The viral particles within infected keratinocytes enter the skin by direct inoculation induced by biomechanical and occupational trauma, friction over pressure points, nail biting, and scratching. Clusters of warts are sometimes found on adjacent moist toe web surfaces. Warts may be transmitted by close physical contact between susceptible hosts, but the long incubation period and variations in host resistance prevent a clear-cut determination of epidemiologic patterns.[37]

Clinical verrucae morphology was previously believed to be primarily a function of anatomic location, host resistance, and age of the verrucae. It was previously thought that verrucae were caused by only one common human papillomavirus. Presently, there are dozens of antigenically distinct human papillomavirus serotypes just as there are many different influenza viruses. Several of the human papillomavirus serotypes produce a variety of different clinical appearances and variation in response to treatment (Table 19–6).

The incidence of warts has been increasing over the past 20 to 30 years in both the United States and Europe, with about 10% of the population being affected. Verrucae are rare in children younger than 5 years of age. Peak incidence is during the school years, from age 5 to 20 years, with decreasing frequency thereafter. Warts are rarer in the elderly but can occur at any age.[38]

Spontaneous regression of warts occurs, with 30% resolving over 3 to 6 months and 50% clearing over 24 months. This phenomenon may account for apparent successful wart treatment with folk cures and old wives' tales. The actual mechanism of spontaneous regression is still unknown, but it probably represents a resurgence of the cell-mediated immune response to recognize, attack, and destroy the foreign viral protein cloaked in host epidermal cells. Although warts normally exhibit some petechial hemorrhage within them, these black dots increase in number and become widespread as the regression process progresses. The regressing wart dries up and eventually peels away.

Deep plantar warts tend to be endophytic or ingrowing and usually appear as a single plan-

---

TABLE 19–6. **Types of Pedal Verrucae**

Type of Verruca	Causative Human Papillomavirus
Deep plantar warts	HPV type 1
Mosaic plantar warts	HPV types 2 and 4
Flat warts	HPV types 3 and 10
Common (papilloma) warts	HPV types 1, 2, and 4

HPV, human papillomavirus.
Data from Fine JD, Arndt KA: Pathophysiology of certain viral infections of the skin. In Baden H, Soter N (eds): Pathophysiology of the Skin. New York, McGraw-Hill Book Company, 1983; and Rogers JA, O'Keefe EJ: The biology and treatment of warts. Compr Ther 13:34–40, 1987.

tar or palmar growth rarely found on other body surfaces. The diameter is best appreciated after paring, which reveals a wider than first expected lesion that somewhat resembles an ant hill, the so-called myrmecia. There is often central hypertrophied papillae within soft macerated keratin surrounded by a horny ring.[39] Deep plantar warts enlarge to become painful, especially if they occur on a weight-bearing area. Their peak incidence is between 12 and 15 years of age.

Mosaic plantar warts represent 26% of all plantar warts and despite their more superficial nature are clinically more resistant and recurrent than other pedal verrucae. They tend to be slightly raised with a dry hyperkeratotic surface. As with all verrucae, they seem to erupt from between the epidermal papillae and obscure the normal dermatoglyphic lines of the skin. Mosaic warts start as individual papules that coalesce into confluent polygonal plaques (Fig. 19–19). They are easily differentiated from solitary endophytic human papil-

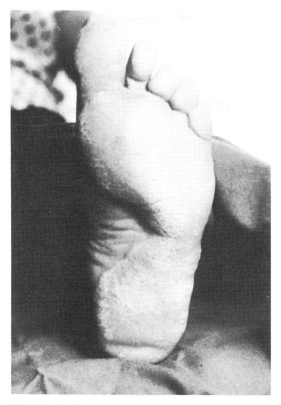

FIGURE 19–19. Extensive, thick plaques of mosaic plantar verrucae. No immune compromise could be detected. All lesions spontaneously resolved without treatment after 3 years.

TABLE 19–7. **Common Cryosurgical Agents**

Liquid nitrogen:	−195° C
Dry ice (Kiddie Kit):	−78.5° C
Nitrous oxide:	−89.5° C

lomavirus type 1 verrucae and are less painful. They are often present concurrently with common hand warts.

Nonplantar pedal verrucae occur less frequently than plantar warts and can appear as common raised papillomas, mosaic plaques, or flat human papillomavirus type 3 warts.[39] These warts are sometimes difficult to differentiate from dermatofibromas, senile keratoses, lipomas, or even helomas.

Management. Benign cutaneous growths should receive benign treatment. The goal of verrucae management is resolution without scarring and minimal pain. In resistant cases, curative zeal must be curbed and the goal of resolution can be modified to a treatment goal of producing a nonpainful lesion. There are many ways to treat warts because all common methods are about 80% effective, and the choice of treatment modality depends on the experience of the podiatrist and the preferences of the patient.

Cryosurgery is a common method of wart destruction that utilizes several different agents on usually non–weight-bearing warts (Table 19–7). Skin freezes at 0°C to −2°C while destruction of benign or malignant tissue occurs at −50°C. Achieving thorough freezing of plantar lesions is difficult with the conventional applicator dipstick method. Goldman has been experimenting with liquid nitrogen utilizing a continuous delivery system under pressure to ensure the required 5-mm lateral extent of freeze that ensures adequate destructive depth for plantar verrucae. He uses an especially designed probe and handpiece with an initial freeze cycle of 90 seconds, then a short 40-second thaw period, followed by a final application of 60 seconds. Local infiltration anesthesia should be avoided because its freezing may increase unwanted tissue destruction. An appropriate topical antibiotic and bandaid dressing is used until the third post-treatment day, when the hemorrhagic blister is drained. Some pain or tenderness on ambulation is to be expected. In 80% of about 50 patients with about 150 warts the lesions resolved with one application (Goldman EP: personal communication, December, 1992).

Keratolytic therapy utilizes many different agents and concentrations to destroy wart tissue and perhaps stimulate host immune response to resolve verrucae.[40] Agent potency can be thought of in two broad groups (Table 19–8): one group for patient-applied agents used as primary therapy for superficial lesions or follow up of surgically treated warts that are nearly resolved, and a second group of chemical agents used by the podiatrist, along with debridement, as primary therapy.

Keratolytic podiatric treatment starts with cleansing and paring of the verruca to a point just before pinpoint bleeding is anticipated. Then a hypoallergenic skin adherent is applied. Depending on the age of the patient, the reactivity potential of the skin, the location of the wart, and the number and depth of the lesions, an appropriate vesicant is chosen and applied sparingly for 48 to 72 hours under occlusion. There are many different regimens used to produce a hemorrhagic blister that is deep enough to destroy the wart yet painless enough to allow nearly full ambulatory function.[41] Eighty percent monochloracetic acid can be coupled with 60% salicylic acid ointment filling a felt aperture pad and covered with occlusive tape to produce a painless mass of keratin that can be debrided weekly until the verruca resolves. A minimum of three treatments is usually required. Follow up with a home care program of paring and application of less potent topical acids nightly for 2 weeks as tolerated both decreases recurrence and increases patient involvement in the treatment program.

Enucleation by blunt dissection or curettage is often used to treat solitary to a few endophytic plantar warts. This requires local plantar anesthesia, which can be uncomfortable to some adults and most children. After excision, bleeding is controlled and further tissue destruction ensured with either electrocautery, chemical cautery, or laser. This method requires pathologic examination of the excised tissue and usually results in a thin, soft, nonpainful plantar scar. As Lemont[42] points out, wart surgery requires lesion excision to the level where the superficial fascia is visible. Many clinicians inappropriately refer to their extent of dissection as the "basement membrane," "fibrous capsule," or "dermis," when actually these are microscopic landmarks superior to the superficial fascia. All wart surgical techniques produce scars, albeit usually nonpainful ones, by destroying all the layers of the epidermis and dermis. Penetration of the superficial fascia, heralded by the protrusion of subcutaneous fat, most easily accomplished at second operations or in excision of particularly older warts, just produces larger scar formation.

Recalcitrant pedal verrucae are inevitable, with 20% of treated verrucae recurring due to host immune anergy. Several tertiary treatment center modalities are available. First is dinitrochlorobenzene (DNCB), a contact allergen with an 80% cure rate. It is not approved by the Food and Drug Administration for verrucae therapy. Unfortunately, DNCB is a potential mutagenic agent and can be found in the photographic industry, thus being a potential potent source of iatrogenic contact dermatitis.[43]

Another treatment appropriate for experienced dermatology referral is the injection of bleomycin intradermally. Bleomycin is cytotoxic to all cells, including human papillomavirus–infected epidermal cells, by inhibiting DNA synthesis. One-tenth milliliter of 0.1% solution is injected, but it is important to limit the total lifetime dose to 5 mL because of potential toxicity. Shumack and Haddock[44] cured 99.23% of 1052 warts with intralesional bleo-

---

TABLE 19–8. **Topical Wart Treatments**

Patient-Applied Treatments
Salicylic acid, 16.7%; lactic acid, 16.7% (Salactic Film)
Salicylic acid, 20%; Lactic acid, 20% (Lactisol-Forte)
Salicylic acid, 27% (Sal-Plant Gel)
Salicylic acid, 26% (Occlusal-HP)
Salicylic acid plaster, 50% (Sal-Acid Plasters)
Salicylic acid plaster, 40% (Mediplast)
Formaldehyde, 10% (Formalyde-10 Spray)

Physician-Applied Treatments
Salicylic acid ointment, 60%
Monochloracetic acid, 80%
Bichloroacetic acid kit
Trichloroacetic acid, 80%
Salicylic acid, 30%; podophyllum, 10% (Verrex)
Salicylic acid, 30%; podophyllum, 5%; cantharidin, 1% (Verrusol)

mycin. The drug is somewhat painful on injection and very expensive, with a short reconstituted shelf life.

A third consideration for recalcitrant painful warts is the topical use of a drying agent such as formalin with 5% 5-fluorouracil. This drug is a false uracil that disturbs DNA and RNA coding, thereby disrupting protein synthesis. I found 5-fluorouracil to be only 50% effective topically when tried on four patients with resistant pedal verrucae. Intradermal injection has been tried by McCarthy and Tate[45] and resulted in a higher cure rate.

Ultrasonic therapy, 0.5 watt/cm² for 10 minutes over 10 treatments, resulted in 15 of 21 patients (71%) being cured. It is thought that this therapy may work by producing marked lesion temperature elevations.[46]

The ''charming'' of warts in susceptible children has been reported.[47] I have found that positive thinking on my part and the patient's imagining his or her white blood cells attacking and killing the warts contributes to helpful mindsets, but whether this actually resolves warts at a rate significantly higher than the rate of spontaneous resolution remains to be proven. Controlled studies are necessary to validate the success of any treatment modality.[48]

It is important for the podiatrist to recognize the light microscopic features of warts. The diagnostic histologic sign of verrucae, wherever they are located and whichever clinical form they take, is the presence of spherical basophilic inclusion bodies in the upper epidermis that represent DNA viral particles. Verrucae also feature a well-defined stratum granulosum and papillomatosis.[37] It is difficult to appreciate on a single cross section the centripetally arranged rete ridges that appear like the petals of a rose. Acanthosis, which is a diffuse hyperplasia of the granular cell layer, is a prominent feature but not specific for warts because it is found in other skin lesions such as psoriasis (Fig. 19–20). The elongated fragile vascular rete pegs account for the clinical appearance of pinpoint bleeding on paring that is a differentiating characteristic of plantar warts.

EPIDERMODYSPLASIA VERRUCIFORMIS

Epidermodysplasia verruciformis is a rare disease that is quite interesting because it man-

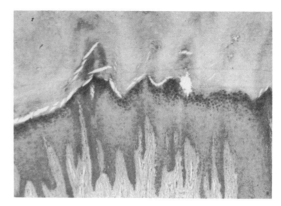

FIGURE 19–20. Histologic study of plantar verrucae.

ifests as widespread eruptions of all varieties of wart serotypes and clinical forms. The extremities, trunk, and face are favored, but any skin surface can be affected with widespread warty papules. Epidermodysplasia verruciformis was previously thought to be a genodermatosis but is actually an autosomal recessively inherited defect in the cell-mediated immune response. The persistent warty lesions erupt in early childhood and persist throughout life. Spouses of heavily infected patients rarely become infected. Squamous cell carcinomas develop within sun-exposed verrucae before age 20 in 20% to 30% of the patients, representing a rare example of malignant transformation of warts in an immunocompromised host.[49]

Common Pedal Eczematous Diseases

Eczema is not a specific diagnosis but only a physical description of a clinical skin reaction pattern that can be acute, chronic, or in between. The term *eczema* describes a morphologic and histologic pattern and does not describe the cause of the skin problem. It literally means ''boiling over of the skin,'' manifesting as bubbles or vesicles in the acute stages of skin inflammation (dermatitis). Many physical, chemical, and immunologic causes account for the many different clinical forms of eczematous dermatitis.[50]

CONTACT DERMATITIS

Contact dermatitis implies physical direct skin contact with an offending agent and can be thought of as occurring as two different types. First is a primary irritant type of contact dermatitis that results from skin contact with a toxic irritant, such as an over-the-counter corn remover, that will always produce a dermatitis in all members of a population if the contact is long enough and the concentration of the agent is high enough. The second type of contact dermatitis is allergic contact dermatitis that is an eczematous response to an allergen, usually a hapten, that the patient was previously exposed to and now develops an immune-mediated hypersensitivity reaction to the challenging protein. Few persons in the general population experience this reaction to the offending agent. There is an induction period of time required between the first exposure to the agent and the subsequent challenge that produces the rash. A good example might be tincture of benzoin used as a skin adherent causing an acute allergic contact dermatitis in a previously sensitized patient (Fig. 19–21).

Contact dermatitis will have a similar clinical appearance whether it is a primary irritant or allergic. From a problem-solving viewpoint it is important to determine if the rash is acute or chronic to determine the most effective anti-inflammatory measures to prescribe (Table 19–9). Lesions of pedal contact dermatitis are often bilaterally symmetric and localized to points of friction and moisture while, in general, sparing the toe web spaces. Web space involvement can occur, however, if the offending agent is a medication component. Determining the origin of the offending agent is

TABLE 19–9. Physical Signs of Dermatitis

Erythema
Edema
Papulation
Vesiculation
Oozing
Scaling (later sign)
Pruritus
Scaling
Hyperkeratosis
Thickening
Fissuring
Lichenification
Hyperpigmentation
Hypopigmentation

often difficult, with many possible sources to consider (Table 19–10). Probably the most common scenario is a hyperhidrotic foot contacting a shoe with a rubber component, exposing the patient to the common sensitizers monobenzyl ether of hydroquinone, 2-mercaptobenzothiazole, or tetramethylthiuram monosulfide. Patch testing proves the diagnosis.

Histologic changes in eczema are generally nonspecific. However, specimens from acute contact dermatitis can demonstrate spongiosis, intraepidermal vesiculation, infiltration of inflammatory cells, and vascular dilation within the upper dermis. The presence of increased numbers of immunologic processing lymphocytes supports the histologic diagnosis of allergic contact dermatitis. The histologic signs of chronic contact dermatitis include acanthosis (hyperplasia of the stratum spinosum), hyperkeratosis, and areas of parakeratosis (persistence of nucleated keratinocytes in the stratum corneum).[51]

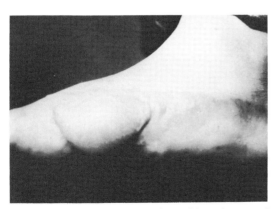

FIGURE 19–21. Allergic contact dermatitis to tincture of benzoin used as a skin adherent for a low dye taping for plantar fasciitis.

TABLE 19–10. Potential Sources of Pedal Contact Dermatitis

Allergic Dermatitis
Shoes, sandals, bedroom slippers
Sock liners, inner soles, arch supports
Socks, stockings, elastic hose
Temporary foot covers (urethane)
Boots, galoshes

Contact Dermatitis
Wearing apparel and jewelry
Chemical components of shoes and stockings
Topically applied medications
Appliances
Occupational exposure (oils, solvents, reagents)

From Samitz MH, Dana AS: Cutaneous Lesions of the Lower Extremities, p 132. Philadelphia, JB Lippincott, 1971.

ASTEOTIC ECZEMA (ECZEMA CRAQUELÉ)

Elderly patients often present with dry, scaling lower extremities, especially in the winter in climates where central heating is necessary. Loss of water in skin, nails, and hair accompanies aging. Itching is a very common complaint. The skin is often fissured superficially with a wrinkled, pavement-brick appearance. Excessive cleansing with strong pure soaps and friction from clothes also contribute to asteatotic eczema. Xerosis is simply dry skin, but symptomatic pruritic inflamed dry skin can be called asteatotic eczema. Management focuses on replacing skin water by hydration followed by emollients. The least expensive agent that the patient will use on a daily basis is most appropriate for prophylaxis. In the eczematous stage a low-potency anti-inflammatory agent in an ointment base is a good idea (Table 19–11). Lactic acid–based topical agents seem more effective than even 20% urea compounds.

LICHEN SIMPLEX CHRONICUS (CIRCUMSCRIBED NEURODERMATITIS)

Normal skin that is repetitively rubbed or scratched becomes a thickened pruritic patch called lichen simplex chronicus. Lichen means mosslike. The skin is raised and palpable with prominent dermatoglyphic lines producing a localized elephant-hide appearance (Fig. 19–22). The patient often complains of intense

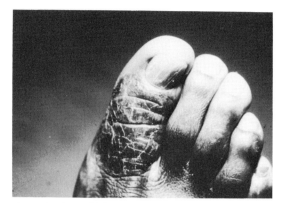

FIGURE 19–22. Lichen simplex chronicus with lichenification.

chronic pruritus that with the subsequent scratching perpetuates the dermatitis. Favored areas are basically any spot that the patient can reach, such as the anterolateral ankle and lower leg.[52] High-potency topical corticosteroid ointments are needed and should be gently applied twice daily or whenever the patient is tempted to scratch. An occlusive or protective dressing may be needed. It is important with any topical prescription for the podiatrist to actually apply a sample agent, which effectively demonstrates to the patient the appropriate areas for treatment, the appropriate amount to be applied, and the podiatrist's concern for the patient's problem.

Rook[53] reports that some persons are genetically predisposed to itching. There is a higher incidence of pruritus-induced scratching in patients with Down's syndrome and diabetes. On the other hand, not all patients are capable of developing lichenification. In predisposed patients, emotional tensions and anxiety exacerbate and perpetuate lichen simplex chronicus.

NUMMULAR ECZEMA

Nummular eczema is a coin-shaped or discoid dermatitis that represents a reaction pattern to various stimuli such as irritants, allergens, soaps, or microbial organisms. It can affect any part of the body, including the foot. It presents primarily as papules and vesicles coalescing into dime-sized to palm-sized plaques. There may be peripheral papules, vesicles, or erythema, with secondary oozing and crusts. The dorsal hands and feet are favored sites. The podiatrist should also consider a di-

TABLE 19–11. **Some Topical Anti-inflammatory Agents**

Generic Name	Brand Name
High Potency	
Betamethasone dipropionate	Diprosone Ointment 0.05%
Fluocinonide	Lidex Cream 0.05%
Desoximetasone	Topicort Cream 0.25%
Medium Potency	
Betamethasone valerate	Valisone Ointment 0.01%
Triamcinolone acetonide	Kenalog Ointment 0.1%
Desoximetasone	Topicort LP Cream 0.05%
Low Potency	
Hydrocortisone	Hytone Cream 1%
Hydrocortisone	Cortaid 0.5%

agnosis of impetigo, ecthyma, or tinea. Moderate to strong topical corticosteroids for the first week followed by pulsed lower-potency agents should be helpful.

JUVENILE PLANTAR DERMATOSIS

Juvenile plantar dermatosis is symmetric fissuring dermatitis favoring the weight-bearing surfaces of the forefeet of prepubertal children.[53] Patients present with recurrent, painful, superficial and deep fissures and cracks (Fig. 19–23). There are areas of erythematous, scaling and peeling skin that may be excoriated, as well as areas of smooth, puffy skin with superficial crazing of the surface. Synonymous terms for juvenile plantar dermatosis include atopic winter feet of children, forefoot eczema, peridigital dermatosis, and recurrent juvenile eczema of the hands and feet. Histologic findings have been nonspecific. Juvenile plantar dermatosis has been found to be a distinct entity and not just a variant of atopic dermatitis.[54] Tinea pedis should be considered but is uncommon in the relatively thin plantar skin of children. Steck[55] has suggested a pathologic mechanism of juvenile plantar dermatosis that involves wet feet that are dried out too quickly on exposure to especially dry dehumidified air, causing loss of skin pliability and subsequent cracking of plantar skin. It has been shown that if the water content of skin is less than 10%, it will crack like old leather.

Management involves topical corticosteroids in the acute phase and prevention of excessively quick dehydration of the pedal skin for

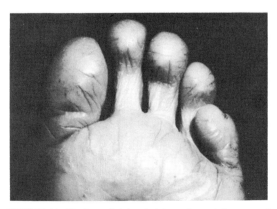

FIGURE 19–23. Superficial painful cracks and fissures of juvenile plantar dermatosis. This disorder is usually bilaterally symmetric.

long-term prevention.[55] As soon as the child removes his or her shoes a thin layer of petrolatum is applied to slow the evaporation process. Juvenile plantar dermatosis is often seen in the winter when indoor humidity is at its lowest. During the summer, children who swim frequently seem to be affected.

DYSHIDROSIS

Despite what the name implies, dyshidrosis has not been found to be an abnormality of sweating or the sweat glands. It is better thought of as a form of stress-induced eczema localized to the palms and soles. Dyshidrosis or pompholyx presents as characteristically recurrent and persistent eruption of deeply seated, tense vesicles, often associated with anxiety. Patients can feel small prevesicle inflammatory papules erupting especially along the lateral edges of their feet and fingers. The lesion can progress to wide zones of acute to chronic eczema. Some patients describe the lesions as itchy nits that must be dug out and thus can become quite excoriated. Some patients may be convinced they are infested or infected. Histologic studies have failed to demonstrate a sweat retention vesicle. Perhaps dyshidrosis is an eczematous reaction to excess sympathetic vasomotor tone. The incidence of familial atopy and other areas of atopic dermatitis may suggest that this is atopic disease in a particular location.[56] Treatment requires patient education about, and identification of, precipitating factors such as excess caffeine ingestion through coffee, tea, and colas or a stressful environment. Biofeedback to control the excess sympathetic tone and subsequent sweating along with general relaxation techniques can be helpful. High-potency topical corticosteroids, sometimes under occlusion, are often required, along with cool soaks to manage the acute flares.

ATOPIC ECZEMATOUS DERMATITIS

Atopic eczematous dermatitis is a genetically determined disorder of sensitive, reactive skin. It is often associated with asthma, hayfever, and allergic rhinitis, with patients having positive findings on multiple scratch or pinprick tests. Thirty-five percent of the patients have a family history of atopy, and serum IgE levels

are elevated. Atopic dermatitis usually starts in infancy with facial rashes and clinical hypersensitivity to the physical and chemical environment. Clearing often occurs after age 2 to 6 years. There are also childhood, adolescent, and adult forms of atopic eczematous dermatitis. The favored sites of involvement include face, scalp, diaper areas, buttocks, hands, and antecubital and popliteal fossae. It may even occur in a generalized form.[57]

Atopic patients are often susceptible to viral infections, including warts, molluscum contagiosum, herpes, and vaccinia, as well as to bacterial infections caused by staphylococci. Aggravating factors that can initiate or exacerbate atopic dermatitis include extreme environmental temperature changes, sweating, soaps, detergents, alkalis, scratchy fabrics such as wool, and friction. Treatment may require antibiotics for secondary infection, antihistamines to control the pruritus, topical corticosteroids of appropriate potency, and avoidance of precipitating factors.[58]

Pedal Hyperkeratotic Disorders: Special Mechanical Lesions

POROKERATOSIS PLANTARIS DISCRETA

Porokeratosis plantaris discreta of Steinberg is seen as a painful hyperkeratotic plantar papule or horny plug resembling a plantar wart but is not virally induced (Fig. 19–24). The

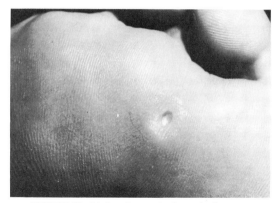

FIGURE 19–24. Porokeratosis plantaris discreta.

lesions are 1 to 3 mm in diameter and do not usually bleed on paring as warts do. The differential diagnosis of plantar keratoses can be challenging at first (Table 19–12). Most often they are found on the weight-bearing aspects of the forefoot, but they can also occur on the arch and heel. The dense, hard, central keratin core is conical and penetrates all the layers of the skin, with some becoming 3 to 5 mm deep.[59]

Previously it was thought that porokeratosis plantaris discreta represented a plugged eccrine duct or was a cyst. This is not the case, because the histologic features resemble those of an invaginated corn, keratoma, or heloma. Underlying dilated eccrine ducts previously believed to be etiologic are a nonspecific finding common to many pressure-induced le-

TABLE 19–12. **Distinguishing Clinical Features of Common Plantar Hyperkeratotic Lesions**

	Usual Location	Relative Diameter	Presence of Pinpoint Bleeding on Paring	Skin Lines
Tyloma	Plantar forefoot over metatarsophalangeal joints	2–3 cm	No	Centrally accentuated
Intractable plantar keratosis	Plantar to prominent metatarsal head	1 cm	No	Surrounding lines accentuated; central lines atrophied
Porokeratosis plantaris discreta	Any plantar area; often near metatarsal head	1–3 mm	No	Central lines lost; few changes in adjacent lines
Verruca	Any area possible	2 mm–1 cm	Yes	Lines do not extend through wart but go around lesion

sions. Loss of the granular cell layer occurs in porokeratosis plantaris discreta and other mechanically induced punctate keratoses such as intractable plantar keratomas, while the granular cell layers are maintained in nonmechanical plantar keratodermas.[60]

Treatment of porokeratosis plantaris discreta is, as always, proportional to the degree of pain and disability. Periodic debridement with careful enucleation followed by application of a keratolytic agent often controls the lesions for long periods. Balance padding with chairside orthotics based on antifriction insole materials also helps.

In a few deep recalcitrant lesions, surgical excision may be necessary but can result in a scar painful on weight bearing.

HEEL FISSURES

Painful cracks within thick hyperkeratotic heel rims are recurrent keratoses that occur symmetrically. Obese, middle-aged women are most frequently affected. A thick plantar heel fat pad architecture that abuts or pinches the heel counter of the shoe seems to be responsible for most cases. They may be localized to the medial or the lateral aspects of the heel. A pressure-induced calcaneal hyperkeratosis that dries out and cracks like an expansion joint in concrete produces a keratin fracture line that can extend into the tender dermis.

Management of painful heel fissures involves hydration of the hyperkeratosis and paring away of the thickened sides of the fissure to flatten it. A bead of topical lidocaine ointment can be applied along the fissure line and then covered with a moleskin patch, secured by skin adherent. The moleskin is stiff enough to stabilize the fissure edges and help heal the fissure line by preventing excess motion. A stiff polyethylene heel protector or cup along with daily lubrication often prevents recurrence of the painful fissures.

PIEZOGENIC PAPULES

Pressure-induced herniation of subcutaneous fat through windows within the superficial fascia of the heel produces benign yellow papules or nodules, which are sometimes alarming to patients (Fig. 19–25). In non–weight bearing, the papules are skin colored

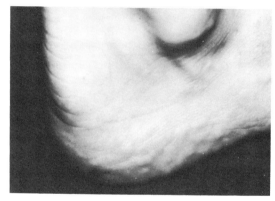

FIGURE 19–25. Piezogenic papules.

and difficult to see, while on weight bearing they become evident but seldom painful. Apparently, septal and or fascial defects allow subcutaneous heel fat to protrude against dermal skin. Most patients are young and athletically active without thick layers of subcutaneous fat. Piezogenic papules are usually found on the medial or lateral aspects of the both heels and also have been observed on the lateral edge of the palms.[61]

Dockery and Diana[62] found that 62 of 100 podiatric patients aged 15 to 72 years had piezogenic papules. The diameter of the papules was between 4 and 8 mm, with only two patients having any associated symptoms. Observation and patient reassurance are appropriate management. Painful piezogenic papules are more likely to be associated with obesity and prolonged standing. They often respond to rigid polyethylene heel protectors or shoe modification and padding. Surgical excision might be necessary in severe causes in which neurovascular elements become entrapped in the herniated fibrofatty tissue.

LYMPHEDEMA-INDUCED KERATODERMA (MOSSY FOOT)

Chronic lower extremity edema may produce thickened skin about the ankles, feet, and toes. Plantar skin, because of its firm attachment to the deep fascia, seems spared. The chronic edema may be due to postphlebitic syndrome, trauma, lymph accumulation, filariasis, or excess fat deposition as in obesity and is not inherited. First the skin becomes diffusely thickened and chronically stretched over the subcutaneous edema; then velvety papillomatosis develops. Later, irregular warty projections, nodules, and tumors can occur. Definitive therapy is not available, while lubrication and support stockings, if tolerated, seem appropriate.[63]

KNUCKLE PADS

Pressure-induced skin changes are often seen overlying multiple interphalangeal joints of the toes. They frequently affect each interphalangeal joint of all eight lesser toes. They resemble helomas but have little hyperkeratosis associated with them (Fig. 19–26). Often the patient is particularly zealous in cosmetic reduction of dead skin. Lesions are often hyperpigmented with zones of hypopigmentation within the older larger lesions. The skin lines are lost, while there is noticeable thickening of skin over the joint. The plaques of postinflammatory hyperpigmentation are due to pressure and friction from particularly ill-

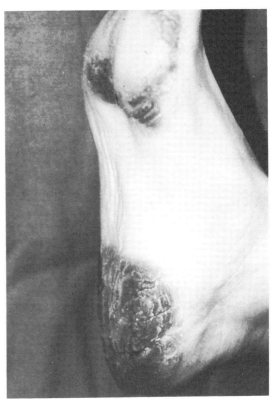

FIGURE 19–27. Psoriatic plantar keratoderma.

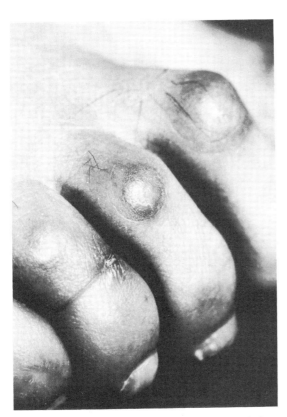

FIGURE 19–26. Knuckle pads at the proximal interphalangeal joints. Note hair-induced digital constriction of the fourth toe.

fitting shoes. Patients may request podiatric paring, which seems inappropriate because of the lack of hyperkeratosis. Limited paring, emollients and control of pressure from shoes are appropriate.[64]

Pedal Papulosquamous Diseases

PSORIATIC KERATODERMA

Plantar psoriasis may occur alone, without other areas of more characteristic psoriatic involvement, such as knees, elbows, or scalp. Plantarly it becomes modified in clinical appearance by chronic weight bearing on structurally different plantar skin (Fig. 19–27). Massive, progressive, yellow to white hyperkeratosis appears atop large erythematous plaques that can crack and present as painful fissures. Characteristically, weight-bearing and non–weight-bearing areas are affected, with extension often seen to lateral pedal skin.

The differential diagnosis includes chronic hyperkeratotic tinea pedis, chronic contact dermatitis, lichen planus, inherited palmoplantar keratodermas, and secondary syphilis.

Management can be difficult in view of the chronic relapsing nature of psoriasis. The painful fissures can be hydrated by hydrotherapy and debrided. Topical corticosteroid ointments under occlusive wrapping used at night may slow down the proliferation of keratin. Pulsed topical corticosteroid therapy should be used to avoid tachyphylaxis or corticosteroid-induced atrophy and hypopigmentation. Salicylic acid ointment, 25%, or urea, 20%, may be used during periods of rest from corticosteroid treatment. Plantar psoriasis characteristically follows a course of months-long flares followed by long periods of clearing. This can be frustrating to the patient and requires that the podiatrist be patient, reassuring, and optimistic.

PUSTULAR PSORIASIS

The first clinical form of persistent pustular psoriasis of the hands and feet is acropustulosis, which is often initiated by trauma or a trivial infection such as of an ingrowing toenail. Acropustulosis is probably a variant of psoriasis and has been called pustular acrodermatitis, acrodermatitis continua, and dermatitis repens by various authors. The disorder is characterized by sterile pustular eruptions and crusts that affect the distal fingers and toes, producing an erythematous glazed skin. The lesions encircle the digit, extend locally, and in some cases become generalized. This pustulosis runs a chronic and recurrent course much like psoriasis vulgaris.

The second pedal form of pustular psoriasis affects the palms, soles, and heels. Palmoplantar pustulosis presents as chronic, persistent pustules occurring symmetrically in fields of intense erythema (Fig. 19–28). It has been debated whether it is a variant of psoriasis. Management is challenging, with coal tars, topical corticosteroids under occlusion, and methotrexate soaks all yielding poor results. Oral administration of tetracycline did result in improvement in 15 of 40 patients in one trial.[65]

LICHEN PLANUS

Another relatively common papulosquamous disease that can affect the feet and nails is lichen planus. It presents as symmetric, pru-

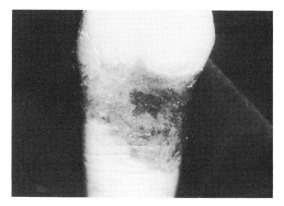

FIGURE 19–28. Palmoplantar pustulosis. This plantar form of pustular psoriasis was intensely erythematous. (Courtesy of Donald Kushner, DPM, Ohio College of Podiatric Medicine.)

ritic, purple (violaceous), polygonal, flat-topped papules with possible pterygium nail dystrophy. The surface of the lesions may demonstrate a delicate scaling or grayish white cross hatching known as Wickham's striae.[66] Scratching may produce a linear pattern on the lower legs and ankles. Lichen planus favors the development of lesions on the anterior wrists and ankles, on the inner thigh, on the sacral region, under the breasts, and on the buccal mucosa. Hypertrophic lichen planus usually develops on the anterior lower legs (Fig. 19–29). The nail dystrophy affects between 1% and 10% of the patients with lichen planus. Affected nails demonstrate pitting, linear lines, subungual keratosis, and sometimes a scarring of the proximal nail fold that produces a wing-shaped overgrowth called pterygium. The histopathology of lichen planus is characteristic in the acute phase. There is immunoglobulin deposition below the basement membrane. A variety of drugs such as gold, antibiotics, thiazide diuretics, and many others have been associated with lichen planus.

Treatment of lichen planus depends on the extent and type of lesions. Topical and intralesional corticosteroids are usually effective in localized lesions while oral prednisone may be needed for generalized lichen planus. Griseofulvin and psoralens and ultraviolet light therapy (PUVA) have also been used successfully.[67]

PITYRIASIS RUBRA PILARIS

A rarer papulosquamous disease, pityriasis rubra pilaris is of concern only because of the

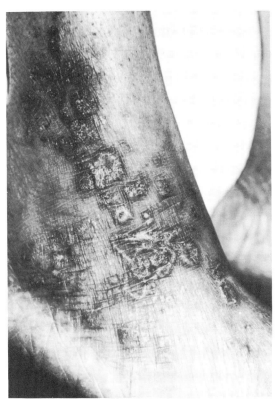

FIGURE 19–29. Linearly arranged polygonal papules and plaques of lichen planus about the ankle and foot.

palmar plantar keratoderma that accompanies it. Its characteristic lesions are acuminate or pinpoint follicular papules and yellow-to-pink scaly plaques that favor the extensor extremities, neck, and trunk. Pityriasis rubra pilaris seldom occurs without palmar plantar involvement. The plantar lesions are generally referred to as the "keratodermic sandal" of pityriasis rubra pilaris with massive cracked and fissured hyperkeratosis on a field of reddened skin often covering the entire plantar aspect of the feet.[68]

The etiology of this disorder is unknown. It has been reported to be both acquired and familial, with an autosomal dominant mode of inheritance. Clinically it may be impossible to distinguish pityriasis rubra pilaris from psoriasis, especially if the keratoderma is the presenting form of the disease. The toenail involvement, which occurs in about 19% of patients, also resembles psoriasis. Plugged hyperkeratotic hair follicles are the clinical key to diagnosis.[66]

Treatment seldom resolves pityriasis rubra pilaris, but topical corticosteroids, keratolytic

gels, and vitamin A acid (0.1% to 0.5%) under occlusion reportedly help symptomatic areas.[69] Vitamin A and isotretinoin have been also used by dermatologists with limited success.

Inherited Palmoplantar Keratodermas

The inherited palmoplantar keratodermas all have hyperkeratosis of the palms and/or soles as a clinical component whether the plantar keratoderma is diffuse or punctate. There have been many syndromes described with different modes of inheritance, various associated defects, and varying prognoses. One should also consider the large degree of interfamily variations in penetrance, phenotypic expression, age at onset, and severity of the individual case. In general, it is easiest to classify this group of disorders by mode of inheritance (Table 19–13). A selected few will be discussed as more common or prototypical representatives of this group.

DIFFUSE PALMOPLANTAR KERATODERMA

The diffuse form of inherited keratoderma is also known as Unna-Thost syndrome. All races are affected, with an incidence of 1 in 40,000 persons. The smooth, uniform hyperkeratosis of weight-bearing and non–weight-bearing areas of the palms and soles begins in early infancy and is fully expressed by 6 months of age. Clinical features include sharp peripheral margins, hyperhidrosis, painful fissures, and, occasionally, nail dystrophy.[63] The thickening may be locally accentuated by biomechanical trauma, while the thin toe-web

TABLE 19–13. **Classification of Palmoplantar Keratodermas**

Autosomal Dominant
 Diffuse keratodermas
 Mutilating keratoderma of Vohwinkel
 Progressive keratoderma (Greiter's syndrome)
 Punctate keratoderma (most common)
 Striate keratoderma

Autosomal Recessive
 Mal de meleda
 Papillon-LeFevre syndrome
 Circumscribed palmoplantar keratoderma

skin is characteristically spared. The palmar involvement is uniformly less intense.

PUNCTATE KERATODERMA

The punctate form seems to be the most common form of palmoplantar keratoderma and is most easily recognized by careful inspection of the palms and soles for 2- to 10-mm diameter horny plugs. The palmar punctate keratoses cluster along the dominant dermatoglyphic lines while plantarly they occur on the weight-bearing and non–weight-bearing areas of the forefoot, arch, and heels (Fig. 19–30). The onset of the lesions may be at any time; however, it is usually between 10 and 45 years of age. Concurrent nail dystrophies are not specifically associated with the keratoderma.[68]

Podiatric primary care for the inherited keratodermas, in general, is nonspecific and involves acute fissure care of symptomatic cracks and paring reduction and enucleation of the hyperkeratotic lesions and plugs after prepar-

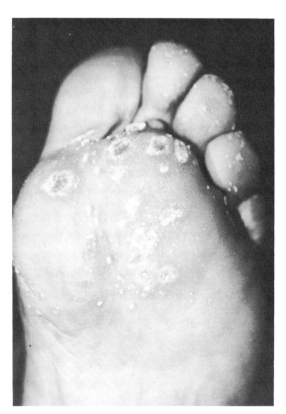

FIGURE 19–30. Punctate keratoderma of the forefoot that is bilaterally symmetric and also affects the palms, but to a lesser degree.

atory hydrotherapy. Avoidance and control of mechanical repetitive trauma can be helpful by utilizing shock-absorbing insoles or chairside orthotics and shoe evaluation. Drying agents may be needed to control commonly accompanying hyperhidrosis. Keratolytics such as Whitfield's ointment, salicylic acid ointment (25% to 40%), and salicylic acid plasters may be necessary to chemically control painful lesions.

Pedal Perspiration Problems

HYPERHIDROSIS

Excessive perspiration is termed *hyperhidrosis* and affects the palms and soles in about 0.25% of the population. Idiopathic hyperhidrosis, which is due to excessive sympathetic vasomotor stimulation of the eccrine glands, is different from pathologic hyperhidrosis, which may be secondary to a febrile process, diabetes, hyperthyroidism, or a lesion of the central or peripheral nervous system.[70]

Eccrine glands are the only skin appendages on the soles since there are no plantar sebaceous glands or hair follicles. There are more than 600 sweat glands per square centimeter on the sole.[71] They respond rapidly, but only weakly, to thermoregulatory stimulation while profoundly responding to mental or emotional stimuli. This is most likely to be a manifestation of the "fight or flight response," producing a better hand grip and increasing the coefficient of friction of the soles. Sweat is normally an odorless solution containing sodium chloride, potassium, urea, and lactate.

The clinical appearance of hyperhidrosis includes usually pinker, moist skin that is vasodilated yet cool to the touch. Although the patient is awake and stimulated, his or her feet feel cool and clammy. White macerated soggy skin is often evident especially between the toes. Either sex can be affected, with onset occurring after puberty and decreasing after age 25 in some patients. Some patients can experience burning, itching, and blister formation. Occasionally the hyperhidrosis can be so severe that drops of sweat can run off the foot. The shoe is often damp, moldy, and prematurely broken down. Hyperhidrosis is often accompanied by tinea pedis, pitted keratolysis, or the odor of bromhidrosis.

BROMHIDROSIS

Foul-smelling sweat occurs when the normally odorless pedal perspiration becomes overgrown with bacteria-decomposing surface protein debris, producing malodorous biochemical wastes.[72] No one bacterial species seems responsible, with many of the resident flora capable of generating volatile acids (Fig. 19–31). Isobutyric acid produces a dirty sock odor, and isovaleric acid smells like "sweaty feet."[73] *Brevibacterium* colonizing human skin produces methanethiol gas, which smells like cheddar cheese. It has also been found that tinea pedis can actually increase *Brevibacterium* counts. The *Trichophyton* species often produce penicillin. The odor-producing *Brevibacterium* are less susceptible to penicillin than other toe-web floral organisms with which they compete.

Management of both hyperhidrosis and bromhidrosis centers first on the reduction of sweat. Several preventive measures should be taken first. The patient should not wear occlusive shoes or synthetic or wool socks. The patient should use leather or fabric shoes or perhaps open sandals, if practical. Cotton socks are absorbent, fungistatic, and bacteriostatic. They can be changed at midday or at least when the patient gets home from work. Pairs of shoes should be alternated daily to allow enough time for thorough drying out. Absorbent powders such as Zeasorb are useful during the day. Talcs, such as baby powder, are four times less absorbent than cellulose-based Zeasorb but are good in reducing friction.

Reduction of perspiration can be achieved by the use of topical antiperspirants such as Drysol (20% solution of aluminum chloride in anhydrous ethyl alcohol). These agents are applied nightly to dried plantar skin under occlusion for 1 week and then tapered to twice weekly for control. Topical glutaraldehyde in a 10% solution can also be used without occlusion but produces some transitory browning of the skin and nails.[74] The use of tap water iontophoresis has been reported to control excess perspiration by possibly electrically stimulating epidermal keratinization and subsequent blockage of the sweat duct orifices.[75] This may require repeated treatments or continued use of a Drionic device (General Medical Company, Los Angeles, CA) at home to maintain the anhidrotic effect.[76]

Reduction of the resident bacterial population can be accomplished using povidone-iodine soap to scrub the feet while bathing each day as needed. A broad-spectrum topical antifungal agent of the imidazole class may be used concurrently to additionally suppress both the fungi and bacteria. A topical antibiotic such as erythromycin in a penetrating gel vehicle (Erygel) may also be useful.

Other factors tend to produce greater pedal perspiration in some patients. Caffeine in coffee, tea, or colas stimulates sympathetic outflow and thus the eccrine gland's sweat production. In addition, many patients are obviously anxious, with psychically initiated sweating of the palms and soles being a significant cause of their hyperhidrosis. Stress reduction and practicing relaxation and biofeedback techniques can be helpful.[77]

Pedal Dermatologic Manifestations of Diabetes

There are many significant general dermatologic manifestations of diabetes. In fact, nearly all diabetics have skin manifestations related to their diabetes.[78] Within the lower extremity there are also skin disorders that have been associated with diabetes, some certainly more common than others (Table 19–14). It is interesting to note that some investigators

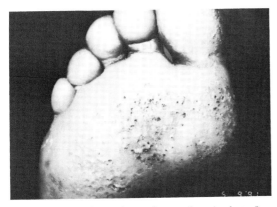

FIGURE 19–31. Maceration and soggy keratin that often accompany hyperhidrosis, bromhidrosis, and pitted keratolysis. (Courtesy of Donald Kushner, DPM, Ohio College of Podiatric Medicine.)

TABLE 19–14. Lower-Extremity Dermatologic Associations With Diabetes

Anhidrosis and oligohidrosis
Bullous diabeticorum*
Candidiasis*
Cellulitis
Diabetic shin spots*
Gangrene
Hemorrhagic callus*
Necrobiosis lipoidica*
Neuropathic ulcer or joint
Paronychia*
Plantar palmar rubeosis
Tinea pedis*
Vitiligo
Yellow skin and nails*
Xerosis and pruritus*

*Discussed in text.

have questioned whether tinea is more common in patients with diabetes. They found that 31% of their diabetic population had culture-proven fungal infections (mostly tinea pedis) compared with 33% of their controls.[79] Several diabetes-associated conditions have already been discussed, such as tinea pedis, nail dystrophies secondary to peripheral vascular insufficiency, and erythrasma. Here three particular diabetes-associated conditions are discussed that need some clarification and additional description.

DIABETIC SHIN SPOTS (DIABETIC DERMOPATHY)

As in all diabetes-associated conditions, the mere presence of brown or red circular to oval macules and papules over the pretibial areas does not in itself mean the patient is diabetic or will develop diabetes at a later date. These acute lesions are 0.5 to 1.0 cm in diameter and over a period of several years evolve to atrophic hyperpigmented patches (Fig. 19–32). They rarely ulcerate and have also been reported to occur on the forearms, the anterior thighs, and even the scalp. These lesions are seen in both insulin-dependent and non–insulin-dependent diabetic patients. However, they are also observed in 1.5% of healthy non-diabetic persons and 20% of patients with various endocrinopathies who have normal glucose tolerance.[80] Diabetic shin spots are found

more often in male diabetics (65%) than in female diabetics (10% to 30%).[81] Some investigators have attempted to link these skin changes to a microangiopathic process such as retinopathy, neuropathy, or nephropathy, but histologic analysis only demonstrates chronic inflammatory changes.[82] The incidence of diabetic shin spots is greatest in patients with diabetic neuropathy and is independent of renal or eye involvement. The lesions are asymptomatic, seldom ulcerate, and do not respond to control of hyperglycemia. The patient should be reassured and educated about these benign skin changes.[83]

NECROBIOSIS LIPOIDICA

Necrobiosis lipoidica presents as a sharply demarcated pretibial plaque that measures between 0.5 cm and 25 cm in diameter (Fig. 19–33). The active border remains erythematous, but the center becomes telangiectic and yellow as lipids are deposited. Ulceration occurs in 35% of cases and is characteristically painful, bilateral, and slow to heal.[77] Although strongly associated with diabetes, necrobiosis lipoidica is rare, with only about 0.3% of diabetics developing the disease. The female-to-male ratio is 3:1, with the age at onset ranging from birth to 76 years and the average age being 30 years.[84]

A consistently effective treatment for necrobiosis lipoidica has not yet been found, and it is well accepted that progression of the disorder does not relate to hyperglycemic control.[85] Potent topical corticosteroids applied to early lesions or the inflammatory rim surrounding

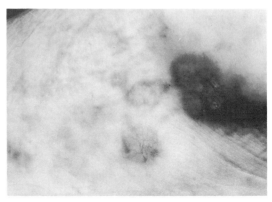

FIGURE 19–32. Diabetic dermopathy at the lateral ankle.

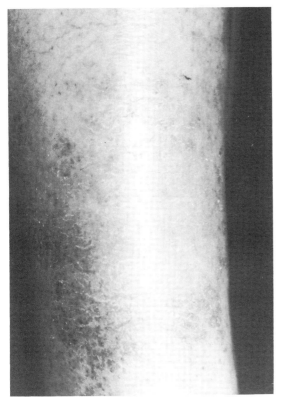

FIGURE 19–33. Necrobiosis lipoidica of the lower anterior leg.

developed lesions are believed to be helpful in blocking the immune-mediated process, but no controlled studies have been published.[81] Pentoxifylline, 400 mg three times a day, has been tried, reportedly with good results.[86] In addition, aspirin, topical heparin, dipyridamole, and even surgical excision have all been tried, with limited and highly variable results.[83]

BULLOUS DIABETICORUM

Bullous diabeticorum clinically presents as large, spontaneously appearing, nontraumatic blisters of the toes, feet, and lower legs in patients with long-standing diabetes (Fig. 19–34). The bullae are sterile unless secondarily infected and resolve spontaneously, usually without scar formation. The lesions are relatively painless and develop overnight without any history of trauma even in diabetics with intact sensation.[87]

Histopathologic studies show inconsistent levels of epidermal separation. Some patients have intraepidermal bullae, while others have subepidermal bullae. No clear-cut differentiation can be made between patients with intraepidermal bullae and those with subepidermal bullae as to age, duration of diabetes, angiopathy, or localization of the lesions.[88]

The etiology of bullous diabeticorum is not known. Hypothetical causes include neuropathy, nephropathy-induced imbalance in calcium and magnesium with subsequent weakness in skin structure, vascular disease, stasis-triggered immune reaction to the skin, or an unknown biochemical disturbance in carbohydrate metabolism.[89] On rare occasions spontaneous blisters have occurred in patients undergoing renal dialysis. Bernstein and associates reported[90] a reduced threshold to suction-induced blister formation in insulin-dependent diabetics as compared with age-related controls.

Successful treatment of the bullae consists of syringe aspiration and drainage of the large bullae followed by povidone-iodine flushing and dry sterile dressing. A surgical shoe helps to reduce footwear irritation and accommodates dressings. Healing occurs within several weeks with transitory hypopigmentation and usually without secondary infection or scarring. Acral bullous pemphigoid should be considered in the differential diagnosis and may require biopsy to look for histologic evidence of subepidermal cleavage characteristic of this progressive disease.[91]

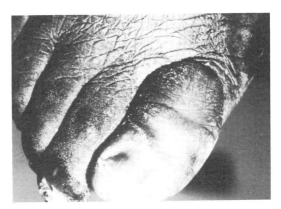

FIGURE 19–34. Bullous diabeticorum of the great toe. (Courtesy of Donald Kushner, DPM, Ohio College of Podiatric Medicine.)

REFERENCES

1. Dawber RPR, Baran R: Structure, embryology, comparative anatomy and physiology of the nail. In Baran R, Dawber RP (eds): Diseases of the Nails and Their Management, pp 2–10. Boston, Blackwell Scientific Publications, 1984.
2. Zaias N: Psoriasis of the nail unit. Dermatol Clin 2:493–505, 1984.
3. Terry RB: The onychial dermal band in health and disease. Lancet 1:179–181, 1955.
4. Wallis MS, Bowen WR, et al: Pathogenesis of onychoschizia (lamellar dystrophy). J Am Acad Dermatol 24:44–48, 1991.
5. Columbo VE, Gerber F, et al: Treatment of brittle fingernails and onychoschizia with biotin: Scanning and microscopy. J Am Acad Dermatol 23:1127–1132, 1990.
6. Baran R, Dawber RPR: Physical signs. In Baran R, Dawber RP (eds): Diseases of the Nails and Their Management. Boston, Blackwell Scientific Publications, 1984.
7. Yinnon AM, Matalon A: Koilonychia of the toenails in children. Int J Dermatol 27:685–687, 1988.
8. Pierre M: The Nail, p 21. New York, Churchill Livingstone, 1981.
9. Baran R, Kechijian P: Longitudinal melanonychia (melanonychia striata): Diagnosis and management. J Am Acad Dermatol 21:1165–1175, 1989.
10. Bodman MA: Onychomycosis update. Curr Podiatry 35:14–15, 1986.
11. Abramson C: Culture identification and therapy of fungal infections of foot and nails. Podiatric Pathology Prints 9:2, 1991. Baltimore, Podiatric Pathology Laboratories.
12. Norton LA: Nail disorders. J Am Acad Dermatol 2:451–467, 1980.
13. Dompmartin D, et al: Onychomycosis and AIDS: Clinical and laboratory findings in 62 patients. Int J Dermatol 9:337–339, 1990.
14. Zaias N: Psoriasis of the nail unit. Arch Dermatol 99:567–579, 1969.
15. Baran R, Dawber RPR: The nail in dermatological diseases. In Baran R, Dawber RP (eds): Diseases of the Nails and Their Management. Boston, Blackwell Scientific Publications, 1984.
16. Fenton D, Wilkinson JD: The nail in systemic diseases and drug-induced changes. In Baran R, Dawber RP (eds): Diseases of the Nails and Their Management. Boston, Blackwell Scientific Publications, 1984.
17. Ward PE, McCarthy DJ: Periungual fibroma. Cutis 64:118–124, 1990.
18. Haneke H, Baran R, Bureau H: Tumours of the nail apparatus and adjacent tissues. In Baran R, Dawber RP (eds): Diseases of the Nails and Their Management. Boston, Blackwell Scientific Publications, 1984.
19. Zaias N, Baden H: Nails. In Fitzpatrick TB, Eisen AZ, Wolff K, et al (eds): Dermatology in General Medicine. New York, McGraw-Hill Book Company, 1979.
20. Laine W: Benign neoplasia of the foot. In McCarthy DJ, Montgomery R (ed): Podiatric Dermatology. Baltimore, Williams & Wilkins, 1986.
21. Sullivan K, Williams J, Lantz DM, et al: Squamous cell carcinoma of the great toe in a black man. J Am Podiatr Med Assoc 80:548–551, 1990.
22. Kegel MF, Scher RK: Metastasis of pulmonary carcinoma to the nail unit. Cutis 35:121–124, 1985.
23. Hodson SB, Henslee TM, Tachibana DK, et al: Interdigital erythrasma: A review of the literature. J Am Podiatr Med Assoc 78:551–557, 1988.
24. Henslee TM, Tanaka TJ, Hodson SB, et al: Interdigital erythrasma: An incidence study. J Am Podiatr Med Assoc 78:559–562, 1988.
25. Rook A, Wilkinson DS, Ebling FJG: Textbook of Dermatology. Boston, Blackwell Scientific Publications, 1979.
26. Gill KA, Buckels LJ: Pitted keratolysis. Arch Dermatol 98:7, 1968.
27. Kates SG, Nordstrom KM, McGinley KJ, et al: Microbial ecology of interdigital infection of toe spaces. J Am Acad Dermatol 22:578–582, 1990.
28. Page JC, McCarthy D, Williams D, et al: Athlete's Foot: Evolving Concepts in the Diagnosis and Treatment of Pedal Infections. South Norwalk, CT, Ortho Pharmaceutical Company, 1990.
29. Johnson ML, Stern RS: Prevalence and ecology of skin disorders. In Fitzpatrick TB, Eisen AZ, Wolff K, et al (eds): Dermatology in General Medicine. New York, McGraw-Hill Book Company, 1979.
30. Elewski BE, Hazen PG: The superficial mycoses and the dermatophytes. J Am Acad Dermatol 21:655–673, 1989.
31. Abramson C: Athlete's foot and onychomycosis caused by *Hendersonula toruloidea*. Cutis 46:128–132, 1990.
32. Abramson C: Athlete's foot caused by *Pseudomonas aeruginosa*. Clin Dermatol 1(1):14–24, 1983.
33. Haroon TS, et al: Antifungal activity of naftifine gel in vivo. Mykosen 30:49, 1987.
34. Kates SG, Myung KB, McGinley KJ, et al: The antibacterial efficacy of econazole nitrate in interdigital toe web infections. J Am Acad Dermatol 22:583–586, 1990.
35. Kotrajaras R: Phaeohyphomycosis. In Jacobs PH, Nail L (eds): Antifungal Drug Therapy. New York, Marcel Dekker, 1990.
36. Savin RC: Treatment of chronic tinea pedis (athlete's foot type) with topical terbinafine. J Am Acad Dermatol 23:786–789, 1990.
37. Bartolemi FJ, McCarthy DJ: Cutaneous manifestations of viral disease. In McCarthy DJ, Montgomery R (eds): Podiatric Dermatology. Baltimore, Williams & Wilkins, 1986.
38. Pass F: Verrucae, including condyloma acuminatum. In Fitzpatrick TB, Eisen AZ, Wolff K, et al (eds): Dermatology in General Medicine. New York, McGraw-Hill Book Company, 1979.
39. Jablonska S, Orth G, Obalek S, et al: Cutaneous warts. Clinical, histologic and virologic correlations. Clin Dermatol 3(4):71–82, 1985.
40. Bunney MH, Nolan MW, Williams DA: An assessment of methods of treating viral warts by comparative treatment trials based on a standard design. Br J Dermatol 94:667–679, 1976.
41. Gibbs RD: Conservative management of plantar warts by gentle chemocautery. J Dermatol Surg Oncol 4:915, 1978.
42. Lemont H, Parekh V: Superficial fascia: An appropriate anatomical boundary for excising warts on the foot. J Dermatol Surg Oncol 15:710–711, 1989.
43. Buchner D, Price NM: Immunotherapy of verrucae vulgaris with dinitrochlorobenzene. Br J Dermatol 98:451–455, 1978.
44. Shumack PH, Haddock MJ: Bleomycin: An effective treatment of warts. Aust J Dermatol 20:41–42, 1979.
45. McCarthy DJ, Tate R: Intradermal use of 5-fluorouracil in human pedal verrucae. J Am Podiatr Med Assoc 69:587, 1979.
46. Tropp BE: Ultrasound in verrucae plantaris. J Am Podiatr Med Assoc 57:326, 1967.

47. Wygant LA: Hypnosis in a case of multiple verrucae. J Am Podiatr Med Assoc 51:660, 1961.

48. Pringle WM, Helms DC: Treatment of plantar warts by blunt dissection. Arch Dermatol 108:79–82, 1973.

49. Nagington J, Rook A: Virus and related infection. In Rook A, Wilkinson DS, Ebling FJG: Textbook of Dermatology. Boston, Blackwell Scientific Publications, 1979.

50. Soter NA, Fitztpatrick TB: Introduction and classification. In Fitzpatrick TB, Eisen AZ, Wolff K, et al (eds): Dermatology in General Medicine. New York, McGraw-Hill Book Company, 1979.

51. Baer RL, Gigli I: Allergic eczematous contact dermatitis. In Fitzpatrick TB, Eizen AZ, Wolff K, et al (eds): Dermatology in General Medicine. New York, McGraw-Hill Book Company, 1979.

52. Samitz MH, Dana AS: Cutaneous Lesions of the Lower Extremities. Philadelphia, JB Lippincott, 1971.

53. Rook A, Wilkinson DS: Eczema, lichen simplex and prurigo. In Rook A, Wilkinson DS (eds): Textbook of Dermatology. Boston, Blackwell Scientific Publications, 1985.

54. Ashton R, Jones R, et al: Juvenile plantar dermatosis. Arch Dermatol 121:225–228, 1985.

55. Steck WD: Wet foot dry foot syndrome. Cleve Clin Q Summer 1983, pp 145–149.

56. Lazar P: Other eczematous disease. In Roenigk HH (ed): Office Dermatology, p 55. Baltimore, Williams & Wilkins, 1981.

57. Champion RH, Parish WE: Atopic dermatitis. In Rook A, Wilkinson DS (eds): Textbook of Dermatology. Boston, Blackwell Scientific Publications, 1985.

58. Arndt KA: Manual of Dermatologic Therapeutics with Essentials of Diagnosis. Boston, Little, Brown & Co, 1983.

59. Lemont H: Histological differentiation of mechanical and non-mechanical keratoses of the sole. In Witkowski JA (ed): Clinics in Dermatology, Vol 1, Diseases of the Lower Extremities. Philadelphia, JB. Lippincott, 1983.

60. Rabinowitz AD: Skin tumors. In Witkowski JA (ed): Clinics In Dermatology, Vol 1, Diseases of the Lower Extremities. Philadelphia, JB Lippincott, 1983.

61. Wilkinson DS: Cutaneous reactions to mechanical and thermal injury. In Rook A, Wilkinson DS (eds): Textbook of Dermatology. Boston, Blackwell Scientific Publications, 1985.

62. Dockery GL, Diana JL: Painful piezogenic papules. J Am Podiatr Med Assoc 68:703–705, 1978.

63. Ebling FJ, Rook A: Disorders of keratinization. In Rook A, Wilkinson DS (eds): Textbook of Dermatology. Boston, Blackwell Scientific Publications, 1985.

64. Costello MJ, Gibbs RC: The Palms and Soles in Medicine. Springfield, IL, Charles C Thomas, 1967.

65. Baker H, Wilkinson DS: Psoriasis. In Rook A, Wilkinson DS (eds): Textbook of Dermatology. Boston, Blackwell Scientific Publications, 1985.

66. Sanders IJ: Psoriasiform disorders. In McCarthy DJ, Montgomery R (eds): Podiatric Dermatology. Baltimore, Williams & Wilkins, 1986.

67. Roenigk HH: "Other" papulosquamous diseases. In Roenigk HH (ed): Office Dermatology. Baltimore, Williams & Wilkins, 1981.

68. Costello MJ, Gibbs RC: The Palms and Soles in Medicine. Springfield, IL, Charles C Thomas, 1967.

69. Samitz MH: Cutaneous Disorders of the Lower Extremities. Philadelphia, JB Lippincott, 1981.

70. Jenkin WM, Craft CF: Management of idiopathic plantar hyperhidrosis. J Am Podiatr Med Assoc 73:475–480, 1983.

71. Grice K: Hyperhidrosis and its treatment by iontophoresis. Physiotherapy 66:43, 1980.

72. Abramson C, Terleckyj B: Bromidrosis, current concepts related to foot pathology. J Am Podiatr Med Assoc 69:252–255, 1979.

73. Amoore JE: Molecular Basis of Odor. Springfield, IL, Charles C Thomas, 1970.

74. Gordon BI: "No sweat." Cutis 15:401–404, 1975.

75. Gordon BJ, Maibach HI: Eccrine anhidrosis due to glutaraldehyde, formaldehyde, and iontophoresis. J Invest Dermatol 53:43, 1969.

76. Peterson JL, Read SI, Rodman OG: A new device in the treatment of hyperhidrosis by iontophoresis. Cutis 29:82–89, 1982.

77. Duller P, Gentry WD: Use of biofeedback in treating chronic hyperhidrosis: A preliminary report. Br J Dermatol 103:143–146, 1980.

78. Goodfile MJD, Millard LG: The skin in diabetes mellitus. Diabetologia 31:567–575, 1988.

79. Lugo-Somolinos A, Sanchez JL: Prevalence of dermatophytosis in patients with diabetes. J Am Acad Dermatol 26:408–410, 1992.

80. Feingold KR, Elias PM: Dermatologic complications: Associations with diabetes. Diabetes Spectrum 3:282–287, 1991.

81. Tadlock LM, Feingold KR: Dermatologic complications of diabetes: II. Clin Diabetes 5:91–92, 1987.

82. Gouterman IH, Sibrack LA: Diabetes. Cutis 25:45–53, 1980.

83. Aagenaes O, Moe H: Light and electron microscopy study of skin capillaries of diabetics. Diabetes 10:253, 1961.

84. Lowitt MH, Dover JS: Necrobiosis lipoidica. J Am Acad Dermatol 25:735–748, 1991.

85. Muller SA, Winkelmann RK: A clinical and pathological investigation of 171 cases. Arch Dermatol 93:272–281, 1966.

86. Littler CM, Tschen EH: Pentoxifylline for necrobiosis lipoidica diabeticorum. J Am Acad Dermatol 17:314–316, 1987.

87. Toonstra J: Bullosis diabeticorum: A report of a case with a review of the literature. Clin Rev 5:799–803, 1985.

88. Bodman MA, Friedman S, Clifford LA: Bullosis diabeticorum: A report of two cases with a review of the literature. J Am Podiatr Med Assoc 81:561–563, 1991.

89. Berstein JE, Medenica M, Soltani K, et al: Bullous eruption of diabetes mellitus. Arch Dermatol 115:624–326, 1979.

90. Bernstein JE, Levine LE, Medenica MM, et al: Reduced threshold to suction-induced blister formation in insulin-dependent diabetics. J Am Acad Dermatol 8:790, 1983.

91. Chuang T, Korkij W, Soltani K, et al: Increased frequency of diabetes mellitus in patients with bullous pemphigoid: A case-control study. J Am Acad Dermatol 11:1099, 1984.

CHAPTER 20

PODIATRIC PERIPHERAL VASCULAR DISEASES

Howard Darvin
Jeffrey M. Robbins
Corliss L. Austin
Jeffrey Lynn

HISTORY AND PHYSICAL EXAMINATION

The podiatrist should be able to recognize various vascular syndromes on the basis of symptoms and physical signs. Deciding if a patient has arterial, venous, or lymphatic insufficiency entails using all the integral parts of the history and physical examination as well as diagnostic and therapeutic maneuvers. The vascular examination is only a part of the overall clinical evaluation of the patient and must be considered in context with the remainder of the history and physical examination. Valuable historical clues that can help determine the severity of the disease process include mode of onset, characteristics, chronologic sequence, associated symptoms, and progression of pain. Pertinent symptoms include ischemic pain, intermittent claudication, rest pain, edema, tissue breakdown, and color and temperature changes.[1, 2]

On examination of the lower extremities the following should be noted: size and symmetry; color and texture of the skin and nail beds; hair distribution on the lower legs, feet, and toes; pigmentation; rashes; scars; ulcers; venous pattern; venous enlargement; and edema. The pulses should be palpated and evaluated for symmetry, regular rhythm, and amplitude. Amplitude varies with the size of the artery and should vary from beat to beat. The radial, brachial, femoral, popliteal, dorsalis pedis, and posterior tibial peripheral arteries are most routinely evaluated. Pulse character should not be bounding or thready. The description of the pulse amplitude is most important. The following grading system is the most accepted: 0 = absent, 1 = diminished, 2 = normal, 3 = increased, and 4 = bounding.

The temperature of the feet and legs is noted by using the backs of the fingers. Unilateral coldness suggests inadequate arterial circulation. Bilateral coldness is usually due to a cold environment or anxiety. Pitting edema is checked by pressing firmly with the thumb for at least 5 seconds behind each medial malleolus, on the dorsum of each foot, and over the shins. Deep phlebitis is palpated for by compressing the calf muscles against the tibia while the knee is flexed and relaxed, and any tenderness, increased firmness, or muscle tension is sought. Signs of superficial phlebitis include tender, indurated, subcutaneous cords with warmth, redness, or discoloration. The patient is asked to stand while the examiner inspects the saphenous system for varicosities. The standing posture allows any varicosities to fill with blood and makes them visible. Any varicosities are then felt for signs of thrombophlebitis.

Valvular competency in communicating veins and the greater saphenous vein is assessed by means of the retrograde filling (Trendelenburg) test. This test entails elevating the patient's leg to 90° to empty it of venous blood. A tourniquet is placed around the upper thigh tightly enough to occlude the great saphenous vein without occluding the femoral artery. The patient is asked to stand, and the examiner watches for venous filling. Normally the saphenous vein fills slowly from below, taking about 35 seconds. Then the tourniquet is released and the rate of venous filling is noted after the patient has stood for 20 seconds. Normally there is none, because competent valves block retrograde flow.

The elevation dependency test is used to assess chronic arterial insufficiency. If pain or diminished pulses suggest arterial insufficiency, then the examiner should look for marked pallor on elevation and rubor on dependency. Both of the patient's legs are raised to about 60° for approximately 1 minute. Slight pallor is normal in light-skinned persons. Color changes may be more difficult to see in black persons. The plantar aspects of the feet should be checked if necessary.[3]

Arterial disease is usually asymptomatic until a patient undergoes acute circulatory catastrophe or develops chronic regional symptoms that announce the presence of systemic disease. Symptoms of lower extremity arterial insufficiency include pain, numbness, coldness, burning, pallor, tingling, and paresthesias. Arterial ischemic disease in the legs often causes hair loss, dystrophic nails, and dryness, which may appear as pruritus. Ischemic ulcers are painful and have a "punched out" appearance. They have discrete edges and are often covered with crust.

Patients with arterial insufficiency may also describe pain, tightness, pressure cramps, aches, and a deep pulling that is reproducible after walking a certain distance. These symptoms are known as intermittent because they occur with exercise and as claudication from the Latin *claudicatio,* meaning "to limp." Chronic arterial occlusion causes intermittent claudication. Ischemic complaints in order of frequency are pain, numbness, coldness, tenderness, burning, fullness, and pallor; they are more severe during exercise.

The podiatrist should be able to evaluate whether there is sufficient blood flow entering the foot and leg to maintain its normal nutrition, to heal, and to sustain nutrition following surgery. Inadequate nutrition, such as lack of protein intake, citrus fruits, and B vitamins, can inhibit the patient's ability to heal. Medical conditions that should be explored include anemia, alcoholism, connective tissue diseases, vasospastic disorders, poor nutrition, and sickle cell anemia. The patient should be asked if he or she heals when cut or bruised. If blood flow is severely diminished, the patient should be referred to a vascular surgeon for further evaluation.[1, 2]

Venous disorders of the lower extremity are due to either obstruction or insufficiency. Venous ulcers develop slowly. These ulcers classically present as a diffusely reddened, thickened area over the medial or lateral malleolus. This frequent site of ulceration is known as the "gaiter" area. The skin has a cobblestone appearance, which has resulted from fibrosis and venous stasis.[1]

The venous obstructive disorders to be discussed are deep and superficial thrombophlebitis. Venous insufficiency states include varicose veins and postphlebitic syndrome. Venous thrombosis may acutely cause morbidity and mortality from pulmonary embolism. In the United States, an estimated 200,000 persons die annually of these complications. Venous conditions will be compounded in the future owing to the increased use of cardiac monitoring, dialysis, and pacing devices that are placed in the upper extremity veins.[1]

Lymphatic disorders also adversely affect the lower extremity. Chronic lymphedema causes the skin to thicken and take on a rough consistency similar to pigskin. The lymphatic system returns proteins that escaped from the capillaries into the circulation. When abnormal lymph flow exists, protein accumulates in tissues and organs, leading to the manifestation of several disease states.[1, 2]

LABORATORY TESTS

Noninvasive Laboratory Tests

DOPPLER STUDIES

Arterial. The Doppler device is an ultrasonic flow detector that emits a beam of a certain frequency (5 mHz in venous studies, 8 to 10 mHz in arterial studies). Objects (e.g., blood flowing in a vessel) moving faster than 6 cm/s alter the frequency of the emitted beam. The reflected beam is received by the probe and compared with the emitted beam. Sound is filtered by an amplifier that gives a flow signal (sound) or a tracing that is proportional to the blood flow velocity. The slower the flow, the lower is the pitch.

The faster the blood flow, the steeper the recorded waveform. There are two types of continuous wave Doppler signals: unidirectional and bidirectional. These Doppler signals produce the same sound. The difference between them is that the unidirectional Doppler signal records both forward and backward flow as a waveform above the baseline. The bidirectional Doppler signal records the forward flow above the baseline and the backward flow below the baseline. Unidirectional Doppler signals should be more than adequate for podiatric assessment.

The normal arterial pattern formed by the qualitative audible Doppler signal is a triphasic picture with full, sharply peaked waves that reflect high velocity and normal volume. In normal arteries, three distinct sounds are produced. The first sound represents forward flow, the second sound represents backward flow, and the third sound represents vessel rebound. Blood flow is usually pulsatile and flows both forward and backward. Only digital arteries have forward flow alone because of their small diameter. In normal digital arteries only one high-pitched sound is heard. Each toe contains two plantar and two dorsal digital arteries. Digital arteries are heard by holding

the Doppler probe at 90° to the toe lightly at the medial and lateral base, both plantarly and dorsally.

In organic occlusive arterial disease the intima is disrupted and the vessels are calcified. As a result, blood flows slower, and backward flow may not occur because of higher resistance. With an audible Doppler signal, abnormal blood flow is represented by a lower pitch and a monophasic sound, which denotes collateralized flow. The waveforms are characteristically broad and flatter, with low amplitudes reflecting lower velocity and decreased volume.[1]

Venous. The flow in extremity veins can be evaluated directly with Doppler studies. The Doppler device can also be used to detect venous valvular insufficiency. The patient is placed in the supine position with the head slightly elevated. A bilateral examination should always be done. Asymmetric findings may indicate early or limited pathologic processes. Deep veins are found adjacent to the accompanying arteries, and the greater saphenous vein can usually be seen under the skin at the medial malleolus.

There are five facets to the venous Doppler signal that should be evaluated:

1. *Spontaneity* refers to venous flow signals that are always present. The absence of these signals represents venous obstruction.
2. *Phasicity* refers to changes in the flow signal with respiration. A normal vein has spontaneous flow with a phasic variation with respiration. Breath holding or Valsalva's maneuver decreases or abolishes flow; with release there is a transient augmentation of the signal. With inspiration, venous flow decreases; and with expiration, venous flow increases. With venous obstruction, this respiratory variation decreases.
3. *Augmentation* refers to changes in venous flow by compression of the tissue proximal and distal to the examining probe. A quick compression of the extremity distal to the probe produces a brisk augmentation, often followed by a transient decrease on release. Proximal compression decreases or abolishes the flow signal, with augmentation coming on release. With incompetent valves, proximal compression produces augmentation owing to the retrograde flow.

These changes disappear with venous obstruction.

4. *Competence* refers to the state of the venous valves in relationship to flow signals and the various maneuvers that are involved in the examination. For example, a thrombosed segment of vein will not show flow, and adjacent collateral veins will have a high-pitched signal. The patent portion of the vein distal to an obstruction will have a continuous flow with no respiratory variation, and the Valsalva maneuver does not produce change. Limb compression may produce limited augmentation, but clearly less than in the normal vein.

5. *Pulsatility* refers to situations, such as congestive heart failure, in which with elevated venous pressure, the venous sounds may be difficult to distinguish from arterial sounds; and instead of varying with respiration, pulsations can be appreciated.[4, 5]

PULSE VOLUME STUDIES

The pulse volume recorder is a system that is based on a recording air-plethysmograph system using standard blood pressure cuffs applied at the toe, midfoot, and ankle; below the knee; above the knee; and at high thigh regions. The cuffs are inflated to a pressure of 65 mm Hg for the recordings so that the cuff will optimally contact the extremity. The sensitive transducer detects the small increase in pressure within the cuff that results during systole. The pulse volume recorder is a qualitative, not quantitative, representation of arterial flow. A tracing of the pulse wave is provided by the recorder. The tracing from each level is categorized as normal, mildly abnormal, moderately abnormal, or severely abnormal. The normal waveform has a brisk, sharp rise to the systolic peak ("teepee"-shaped) and usually displays a prominent dicrotic notch. Fast flow is represented by a narrow "teepee"-shaped peak, whereas slow flow is represented by a rounded ("igloo"-shaped) tracing. Early disease is characterized by the absence of a dicrotic notch and a more gradual, prolonged downslope. Moderate disease is characterized by the rounded systolic peak. Severe occlusion is represented by a flattened wave with a slow upstroke and downstroke. The pulse volume recordings should correlate with results of Doppler studies. Amplitudes should be compared from one side to the other to assess unilateral disease.[4, 5]

PHOTOPLETHYSMOGRAPHY

Photoplethysmography is used to indicate skin blood flow. An infrared frequency is emitted and reflected by hemoglobin molecules located in the cutaneous microcirculation. A photoelectric detector measures this reflected beam, and the signal is transformed and recorded as a waveform. This waveform is representative of pulsatile flow in the subpapillary venous plexus of the skin. Photoplethysmography should be used to record skin flow around ulcerations and is essential if lower extremity surgery is a consideration. Waveforms recorded from the plantar tufts of the digits are much larger than those recorded from other places on the skin.

Normal rapid flow looks like a narrow "teepee"-shaped waveform. Lesser backward flow is represented by a much smaller peak on the downslope of the first. The notch between the two peaks, the dicrotic notch, denotes blood flow in a forward and backward fashion. The presence of the dicrotic notch implies that there is no significant obstruction in any proximal connecting artery. However, blood flow can still be normal in the absence of the dicrotic notch in skin because the vessels are so small. Discrepancies between the dicrotic notching and audible sounds of digital arteries should be rechecked.[4]

DUPLEX SCANNING

Duplex scanning is a noninvasive, direct, functional test for peripheral artery stenosis. Peripheral arterial stenosis can be localized and classified with this modality nearly as well as angiography. It is particularly used for the diagnosis of aortoiliac disease and is ideally suited for follow-up after angioplasty or other forms of revascularization. Duplex scanning can identify lesions that are amenable to percutaneous transluminal angioplasty. Duplex examinations guide the angiographer to diseased segments. This test has also been used to identify grafts at risk for sudden thrombosis.

B-mode imaging is combined with pulsed Doppler ultrasonography to obtain arterial imaging and velocity information from the actual sites of stenosis. The image is used to direct the pulsed Doppler sample volume to a specific location in the arterial segments and to determine the incidence angle of the Doppler beam with the vessel axis. Velocity information is recorded graphically with time on the abscissa and velocity on the ordinate, and the amplitude of the velocity signal is indicated by shades of gray.[6]

OXIMETRY

Oximetry is used to measure arterial oxygenation with the inherent advantage of depending on transillumination and optical analysis at two wavelengths rather than transcutaneous flow of oxygen. It is a noninvasive means of monitoring oxygenation primarily in adults. It requires a low temperature of about 39°C, which diminishes the danger of local burning. The pulse oximeter has a built-in signal of inaccuracy when blood flow is low.[7]

Arteriography

Arteriography is used primarily in the extremities to image the effects of atherosclerosis. Its serves as a road map for surgical or percutaneous angioplasty and is invaluable in the evaluation of vascular integrity after trauma. It has also been used to demonstrate the vascular supply to tumors and to detect arteriovenous connections.

Arteriograms involve isolation of a vessel for placement of the arteriogram catheter. The femoral artery is commonly used. If the iliac system is patent on the side of the arterial puncture, the catheter can be advanced into the aorta to give bilateral runoff arteriograms, or the catheter may be advanced into the contralateral iliac and thus the femoral system and below to give more selective views. Aortograms are typically used to demonstrate the aorto-iliac, femoral, popliteal, and distal circulation. Common complications include dye reactions, contrast material–induced changes in renal function, and localized hematoma.[4, 8]

ARTERIAL DISEASE
Atherosclerosis

Atherosclerosis is a degenerative process of the arteries and is characterized by the deposition of fatty substances and fibrous thickening of the intimal layer of the artery, resulting in the narrowing of the vessel lumen and hardening and loss of elasticity of the vessel wall.

As part of the normal aging process, the arteries undergo a process commonly referred to as "hardening of the arteries." This process is characterized by increase in the intimal area, a loss of the elasticity of the vessel wall, and an increase in both calcium content and diameter of the vessel. Studies by various authors determined that the lesion of atherosclerosis is an intimal proliferation of smooth muscle cells that occurs mainly at vessel branch points in arteries.[3, 9] These cells will proliferate initially when no free fat is demonstrable in the cells. With time and advancement of the atherosclerotic process, free fat appears in the intimal cells and later in the extracellular space. The fatty deposits accumulate along the intimal layer and may eventually occlude blood flow or become a complicated lesion, leading to thrombosis, calcification, or aneurysm formation.

Atherosclerosis of the lower extremity may go undiagnosed because the process may remain asymptomatic. When the initial symptom of intermittent claudication presents there is already significant disease and a greatly increased morbidity from coronary and cerebrovascular disease.

PATHOGENESIS

Before the theory of Juergens, Spittell, and Fairbairn,[10] two hypotheses were considered regarding the etiology of atherosclerosis. The "imbilution hypotheses" by Virchow (later modified as the lipid hypothesis) stated that lipids in the arterial wall represent a transduction of blood lipids that form complexes with acid mucopolysaccharide. The arterial accumulation occurs because of the lack of a mechanism for removing the lipids. The "incrustation theory" of Robitansky suggested that intimal thickening results from fibrin deposition with subsequent organization of fibroblasts with secondary accumulation of lipids. Recently this theory has been modified, suggesting that endothelial cell injury with deposition of platelets initiates the intimal proliferation. Juergens, Spittell, and Fairbairn[10] integrate both of these theories and state that "the pathogenesis of atherosclerosis depends upon a complex sequence of critical events occurring in the interaction of blood elements with the arterial wall and each event may be modified by a different risk factor." These researchers indicate that both lipid transport and platelet interaction with the arterial wall play important roles in this sequence. Based on experimental evidence, the major critical events in the development of atherosclerosis appear to be the following:

■ Hemodynamic stress
■ Endothelial injury
■ Arterial wall–platelet interaction
■ Smooth muscle cell proliferation
■ Lipid and lipoprotein entry and accumulation
■ Altered mechanisms of lipid removal
■ Fibrosis and the development of fibrin thrombi
■ Ulceration, calcification, and formation of aneurysms

ETIOLOGY

Various risk factors have been established for the development of atherosclerotic disease.[10-12] These risk factors include age and gender, diabetes mellitus, hypertension, hyperlipoproteinemia, cigarette smoking, and a positive family history.

Age and Gender. Atherosclerosis occurs predominantly among men between the ages of 50 and 70 years. The disease tends to become symptomatic 5 to 10 years earlier in men. Women tend to become affected at a later age and have an increased incidence after the age of 60 years. This is probably due to the postmenopausal loss of the protective effect of estrogen. Clinical trials have shown that administration of estrogen to men who had previous coronary thrombosis decreased the number of secondary coronary attacks.

Diabetes Mellitus. Diabetes is a significant risk factor for the development of atherosclerosis. In general, the mechanisms involved are poorly understood. The severity and extent of atherosclerosis is increased in patients with diabetes. Studies by Kannel and McGee[13] indicated that patients with impaired glucose tolerance were at increased risk for developing atherosclerosis obliterans. Diabetics have a higher incidence of below-the-knee disease (trifurcation disease),[12] a similar incidence of femoropopliteal disease, and a lower incidence of aortoiliac disease than nondiabetic patients. Atherosclerosis affecting the diabetic usually involves the smaller arteries, beginning at the knee and including the anterior tibial, posterior tibial, and the peroneal arteries.

Levin and O'Neal[11] stated that "it is the accelerated and more pronounced atherosclerosis of the arterioles that differentiates the peripheral vascular disease of the diabetic from that of the non-diabetic." Control of serum glucose levels has not been found to reduce the risk of or slow the rate of atherosclerosis. In a 25-year study, Pirart[14] concluded that serum glucose control does not slow the acceleration of atherosclerosis. Good control may prevent or stabilize the microangiopathies such as retinopathy or nephropathy; however, this has not been proven to reduce the risk of peripheral vascular disease.

Hypertension. Hypertension has been shown to increase the development of coronary artery disease; however, a correlation between hypertension and atherosclerosis of the extremities has yet to be proven.

Patients with hypertension have been shown to have an increased incidence of coronary artery disease, as well as cerebrovascular disease. Evidence suggests that increased turbulence of blood flow particularly in hypertensive patients at selected anatomical sites within the arterial tree may result in endothelial cell damage and in the development of atherosclerotic lesions. Increased pressure within the arteries causes sclerosis of the vessel wall. Damage to the vessel wall can result in thrombosis or rupture. The earliest stage in the development of these atheromatous plaques on the inner surfaces of the arteries is damage to the endothelial cells and underlying intima. The damage may be caused by the physical abrasion of the endothelium by the pulsating arterial pressure on the vessel wall.[15] Once a plaque has developed on an arterial wall of a hypertensive patient, the blood flow becomes turbulent. This will aggravate the situation, causing more damage to the endothelial cell lining, and the process continues.

Hyperlipidemia. Hyperlipidemia has also been proven to be a causative factor in coronary artery disease; however, no clear-cut data show evidence of hyperlipidemia as a cause of peripheral vascular disease.

Elevations of lipoproteins of low density and lipoproteins of very low density are associated with atherosclerosis. Hyperlipoproteinemia has specifically been associated with atherosclerosis in young patients.[9] The lipids of atherosclerotic plaques are derived from plasma lipoproteins. Circulating lipoproteins therefore play an important role in the pathogenesis of atherosclerotic vascular disease.

Lees and Frederickson[16] classified primary lipid disorders into five basic types using a paper electrophoretic technique to separate and identify the major lipoprotein classes. Types II, III, and IV are associated with premature atherosclerosis. Types I and V, which are fat-induced hyperlipidemias, are not associated with premature atherosclerosis. The development of atherosclerotic plaques depends in large part on the presence of certain lipids and lipoproteins in the vessel lumen at the time of endothelial injury.[11] The lipids travel through gaps between endothelial cells in the vessel wall, where they accumulate and serve as irritants stimulating more scar tissue formation along the vessel wall.

Cigarette Smoking. Cigarette smoking has also been shown to increase the incidence of atherosclerotic heart disease and peripheral vascular disease. Cigarette smoking has been determined to decrease high density lipoprotein cholesterol levels, alter platelet functions, and directly injure endothelial cells, thereby causing proliferation of arterial smooth muscle cells. Smoking causes intimal layer injury and platelet defects. This combination may lead to an increased tendency for thrombus formation.

Because cigarette smoking increases the carboxyhemoglobin levels in the blood, it decreases the oxygen-carrying capacity of the red blood cells, which leads to a hypoxic state. Couch[17] has demonstrated the effects of cigarette smoking as a cause of atherosclerosis. He stated that intimal injury may be caused by increased levels of carboxyhemoglobin or by platelet dysfunction leading to an increased tendency toward thrombus formation. Studies by Nadler and associates[18] have revealed that cigarette smoking inhibits prostacyclin forma-

tion. An important effect of smoking is its possible influence on prostacyclin formation by the endothelium.[19] Prostacyclin is an important prostaglandin that promotes vasodilation. These adverse effects are compounded by the vasoconstrictive properties of nicotine.

Family History. Genetics play a major role in the etiology of various lipid disorders. Genetic dyslipidemias may be associated with atherosclerosis. This may be due to an inherited familiar hypercholesterolemia. The abundant cholesterol occurs almost entirely in the low density lipoproteins. This often results from lack of low density lipoproteins receptors on cell membranes. Patients with hereditary atherosclerosis may have normal serum cholesterol levels, but other factors may lead to disease.

PATHOPHYSIOLOGY

Atherosclerosis most often occurs at the origin of arteries or at sites of bifurcation. A common area of involvement is the superficial femoral artery at Hunter's canal. Atherosclerotic plaques tend to involve the arteries in a circumferential pattern; however, in the lower extremity, they frequently occur on the posterior aspect of the arteries.

With progression of the disease process, segmental occlusion of the arterial supply develops. Tissues distal to the obstruction undergo ischemic changes, although the degree of ischemia depends on the location and extent of the occlusive process and on the development of collateral channels.[12]

SIGNS AND SYMPTOMS

The symptoms of atherosclerosis are usually gradual as a result of a slowly progressive obliteration of the arterial lumen. The various symptoms affecting patients are sometimes subtle and at other times may be quite evident. A common complaint of patients with arteriosclerosis obliterans is intermittent claudication. Classically, the patient will complain of pain, ache, cramping, or a sense of fatigue in a distinct muscle group that is brought on by a definite amount of walking and is relieved by rest. This is readily reproducible. Intermittent claudication most commonly results from atherosclerosis but may result from other types of occlusive arterial disease. In chronic occlusive arterial disease, intermittent claudication is usually the earliest symptom. It may be unilateral at first, with subsequent involvement of the contralateral leg. The most common part affected is the calf. However, it may also occur in the lower back, hip, thigh, and foot. The distance that the patient is able to walk before symptoms develop varies with the severity of the arterial occlusion.

As the atherosclerotic disease progresses, patients will often complain of rest pain, usually occurring at night. The symptoms of rest pain indicate that the disease process is more severe and has advanced to the point at which the tissues are poorly oxygenated without the stress of muscle use. The patient will often complain of having night pain occurring in the toes that is relieved by placing the limb in a dependent position. Dependency allows for increased tissue perfusion distally. The affected foot usually demonstrates pallor when the limb is placed in the elevated position, and rubor is apparent on dependency. As stated before, the patient will usually experience pain at the distalmost part, in this case, the digits. But pain may also occur in the foot or leg. The pain most commonly occurs at night and is a dull, persistent, aching type of pain that may interfere with sleep. Rest pain may be the result of gradual, chronic, and progressive arterial occlusion. It also often follows acute arterial occlusion. When ischemia becomes so severe that the tissues are hypoxic, they begin to necrose and ulcerate.

When the arteriosclerosis obliterans progresses to this stage, the pain can be moderate to severe. The pain is usually worse at night and persists for a long period of time. Diabetics or patients with peripheral neuropathies of other causes may not have pain associated with the clinical picture of severe vessel disease. The pain is aggravated often by elevation of the limb, which would reduce arterial flow to the distal tissues and make the ischemic situation worse.

Eventually, ischemia will lead to tissue necrosis. Ulcerations or dry gangrene may develop at the distal aspect of the digits or over areas of constant pressure. Patients with arterial insufficiency will often describe cold sensitivity of the foot.[20] Other patients complain of dysesthesias such as burning, tingling, or numbness of the feet and toes. These are common symptoms in patients with neuropathies secondary to diabetes and alcohol abuse even in the presence of adequate arterial perfusion.

Patients with severe arterial insufficiency often develop sedentary lifestyles owing to pain and cramping. Eventually, diffuse atrophy occurs, evident by muscle weakness, muscle atrophy, and osteoporosis of the lower limb. Pain associated with ischemic neuropathy is usually quite severe and can occur as numbness, tingling, or a burning sensation. This type of pain usually occurs in the digits but can be more proximal.

PHYSICAL EXAMINATION

The physical examination in the assessment of atherosclerosis obliterans is of utmost importance and can be used to differentiate it from other vascular disorders. The examination should consist of a systematic approach. The examiner should compare one lower extremity with the other, because one limb is usually affected more severely than the other. The first examination should be observation of the lower extremity. Important observations, which are signs of atherosclerosis obliterans, are trophic changes such as atrophy of the digits, dystrophic nails, color changes, and alterations. Skin changes such as cracking or dryness and poor skin turgor are also a possible sign of arterial disease. The absence of hair growth is not an accurate indicator of disease, since it may decrease normally with advancing age. The skin may often appear tight, shiny, and thin. The classic color changes associated with atherosclerosis obliterans vary based on the severity of the disease. In advanced disease, gangrenous changes and possibly ulceration may be present. In severe cases, the feet are ruborous. The patient may have pallor on elevation and rubor on dependency. This finding indicates long-standing arterial disease.

The pulses of the lower extremity should be palpated. These include the femoral, popliteal, posterior tibial, and dorsalis pedis arteries. Assessment of capillary refill in the digits is important and should be done while the leg is still in the elevated position by pressing and releasing the distal pulp of the toe. The normal capillary refill time should be between 3 and 5 seconds. The absence of the pedal pulses should raise the suspicion of proximal occlusion, stenosis, or severe atherosclerosis. Both the strength and regularity of the pulses should be noted. In a case of arterial insufficiency, the patient's feet may also appear cyanotic or with pallor of the digits and possibly more color changes in severe cases.

Temperature differences may be evident when both extremities are compared. Extremities with arterial insufficiency may feel cool to palpation, and often an obvious area of demarcation and temperature gradient may be noted. The Brodie's Trendelenburg test consists of elevating and exsanguinating the limb, placing a tourniquet on the calf, and situating the limb in a dependent position. The tourniquet is then removed. Following removal of the tourniquet, filling of the previously marked vein on the foot that takes more than 35 seconds indicates arterial insufficiency. This test may also be used to assess the superficial venous system.

LABORATORY TESTS

The history and physical examination can give the practitioner important information regarding the circulatory status of a patient. To quantify this information, various noninvasive modalities may be used. A simple vascular laboratory test is the ankle-arm systolic blood pressure index. Other tests using the noninvasive Doppler instrumentation are segmental pressures and segmental volume photoplethysmography. Transcutaneous oxygen measurement assesses tissue perfusion and has been thought to yield a more accurate degree of ischemia. Duplex ultrasonography has been implemented in the evaluation of lower extremity arterial occlusive disease. This modality has been utilized for assessment of larger vessels of the thigh and popliteal region. A relatively new modality in the evaluation of the patient with vascular disease is positron emission tomography. The use of this technique in the study of vascular disease appears valuable in the area of regional blood flow, regional oxygen extraction ratio, and local metabolic rate for oxygen. Arteriography is the gold standard for visualizing the lower extremity arterial tree if surgical treatment is a consideration.

Embolism and Thrombosis

An arterial embolus is a clot that has traveled from a distant site and is forced into a smaller artery. Emboli may detach from any location in the heart or arterial tree and progress through the bloodstream to lodge in any artery in the body. Arterial emboli may also originate from proximal ulcerated arterial plaque or thrombus. Small embolic occlusion of the digital vessels and other small end-arteries is known as blue toe syndrome or atheromatous emboli syndrome. The patient may present with digital necrosis and ecchymotic areas that may progress to gangrenous areas. It is important for the physician to realize that this may be caused by an embolus from a more proximal site.

The signs of acute arterial occlusion vary from the time of occlusion to the time of presentation. For instance, if the patient is examined within 8 hours of acute occlusion, the extremity will appear pale secondary to acute spastic reaction of the distal arteries. At 12 to 24 hours following occlusion, the involved extremity may appear cyanotic and mottled. The spasm that caused the pallor now resolves, and a rebound vasodilatation occurs. The limb may feel soft initially and, later, if allowed to remain ischemic, the muscles become firm and rigid.

The Doppler device may be used to detect the site of the embolus and confirm the absence of pulses. Both limbs need to be elevated, and the Doppler study is performed to obtain segmental pressures and pulse waveforms that may indicate the area of occlusion. Angiography may be used when the presentation is somewhat ambiguous and may also aid in the differentiation between embolic occlusion from thrombotic occlusion. Other advantages of arteriography include its use in localizing the occlusion and in diagnosing atypical causes of acute ischemia, such as dissecting aneurysms and giant cell arteritis. Angiography is invasive and therefore not without potential complications. In most cases of an acute occlusive event, the clinical picture alone is enough to make the diagnosis of an embolic event.

TREATMENT

The initial management of acute arterial occlusion is anticoagulation therapy with heparin. A bolus of heparin is given followed by a heparin infusion to maintain therapeutic anticoagulation.

The surgical treatment varies depending on whether the occlusion is embolic or thrombotic. In embolic events, surgical embolectomy is indicated to reperfuse the limb. In cases of thrombosis, surgical thrombectomy in conjunction with a definitive reconstructive procedure has been proven to reduce morbidity and mortality rates.[21]

In the diagnosis of an arterial embolus, the "five Ps" (pain, pallor, paresthesia, pulselessness, and paralysis) may be found. The onset of pain is sudden, since the patient is able to pinpoint the onset of the pain that is caused by the rapid ischemic event. The pain is most intense in the distal part of the extremity. Paresthesia is usually the next symptom. Pallor or decrease in local temperature may be the next manifestation. All pulses distal to the occlusion are absent, and the pulse above the site of lodgment of the embolus may be strong, caused by increased resistance secondary to the clot. It is important to note the level of the ischemic change by detecting temperature change using the back of the hand. Sensory changes should also be recorded carefully. Paresthesia and hyperesthesia are signs of advancement of ischemia. If the situation advances to the point of paralysis, then irreparable damage has usually been done. The muscles, especially those of the calf, are at first soft but later become indurated. When they become firm and tight, the changes are considered irreversible.

The diagnosis of acute emboli should be established by the findings of the history and physical examination. Instrumentation such as the Doppler sensor can be used to detect the site of the embolus and confirm the absence of pulses. Arteriosclerotic heart disease and myocardial infarction are the most frequent source for arterial emboli.[22] Emboli may also originate from prosthetic heart valves, aortic atheromatous plaques, and aortic aneurysms.

Aneurysms

An aneurysm is a permanent dilatation of an artery. Once the initial process begins, an aneurysm enlarges gradually and a thrombus usually develops within the aneurysm. The increasing size may lead to multiple complications such as compression of adjacent structures, hemorrhage, rupture of the artery, thrombosis, and embolization. Aneurysms have a tendency to develop at areas where the artery is not supported by skeletal muscle and is therefore subject to bending forces.

Various types of aneurysms exist. A fusiform aneurysm is one in which there is a uniform diffuse dilatation of a segment of an artery. In a saccular aneurysm there is an "outpouching" of an artery resulting from stretching and a thinning of the medial layer. A dissecting aneurysm is a cavity formed by dissection of blood that forms between layers of the vessel wall. A false aneurysm is defined by the development of a sac surrounding a hematoma that maintains a communication with the lumen of an artery whose wall has been ruptured.

The most common cause of an aneurysm is atherosclerosis. Other less common causes include congenital defects of the vessel wall, vascular trauma (including both blunt and penetrating types), infection (specifically syphilitic and mycotic), and polyarteritis.

Aneurysms are more common in older men, usually appearing after the age of 50. Clinical signs of aneurysm may be detected in the foot. Thromboembolism from an abdominal aortic aneurysm, for example, may manifest itself in the foot. The patient may present with multiple emboli from a proximal site. This is commonly referred to as "shower emboli" or "blue toe syndrome."

Popliteal artery aneurysms commonly occur just distal to the knee where the artery bends frequently. There is a 60% incidence of bilateral popliteal artery aneurysms. Popliteal aneurysms are associated with aneurysms of other larger vessels, such as the abdominal aorta or femoral artery.[23]

The diagnosis of aneurysms of the lower extremity, specifically the femoral and popliteal arteries, can be made by means of a careful physical examination. A pulsating mass can be detected by palpation using a thumb and index finger. Expansion of the artery on pulsation can be felt if the thumb and forefingers are placed on each side of the mass. A systolic bruit can often be heard with the use of the "bell end" of the stethoscope.

The use of B-mode ultrasonography is a reliable means of diagnosis of popliteal and femoral aneurysms. This procedure can differentiate an aneurysm from a cyst or tumor within the popliteal fossa area.

Complications of femoral and popliteal artery aneurysms include thrombosis and distal embolization.[23] These complications can lead to ischemia, ranging from claudication to superficial infarction of tissues of the forefoot to digital artery occlusion. These thrombotic or embolic events may ultimately cause gangrene of the toes, foot, or leg. Complications of aneurysms may result in severe ischemic situations. The detection of this anomaly is critical, and repair before embolic or thrombotic symptoms become evident is crucial to prevent limb or digit loss.

Mönckeberg's Medical Calcific Sclerosis (Senile Medial Calcinosis)

In the early 1900s, Mönckeberg, a German pathologist, studied vascular disease in the elderly. He found that elderly and middle-aged persons, especially men, may have extensive finely divided calcinosis of the aorta and large arteries of the extremities. This calcinosis occurring in the medial layer of the artery is known as medial calcinosis or medial calcification. Medial calcinosis may involve the large and medium-sized arteries of the extremities with extensive changes in the medial layer of the vessel and minimal involvement of the intimal layer. The vessel layer changes consist of fragmentation, degeneration, and actual disappearance of muscle and elastic fibers and replacement with fibrous tissue. Calcium deposits and focal hemorrhage are usually seen as secondary manifestations. The medial layer may be either thickened or thinned by this process. There may be irregular increases in the diameter of the vessels as well as increases in the vessel length, leading to tortuosity. The biomechanical changes in the arteries do not differ from those resulting from mechanical injury and repair of other connective tissues. The disease process of medial calcific sclerosis according to Mönckeberg is of little clinical significance and does not in itself indicate arterial occlusive disease or weakness of the vessel walls.

Fibromuscular Dysplasia (Hyperplasia)

Fibromuscular dysplasia is a segmental, nonatherosclerotic vascular disease of unknown cause that primarily affects arteries of intermediate size. Fibromuscular dysplasia was first described in 1938 by Leadbetter and Burkland. Arteriography has made it possible to make this diagnosis since this process is seen on the arteriogram as a "string of beads" appearance of the affected vessel. Fibromuscular disease most commonly occurs in the renal artery of young and middle-aged women; however, it may be seen in multiple arteries. Hypertension is usually the dominant symptom of the disease.

In symptomatic patients, obstruction usually results from intraluminal impingement by the deranged and protuberant media or by constrictive fibrosis of the vessel wall. The diagnosis of fibromuscular dysplasia is made on the basis of angiographic findings. A classification of fibromuscular dysplasia was proposed and formulated by Harrison and McCormack. Intimal fibromuscular dysplasia causes a rarely seen concentric narrowing of the arterial lumen owing to an intimal proliferation different from an organized mural thrombus. Medial disease causes a narrowing of the arterial lumen because of an increase in fibroelastic tissue and in deranged muscular elements of the tunica media.

Adventitial fibromuscular dysplasia is the least common of the various types within the classification scheme. In this type there is an increase in the fibrous elements surrounding the artery that cause a narrowing of the arterial lumen.

Cystic Medial Necrosis

Cystic medial necrosis was first described by Erdheim in 1929 and is characterized by noninflammatory focal accumulations of mucoid material in the media of the artery. These cystic lesions lie parallel to the medial fibers and are usually found in the middle and outer thirds of the media layer. The lesions are seen most commonly in the aorta but have been found in various other arteries. Disruption of the media involves the elastic collagen, smooth muscle cells, and ground substance. The disruption is related to the aging process and occurs prematurely in patients with Marfan's syndrome. According to Lie and Jeurgens,[13] the disruption is not cystic because the space represents a collection of gel-like ground substance without a distinct lining. It is not necrosis, as originally thought, but rather structural faults in the media layer resulting from degeneration of the elastic tissue and smooth muscle cells.

VASOSPASTIC DISORDERS

Raynaud's Syndrome

Raynaud's syndrome is a collection of symptoms caused by vasospastic changes that usually occur in the fingers and toes. This vasospastic mechanism can be exacerbated by poor blood circulation, but the exact pathogenesis is unclear. Attacks of threefold color change are brought on by exposure to cold or emotional upset. White (digital arteriolar vasospasm) is followed by blue (blood desaturation) and then by red (hyperemia). Color changes may occur in the sequence just described, in isolation (one or two of the three), or, on occasion, simultaneously in different parts of a single extremity. Changes may vary from finger to finger. Thumbs are often spared. Bilateral, symmetric involvement of the hands occurs, and normal pulses are present. Symptoms have persisted for at least 2 years without identification of any underlying cause. Digital gangrene is only limited (superficial) or nonexistent. Varon and colleagues discussed three mechanisms that compromise digital blood flow: (1) decreased perfusion pressure, (2) decreased digital artery radius, and (3) increased blood viscosity.[24, 25]

Raynaud's symptoms are associated with several diseases. Ninety-five percent of patients with scleroderma, 91% of patients with mixed connective tissue disease, and 40% of patients with systemic lupus erythematosus have presented with Raynaud's symptoms. According to Goodfield, less than 10% of patients with primary *Raynaud's phenomenon* associated with 20

systemic diseases develop connective tissue disease later in life, so the outlook is very good. If symptoms of Raynaud's syndrome begin before the age of 20 years, the likelihood of an associated connective tissue disease decreases. However, a positive antinuclear antibody test or severe onset of symptoms is indicative of an associated connective tissue disease. Internal Raynaud's syndrome affects the organs with or without concurrent cutaneous digital vasospasm. This may cause clinical problems such as angina and nephropathy. Renal involvement is the most important predictor of prognosis in patients with connective tissue disease.[24, 26]

Raynaud's syndrome affects women nine times more than it affects men. The initial benign episodes usually appear in the second or third decade of life. The fingers and toes are most commonly affected. Unusual sites affected include the tongue, throat, penis, vulva, and pinnae of the ears. Skin overlying the knees, elbows, and heels is usually affected in slender persons. Complaints may include numbness of the fingers; dysfunction, lessened dexterity, and decreased sensation in the hands; ulceration of the fingertips; and, rarely, gangrene.[24]

Raynaud's disease is thought to be caused by digital artery vasospasm and refers to symptoms occurring in the absence of underlying conditions. It is mainly a disorder of women who are younger than 40 years of age. The prognosis is excellent. Mild cases respond to simple preventive measures such as the use of heavy gloves and socks and avoidance of cold exposure and sympathetic agonists, such as caffeine, nicotine, or antihistamines. Sympathectomy has a more lasting benefit in Raynaud's disease than in scleroderma.[25, 27]

Raynaud's phenomenon has been used to describe digital changes occurring in association with other diseases. It may occur as a primary disorder (Raynaud's disease) or secondary to a number of underlying conditions (secondary Raynaud's phenomenon). All the secondary forms of Raymond's phenomenon must be ruled out to make a diagnosis of the primary disorder. Spittell and coworkers[27] suggest that propranolol precipitates this phenomenon and that increased incidence has been found in men receiving combination chemotherapy for testicular cancer.

The key to diagnosis is in the patient's history. The interview and physical examination can be used to identify associated conditions, primarily connective tissue disorders. Symptoms and signs include joint swelling, skin changes, telangiectasias, dysphagia, and conjunctivitis, as well as decreased lacrimation and dry mouth.[25]

On examination of the skin, physical findings include one or more of the symptoms of pallor, cyanosis, and rubor. These changes may be elicited by a cold challenge, classically done by immersing the hands in cold water. The nail fold capillaries can be examined by applying immersion oil to the nail folds and then using a widefield microscope. Abnormal findings suggest that a significant associated condition may be present. For example, dilated, tortuous capillaries and dropout of capillaries may be the earliest indicators of the subsequent appearance of scleroderma. Peripheral pulses should be assessed. The Allen test is used to determine patency or occlusion of the ulnar artery or radial artery in the hand, occlusion of the superficial palmar arch or digital arteries, or both. Asymmetric symptoms suggest vascular compromise, such as atherosclerosis, thoracic outlet syndrome, or occupational injury. Tests for thoracic outlet compression are particularly indicated in the examination of patients with unilateral symptoms. Symmetric symptoms suggest primary Raynaud's disease or an association with connective tissue disease.[24, 25]

Laboratory assessment should include a complete blood cell count, urinalysis, erythrocyte sedimentation rate, chemistry profile, antinuclear antibody tests, and rheumatoid factor determination. If antinuclear antibody is positive and other features of scleroderma or CREST syndrome are present, an anti-topoisomerase I and anticentromere antibody assay may confirm CREST syndrome and primary systemic scleroderma, respectively. Digital arteriography and thermography are considered research tools only. However, Doppler ultrasonography, digital subtraction angiography, and digital plethysmography may be helpful in the diagnosis if disease of the larger vessels is suspected.[24, 25]

There is no cure for Raynaud's syndrome. All cases do not require therapy. Pharmaco-logic therapy is necessary if vasospasm causes pain, dysesthesia, or dysfunction or if digital ulceration or gangrene is incipient. Patients should be advised to avoid tobacco use and passive smoke from any source. They should limit their intake of caffeine and switch to de-caffeinated drinks. Sources of vibrational injury, such as jackhammers and chain saws, should be avoided. Treatment includes avoidance of precipitating factors, biofeedback (a self-hypnosis, relaxation, meditation, and visual imagery technique that rewarms skin), and pharmacologic therapy. Vardon and colleagues[25] relate calcium channel blockers as the most successful pharmacologic therapy. Diltiazem, nifedipine, and nicardipine (but not verapamil) decrease the severity and frequency of attacks, but in most cases digital blood flow and temperature were not significantly changed. These drugs promote digital arteriolar vasodilation. They are widely used as antihypertensives and antianginals and are tolerated well by most patients. Side effects include orthostatic hypotension, diarrhea, and flushing. Stanley and associates listed several pharmacologic agents but advised that risks, benefits, and cost should be carefully considered. Hyperbaric oxygen may be helpful if digital ulceration is a factor. Surgical therapy entails digital sympathectomy.[24, 28]

Acrocyanosis

Acrocyanosis is a rare disorder of the peripheral vascular circulation that is characterized by a purple/blue discoloration of the hand, feet, and face. The discoloration is not an intermittent problem, and this distinguishes acrocyanosis from Raynaud's phenomenon. Sufferers seem to have a low resting blood flow, probably coupled with venous stasis, so that blood becomes much more deoxygenated in the extremities than normal. Patients complain of coldness and color of the affected part. The onset is most common during adolescence and early adult life. The ratio of female-to-male cases is on the order of 6:1. Treatment is not beneficial.

Acrocyanosis has been associated with anorexia nervosa, Asperger's syndrome, and palmoplantar keratoderma.[29] Why acrocyanosis occurs in anorexia nervosa is uncertain. Bhanji and Mattingly[20] found 32 anorectics (21%) of 155 anorectic subjects to have acrocyanosis. Acrocyanosis was more prevalent among the more severe anorectic subjects. It was associated with facial and trunk pallor, slower pulse rates, and higher fasting plasma glucose levels. Hand and calf blood flow was found to be reduced as compared with healthy controls. The body's core temperature has been poorly maintained, and bradycardia has frequently been present in anorectics.

Rustin and colleagues[30] reported two patients with anorexia nervosa with associated acromegaly to have acrocyanosis. These subjects developed soft tissue swelling of their hands, worsening of their peripheral vascular disease, evidenced by the appearance of acrocyanosis and Raynaud's phenomenon, and a worse prognosis following the onset of their anorexia nervosa. Oral nifedipine significantly improved the chilblains and Raynaud's phenomenon but had no effect on the acrocyanosis. However, ketanserin improved the acrocyanosis in one of the subjects.[20, 26, 29–31]

Livedo Reticularis

Livedo reticularis is a disorder of vasoconstriction that involves the subpapillary venous plexus of the dermis. The etiology is unknown, but the presumed mechanism includes arteriolar constriction followed by stasis and dilation of capillaries and veins. The capillaries fill with unsaturated blood, resulting in a netlike marbled bluish or reddish appearance of the skin. This local area of mottling or reticular blue discoloration generally occurs on the shins and feet. This disorder usually begins before the ages of 20 and 30. The incidence in men versus women is the same. Livedo reticularis has an idiopathic and a secondary form.

The idiopathic form has two variants: cutis marmorata and livedo reticularis idiopathica. Cutis marmorata is a physiologic response of normal dermal arterioles to cold exposure that disappears with warming. It is a benign and transient mottling seen most often in swimmers or others whose skin is exposed on a cool day. Livedo reticularis idiopathica has a more intense mottling that is persistent and does not disappear in warm environments. A high incidence of hypertension is present in the idiopathic form.

Secondary livedo reticularis may be the initial manifestation of systemic lupus erythematosus and polyarteritis nodosa. In the Sneddon syndrome, livedo reticularis is associated with cerebrovascular pathology (strokes and nerve palsies), which may be fatal. When secondary to therapy with amantadine hydrochloride, livedo reticularis will disappear 2 to 4 weeks after the drug is discontinued. In its secondary form, the reticular discoloration usually persists no matter what changes occur in environmental temperature.[1, 26, 27, 32]

Livedo reticularis is usually a benign disorder, but occasionally ulceration and gangrene occur. Ulcerations usually appear in winter and heal in summer. Abstinence from smoking and protection from cold may be helpful. Treatment is usually not required. Some patients note aching, coldness, and soreness that may be disabling. Lumbar sympathectomy may provide a great deal of symptomatic relief in these cases.[1, 26, 27, 32]

Erythermalgia

Erythermalgia is a rare disorder in which episodes of symptomatic intense vasodilation occur in the hands and feet. Erythema is accompanied by increased skin temperature and pain. The increased cutaneous blood flow tends to persist even in cold environments. The idiopathic form of this disorder is not well understood but is related to decreased vasomotor tone. The secondary form of this disorder may be due to obstructive arterial disease, myeloproliferative disorders, polycythemia, hypertension, or a successful arterial bypass graft. Occasionally, erythermalgia is hereditary. There is no sex predilection, and the disease may occur at any age.

The onset of this disorder is insidious, but the frequency and duration of attacks may become more pronounced. Symptoms may eventually become almost continuous, causing total disability. During an attack, patients will complain of burning pain usually in the balls of the feet and tips of the toes and less commonly in the corresponding parts of the hands. The attacks are usually provoked by elevation of skin temperature, whether by environmental heat, exercise, or dependency; they are relieved by elevation or cool of the affected extremity. Trophic changes, ulcerations, and gangrene are rare.

Treatment is symptomatic and includes avoidance of heat exposure.[32] Elevation of the extremity and cold applications may terminate an attack. Aspirin (650 mg) is usually effective. Calderone and Finzi reported successful results with piroxicam (10 to 20 mg) in patients with aspirin allergy.[33] Vasoconstrictive agents, such as methysergide or epinephrine, or β-adrenergic blocking agents, such as propranolol, have also been effective in some patients. Secondary cases may be managed by treating the primary disorder.[1, 32, 33]

COLD-RELATED DISORDERS

Chilblains (Perniosis)

Chilblains presents as inflammatory, usually bilateral, symmetric lesions of the skin that occur as an abnormal reaction to a moderate degree of cold. Chilblains is rare in bitterly cold climates. It is more commonly associated with continued exposure to damp, cold, above-freezing environments. Although the exact pathophysiology is unknown, several authors have suggested a vascular basis. This condition occurs in all ages, in both sexes, and in all races. Children and women younger than the age of 20 are most commonly affected, and there is a familial tendency. Chilblains may become chronic in the elderly with peripheral vascular disease.

Chilblains usually presents acutely as erythematous, mauve or purplish swellings that give rise to throbbing pain and itching. The lesions usually occur at the onset of cold spells in the winter and last 2 to 3 weeks. This condition is usually mild and self-limiting. More symptomatic or persistent cases may include purpura, blistering, or ulceration and should be referred to a medical practitioner. In patients with predisposing conditions, such as globulinemia, dysproteinemias, chronic myelomonocytic leukemia, and lupus erythematosus, chilblains can last for several months and may recur annually. Exposure to cold during work or play, often with inadequate clothing, induces lesions within a few hours after expo-

sure. A special form of perniosis known as kibes (also described as equestrian cold panniculitis) occurs in the winter on the upper lateral aspect of the thighs of women who ride horses or on the buttocks of women who drive tractors.[34]

The extremities are most often affected, particularly the dorsum of the proximal phalanges of fingers and toes, the plantar surfaces of toes and heels, and the ears and nose. Lesions may also occur on the thighs and legs.

A laboratory workup for patients in whom chilblains is suspected should include a complete blood cell count, antinuclear antibody titer evaluation, serum chemical profile, and cryoglobulin and cryofibrinogen analysis.

Therapeutic suggestions for chilblains include prophylactic measures such as use of adequate home heating and clothing, consuming proper food, and getting sufficient exercise and therapeutic measures such as the use of ultraviolet light, topical corticosteroids, and vasodilators.[34] After conducting a randomized, double-blind study, Langtry and Diffey[35] concluded that ultraviolet phototherapy was not valuable in the prophylaxis of chilblains. Fitzgerald[36] "cured" chilblains with a combination regimen of intravenous calcium and intramuscular vitamin K. Nifedipine (20 mg) has been found to be an effective treatment of severe recurrent chilblains.[37] Rustin and coworkers[38] found nifedipine (20 to 60 mg daily) to significantly reduce the time of clearance, pain, soreness, and irritation of the lesions. Nifedipine was also found to prevent the development of new chilblains.[34, 38] Nifedipine is well tolerated by most patients, but sometimes it has caused headaches and facial flushing. When applied to lesions, nitroglycerin (Nitro-Bid) ointment has also been found beneficial.[39] In severe cases, sympathectomy has been helpful.[34] Rustin and coworkers relate unsatisfactory treatments, which included advice to keep affected areas warm, exposure to local ultraviolet light, administration of the vasodilators nicotinic acid and thymoxamine, intravenous calcium and intramuscular vitamin K, corticosteroids, and, in recalcitrant cases, sympathectomy.[35–40]

Trench Foot (Immersion Foot)

Trench foot is the result of prolonged exposure of the extremities to cold (nonfreezing) by wearing wet socks or wet footwear. It was common among soldiers during war but now is seen only in explorers who misjudge the difficulty of their expedition. Haller[41] related that trench foot caused serious attrition among the fighting troops through swollen limbs, impaired sensory nerves, inflammation, and even loss of tissue through gangrene.

Prolonged exposure under cold, wet conditions results in vascular injury. Vasoconstriction and heat loss, facilitated by moisture, cause ischemia, tissue injury, and increased endothelial permeability. Thereafter, extensive extravasation of protein and fluid may cause an increased hematocrit, sludging, and further aggravation of ischemia. Extensive vascular injury and gangrene with periarterial fibrosis and small arterial thickening with possible occlusion are seen in advanced cases. Veins show perivenous fibrosis, inflammatory reaction, and hemorrhage. The nerves may also be affected. Hyperhydration of the plantar stratum corneum may be the only finding at relatively high temperatures.

Three successive stages are used to recognize distinct clinical manifestations: (1) vasoconstrictive phase, (2) hyperemic phase, and (3) late vasospastic phase. The involved extremity becomes pale and cool, and the patient has paresthesias and a feeling of coldness in the vasoconstrictive phase. During the hyperemic phase, the extremity becomes hot and edematous. Pain or paresthesias may be present. The swelling may be aggravated by heat and by placing the limb in a dependent position. Subcutaneous tissue hemorrhages and blebs filled with serous or hemorrhagic fluid may appear. In severe cases, gangrene may intervene. This stage may persist for several days. This condition may be complicated by lymphangitis, cellulitis, and thrombophlebitis. In the late vasospastic phase there is an increased sensitivity to cold and typical secondary Raynaud's phenomenon, with excessive sweating, pain, and paresthesias of the lower extremities. This phase may persist for years. Ahle and associates[42] concluded that subjects who previously had trench foot injuries and nearly 60% of a normal population may be at significant risk for cold injury.

Treatment for the initial vasoconstrictive phase includes bed rest with the extremity in the horizontal position and a warm environment. During the hyperemic phase, the extremity should be placed at heart level and kept cool to diminish edema. To avoid infection the foot should be kept dry and clean. Pain may require use of an analgesic or narcotic. Sympathectomy may also be helpful in the hyperemic stage and in preventing the late vasospastic phase.[1]

Frostbite

Frostbite is tissue freezing that results from exposure to subfreezing temperatures. The body responds to very cold environments by conserving core body temperature at the expense of the extremities. Therefore, the extremities are more difficult to keep warm and the feet are among the parts most prone to frostbite. Predisposing factors include peripheral vascular insufficiency, improper clothing, exhaustion, and previous cold injury. Blacks are more susceptible than whites to frostbite. Superficial frostbite involves skin and subcutaneous tissues, while severe frostbite involves deeper structures, such as muscles, tendons, and bones. Most frostbite is of the slow freezing, superficial type. Only the superficial structures are involved, and affected areas appear as a white patch of frozen skin. Superficial frostbite usually heals in a few days without permanent sequelae. Differentiating superficial frostbite from deep frostbite is difficult because there is little apparent difference initially. The extent of deep tissue damage can be determined only after thawing. Rapid frostbite occurs in a few minutes and takes place at high altitudes with extremely low temperatures. It has a predilection for the extremities rather than the face and ears.

There is a four-part classification system for frostbite. First-degree frostbite involves hyperemia and edema that may develop in 3 hours and last up to 10 days. Superficial skin layers begin to slough after about a week. Second-degree frostbite involves the development of hyperemia, edema, and blisters. The blisters desiccate and develop black eschar in 2 to 4 weeks. Pink skin appears after sloughing of the eschar. Third-degree frost involves full-thickness skin injury with some extension into the subcutaneous tissues. Blisters appear at the edges of this injury, and skin appears hard and features an eschar that takes 2 months to heal. This eschar may produce a tourniquet effect if it is circumferential. Fourth-degree frostbite involves all tissues, including bone. The affected part is completely destroyed. It becomes black and dry and shrivels in a few months. This type of injury usually advances to autoamputation.[43]

The exact mechanism producing cell injury is unknown. Frey[43] suggests that frostbite occurs when extracellular water freezes, resulting in hypertonicity and cellular dehydration. Another damage mechanism is the disruption of cell membranes by intracellular ice crystal formation and cold-induced shifts in the lipid and phospholipid portions in the membranes. Severe vasoconstriction and decreased blood flow is also related to cold-induced tissue damage. Capillaries and arterioles can constrict, leading to thrombus formation with resultant vascular occlusion, tissue hypoxia, and ischemic necrosis resembling a burn.

A frostbitten victim is usually unaware of changes in the affected part. Initially, frostbite presents as a sharp, pricking sensation. Cessation of discomfort in the involved area is a reliable symptom of incipient frostbite in the toes. This is often followed by a pleasant feeling of warmth. The skin initially becomes red and then pale and waxy white. This stage is reversible but will progress to frostbite if left unchecked.

Treatment of an acute event should consist of rapid warming as fast as possible in a 40°C to 44°C environment. Slow rewarming increases crystal size and hence is more damaging. Areas affected by frostbite should never be rubbed with snow or massaged. Exercising to warm the body core temperature may be helpful, but impacts to frostbitten feet should be avoided. A frostbitten victim should not be thawed until he or she has reached shelter and is no longer in danger of refreezing. Strong persons can walk a long way on frozen feet without causing further injury. However, if the victim is permitted to walk on a recently thawed foot or toe he or she will not be able to assist in his or her own rescue. Heavy sedation may be required during rewarming. After rewarming, which usually takes about 20 minutes, the frozen area is exposed to room air at 21°C to 26°C. Smoking should be prohibited. Pressure dressings may be used, but the open method with sterile surrounding is usually preferred. Vesicles, bullae, and eschars should be left untouched. Surgical debridement and escharotomy should be delayed until the eschar starts to separate. Patients should be restricted to complete bed rest until foot edema subsides and blisters are completely dry. Toes may be separated by lamb's wool to prevent maceration of tissue. Sterile procedures should be followed to lessen the risk of infection, and tetanus prophylaxis should be given on hospital admission.[1] Frey[43] suggests that on warming, hypoxia, metabolic acidosis, and hypotension can result and can be treated with oxygen, sodium bicarbonate, warm intravenous fluid, and, occasionally, intermittent positive-pressure ventilation. Mehta and Wilson[44] recommend using the triple-phase bone scan to indicate tissue viability as early as 2 days after cold injury. The perfusion and blood pool images demonstrate the ischemic tissue at risk, while the delayed bone scan images demonstrate the extent of deep tissue and bone infarction. Daum and coworkers[45] did not find buflomedil, a peripheral vasodilator, to improve vascular patency in acutely frozen victims.

VENOUS DISORDERS

The venous system plays an important role in the transport of blood from peripheral tissues back to the heart and, because of capacitance, acts as a reservoir for the circulatory system. The pressure changes within the venous system are mediated by the sympathetic nervous system.

Varicose Veins

Varicose veins are veins that have become elongated, tortuous, and dilated. The veins of the lower extremity can take on these characteristics as late complications of deep venous thrombosis. These veins can develop during pregnancy and are known as secondary varicose veins or they can be primary and of unknown etiology. The prevalence of varicose veins increases with age and is twice as common in women than in men.

Varicose veins can be classified as primary or secondary. Secondary varicose veins have an underlying pathologic process, usually deep venous thrombosis. Primary varicose veins have a normal deep venous system and are due to a defect in the superficial vein valves. In understanding the cause of varicose veins it is important to understand that the deep venous system contains valves that help to pump blood proximally. These valves are considerably weakened following deep venous thrombosis and therefore cause stasis of blood, which backs up into the superficial venous system causing the varicosities.

The calf muscles act as a venous pump mechanism in the lower extremity, thus playing a major role in venous return. The pressure during muscular systole can reach as high as 250 mm Hg in the leg and 115 mm Hg in the thigh. In muscular diastole, the venous pressure in the deep system falls below that of the superficial veins, drawing blood in from them and from the surrounding capillaries of the muscles and distal veins.[15]

Varicosities result from incompetence of the one-way valves that are necessary for the efficient work of the musculovenous pump. Other etiologic theories suggest an inherited weakness in the structure of the vein wall or valves. A positive family history has been reported in 50% of patients. Other factors such as prolonged standing, obesity, pregnancy, age, and being female have all been postulated. According to Benkitt, new studies show that the Western diet, depleted in fiber-rich foods, is an underlying factor. Dilatation of the vein is also considered as a cause that is secondary to intravenous pressures exceeding the ability of the vein wall to withstand deformation.

To understand the varicose vein, the physician also needs to have a basic understanding of anatomy of the venous system. The leg contains three groups of veins: superficial, deep, and perforating. The superficial and deep systems are linked by the perforating veins. The superficial veins have thick muscular walls and are basically considered veins of moderate size, which form most of the prominent superficial varices and the main superficial veins—the greater and lesser saphenous. The greater saphenous vein begins distally as an extension of the dorsal venous arch medially and courses upward through the medial aspect of the leg and thigh and empties into the common femoral vein. The greater saphenous vein has two important pairs of tributary vessels: one pair joins at the knee and the other pair joins at the hiatus saphenous in the thigh.

The lesser saphenous vein originates on the posterolateral aspect of the ankle and passes proximally to pierce the deep fascia in the upper third of the leg. This vein empties into the popliteal vein at the superior popliteal space. The greater and lesser saphenous veins are connected by the posterior medial vein of the thigh along its course.

The deep veins of the lower extremity follow the arteries and are paired directly with the posterior tibial, anterior tibial, and peroneal veins. These veins drain into the popliteal and femoral veins of the thigh.

The perforating veins pierce the deep fascia, and they form a communicating system between the superficial and deep systems. The perforators are prevalent in the lower leg, and they may become incompetent, causing "backing up" and therefore varicosities of the superficial system.

The most common symptom associated with varicose veins is a dull heavy ache that develops after prolonged standing. The ache is relieved by elevation of the legs or with the use of support stockings or bandages. Edema of the legs is a common symptom that may be relieved by elevation. Occasional symptoms of itching, burning, cramps, or fatigue may occur. Not uncommon is the cyclic premenstrual exacerbation of symptoms. The symptoms are not related to the size of the varicose veins or degree of incompetence. Often, patients with severely involved legs may be asymptomatic whereas patients with minimal varicosities may have numerous complaints.

On physical examination, the inspection of the location is important. The location of the varicosities in the legs suggests whether they are associated with the greater or lesser saphenous vein. Inspection of the lower extremity should extend from the level of the groin to the distal foot. Pigmentation of the skin, dermatitis, induration of the skin, subacute cellulitis, and ulceration may be indicative of chronic venous insufficiency. Primary varicosities usually develop at the groin and spread inferiorly. Secondary varicosities usually develop at the ankle or leg and extend superiority. Palpation of the varicosity using the pulp of the fingers is most helpful in detecting varicosities. The veins can be tender owing to inflammation or thrombosis, or they may be quite firm or fibrous. A defect felt in the deep fascia suggests that it is most likely an incompetent perforating vein.

Various tests may be performed to clinically diagnose varicosities. The cough impulse test is performed with the patient standing. The examiner places his or her fingers on the greater saphenous vein 4 to 5 inches inferior to the saphenofemoral junction and asks the patient to cough. An expansile impulse in combination with a thrill will indicate incompetence of the end (terminal) saphenous valve at the junction of the femoral veins.

The Perthes test gives the practitioner information regarding the perforating and deep systems. A tourniquet is applied to compress the superficial veins just below the knee. The patient walks for 1 minute while the veins of the foot are observed. Should the veins become less prominent, they are normal. If they remain the same size, the valves of the perforators are incompetent. If the veins become more prominent and the patient complains of leg pain, deep venous insufficiency with perforator incompetence is suspected.

The retrograde filling test (Brodie's Trendelenburg) demonstrates valvular incompetence in the lesser saphenous veins. This test helps to differentiate valvular from perforator incompetence. To perform this test, the patient should lie supine and elevate and exsanguinate the legs. A tourniquet is applied to occlude the superficial venous system below the saphenofemoral junction. The patient stands, and the examiner should note the pattern of superficial filling (refilling). If the superficial veins below the tourniquet fill rapidly, the perforators or lesser saphenous vein is incompetent. If, however, the superficial veins remain empty, filling when the tourniquet is released, the saphenofemoral junction valve is incompetent. Normally, the varicose veins will fill within 30 to 60 seconds.

Treatment of varicose veins as well as chronic venous insufficiency is ideally prophylaxis. Today, however, there are a variety of conservative as well as surgical treatment options.

Elastic compression stockings may relieve symptoms. The support needs to be of adequate pressure distribution, which decreases distally to proximally. These supports are most effective when applied in the morning before rising and removed on retiring at night. Ambulation, swimming, or other activities are encouraged to promote venous return of the calf muscle pump system. Elevation of the legs when not exercising is recommended.

Sclerotherapy has gained popularity in recent years owing to advancements in techniques. With the use of sodium tetradecyl sulfate (3% solution) the varicosities can be sclerosed by localized destruction of the venous intima. This agent has a thrombogenic effect on the involved vein. Contraindications to sclerotherapy are allergy to the agent, excessive obesity, pregnancy, disease with a poor prognosis, limb eczema, or infections of the limb or conditions that cause the patient to be immobile following injection.

Surgical treatment is recommended for incompetence of either the long or the short saphenous vein. Local excision or ligation treatment of varicose veins is a surgical option.

Deep Venous Thrombosis

INCIDENCE

Deep venous thrombosis is a major cause of morbidity and mortality. Studies show that many more patients have deep venous thrombosis than would be predicted based on signs and symptoms. Approximately 50% of venous thromboses are clinically asymptomatic. The incidence of thrombosis in the surgical patient is reported to be between 20% and 50%. Prophylaxis is therefore crucial.

PATHOPHYSIOLOGY

Classically, Virchow's triad has been associated with deep venous thrombosis. This is the triad of intimal damage, hypercoagulability, and a reduction in blood flow or stasis. Intimal damage may initiate the coagulation cascade by releasing substances from the vessel wall. Venostasis is associated with immobilization, bed rest, sitting, and prolonged standing. Slowing of the blood flow allows activated clotting factors to accumulate and diminishes naturally occurring anticoagulants. This allows platelets to eventually aggregate. Patients with previous attacks of deep venous thrombosis no longer have unidirectional blood flow because of destruction of their vein valves. This may cause a slowing of their blood flow. Oral contraceptives and pregnancy have been associated with alterations in clotting factors that promote coagulation.

PROPHYLAXIS

Avoidance of venostasis is best maintained by remaining active during the perioperative period. Leg elevation, elastic compression hose, and sequential pneumatic compression devices have all been shown to diminish venous stasis.

MANAGEMENT

Patients suspected of having deep venous thrombosis should be evaluated expeditiously. In physical examination the involved extremity may have varying degrees of edema. Homan's sign, the production of calf pain with passive dorsiflexion of the ankle, may or may not be present.

Definitive diagnosis should be made in the patient with suspected deep venous thrombosis. This is best accomplished with a duplex ultrasound examination of the affected limb. Barring this, a venogram remains the "gold standard." However, venography is associated with causing deep venous thrombosis in approximately 10% of the cases in which it is performed.

Once the diagnosis has been ascertained the patient should be anticoagulated with intravenous heparin. Heparin inhibits coagulation and enables thrombolysis to occur. If there are no contraindications, the patient should receive 5000–10,000 units of heparin as a bolus. This should be followed with a constant heparin infusion sufficient to maintain the activated partial thromboplastin time between 60 and 80 seconds. Following approximately 1 week of heparinization the patient is changed to oral warfarin therapy, and this is used for 3 to 6 months. Several adverse reactions to heparin are possible. These include heparin-induced thrombocytopenia, which is recognized by an increasing heparin dose and a decreasing platelet count.

Outpatient anticoagulation with warfarin inhibits the hepatic synthesis of the vitamin K–dependent clotting factors. The dose of warfarin should maintain the patient's prothrombin time at approximately two times the control prothrombin time. The complications of warfarin, other than hemorrhage, are relatively few. A rare dermal gangrene is reported in the literature.

Streptokinase, urokinase, and tissue plasminogen activator are agents used for thrombolysis of clot. Use of thrombolytic agents appears to be most beneficial in cases in which venous gangrene is impending. Several controlled clinical trials have shown some benefit with these agents, but because of their cost they are generally not used to treat all episodes of deep venous thrombosis.

In certain circumstances anticoagulation cannot be continued. In patients who develop a bleeding complication, who have undergone major surgery, or who have had a hemorrhagic cerebrovascular accident, an alternative therapy must be used.

Pulmonary embolism is a potentially life-threatening complication of deep venous thrombosis. When anticoagulation cannot be maintained, interruption of the inferior vena cava with a filter is effective prophylaxis against pulmonary embolism.

In the pregnant patient who develops deep venous thrombosis, warfarin cannot be used for outpatient treatment because of its teratogenic effect. These patients are usually maintained on subcutaneous heparin therapy until after delivery.

Superficial Phlebitis

Inflammation of a superficial vein can result from several causes. Most commonly, an area of varicosity sets up blood flow for relative stasis. Subsequently, a thrombus forms and an inflammatory response ensues. Although this can be quite painful and incapacitating, superficial phlebitis does not have the severe complications of deep venous thrombosis, namely, pulmonary embolism.

Superficial phlebitis is usually a benign and self-limiting entity. Treatment is aimed at relief of the painful inflamed areas with oral medications. Symptomatically the patient often feels better following application of a heating pad or an alcohol-moistened washcloth, which leaves the skin feeling cool. Usually the acute attack lasts for several days before subsiding, leaving the patient with a hardened thrombosed area where the inflammatory nidus began.

On rare occasions the area of phlebitis may migrate up the saphenous vein and approach the saphenofemoral junction. Here surgery would be indicated for interruption of the saphenous system before the clot could spill into the deep venous system, initiating a deep venous thrombosis.

Less commonly, suppurative thrombophlebitis can be seen in the veins of the arms. This is most frequently observed in the patient recuperating from extensive burns, but this can occur in any patient with an indwelling catheter. For that reason, catheter sites are frequently rotated every third day. Should an area of suppuration be noted, the appropriate treatment is complete excision of the affected vein while leaving the operative incision open and allowing this to granulate.[46]

LYMPHATIC DISORDERS

Prolonged sitting or standing will cause edema in almost everyone. Excessive intake of sodium and hot weather exacerbate swelling. Persons with rheumatoid arthritis who are paralyzed or who are confined to chairs or wheelchairs are especially prone to this condition. This physiologic edema can be helped by restricting salt consumption, using support stockings, and using diuretics when necessary.

Swelling needs to be distinguished from edema of cardiac, hepatic, renal, and lymphatic origins. General causes of leg swelling include congestive heart failure, hepatic cirrhosis, nephrotic syndrome, and hypoproteinemia secondary to malabsorption or malnutrition. Persons with edema caused by congestive heart failure usually have a history of dyspnea on exertion, orthopnea, and paroxysmal nocturnal dyspnea. Examination reveals lung rales, distended neck veins, tachycardia, car-

diomegaly, hepatomegaly, and ventricular gallop. Chest roentgenography is usually diagnostic of cardiomegaly and pulmonary congestion.

Blood tests and liver biopsy can confirm a suspicion of hepatic cirrhosis. Suspicion of hepatic cirrhosis should be heightened when jaundice, gynecomastia, hepatosplenomegaly, ascites, palmar erythema, and spider angiomas are present.

Hypoalbuminemia, proteinuria, and hypercholesterolemia are often used to establish the diagnosis of nephrotic syndrome. When these conditions are present, the cause can often be established by renal biopsy.

Lymphedema is a painless, insidious swelling of the soft tissues owing to malformation or malfunction of the lymphatic system. The edema may be either soft and pitting or firm and difficult to pit, depending on its duration. The first sign of lymphedema is classically a puffiness on the dorsum of the foot or about the ankle. Over several months, however, the swelling increases and extends up the calf and occasionally into the thigh. The swelling becomes firmer and resists pitting. Bed rest may reduce but not eliminate the swelling.

Lymphedema may be classified into idiopathic (primary) and secondary types. Primary lymphedema is caused by an inherited defect in the lymphatic system with aplasia, hypoplasia, or varicose dilatation of the lymphatic vessels. Clinically, idiopathic lymphedema affects women more than men at a ratio of 10:1. The extremities are usually involved, but other parts of the body may be affected, such as the face and genitalia. Congenital lymphedema is so severe that swelling of the legs may be present at birth. The congenital form may occur sporadically or in several siblings of a family over several generations. This familial form of idiopathic lymphedema is called Milroy's disease. Lymphedema praecox is less severe, and the edema does not begin until 10 to 25 years of age. Lymphedema tarda is a late form of idiopathic lymphedema that does not appear until after the age of 35 years.[10]

Secondary lymphedema may be due to carcinoma, infection, radiation, surgical removal of lymph nodes, local tissue injury or inflammation, filiariasis, or retroperitoneal fibrosis. Prostate cancer and malignant lymphoma are the most common causes of secondary obstructive lymphedema in men and women, respectively. Any tumor that invades or obstructs the lymphatic system can cause secondary lymphedema, such as carcinoma of the bladder, testis, and skin.

Other causes of secondary lymphedema include repeated episodes of cellulitis and lymphangitis, usually caused by streptococci. Streptococci enter the lymphatic system through macerations of the skin or interdigital fissures in areas involved by cutaneous trichophytosis. Filiariasis is very common in the tropical climates but is rarely a cause of lymphedema in North America.[3, 6]

LIPEDEMA

Lipedema is a common, chronic condition in which there is a bilateral and symmetric deposition of fat in the lower extremities. This condition is often mistaken for lymphedema or venous insufficiency. It affects women almost exclusively and may be familial. Patients may complain of swollen legs, but they do not often associate it with a gradual increase in weight. The condition is painless. Some patients may, however, have mild to moderate tenderness in the legs. Characteristic findings include marked obesity from the waist down. The legs are nonpitting and symmetric, and the skin and underlying structures feel like adipose tissue. The distinguishing diagnostic feature of lipedema is that the foot is never involved.

Treatment includes support stockings, which are often uncomfortable. Diuretics are of no value. Patients should be counseled on the importance of weight loss. Weight loss is typically slow from the waist down and first occurs elsewhere. With prolonged consistent weight loss, the condition may improve.[1, 27]

CASE EXAMPLES

Case 1: Occlusive Vascular Disease

A 33-year-old black man presented to the Cleveland Foot Clinic with a chief complaint of a painful fifth digit on his right foot. The patient stated that his fifth toe on his right foot had been bothering him for 2 weeks and that he noticed some "spots" under the skin. He related diffuse pain and numbness dorsally and plantarly about the fifth digit and the fifth metatarsophalangeal joint. The onset of the pain was sudden. The pain is exacerbated with prolonged weight bearing, and this is when the digit becomes numb. Extremes of both hot and cold temperatures aggravate the symptoms.

The patient denied any general medical conditions or allergies. He was not taking any medications. On further questioning the patient stated he takes garlic and water for hypertension, although he has never been diagnosed as having hypertension. There is a history of hypertension, alcoholism, and tuberculosis in his family.

The patient is a railroad trackman who has been laid off. He has smoked one pack of cigarettes a day for the past 17 years. He drinks caffeinated beverages and approximately a fifth of liquor per week.

On physical examination his blood pressure was 155/110 mm Hg, his temperature was 99°F, and his respirations were 18/min. He was 5 feet, 11 inches tall and weighed 260 pounds.

Noninvasive vascular examination showed nonpalpable right and left dorsalis pedis and posterior tibial pulses. Skin temperature was warm to warm from leg to foot and warm to cold from foot to toes (colder on right). On elevation, pallor with a mottled appearance was noted on his right foot, and no pallor was evident on the left foot. The capillary filling time was 8 seconds on the right foot and 4 seconds on the left foot. Dependency showed a dusky red rubor on digits 1 through 5 on the right foot and no color change on the left foot. The ankle-arm index was 1.06 (left) and 0.50 (right).

All of the Doppler waveforms on the right side were pulsatile, were multiphasic, and had a good amplitude. The waveforms on the left were pulsatile, showed a complete loss of reverse flow, and were smaller in amplitide than those of the left. In pulse volume recording, the waveforms were normal on the right and abnormal on the left, with a complete loss of the dichrotic notch and a rounding of the waves. This was demonstrated in all levels of the leg.

Segmental blood pressures revealed a probable occlusive process above the high thigh level as evidenced by the .92 high thigh/arm index:

	Left	Right
Brachial	153	153
High thigh	141 0.92	196 1.28
Above knee	132 0.86	210 1.37
Below knee	98 0.64	172 1.12
Ankle (posterior tibial)	83 0.54	159 1.04
Ankle (dorsalis pedis)	77 0.50	162 1.06

Photoplethysmographic waveforms on the left were normal in size and shape. The waveforms on the right side were rounded and irregular.

The patient was immediately referred to a vascular surgeon for evaluation and treatment. An arteriogram revealed a thrombosis of the right superficial femoral artery. Treatment consisted of infusion of urokinase and angioplasty.

DISCUSSION

This was an unusual presentation for occlusive arterial disease. An ankle-arm index of 0.50 on the affected side in a young, nondiabetic man would not usually be expected to be associated with symptoms such as local pain and numbness. It is apparent that shower emboli from the superficial femoral thrombosis were responsible for the fifth digit pain and numbness.

The most important point to be made from this patient presentation is that not all patients are typical. Here is a 33-year-old nondiabetic with significant peripheral vascular disease who presents in an atypical fashion. The early diagnosis of his underlying disease enabled him to be treated with less invasive therapies than bypass surgery.

Case 2: Occlusive Vascular Disease

An 84-year-old man presented to the Cleveland Foot Clinic with a chief complaint of painful ulcers on both halluces. He admitted to having been diagnosed with hypertension for 1 year and having had vascular surgery on his right leg. He has a 60 pack/year history of cigarette smoking and continues to smoke. He also stated he has headaches.

Physical examination revealed limb hair loss, skin color changes, trophic nails, ulcerations, and rubor.

Noninvasive vascular examinations showed nonpalpable right and left posterior tibial and dorsalis pedis pulses. His ankle-arm index was 1.11 (right) and 1.12 (left).

All of the Doppler waveforms were pulsatile but extremely irregular with no discernible wave pattern. This is probably indicative of collateralized flow and represents chronic arterial disease. In pulse volume recording the wave patterns were abnormal in that they were irregular and rounded with no discernible wave pattern. Photoplethysmographic digital waveforms were absent at the highest sensitivity, indicating severe arterial disease.

The patient was immediately referred to a vascular surgeon for evaluation and treatment.

DISCUSSION

Findings on physical examination of loss of limb hair, trophic nails, and ulcerations clearly indicate the presence of significant ischemic disease. The ankle-brachial index of greater than 1 bilaterally with irregular Doppler waveforms is significant for calcific changes in the vessel giving an artificially elevated index. Based on the patient's clinical presentation he underwent arteriography, which demonstrated multilevel occlusive disease involving the superficial femoral, popliteal, and tibial vessels. The patient had an in situ femoral popliteal artery bypass with a popliteal to dorsalis pedis in situ bypass segment as well. Postoperatively the patient did well. He immediately noted a resolution of his rest pain, and his ulcers had healed within 1 month.

Case 3: Vasospastic Disease

A 52-year-old white woman presented to a peripheral vascular surgeon with a chief complaint of her fingers becoming painful with color change on an intermittent basis. The patient was in her usual state of good health until 1 week before presentation when after brushing snow off her car windshield she noted her fingers turned white and became quite painful. Subsequently she noted her fingers became "flaming pink," before returning to their usual color and becoming pain free after

3 to 4 hours. In the coming week she noted recurrences after opening the freezer and after exposure outdoors, as well as after smoking a cigarette. Her medical history was unremarkable except for frostbite of her toes as a teenager. She is a housewife. She has smoked one pack of cigarettes per day for the past 30 years.

Pulse evaluation showed the following:

	Carotid	Brach- ial	Radial/ Ulnar	Femoral	Pop- liteal	Dorsalis Pedis/ Proximal Tibial
Right	2+	2+	2+/2+	2+	+	2+ /2+
Left	2+	2+	2+/2+	2+	+	2+ /2+

Laboratory studies showed a negative antinuclear antibody test and a negative rheumatoid factor.

DISCUSSION

Raynaud's disease and Raynaud's phenomenon are often grouped together under vasospastic conditions. Classically, Raynaud's disease is used to define an idiopathic vasospastic condition without any associated disease process. Raynaud's syndrome is typically used to define a cold or emotion-induced episode of digital ischemia. In most patients the hands and fingers are involved, although feet and toes and occasionally nose, cheeks, and ears may be affected. Classically, the hand or digit undergoes blanching, with the feeling of numbness. After the patient leaves the cold environment for warmer surroundings the digits become cyanotic after 10 to 30 minutes and finally become red, reflecting a reactive hyperemia. The basis of treatment for patients with Raynaud's disease is palliation since no cure is available. The first step in treatment is avoidance of cold, tobacco products, birth control pills, β-adrenergic blocking drugs, and ergotamine preparations. At present the calcium channel blocking drug nifedipine, 10 mm three times a day, produces excellent results in the majority of patients.

Case 4: Superficial Thrombophlebitis

A 27-year-old man noted a painful area at the medial aspect of his left calf. He was re-ferred to a vascular surgeon. The patient was in his usual state of excellent health and had awakened that morning with pain in his left calf. His history was unremarkable. He did not use tobacco products and drank alcoholic beverages occasionally.

Physical examination showed palpable pedal pulses, a 2 × 4-cm area of erythema, tenderness at the left medial calf, and a palpable cord. A duplex scan of the leg showed a clot in the greater saphenous vein.

DISCUSSION

Superficial thrombophlebitis is a benign and self-limiting process. Typically, treatment revolves around alleviation of the symptoms. This includes the administration of oral nonsteroidal anti-inflammatory medications and the topical use of heat. Surgery is usually not indicated; however, should the clot extend proximally up the saphenous vein toward the saphenofemoral junction, ligation of the vein to prevent the spillage of the clot into the deep venous system is recommended.

Case 5: Deep Venous Thrombosis

A 45-year-old man noted a swollen, tender right leg following a transatlantic airline flight. He was referred to a vascular surgeon. The patient was in his usual state of good health. Following the flight from Paris to New York, he noted swelling and pain in his right leg. He had no history of trauma or any similar previous episodes. The patient did have a history of hypertension. He had smoked one third of a pack of cigarettes per day for the past 20 years.

Physical examination demonstrated palpable femoral, popliteal, and pedal pulses in both legs. The right leg had 2+ edema from the dorsum of the foot proximally to the lower thigh. The left leg was without ulcers or lesions. Homan's sign was present. Noninvasive studies showed a positive impedance plethysmograph with prolonged emptying. The duplex scan showed a clot in the saphenofemoral vein.

DISCUSSION

Deep venous thrombosis is a potentially life-threatening disease. If untreated, the clot may extend and break off, becoming a free floating embolism in the venous system and eventually lodge in the lungs as a pulmonary embolism. Late complications, although not life threatening, can be terribly debilitating. These include chronic venous insufficiency and ulcer formation, as well as intractable edema. The basis of treatment for an acute deep venous thrombosis revolves around anticoagulation. This is done with intravenous heparin with a change to oral warfarin for outpatient therapy. This therapy is usually continued for 3 to 6 months. Should the patient have a contraindication to continuation of anticoagulation, such as bleeding or continued pulmonary embolism occurrence despite adequate anticoagulation, then interruption of the vena cava with a filter is indicated.

REFERENCES

1. Young JR: The swollen leg. Cardiol Clin 9(3):443–456, 1991.
2. Horwitz O, McCombs PR, Roberts B: Diseases of Blood Vessels, pp 51–60, 79, 205–210, 359. Philadelphia, Lea & Febiger, 1985.
3. Bates B: A Guide to Physical Examination and History Taking, pp 414–418. Philadelphia, JB Lippincott, 1987.
4. Zier BG: Essentials of Internal Medicine in Clinical Podiatry, pp 51, 64–74, 86–93. Philadelphia, WB Saunders, 1990.
5. Moore W: Vascular Surgery: A Comprehensive Review, ed 2, pp 221–227. Orlando, FL, Grune & Stratton, 1986.
6. Bergan JJ, Yao JST: Arterial Surgery: A New Diagnostic and Operative Technique, pp 438–445, 467–472. Orlando, FL, Grune & Stratton, 1988.
7. Gloviczki P, Calcagno D, Schirger A, et al: Noninvasive Evaluation of the Swollen Extremity: Experiences with 190 Lymphoscintigraphic Examinations. J Vasc Surg 9:683–690, 1989.
8. Putman CE, Ravin CE: Textbook of Diagnostic Imaging, pp 1410–1411. Philadelphia, WB Saunders, 1988.
9. Barndt R, Blakenhorn PH, Crawford DW: Prevalence of asymptomatic femoral artery atheromas in hyperlipoproteinemic patients. Atherosclerosis 20:252–262, 1974.
10. Jeurgens JL, Spittell JA Jr, Fairbairn JF: Peripheral Vascular Diseases, pp 218–230. Philadelphia, WB Saunders, 1980.
11. Levin ME, O'Neal LW: The Diabetic Foot, ed 2. St. Louis, CV Mosby, 1977.
12. Young JR, Graor RA, Olin JW, Bartholomew JR: Peripheral Vascular Diseases. St. Louis, Mosby–Year Book, 1991.
13. Jeurgens JL, Bernatz PE: Atherosclerosis of the extremities. In Jeurgens JL, Spittell JA Jr, Fairbairn JF (eds): Peripheral Vascular Disease, pp 253–294. Philadelphia, WB Saunders, 1980.
14. Pirart J: Why don't we teach and treat diabetic patients better? (Editorial) Diabetes Care 1(2):139–140, 1978.
15. Guyton AC: Textbook of Medical Physiology, ed 7. Philadelphia, WB Saunders, 1986.
16. Lees RS, Frederickson DS: Use of paper electrophoresis in the diagnosis and study of hyperglyceridemia. Circulation 30:20, 1964.
17. Couch NP: On the arterial consequences of smoking. J Vasc Surg 3(5):807–812, 1986.
18. Nadler JL, Velasco JS, Hurton R: Cigarette smoking inhibits prostacyclin formation. Lancet 1:1248–1250, 1983.
19. Ellenberg M, Rifkin H: Protein metabolism. In Rifkin H, Porte D, Jr (eds): Diabetes Mellitus: Theory and Practice, ed 4. New York, Elsevier Science Publishing, 1990.
20. Bhanji S, Mattingly D: Acrocyanosis in anorexia nervosa. Postgrad Med J 67:33–35, 1991.
21. Jivegord L, Holm J, Scherster T: The outcome in arterial thrombosis misdiagnosed as arterial embolism. Acta Chir Scand 152:251, 1986.
22. Darling RC, Austin WG, Linton RR: Arterial embolism. Surg Gynecol Obstet 124:106, 1967.
23. Wycholis AR, Spittel JA Jr, Wallace RB: Popliteal aneurysms. Surgery 68:942, 1970.
24. Marcus S, Wiener SR, Suzuki SM, Kwan L: Raynaud's syndrome. Postgrad Med 89(4):171–187, 1991.
25. Vardon J, Gasman JD: Raynaud's disease: An update. Hosp Pract 26(1):157–159, 1991.
26. Goodfield M: Cold-induced skin disorders. Practitioner 15:1616, 1618–1620, 1989.
27. Spittell JA Jr: Clinical Vascular Disease, pp 75–83, 293–298. Philadelphia, FA Davis, 1983.
28. Van Lith JMM, Hoekstra HJ, Boeve WJ, Weits J: Lymphedema of the legs as a result of lymphangiomyomatosis: A case report and review of the literature. Neth J Med 34:310–316, 1989.
29. Carpenter PK, Morris D: Association of acrocyanosis with Asperger's syndrome. J Ment Defic Res 34 (Pt 1):87–90, 1990.
30. Rustin MHA, Forman JC, Dowd PM: Anorexia nervosa associated with acromegaloid features, onset of acrocyanosis and Raynaud's phenomenon and worsening of chilblains. J R Soc Med 83(8):495–496, 1990.
31. Nielsen PG: Diffuse palmoplantar keratoderma associated with acrocyanosis. Acta Derm Venereol 69(2):156–161, 1989.
32. Friedman SA: Vascular Diseases, pp 82–84. Littleton, MA, John Wright & Sons, 1982.
33. Calderone DC, Finzi E: Treatment of primary erythromelalgia with piroxicam. J Am Acad Dermatol 24:145–146, 1991.
34. Goette KD: Chilblains (perniosis). J Am Acad Dermatol 23(Pt 1):257–262, 1990.
35. Langtry JA, Diffey BL: A double-blind study of ultraviolet phototherapy in the prophylaxis of chilblains. Acta Derm Venereol 69:320–322, 1989.
36. Fitzgerald KJ: Cure for chilblains. Med J Aust 13:676, 1980.
37. White AD: Chilblains. Med J Aust 154:406, 1991.
38. Rustin MHA, Newton JA, Smith NP, Pauline MD: The treatment of chilblains with nifedipine: The results of a pilot study, a double-blind placebo-controlled randomized study and a long-term open trial. Br J Dermatol 120:267–275, 1989.
39. Klaponan MH, Johnston WH: Localized recurrent postoperative pernio associated with leukocytoclastic vasculitis. J Am Acad Dermatol 24(5):811–812, 1991.
40. Lacroix HR, Gruwez JA, Casteels-Van Daele MC, Dequeker J: Lymphedema of the leg associated with rheumatoid arthritis. Lymphology 24:68–70, 1991.
41. Haller JS: Trench foot: A study in military-medical re-

sponsiveness in the Great War, 1914–1918. West J Med 152:729–733, 1990.

42. Ahle NW, Buroni JR, Sharp MW, Hamlet MP: Infrared thermographic measurement of circulatory compromise in trenchfoot-injured Argentine soldiers. Aviat Space Environ Med 61:247–275, 1990.

43. Frey C: Frostbitten feet. Physician Sports Med 20(1):67–76, 1992.

44. Mehta RC, Wilson MA: Frostbite injury: Prediction of tissue viability with triple-phase bone scanning. Radiology 170:511–514, 1989.

45. Daum PS, Bowers WD Jr, Tejada J, et al: An evaluation of the ability of the peripheral vasodilator buflomedil to improve vascular patency after acute frostbite. Cryobiology 26:85–92, 1989.

46. Rutherford R (ed): Vascular Surgery, ed 2. Philadelphia, WB Saunders, 1984.

BIBLIOGRAPHY

Abramson DI, Miller DS: Vascular Problems in Musculoskeletal Disorders of Limbs. New York, Springer-Verlag, 1981.

Athreya BH, Ostron BE, Eichenfield AH, Goldsmith DP: Lymphedema associated with juvenile rheumatoid arthritis. J Rheumatol 16:1338–1340, 1989.

Bastien MR, Goldstein BG, Smith JG: Treatment of lymphedema with a multicompartmental pneumatic compression device. J Am Acad Dermatol. 23:951–952, 1990.

Brostrom LA, Nilsonne U, Kronberg M, Soderberg G: Lymphangiosarcoma in chronic hereditary oedema (Milroy's disease). Ann Chir Gynaecol 78:320–323, 1989.

Burnard KG, et al: The relative importance of incompetent communicating veins in the production of varicose veins in venous ulcer. Surgery 82:9, 1977.

Caleffi E, Bocchi A, Villani LC, Banchini E: Successful treatment of an impressive primary lymphedema of the extremities. Int Angiol 9:288–291, 1990.

Caputo R, Gianotti R, Grimalt R, et al: Soft fibroma-like lesions on the legs of a patient with Kaposi's sarcoma and lymphedema. Am J Dermatopathol 13:493–496, 1991.

Dacre JE, Scott DL, Huskisson EC: Lymphoedema of the limbs as an extra-articular feature of rheumatoid arthritis. Ann Rheum Dis 49:722–724, 1990.

Ernst CB, Stanley JC: Current Therapy in Vascular Surgery, ed 2, pp 581–584. Philadelphia, BC Decker, 1991.

Fishman AB: Pulmonary Diseases and Disorders, ed 2, vol 3, p 236. New York, McGraw-Hill, 1988.

Fritz RL, Perrin DH: Cold Exposure Injuries: Prevention and Treatment. Clin Sports Med 8:111–128, 1989.

Grillet B, Dequeker J: Rheumatoid lymphedema. J Rheumatol 14:1095–1097, 1987.

Intenzo CM, Desai AG, Kim SS, et al: Lymphedema of the lower extremities: Evaluation by microcolloidal imaging. Clin Nucl Med 14:107–110, 1989.

Kannel WB, McGee DL: Update on some epidemiologic features of intermittent claudication: The Framingham study. J Am Geriatr Soc 33:13, 1985.

Kempczinski RF, Yao JST: Practical Noninvasive Vascular Diagnosis, ed 2. Chicago, IL, Year Book Medical Publishers, 1987.

Kinmouth JB: The Lymphatics, ed 2. London, Edward Arnold, 1982.

Levine PH: An acute effect of cigarette smoking on platelet function: A possible link between smoking and arterial thrombosis. Circulation 48:619–623, 1973.

McNeill GC, Witte MH, Witte CL, et al: Whole-body lymphangioscintigraphy: Perferred method for initial assessment of peripheral lymphatic system. Radiology 172:495–502, 1989.

Moore WX: Vascular Surgery: A Comprehensive Review, pp 688–689. Philadelphia, WB Saunders, 1991.

O'Brien BM, Khazanchi RK, Kumar PAV, Dvir E, Pederson WC: Liposuction in the treatment of lymphedema: A preliminary report. Br J Plastic Surg 42:530–533, 1989.

Richards TB, McBiles M, Collins PS: An easy method for diagnosis of lymphedema. Ann Vasc Surg 4:255–259, 1990.

Robbins JM, Harkless LB: Peripheral vascular disease in the lower extremity. Clin Podiatr Med Surg 9(1):139–164, 1992.

Scurry JP, Cowen PS: Necrobiotic pernio. Austr J Dermatol 30:29–31, 1989.

Vaughn BF: CT of swollen legs. Clin Radiol 41:24–30, 1990.

CHAPTER 21

PODIATRIC RHEUMATOLOGY

Eugene P. Goldman

There are many excellent books on the subject of podiatric rheumatology. This chapter is intended not to replace these books but merely to act as a ready reference for the busy primary care podiatrist who is confronted with a patient presenting with joint pain. The focus of treatment for each of the sections in this chapter is conservative. We all recognize the role of surgery in alleviating the suffering of these patients, but that approach is best left to a text dedicated to the complexities of surgical intervention.

The rheumatologist and podiatrist share many patients. The rheumatologist makes or confirms the diagnosis of the disease entity and begins systemic therapy, while the podiatrist may also make the primary diagnosis and often is consulted to help achieve maximum function for the increasingly dysfunctional patient. As an expert in the administration of palliative care, rehabilitation therapies, and orthotic devices and, in many cases, as a skilled surgeon, the podiatrist joins the team called together to improve the life of the patient with arthritis.

OSTEOARTHRITIS

CLINICAL PRESENTATION

Degenerative joint disease, known as osteoarthritis, is the most common form of arthritis. Typical presentations include pain with motion of a joint, stiffness, and joint enlargement as the deposition of bone matrix around the damaged joint slowly progresses. One of the key differentiating points about the presentation of osteoarthritis is that pain occurs typically *with* activity, not before, and it resolves with rest. The etiology includes trauma, long-term wear and tear associated with repetitive motions, and misaligned joints due to either congenital or acquired causes (e.g., a progressive hallux abductovalgus deformity or congenital hip dysplasia).

Direct trauma is an obvious and an unquestionably frequent cause of this type of arthritis. When we think of runners, an image of knees

345

and ankles gnarled by osteophytes and degenerated cartilage can be summoned, but the reality is that male runners do not show a higher incidence of osteoarthritis than does the general population of a similar age. A true traumatic origin of osteoarthritis could be an intra-articular fracture, a joint scarred by infection, or a joint surface defaced by a foreign object.

Repetitive motions can cause microstresses on joint surfaces, which may lead to degeneration and may be seen in certain workers such as meat cutters (wrists), ballet dancers who go "en pointe" (metatarsophalangeal joints), and migrant field hands (spines). This type of trauma may not be recognized as early as frank trauma and thus may continue for longer periods, eventually resulting in similar degenerative changes.

The average age at onset is during the sixth decade. The pattern for presentation is indefinite: it can be unilateral or bilateral, symmetric or asymmetric. In general, this is a noninflammatory process, but secondary synovitis, due to the misshapen joint, is not uncommon. The earliest change in this disorder is the fissuring or cracking of the cartilage surface of the joint. This leads to thinning of the cartilage and eventually to joint space narrowing. The underlying bone is put under pressure and responds to these forces by producing new bone, hence the osteophyte formation associated with osteoarthritis. Eventually, the new bone formation impedes the motion of the joint and further damage to the joint surface occurs until there is bone-on-bone contact within the joint, producing pain with motion that is alleviated with rest.

DIAGNOSIS

Physical examination of the joint is paramount to making the proper diagnosis. Pain with passive motion, retrograde force into the joint, and joint crepitus are key findings. Joint enlargement found with joint palpation is quite common, owing to periarticular osseous proliferation; when found at the proximal interphalangeal joint level, it is called Bouchard's nodes. Fluid accumulation that can be present in or around the joint is caused by synovitis from osseous irritation or bursae formation from subcutaneous bony prominences. In the foot and ankle, the primary sites of generalized osteoarthritis are the proximal interphalangeal and metatarsophalangeal joints, the subtalar and midtarsal joints, and the tibiotalar articulation. A secondary variant is diffuse idiopathic skeletal hypertrophy. Although this is primarily diagnosed by radiographic examination of the spine, the foot can be the primary site of involvement, and this is also a radiographic diagnosis. Here, osteophytic proliferation is extensive, mostly at ligament and tendon attachment sites, and the calcaneus is usually heavily affected. The exact cause is unknown, and there is no treatment.

Radiographic changes range from barely noticeable in the very early stages of degeneration to marked joint space narrowing and subchondral eburnation along with significant periarticular osteophyte formation (Fig. 21–1) to diffuse idiopathic skeletal hypertrophy (Fig. 21–2).

TREATMENT

Support of the affected joint(s) along with protection is the conservative treatment goal. Modalities useful here include ultrasound therapy for reduction of synovitis or bursitis, motion therapy to reduce stiffness and keep the parts mobile, paraffin baths, hot water soaks, orthotic devices and molded shoes to accommodate bony prominences, and the use of anti-inflammatory drugs, moving from low doses of aspirin along the spectrum of the nonsteroidal anti-inflammatory medications. Occasional intra-articular and periarticular injections with a corticosteroid agent may temporarily alleviate the restrictions of the joint degeneration and provide, in some cases, lasting relief. A maximum of three injections per joint in the span of a year should be the rule, and if the effect is not completely satisfactory, the risk–benefit equation must be solved before proceeding with this modality.

On the horizon are approaches that may include the use of human growth hormone to induce new cartilage formation and other injectable agents designed to stimulate new cartilage growth and stabilize the existing joint surface.

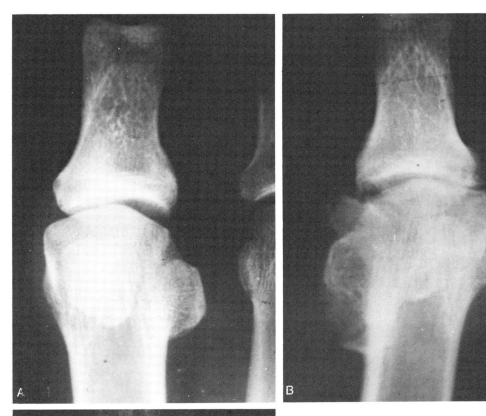

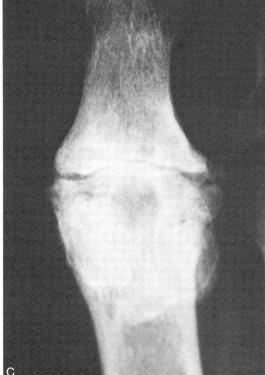

FIGURE 21–1. *(A)* Medial focal joint space narrowing of first metatarsophalangeal joint. (Courtesy of Larry Osher, DPM.) *(B)* Focal lateral joint space narrowing of the first metatarsophalangeal joint with lateral marginal joint osteophyte formation and mild subchondral sclerosis. Note sesamoidal involvement. *(C)* Extensive osteophyte formation along with concentric loss of joint space. Note the large, central subchondral cyst within the first metatarsal head.

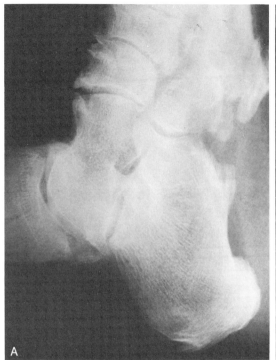

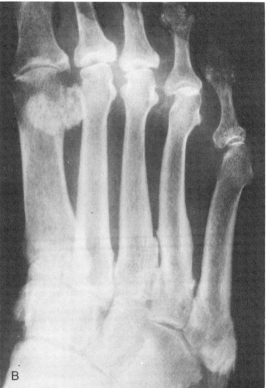

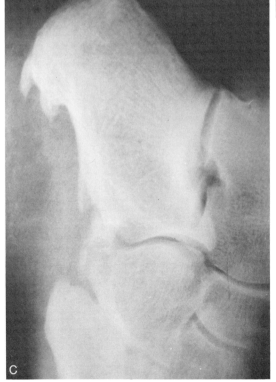

FIGURE 21–2. *(A)* Lateral study of the foot of a patient with diffuse idiopathic skeletal hypertrophy, displaying proliferative enthesophytes of the retrocalcaneal and infracalcaneal zones and the base of the fifth metatarsal. Dorsal midfoot spurring is also apparent, but without other evidence of joint arthrosis. *(B)* Medial oblique study of the foot of same patient. Osseous apposition of the anterior tibial and peroneus brevis attachment zones can be seen. *(C)* Lateral pedal view of a different patient displays large and somewhat poorly defined infracalcaneal ''spurs.'' Notice the unusual involvement of the short plantar ligamentous zone. (Figures courtesy of Larry Osher, DPM.)

CRYSTAL-INDUCED MONOARTICULAR ARTHROPATHY

Gout

CLINICAL PRESENTATION

A mostly male disease until the age of menopause for females, gout presents initally at the first metatarsophalangeal joint in the foot over 90% of the time. The alternative term for a gouty presentation at this site is *podagra*. Boys remain unaffected until puberty.

The classic time for an attack of gout is early morning or late night. The underlying cause for this is reabsorption of excess joint fluid at night that results in precipitation of uric acid crystals. The blood saturation of uric acid is 6.4 mg/dL. Hyperuricemia, which is defined as serum urate concentration more than 2 standard deviations above the laboratory standard for the age and sex of the patient, may result in gout or it can be asymptomatic. In those cases in which the high level of uric acid is pathogenic, the mechanism of disease is related to the saturation point of blood for the urate crystals. In the extremities, especially the foot, the temperature is lower than the core temperature. As the temperature drops, the solubility of the crystals decreases, eventually causing precipitation according to the laws of chemical equilibria. If the joint contains excess fluid due to repeated daily microtrauma, such as the first metatarsophalangeal joint would be subject to, or due to previous frank trauma, the nightly reabsorption combined with the lower solubility in a person with hyperuricemia will precipitate significant quantities of the crystal into the joint.

The precipitated monosodium urate crystals are engulfed by the joint phagocytes. The phagocytes attempt to dissolve the crystals with endogenous lysozymes, which are unsuccessful, and the enzymes spill into the joint itself and greatly inflame the synovium, causing the acute joint pain, effusion, and erythema associated with gout.

Hyperuricemia can be a multisystemic disease associated not just with gout and gouty arthritis but also with increased cholesterol levels, increased serum hemoglobin levels, and increased white blood cell counts. Persons with gout have higher associations with hypertension, stroke, arteriosclerosis, heart disease, and kidney failure.[1]

CAUSES

Gout can be caused by metabolic mechanisms, accounting for 20% of cases, and renal mechanisms, accounting for 80% of cases. In normal persons, the pathway for purine metabolism involves the breakdown of purines to phosphoribosylpyrophosphate (PRPP). Xanthine oxidase converts the PRPP substrate to xanthine, which becomes uric acid. Normally, if too much xanthine is produced, the PRPP level rises through negative feedback inhibition, and the enzyme hypoxanthine guanine phosphoribosyltransferase (HGRPT) converts the purines to guanidylic acid through an ancillary pathway.

In patients with gout, the lack of HGRPT causes high levels of uric acid because there is no inhibitory pathway; the excessive PRPP causes overactive xanthine oxidase, and the result is the overproduction of uric acid. Lesch-Nyhan syndrome is the rare recessive sex-linked genetic total lack of HGRPT and is characterized by huge production of uric acid, mental retardation, compulsive mutilation, impaired renal function, and severe attacks of gout.

The renal mechanism results in the underexcretion of uric acid due to (1) decreased clearance of uric acid in the microtubules; (2) competition of the uric acid in the tubules with certain medications, such as aspirin in low doses and thiazide diuretics; and (3) lactic acidosis inhibiting uric acid excretion in the tubules, as occurs with binge drinking of alcohol or surgery.

CLASSIFICATION

Gout can be classified as primary or secondary. Primary gout is a congenital metabolic or renal defect. It is autosomal dominant and can be found in a family history. It mostly affects males. Females may have it too, but estrogen has a protective effect. Boys are prone to develop the disorder after puberty owing to the associated rise in testosterone levels. Secondary gout is a common sequela of myeloproliferative diseases such as lymphoma, chronic myelogenous leukemia, and polycythemia vera and of conditions such as psoriasis and sarcoidosis that feature rapid turnover of tissue. Chemotherapy causes massive cell death and rapid release of purines, which overwhelms the kidneys and blocks renal excretion. Patients with these myeloproliferative diseases and cutaneous conditions are pretreated with allopurinol to block the enzymatic conversion of the purines to uric acid.

We further classify patients with gout into two more categories: the overproducers vs. the underexcretors. In the 20% of patients who can be classified as overproducers, the primary cause is the enzyme defect described earlier. The secondary causes are the myeloproliferative diseases and psoriasis. A 24-hour urine collection would show greater than 600 mg of uric acid. Treatment is aimed at slowing the production with enzyme blockers.

The other 80% of patients are the underexcretors. The primary cause here is the decreased clearance in the kidney of the uric acid. Medications that cause the inhibition of excretion of uric acid are the secondary cause. A 24-hour urine collection will show less than 600 mg of uric acid. Treatment is with uricosuric agents designed to increase excretion, such as probenecid or sulfinpyrazone. These agents are used only after the acute phase of the gout attack is over.

DIAGNOSIS

Acute Gouty Arthritis. The clinical picture is one of acute pain, swelling, redness, and heat over the affected joint. The attack lasts from 3 to 10 days without treatment. When the acute inflammatory phase is over, there is reduction of swelling, peeling of the skin over the involved joint, and a lessening of the pain. Following complete resolution, the next attack may occur within weeks or months or not for years. The more acute the episode, the more likely the patient will be to have another.

The steps in making the definitive diagnosis include obtaining a serum monosodium urate level and performing a joint aspiration. A serum level of 11 mg/dL or higher gives a greater than 80% chance of gout. However, in about 20% of patients with gout, the level is 7 mg/dL or less, which is considered normal. The joint tap in a gout attack will show negatively birefringent crystals under polarized light (a yellow color). An important point to remember is that the joint fluid sample should be sent for culture and sensitivity and Gram's stain to absolutely rule out an infectious source of the problem. This means that the tapped fluid must be handled in a completely sterile fashion. Another clinical point to be aware of is that a polarized microscope is not absolutely necessary to make a certain diagnosis of gout. Needle-shaped crystals seen in macrophages are diagnostic of gout, too (Fig. 21–3). In addition, the white blood cell count will be 15,000 to 20,000/mm^3 since gout is an inflammatory process.

Intercritical Gout. The next phase is called intercritical because the patient is usually symptom free. The serum uric acid level often remains elevated, and joint crystals can still be aspirated during this stage. The serum level can be confusing because during the actual acute phase the serum level drops to normal or below owing to the sudden precipitation of the monosodium urate crystals into the joint. During the early intercritical phase, the level may rise only to normal levels, and thus a clear clinical picture may not be established. It is the joint crystal presence that can indicate the definitive diagnosis during this stage.

Chronic Tophaceous Gout. In advanced gout, that which has occurred over a period of about 10 years, deposits of tophi become prevalent and clinically identifiable in at least 50% of patients. The tophi form mostly in areas of lower body temperature where there is a

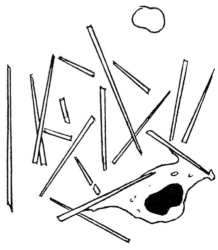

FIGURE 21–3. Needle-shaped uric acid crystals evident from a joint tap in a patient with gout.

greater degree of crystal deposition. These sites include the helix of the ear, the olecranon bursa, the Achilles tendon, and, of course, the synovium of affected joints. Chronic gout with tophi may resemble rheumatoid arthritis, but the asymmetry of the presentation tends to rule out other diagnoses. The tophi may resemble a rheumatoid nodule, and definitive differentiation requires biopsy or excision and pathologic confirmation.

The chronic form of this disease can lead to severe arthritis by destruction of the joint surface by the large and irritating tophi deposits. In addition, 15% to 20% of all patients with gout develop kidney stones, and these urate stones account for 10% of all kidney stone deposits.

RADIOGRAPHIC SIGNS

During the early acute attack, radiographs show only the soft tissue swelling surrounding the affected joint. However, radiographs are still important to rule out other causes of the clinical presentation. In chronic gout, the deposition of the uric acid crystals in the joint leads to punched-out lesions in the intra-articular or periarticular regions (Fig. 21–4). They are well circumscribed with sclerotic margins. More frequently, the articular surface is well preserved until large tophi deposits cause cartilage damage. The extra-articular tophi deposits eventually calcify and thus become visible on the radiographs. One other point to remember is that while rheumatoid arthritis also presents as punched-out lesions and erosions, it usually begins on the fifth metatarsal and progresses medially, while gout usually presents initially on the first metatarsal.

TREATMENT

In the acute phase, drug therapy is the only rational choice for relief of the severe pain. If treatment is begun within the first 24 hours of onset, colchicine, 0.6 mg/h, is given until one of the following happens: A maximum of 10 doses have been given; the attack subsides; or severe nausea, vomiting, or diarrhea occurs. A favorable response to colchicine is considered diagnostic for crystal deposition disease (either gout or pseudogout). Remember, colchicine is not an anti-inflammatory agent. It

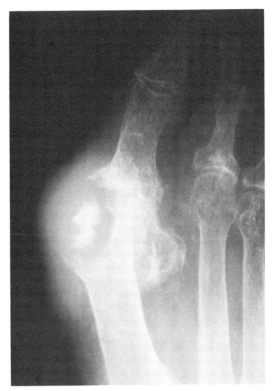

FIGURE 21–4. Punched-out lesions on a radiograph of a patient with gout. (Courtesy of Larry Osher, DPM.)

inhibits the lymphocytes in the joint fluid from engulfing the monosodium urate crystals.

The nonsteroidal anti-inflammatory medications are important in the acute phase. Indomethacin (Indocin) has been the drug of choice for treatment of symptoms lasting past the initial 24-hour presentation stage owing to its proven efficacy in the treatment of this disease. The usual dose is 50 mg three times a day for 2 to 3 days, followed by 25 mg three times a day for the remainder of the 10-day course. Other nonsteroidal agents have also been shown to be effective, and the choice is left to the treating physician.

The current thinking on treatment of chronic gout is that uricosuric and xanthine oxidase inhibition drugs need be given to only those patients who demonstrate frequent painful attacks, those with signs of gouty arthritis with joint destruction, and those with tophi deposits and/or renal urate stones.[2] With the proper combination of these agents, the serum level and the synovial fluid level of the urate crystals can be reduced and the joint fluid can actually be cleared of crystals. The primary care physician should be consulted early in the course of the attack of gout, and a plan should be established for future evaluation to prevent major symptoms from occurring again.

Calcium Pyrophosphate Dihydrate Crystal Deposition Disease

CLINICAL PRESENTATION

Calcium pyrophosphate dihydrate crystal deposition disease (CPPD) is also known as pseudogout because of its goutlike presentation and as chondrocalcinosis articularis because of the calcified appearance of the joint cartilage on radiographs. The asymptomatic deposition of CPPD crystals into the joint fluid and eventually into the cartilage surface progresses into the later decades of life.[3] Autopsy specimens show that 50% of persons who survived into their ninth decade have evidence of chondrocalcinosis.

CPPD crystal deposition–induced arthritis can be considered idiopathic, can be hereditary, or can be associated with metabolic disease such as gout, hyperparathyroidism, amyloidosis, or surgical stress. The process is almost the same as that which initiates the inflammation of the joint in gout. The CPPD crystals attach to the cartilage surface in the joint. Motion causes them to break off into the synovial fluid, and they are phagocytized like the urate crystals. The lysosomal enzymes fail to dissolve the crystals, and they spill into the joint fluid, irritating the synovium and producing the pain associated with the disease. The foot and knee are the most common sites of involvement. Also, CPPD is not uncommonly associated with an enthesopathy involving the foot, especially the heel.

Other conditions simulated by the CPPD disorder include pseudorheumatoid arthritis and pseudo-osteoarthritis. Like pseudogout, these conditions are less severe than their actual counterparts and are usually self-limited. The ability to differentiate the symptoms and establish the correct diagnosis is made difficult by the overlap of signs and presentations. To rule out rheumatoid arthritis, a rheumatoid arthritis latex factor test should be done.

DIAGNOSIS

As in gout, the aspiration of joint fluid is essential for a definitive diagnosis. Here, the crystals are positively birefringent and cast a blue pallor over the microscope slide (see Fig. 21–4), since they are perpendicular to the plane of polarized light.

RADIOLOGIC FEATURES

The presence of chondrocalcinosis is suggestive of CPPD (Fig. 21–5A). Superimposed on this change is degenerative wasting of the cartilage, clouding the true diagnosis. When the joint tap is positive for the CPPD crystals and the radiographs show the typical calcific stippling pattern, CPPD is virtually a certainty. The fibrocartilage of the knee, wrist, and symphysis pubis is a common site for screening. In the foot, fine lineal calcifications of the Achilles tendon may be seen (Fig. 21–5B).

TREATMENT

Although the nonsteroidal agents and colchicine, used in the same fashion and dosages as used with gout, are certainly helpful with the management of pain in the acute episode, both acting to reduce or eliminate the source of inflammation, the other drugs used in gout to clear the joint of crystals will not be of benefit. The only way to clear the joint of CPPD crystals is to perform a thorough aspiration of the joint fluid, followed by deposition of a corticosteroid agent. The long-term management of this disorder is directed at amelioration of the symptoms for each episode.

INFECTIOUS ARTHRITIS

Bacterial Infectious Arthritis

Bacteria are the most important cause of joint infection and must be recognized quickly since joint destruction can occur in a few days. There are two main categories of bacterial joint infections: gonococcal and nongonococcal bacteria. The gonococcal infections are caused by *Neisseria*, whereas most nongonococcal infections are caused by *Staphylococcus*.

Hematogenous spread of bacteria accounts for most of the cases of infectious arthritis,

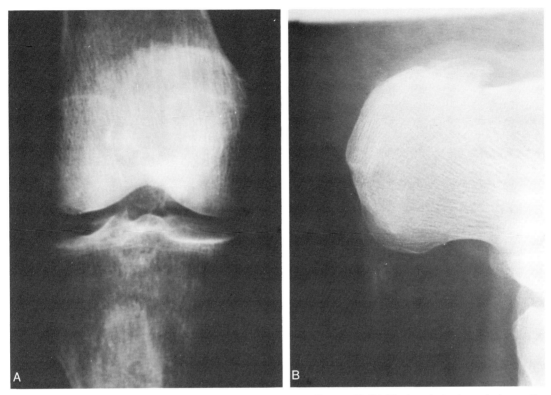

FIGURE 21–5. Calcium pyrophosphate dihydrate crystal deposition disease. *(A)* Calcific deposits in the articular cartilage of the knee. *(B)* Fine lineal calcification of the Achilles tendon.

while the remaining presentations occur in persons with puncture wounds, osteomyelitis adjacent to a joint space, systemic connective tissue diseases, and chronic illnesses and in the debilitated, infants, and the elderly. The mechanism of joint destruction by bacteria centers on the relatively high vascularity of the joint synovial tissue and thus the likelihood of bacteria to enter the joint cavity. Once this happens, the body's defense mechanisms are mobilized and the rapidly multiplying bacteria are engulfed by the endogenous synovial cells and the circulating macrophages, as well as by the phagocytes attracted to the site by chemotaxis. The defense cells secrete proteolytic enzymes into the synovial fluid, which then bathes the entire synovial and cartilage surfaces. The result is a thickening and granulating of the tissue lining with concomitant tissue destruction. The protein content of the cartilage is simultaneously reduced, leading to a severe weakening of its structure and the eventual destruction of each layer at the end of the infectious process. Once the raw subchondral bone is exposed, painful joint motion limitation will

occur, followed by fusion and ankylosis.[4] *Neisseria* and *Streptococcus* groups act more slowly in the joint destruction process, so early treatment can preserve the joint, while *Staphylococcus* and coliforms and other gram-negative bacteria show rapid joint destructive potential. The gram-negative bacteria are more frequently seen in joint infections involving children, while the gram-positive bacteria affect adults with greater regularity.

CLINICAL PRESENTATION

The initial presentation of an infected joint can look much like gout. The area is hot, painful, and swollen. The onset is acute, and the infection is monoarticular or pauciarticular. A low-grade fever is sometimes present. The knee is most commonly affected, followed by the wrist, shoulders, elbows, hips, and feet. As we know, gout is not common in younger persons. So, a single hot joint in a young person must be tapped and should be considered infected unless proven otherwise. Again, delay in the establishment of a proper diagnosis and institution of correct treatment can readily result in the destruction of the involved joint.

The diagnosis of an infected joint requires proof of the existence of bacteria in the joint fluid. This is accomplished through a joint aspiration. The fluid must then be Gram's stained and sent for culture and sensitivity studies. Overall, the causative organism will grow in only 50% of joint taps. In addition, blood cultures taken at this time will be positive in only 50% of cases. It is possible to examine the aspirated joint fluid and, in the absence of positive culture evidence of bacterial infection, surmise the presence of such organisms by the analysis of the contents of the joint fluid. The number of white blood cells usually exceeds 50,000 cells/mm^3 with a shift to the left, and the synovial blood glucose level is lower than a concomitant blood glucose reading. It is also very important to obtain radiographs of the involved joint to establish the condition of the subchondral bone. Usually taking at least 10 days to appear on films, the infection-mediated joint destruction may also be detected earlier by use of the triphasic bone scan. The results of a technetium-99m scan are nonspecific, merely indicating inflamed synovium, but the sensitivity is high, thus permitting early intervention when infection is suspected. A more specific radiopharmaceutical is indium-111. When labeled onto white blood cells, which pool at sites of infection, this test will reveal occult joint infections.

Gonococcal Arthritis

Gonococcal infection is the number one cause of pauciarticular arthritis in the younger age group. Disseminated gonococcal infection is the basis for hematogenous spread of the *Neisseria* organism in young, otherwise healthy adults.[5] Disseminated gonococcal infection occurs in less than 1% of persons who acquire gonorrhea, so the actual incidence of arthritis here is small. Women acquire 71% of cases of gonococcal infection during menses or pregnancy owing to increased blood supply in the genital region at these times. It is also more common in women owing to asymptomatic harboring of bacteria in the vagina. The same presence in the male genitourinary tract would be easily noticed and usually treated without further sequelae.

There are two phases of arthritis caused by disseminated gonococcal infection. In stage I, the *Neisseria* bacteria are disseminating in the bloodstream. The patient has chills and shakes. There are migratory arthralgias throughout the body. Pathognomonic skin lesions appear, congregating around the affected joint(s), most likely the knee, wrist, or ankle. These are hemorrhagic macules with central papules. Usually two to nine macules are present. A joint tap of the affected site is negative at this point. A blood culture is positive about 50% of the time at this stage. Tenosynovitis is common, involving more than one joint, and is especially common in the toes. Interestingly, only one fourth of patients with disseminated gonococcal infection have genitourinary symptoms of the disease, while this same group has over 75% positive cultures for *Neisseria* from swabs of the genital area.

In stage II the gonococci begin to localize on average in one to three joints and a pauciarticular arthritis begins. This is a purulent form of arthritis and is characterized by hot, swollen joints, skin lesions confined to the affected joint(s), and fever. At this stage, blood cultures are usually negative, the joint tap is positive for the organism in 25% to 50% of patients, and the mean synovial leukocyte count exceeds 68,000 cells/mm^3. The skin lesions around the affected joint(s) can be cultured and will usually show gram-negative diplococci on Gram's stain.

Nongonococcal Arthritis

As a general rule, gram-positive bacteria, predominently *Staphylococcus aureus* and *S. epidermidis*, followed by *Streptococcus hemolyticus*, are the major agents of joint sepsis in adults and older children, while gram-negative bacteria such as *Hemophilus influenzae* predominate in children up to age 24 months.[6] Neonates and the elderly commonly show *Escherichia coli* as the causative organism, while debilitated persons, diabetics, and intravenous drug users are infected with *Proteus, Serratia,* and other gram-negative bacteria. Persons with sickle cell disease are prone to *Salmonella* infections.

The source for these infections is usually a puncture wound, open sores on the skin over a joint, adjacent cellulitis or osteomyelitis, or hematogenous spread from a remote site of infection, such as a strep throat or pyelonephritis. About 20% of nongonococcal joint infections follow inadequate treatment of an existing infection, allowing a superinfection to develop and spread hematogenously. Preexisting joint damage, especially in patients with rheumatoid arthritis, predisposes to joint sepsis, usually of the *Staphylococcus* variety.

With the increase in the number of implants used to surgically reconstruct the foot comes an increase in the incidence of joint sepsis. *Staphylococcus* predominates, but the anaerobic bacteria, such as *Peptococcus*, *Peptostreptococcus*, and *Bacteroides*, are also major causes. These infections will often become chronic owing to the "barrier-to-treatment" effect of the implant itself, mainly by the formation of a layer of glycocalix over the device, making antibiotic penetration difficult, if not impossible. These cases usually result in the removal of the implant and revisional arthroplasty of the site with an extended course of antibiotic treatment.

DIAGNOSIS

To summarize, a joint tap is essential but not always diagnostic. Culture swabs of other body sites, the "source" of the infection, may be necessary to firmly establish the causative organism. The aspirate is Gram's stained and sent for culture and sensitivity testing. The fluid is examined and will usually show poor mucin clotting and a poor string test. The synovial fluid can be divided into three categories:

Category I: No white blood cells on microscopy

Category II: Up to 20,000 white blood cells/mm^3

Category III: More than 80,000 white blood cells/mm^3

Categories I and II are associated with gout and rheumatoid arthritides, while infectious arthritis yields a class III synovial fluid. In addition, the glucose level is decreased compared with the blood glucose level, and the protein level is increased.

TREATMENT

As is always the case with bacterial infections, treatment is organism specific, determined by the culture and sensitivity report. For penicillin-susceptible bacteria, such as that involved with disseminated gonococcal infection, penicillin G, 10 million units, given daily intravenously for 10 days is usually sufficient, as is a 10-day course of an oral penicillin covering the gram-negative spectrum. Nongonococcal arthritis bacteria require more complex antibiotic regimens, and an infectious disease consultation is usually advisable. The Gram's stain from the joint aspirate will serve as the guide for the initial drug course, followed by the culture and sensitivity results. Adequate drainage of the infected, suppurative joint is necessary, and surgical consultation is required at the earliest possible moment to avoid irreparable joint damage. Splinting of the joint is very helpful for long-term protection of the joint surfaces, and physical therapy should be started as soon as the infection is brought under control to minimize long-term joint dysfunction.

Bacterial arthritis is a source of chronic joint disability, including pain, stiffness, and loss of function. Over 50% of patients so afflicted will never recover completely.

Viral Infectious Arthritis

The two major viral-induced infectious arthritis categories are rubella and hepatitis B.

Rubella is seen predominently in young women, with 30% of these women developing arthralgias and fewer developing frank arthritis. Fifteen percent of men are so afflicted. The involved joints are the small ones of the feet and hands. The joints are warm, not hot, and are tender with slight effusions. The diagnosis is made by diagnosing the rubella infection, which is characterized by a diffuse maculopapular rash, fatigue, and lymphadenopathy. The arthritis can last for 6 months or longer but will usually resolve with time.

Hepatitis B arthritis shows a triad of (1) urticaria and rashes, (2) pauciarticular arthritis and stiffness of the small joints of the hands and feet, and (3) fever, which may precede the onset of jaundice by up to 1 month. This is not a true joint infection but a result of antibody–antigen complexes activating the lysosomal enzyme system within the joint capsule and causing acute synovitis. Diagnosis is made with virologic confirmation of the hepatitis B infection. Chronic active hepatitis B can lead to chronic, virally induced arthralgias. Otherwise, the course of the disease is self-limited and without long-term joint sequelae.

Lyme Disease

The bite of the *Ixodes* tick may transmit the spirochete *Borrelia burgdorferi*.[7] If this occurs, the first symptom in at least 75% of victims is the appearance, about 1 month after the bite, of a characteristic rash known as erythema chronicum migrans. This large annular lesion appears at the site of the bite, and the ring expands, adding layers of red upon blue before clearing. Associated symptoms include malaise, fever, chills, and arthralgias. In those patients in whom joint pain develops early on, there is over a 50% chance of progression to a full-blown arthritis, lasting months to years, mainly affecting larger joints. Polyarthritis of smaller joints is not uncommon.

After confirmation of the infection with immunologic testing, treatment is directed at eradication of the spirochete with penicillin (or with erythromycin in penicillin-allergic patients). Infectious disease consultation is mandatory.

RHEUMATOID ARTHRITIS

Rheumatoid arthritis is an inflammatory, symmetric, joint-destructive disease that usually presents in the small joints such as the metatarsophalangeal, the talonavicular, and the subtalar joints and at the Achilles tendon insertion into the calcaneus. The tendon surfaces most involved are the flexors, which pull the digits plantarly and laterally. The axial skeleton is usually spared. This is a disorder of the synovium, unlike degenerative joint disease, which affects the cartilage surface. Because rheumatoid arthritis is inflammatory, it has systemic manifestations such as malaise, fever, and morning stiffness usually lasting 45 minutes or more. Women, mostly in the 40- to 60-year age group, are affected three times more often than men, and the overall inci-

dence for all age groups in the United States is about 1% of the population. The initiating cause remains unknown.

The basis for diagnosis is the presence of the rheumatoid factor IgM antibody in the serum that is detected during immunologic surveys. Although a positive test is not specific for rheumatoid arthritis, a positive test combined with radiologic evidence of characteristic joint destruction and a concise clinical history leaves little doubt as to the nature of the disease. Other conditions having the IgM factor present in the serum include systemic lupus erythematosus, polymyositis, sarcoidosis, and leprosy. Conversely, 75% of patients with active rheumatoid disease will show the presence of this antibody.

PATHOGENESIS

The most widely accepted theory for the pathogenesis of rheumatoid arthritis involves the reaction between the IgM antibody and the IgG antigen substrate.[8] For some as yet undiscovered reason, the IgG antibody has become "foreign" to the person's immune system, and it is treated as an invader and thus as an antigen. This complex-forming reaction takes place in the synovial joint fluid and provokes the complement sequence, attracting polymorphonuclear leukocytes into the joint cavity. These cells phagocytize the complexes and release large quantities of prostaglandin precursors and hydrolytic enzymes into the joint fluid, which damage and inflame the synovial joint lining. The consequence of long-term inflammation of the synovium is the formation of pannus, a granulation tissue, across the joint space. This, in turn, creates unfavorable conditions, such as release of proteolytic enzymes into the cartilage surface, for the continued existence of smooth, healthy cartilage, which leads to pain and joint limitation of motion of a cartilaginous origin, in addition to the pain from the originating synovial inflammation. Eventually, the pannus scarifies and the joint undergoes fibrous ankylosis. This is the major reason why rheumatoid arthritis is destructive to the joint.

CLINICAL PRESENTATION

The American Rheumatism Association has established criteria for the diagnosis of rheumatoid arthritis, which can be found in tabular form in Appendix 2 in the *Primer on Rheumatic Diseases* published by the Arthritis Foundation. In this section of the chapter the focus is on the symptoms seen in the foot and the associated extra-articular manifestations.

The normal synovium is very thin. The interior lining is one cell thick, and this is covered by a thin support structure. When a pannus forms, the juxta-articular bone degrades at the synovial attachment sites, and cystic structures develop. The pannus invades the subchondral tissue. The joint ligaments are stretched by the proliferative synovial tissue, and laxity begins, resulting in characteristic joint deviations.

Radiographs show the cysts and cartilage loss clearly and aid in the diagnosis of the disease process. The signs in the feet are erosive changes at the medial aspects of the metatarsal heads, known commonly as "rat bite" erosions. They begin with the fifth metatarsal head, which also shows these changes laterally, and progress medially across the remaining metatarsals (Fig. 21–6). The fibular deviation of the toes is also characteristic of rheumatoid disease, as is dorsal toe contracture with subluxation and dislocation at the metatarsophalangeal joints. Retrocalcaneal bursitis is also common, and the inverted "E" sign at the posterosuperior aspect of the calcaneus is the erosive change in the bone brought about by the pressure from this bursa.

To summarize the radiographic changes seen with rheumatoid arthritis, the stages of progression are

    I. Soft tissue swelling with periarticular osteoporosis
   II. Trabecular thinning at the bone site where the synovium inserts
 III. Joint surface erosion in the "rat bite" fashion or the "dot-dash" pattern
 IV. Loss of joint space with subluxation and fibular deviation

The sclerotic changes, along with osteophytes seen in degenerative joint disease, are absent here. Comparative views of the hand are sometimes taken, and these will show erosive changes at the synovial insertion point in the wrist at the styloid process.

EXTRA-ARTICULAR MANIFESTATIONS

The skin of the foot can show deformities associated with seropositive rheumatoid disease. The most common skin lesion, seen in 10% to 20% of patients, is the rheumatoid nodule. This histologically unique structure can be mistaken for gouty tophi or cysts, but microscopically it is composed of pallisading fibroblasts with central fibrinoid necrosis. The area plantar to the metatarsal heads is a frequent site, as is the area surrounding the distal elbow.

Endarteritis and polyarteritis nodosa are rarer manifestations. Endarteritis presents as periungual infarcts that are red and tender. Polyarteritis nodosa affects medium-sized arteries in the leg and foot. Rheumatoid vasculitis affects medium- to large-sized arteries and can paralyze muscles governing function of the foot. More than one source has reported cases of dropfoot secondary to paralysis of the anterior tibialis muscle due to rheumatoid vasculitis.[9] Other changes that can occur with rheumatoid disease include Sjögren's syndrome, rheumatoid lung disease, and cardiac lesions.

LABORATORY ANALYSIS

Apart from the immunologic assay designed to identify and quantify the IgM antibody level, the erythrocyte sedimentation rate and analysis of the synovial fluid can yield significant findings and help to establish the diagnosis.

The differences between synovial fluid in normal persons versus patients with rheumatoid disease are shown in Table 21–1. Note that the complement, a system of 20 or so proteins normally found in the plasma that mediate inflammatory responses, is low caused by activation (due to inflammation) and then consumption by the IgM–IgG complexes. The plasma level is also low and thus is also a measurement of the disease process.

TREATMENT

The treatment pyramid is a universally accepted scheme for gradually increasing the complexity of therapies. The most conservative measures are on the bottom, with intricate and often experimental drug treatments at the top (Fig. 21–7).

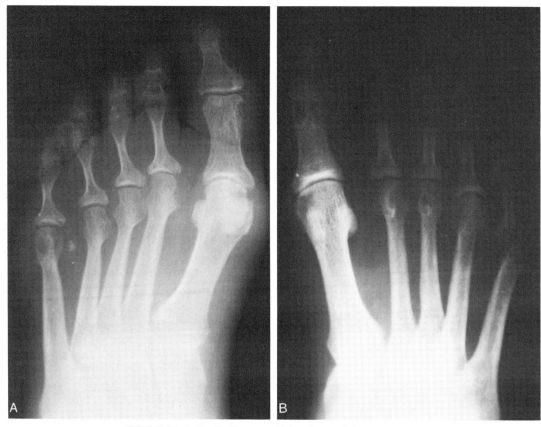

FIGURE 21–6. *(A)*, *(B)* Rheumatoid foot in two different patients.

The salicylates and the nonsteroidal anti-inflammatory agents are the first-line drug therapy in the treatment of rheumatoid arthritis. There are six classes for these drugs. The selection of one type over another should be based on history of use, tolerance to gastrointestinal side effects, overall patient compliance, and cross sensitivities with other medications. The usual precautions apply, such as monitoring of

liver and kidney function for long-term use and adequate warning and documentation of gastrointestinal side effects.

Therapeutic exercises are designed to maintain joint flexibility, retain muscle tone, and preserve the physiologic strength of ligaments and tendons. These should be taught by a physical therapist, and the patient should be observed at regular intervals to assess functional progress. The adjunctive use of accommodative and semirigid orthotics, extra-depth shoes with heat-moldable inlay material, molded shoes, and braces is important in the maintenance of function and in the improvement in the quality of daily life.

The use of corticosteroids is now limited to intra-articular injections and short courses of oral administration for treatment of extra-articular manifestations of rheumatoid disease. The accepted rule is no more than three injections per joint per calendar year.

When the nonsteroidal medications are no longer deemed effective in a patient, another

TABLE 21–1. **Synovial Fluid Analysis: Normal vs. Rheumatoid Arthritis**

	Normal	Rheumatoid Arthritis
Color	Clear	Cloudy
Mucin clot	Good	Poor
Cell count	<200 white blood cells	>200 white blood cells
Protein	<2.0 mg/dl	>2.0 mg/dl
Immune complexes	Absent	Present

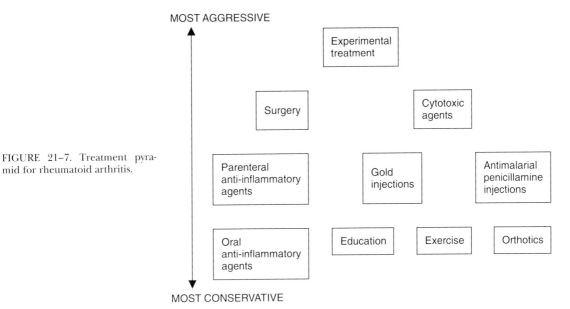

FIGURE 21–7. Treatment pyramid for rheumatoid arthritis.

MOST AGGRESSIVE

Experimental treatment

Surgery

Cytotoxic agents

Parenteral anti-inflammatory agents

Gold injections

Antimalarial penicillamine injections

Oral anti-inflammatory agents

Education

Exercise

Orthotics

MOST CONSERVATIVE

step is taken up the treatment pyramid, and the slow-acting drugs such as penicillamine, gold salts, and antimalarial agents are used. There are numerous side effects associated with these drugs, and close monitoring of the patient is essential.

Cytotoxic agents are used in the treatment of rheumatoid vasculitis, and new experimental medications are being developed that require highly specialized use but offer greater promise for control of this insidious disease.

Surgery is an important adjunct to all the above treatments. Reconstructive procedures, especially with the use of implants, can provide great relief of pain and vastly improve function.

SERONEGATIVE SPONDYLOARTHROPATHIES

Reiter's syndrome, psoriatic and enteropathic arthropathies, and ankylosing spondylitis comprise most of the seronegative spondyloarthropathies. The common factors shared by these entities include the absence of rheumatoid factor (hence the term *seronegative*), the similarities in the distal joint arthropathies, and the involvement of the sacroiliac joints. In addition, the association with the gene position HLA-B27 is significant. Between 5% and 10% of persons with this genetic marker will develop a related arthritis, and up to 50% of

persons who have the marker and who have relatives with an active HLA-B27–related disorder will develop such a condition. The other major association is with *Klebsiella* bacteria. There are theories that *Klebsiella* can transform the cell surface markers of lymphocytes, thus precipitating ankylosing spondylitis in HLA-B27–positive persons. The exact mechanism for this change is unknown.

To summarize, the hallmarks of seronegative spondyloarthropathies are association with the HLA-B27 marker; sacroiliitis; enthesopathies, as opposed to synovitis; asymmetric peripheral pauciarticular arthritis; acute iritis in 50% of these patients; and negative rheumatoid factor.

The sites of attack for this class of arthritides are the tendinous insertions of the axial skeleton, the sacroiliac joint, and the small joints of the hands and feet, thus creating enthesopathies.

Reiter's Syndrome

Although Reiter's syndrome has been classically described as a triad of symptoms, it is truly a tetrad since dermatitis is seen in up to 30% of patients diagnosed with Reiter's syndrome. The complete syndrome presents as arthritis, nonspecific urethritis, and conjunctivitis. It is thought that the etiology is infectious,[10] and the presentation of the initiating infection and subsequent arthritis with no other manifestations has been called the incomplete syndrome by Arnett and coworkers.[11] The infection causing this syndrome arises from either the gastrointestinal or the genitourinary tract. In the former case, *Shigella* and *Yersinia* are major suspect bacteria, and with the latter, *Chlamydia* is a prime candidate.[12] The arthritis that follows is a reactive type and is not septic. One current theory states that the bacteria react with the HLA-B27 markers in the infected person, initiating the arthritis.[13] The exact cause remains unknown, although we do know that 80% of the presentations will be in men and that about 2% of persons with infections caused by the bacteria listed earlier will progress to Reiter's syndrome. It is also known that *Neisseria gonorrhoeae* is *not* the cause of Reiter's syndrome.

CLINICAL PRESENTATION

Arthritis. The arthritis can have an explosive onset. The so-called sausage toe, also seen in psoriatic arthritis, is the hallmark of the foot involvement. The soft tissue insertions within the digit, including the ligaments and tendons, become acutely inflamed, leading to the classic edema in the toe. The distal interphalangeal joint is affected, with radiographic evidence of marginal erosions and periosteal bone formation. The "pencil-in-cup" presentation is seen here radiographically, as well as in psoriatic arthritis (see Fig. 21–8).

This is a chronic disease, and so the cycle of resorptive arthropathy followed by periosteal new bone formation often leads to ankylosis of the affected joint.

The tendinous insertions on the calcaneus are also classically involved. The Achilles and plantar fascial attachments are the two sites that show swelling, acute tenderness, and radiographic changes, including fluffy periosteal bone formation, the so-called lover's heel (Fig. 21–8).

Lastly, low back pain is reported, usually associated with sacroiliitis. This disease progresses to ankylosing spondylitis in 3% of known cases.[14]

Urethritis. In 30% of the patients with Reiter's syndrome, *Chlamydia* will be cultured from the clear, mucoid urethral discharge.

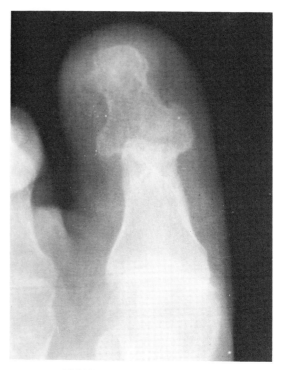

FIGURE 21–8. Reiter's syndrome.

The most common symptom is severe burning on urination. In women there may be cystitis without urethritis, which may go unnoticed.

Conjunctivitis. Conjunctivitis is a mild nonpurulent inflammation of the conjunctiva. It may be unilateral or bilateral and occurs early in the disease process.

Dermatologic Presentations. Balanitis circinata occurs on the penis as shallow ulcers, and keratoderma blennorrhagicum appears as a vesicular eruption on the soles of the feet (Fig. 21–9). Histologically, the foot lesions are identical to pustular psoriasis. The lesions scale and present in a moccasin sole distribution. Overall, the skin lesions occur in about 30% of the patients with Reiter's syndrome.

TREATMENT

The gold standard of therapy is a nonsteroidal anti-inflammatory agent. The choice is left to the treating physician, but indomethacin remains one drug with a reputation for being highly effective. There is no proof that antibiotics are helpful in shortening or "curing" the disease even though Reiter's syndrome has an infective etiology. Tetracycline is

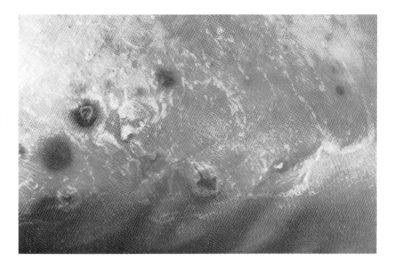

FIGURE 21–9. Skin lesions of pustular psoriasis. (From Gibbs RC: The skin. In Jahss MH [ed]: Disorders of the Foot and Ankle: Medical and Surgical Management, ed 2, p 1552. Philadelphia, WB Saunders, 1991.)

used for the relief of the urethritis early in the disease course. Intra-articular corticosteroid injections offer amelioration of local symptoms, but only temporarily. Systemic corticosteroids are of no use in long-term management. Topical corticosteroids are used in treating the dermatologic and conjunctival inflammations.

For long-term management of the pedal arthritis, accommodative orthotics with appropriate heel padding may be used to control impact forces and alleviate the pull of the plantar fascia and Achilles tendon on their respective insertion sites. The enthesopathies may also be helped by local application of ultrasound, by paraffin baths, and by electrostimulation therapy.

Psoriatic Arthritis

Which comes first, the skin disease or the arthritis? In up to 15% of the affected population, the arthritis precedes the psoriatic extensor surface skin plaques. For most sufferers, however, the skin and nail changes precede the arthritis by months to years. Overall, 7% of patients with psoriasis will have inflammatory arthritis.[15] Psoriatic arthritis in the foot mimics the arthritis of Reiter's syndrome. Therefore, in describing this and other similar clinical presentations, it is proper to state that the patient most likely has a seronegative spondyloarthropathy. There are patterns of presentation, however, and these are more characteristic of psoriatic arthritis than of the other seronegative arthritides.

CLINICAL PRESENTATION

Arthritis Patterns. There are four major types:

1. Asymmetric one- or two-joint involvement with sausage digit formations at the distal interphalangeal joint levels, seen in up to 10% of patients with the disease.
2. Polyarthritis that mimics rheumatoid arthritis, seen in 25% of the afflicted population. In the absence of concomitant rheumatoid disease, the rheumatoid factor would be negative.
3. Spondylitis and sacroiliitis with asymmetry as the typical presentation type associated with the more common psoriatic arthritis presentations in the peripheral joints.
4. Peripheral joint pauciarticular asymmetric arthritis, the most common presentation, in 95% of affected patients.[16]

Dermatologic Patterns. Round skin plaques found over the extensor surfaces of joints composed of white, desquamating remnants of epidermis over a red base with pustules often present, even if only microscopically, and are pathognomonic for psoriasis. The diagnosis of psoriatic arthritis cannot be made in the absence of psoriatic-type skin or nail lesions. Nail changes (usually pitting or ridging) are seen in 80% of patients with psoriatic arthritis but in only 20% of patients with just skin lesions (Fig. 21–10).

RADIOGRAPHIC FINDINGS

The distal interphalangeal joint involvement in the feet is initiated by the presence of an enthesopathy at the attachment sites of ligaments and tendons in the toes. This creates a periostitis, and thus a radiographically discernible change begins (Fig. 21–11). The progression of intra-articular effusions leads to the characteristic whittling of the interphalangeal joint surfaces and the eventual production of the classic "pencil-in-cup" appearance.

TREATMENT

As with most arthritides, the agents of choice are the nonsteroidal anti-inflammatory drugs, combined with appropriate intervals of rest, exercise, and supportive measures, such as properly molded shoes and orthotic inserts to accommodate foot deviations and protect preulcerous skin areas subject to excessive shoe pressure.

For those cases resistant to basic measures,

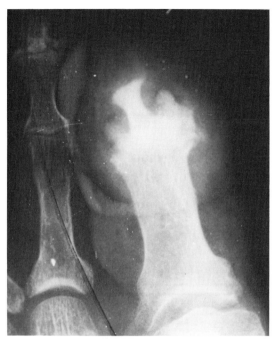

FIGURE 21–11. Osteosclerosis and acrolysis of the distal hallucal phalanx with bony ankylosis of the interphalangeal joint. The blurred appearance is due to periostitis. (Courtesy of Larry Osher, DPM.)

there are stronger medications, such as gold injections, methotrexate, antimalarial agents, and intra-articular corticosteroid injections. In addition, for joints too damaged for conservative treatments, replacement surgery remains a viable option. The skin lesions are treated with topical corticosteroids or psoralen-activated ultraviolet light (PUVA) therapy. In many patients the severity of the skin disease is directly correlated to the severity of the joint inflammation. Therefore, the best prognosis is for the group of patients presenting with asymmetric pauciarticular joint inflammation and thus the group with the fewest skin eruptions. The worst prognosis is reserved for those unfortunate few patients who develop arthritis mutilans, a rapidly progressive form of psoriatic arthritis in which bone resorption occurs rapidly and in which a joint may be totally destroyed in a matter of months. Surgical intervention is likely for these patients.

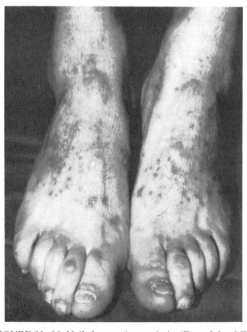

FIGURE 21–10. Nail changes in psoriasis. (From Jahss MH: Disorders of the hallux and first ray. In Jahss MH [ed]: Disorders of the Foot and Ankle: Medical and Surgical Management, ed 2, p 1158. Philadelphia, WB Saunders, 1991.)

Ankylosing Spondylitis

The prototype of the HLA-B27–positive arthropathies is ankylosing spondylitis. Remember, the seronegative spondyloarthropathies are characterized by a negative rheumatoid factor test, a positive HLA-B27 marker test, and sacroiliitis with or without peripheral joint inflammation. The distribution of these arthritides shows a predilection for tendinous insertions (the enthesis) rather than the synovial surfaces of joints. This means the entire axial skeleton will be affected, as well as fibrocartilage surfaces at the sacroiliac joint, the attachments of the plantar fascia, and the Achilles tendon insertion at the calcaneus.

Ankylosing spondylitis affects the sacroiliac joints primarily and the axial skeleton to a lesser extent. Psoriatic arthritis and Reiter's syndrome affects the peripheral joints, especially the distal interphalangeal joints of the toes, and, to a lesser degree, the sacroiliac joints. Rheumatoid arthritis is symmetrically distributed to synovial-lined joint surfaces, and degenerative joint disease affects weight-bearing joints in an uneven pattern.

CLINICAL PRESENTATION

This disease is seen mostly in young men in the 20- to 30-year age group. Initial complaints include low back pain, morning stiffness, and lessening symptoms with activity during the day. There can be involvement of the cervical spine in the form of frequent stiff necks. Clinically, there is loss of the normal lordotic spinal curvature, with decrease in forward flexion, decrease of chest expansion due to costochondritis, and peripheral joint involvement in one fifth of affected patients.

PATHOLOGY

Ankylosing spondylitis tends to occur in the upper two thirds of the fibrocartilaginous joint surface and the lower third of the synovial-lined joint in the sacroiliac joint. The inflammation is in the cartilage itself. The lymphocytic infiltration in the cartilage erodes the subchondral bone, and new bone formation begins to occur with ankylosis of contiguous bone structures. In the hip joint, the most common peripheral site affected, and in the spine, erosions at the enthesis result in periosteal reaction and new bone formation, which, in the spine, gives a squared-off appearance to the vertebral bodies and eventual bony ankylosis with loss of motion.

RADIOLOGIC DIAGNOSIS

The squared-off appearance on the superior and inferior corners of vertebral bodies is seen on a posteroanterior spinal radiograph. In advanced ankylosis, the classic "bamboo" spine appearance is recognized. In the spondylosis of Reiter's syndrome and psoriatic arthritis, the enthesopathy of the vertebral bodies is asymmetric, whereas in ankylosing spondylitis, the appearance is uniform and symmetric. The radiographs of the foot may reveal a vertical spur at the plantar aponeurosis attachment site on the calcaneus along with the spurring of enthesopathy at the Achilles tendon insertion (Fig. 21–12).

TREATMENT

With therapy with anti-inflammatory medication, the sufferer of this disease should lead a fairly active life. With active physical therapy

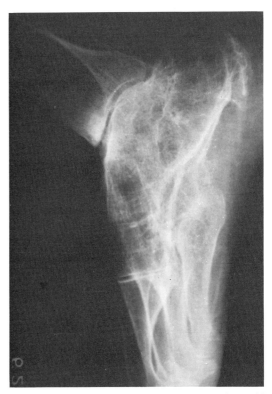

FIGURE 21–12. Extensive tarsal bony ankylosis along with a large, poorly defined calcaneal spur in ankylosing spondylitis. (Courtesy of Larry Osher, DPM.)

and appropriate exercise, a shoe orthosis, and posterior heel protection, the patient, barring extra-articular manifestations that may be life threatening, such as spinal fractures and cardiac conduction defects, can maintain good posture and a comfortable gait.

Enteropathic Arthritis

There are two types of arthritis that can be associated with either ulcerative colitis or Crohn's disease. The first is a pauciarticular large joint arthritis affecting the knee or ankle, and the second is spondylitis (the symmetric variety). With pauciarticular arthritis, the joint inflammation level parallels the degree of bowel inflammation. When the bowel quiets down, the arthritis goes into remission. With the spondylitis, the bowel inflammation and the arthritis are not on parallel courses. With clearing of the bowel inflammation, the enteropathic spondylitis continues, and the course is similar to that of ankylosing spondylitis. In both cases, there is a negative association with the HLA-B27 antigen.

Another variety of enteropathic arthritis is reactive arthritis caused by an enteric infection of *Shigella, Yersinia,* or *Salmonella.* This is a self-limiting arthritis for most sufferers, clearing in 1 to 3 months. Typical presenting complaints include plantar fascial pain and Achilles tendonitis. Plantar heel pain without spur formation is also reported. In some males, resistant strains of bacteria may eventually lead to active Reiter's syndrome.[17]

Treatment is typical of other inflammatory joint diseases and includes nonsteroidal anti-inflammatory agents, rest, physical therapy, and intra-articular corticosteroids. Achilles tendon and plantar fascial rest straps will also benefit the patient until the disease resolves.

REFERENCES

1. Boss GR, Seegmiller JE: Hyperuricemia and gout: Classification, complications and management. N Engl J Med 300:1459–1468, 1979.
2. Wallace SL, Singer JZ: Gout: In Schumacher H (ed): Primer on the Rheumatic Diseases, ed 9. Atlanta, GA, Arthritis Foundation, 1988.
3. McCarty DJ, Kohn NN, Faires JS: The significance of calcium phosphate crystals in the synovial fluid of arthritic patients: The "pseudo-gout" syndrome. Ann Intern Med 56:711, 1962.
4. Goldenberg DL, Reed JI: Bacterial arthritis. N Engl J Med 312:764–771, 1985.
5. O'Brien JP, Goldenberg DL, Rice PA: Disseminated gonococcal infection. Medicine 62:395–406, 1983.
6. Rosenthal J, Bole GG, Robinson WD: Acute non-gonococcal infectious arthritis. Arthritis Rheum 23:889–897, 1980.
7. Steere AC, Grodzicki RL, Kornblatt AN: The spirochetal etiology of Lyme disease. N Engl J Med 308:733–740, 1983.
8. Zvaifler NJ: Immunology of joint inflammation in rheumatoid arthritis. Adv Immunol 16:265–336, 1973.
9. Goldman EP, Stess R: Rheumatoid vasculitis—a case report. J Am Podiatr Med Assoc 74:514–516, 1984.
10. Wilkens RF, Arnett FC, Bitter T: Reiter's syndrome. Arthritis Rheum 24:844–849, 1981.
11. Arnett FC, McClusky OE, Schacter BZ: Incomplete Reiter's syndrome. Ann Intern Med 84:8–12, 1976.
12. Keat AC, Maini RN, Nkwazi GC: Role of *Chlamydia trachomatis* and HLA-B27 in sexually acquired reactive arthritis. Br Med J 1:605–607, 1978.
13. Seager K, Bashir HV: Evidence for specific B27 cell marker in patients with ankylosis spondylitis. Nature 277:68–70, 1979.
14. Lerisalo M, Skylv G, Kousa M: Follow-up study on patients with Reiter's disease and reactive arthritis, with special reference to HLA-B27. Arthritis Rheum 25:249–259, 1985.
15. Wright V: Sero-negative polyarthritis: A unified concept. Arthritis Rheum 21:619–632, 1978.
16. Kammer GM, Soter NA, Gibson DJ: Psoriatic arthritis: A clinical immunologic and HLA study of 100 patients. Semin Arthritis Rheum 9:75–97, 1979.
17. Keat A: Reiter's syndrome and reactive arthritis in perspective. N Engl J Med 309:1606–1615, 1983.

CHAPTER 22

GERIATRIC ASSESSMENT

Robert M. Palmer

Improved social conditions and medical care and the demographic changes during the 20th century have increased the number of older persons in the United States. In 1985, the proportion of the American population aged 65 and older had increased to 12% from 4% in 1900. By the year 2030, an estimated 18.5% of Americans will be 65 years of age or older. Life expectancy in old age is increasing as well. The average additional life expectancy of a community-dwelling 65-year-old woman is 19 years; for a 65-year-old man it is 15 years. Even at age 85, the additional life expectancy is more than 5 years for both men and women.[1]

With the aging of the American population, the prevalence of chronic diseases, illnesses, and related functional disabilities has increased. The loss of functional independence experienced by the frail elderly population places great strain on the economic resources of patients, their families, and society and has led to a crisis in long-term care. A "geriatric imperative" has arisen to address the functional and health care needs of older persons. Health care professionals have developed a systematic process, called comprehensive geriatric assessment, composed of a multidisciplinary evaluation in which the problems of older persons are uncovered, described, and explained, if possible, and in which the resources and strengths of the person are cataloged, need for services assessed, and a coordinated care plan developed to focus interventions on the person's problem.[2] Comprehensive assessment involves the evaluation of the physical, psychosocial, and environmental factors affecting the health of an elderly person. "Functional status" refers to the older person's ability to function independently in the physical, mental, and social activities of daily life. Functional status reflects the personal disabilities and social handicaps that result from impairments (losses or abnormalities of physiologic or psychological function at the organ level). Functional status is often measured in terms of activities of daily living (ADL). It may also be measured in terms of mobility and cognitive functioning.

A growing body of literature attests to the usefulness of a comprehensive assessment of frail elderly patients to identify, evaluate, and treat functional impairments and possibly improve therapeutic outcomes. The goals of a comprehensive geriatric assessment are (1) to improve diagnostic accuracy; (2) to guide the selection of interventions to restore or preserve health; (3) to recommend an optimal environment for care; (4) to predict outcomes; and (5) to monitor clinical change over time.[2] Often the assessment is conducted by a team of health care professionals—geriatricians, social workers, nurse specialists, rehabilitation therapists—with expertise in this area. Both case finding and in-depth approaches are used in the assessment process. The case finding or screening instruments can be easily administered by health care professionals in various settings. When abnormalities are detected, an in-depth evaluation may be conducted by an interdisciplinary team, often in a geriatric assessment unit.

Geriatric assessment differs from the standard medical evaluation in its concentration on frail elderly persons, emphasis on functional status and quality of life (the patient's global perception of life satisfaction), and frequent use of interdisciplinary teams.[3] An assessment may uncover treatable functional impairments that are uncommon in middle-aged patients. For example, compared with a 55-year-old man, an 80-year-old man with foot pain is more likely to be demented, have multiple co-morbid conditions (e.g., arthritis, heart disease, and sensory impairments), be impaired in basic ADL (e.g., bathing and dressing), develop an adverse drug reaction leading to delirium, have fewer social supports (e.g., family caregivers), and require long-term care at home or in a nursing home. A comprehensive assessment of this elderly man would begin with a screening test for functional disabilities coupled with an appropriate referral to a geriatric assessment unit for an in-depth evaluation. Some interventions may reverse or improve the patient's functional disabilities: changing medications to avoid adverse drug reactions (e.g., confusion from psychotropic medications), prescribing exercises to main-

tain joint and muscle function, recommending assistive devices (e.g., hearing aids) to maximize sensory input, identifying caregiver availability and needs in the home, and initiating arrangements for home care (e.g., short-term physical therapy) that may obviate nursing home placement.

Patients who are most likely to benefit from a comprehensive assessment include those who have a living situation in transition (e.g., from home to nursing home), the recent development of physical or cognitive impairments, and inadequate primary medical care.[2] A comprehensive geriatric assessment is also useful when evaluating patient competency or dealing with potential medicolegal issues. A comprehensive assessment linked to interventions can reduce the level of caregiver burden or strain experienced by family members of impaired elderly patients.

Five elements of a comprehensive geriatric assessment have been identified: (1) physical health, (2) mental health, (3) social and economic status, (4) functional status, and (5) environmental characteristics.[2] Although this comprehensive approach is often time consuming and requires a multidisciplinary team, components of the assessment can be performed easily in an office practice. Each element of the assessment process contributes to a better understanding of the elderly patient's health status and prognosis, which helps guide clinical decision-making.

EFFECTIVENESS OF GERIATRIC ASSESSMENT

A comprehensive assessment is most effective when coupled with ongoing interventions. In controlled trials, primarily of medically ill patients, favorable outcomes affected by comprehensive assessment include prolonged survival, reduced medical care costs, reduced use of acute hospitals, and reduced use of nursing homes.[2] Other benefits reported include increased use of health and social services delivered in the home, reduced medication usage, and improved placement location. Improved mood and cognition, diagnostic accuracy, and functional status have also been reported.[2] Studies conducted in hospitalized patients document the effectiveness of geriatric assessment compared with usual medical care to detect cognitive impairment, depression, and functional dependency in older patients.

The importance of functional limitations is demonstrated in studies showing their independent contribution to certain undesirable outcomes: prolonged hospitalization, readmission to hospital, nursing home placement, and mortality.[4, 5] Interventions can favorably affect these outcomes, particularly when targeted at patients who are likely to benefit from the assessment and when there is follow-up and direct clinical control.[3, 6]

The effectiveness of comprehensive geriatric assessment has been most clearly demonstrated in studies of specialized units. The first randomized controlled trial of a geriatric assessment unit was conducted in a Veteran Affairs hospital. In this study, elderly veterans who were convalescing from an acute hospitalization and were functionally impaired were randomized to either a special inpatient unit (and follow-up in a geriatric outpatient clinic) or to usual medical care on the ward and clinics.[7] The patients receiving the intervention were less often discharged to a nursing home and less likely to spend any time in a nursing home following discharge. Hospital readmissions and mortality over the subsequent year were more common in the control group.[7]

A randomized trial of a geriatric assessment and rehabilitation unit, performed within a rehabilitation hospital, also had positive results.[8] Elderly patients recovering from acute hospital care for medical or surgical illnesses were randomized to receive assessment and rehabilitation on the special unit or usual care in the community. Treatment on the special unit resulted in significantly decreased nursing home admissions. Special unit patients had significantly more functional improvement in several basic self-care activities and more were residing in the community 6 months after randomization. There was a trend toward fewer deaths among patients treated in the special unit.[8] The costs of the intervention, however, were considerable in this and the previous study, primarily related to the extended length of hospitalization of the intervention groups. Consequently, current research interest in inpatient geriatric assessment has shifted to innovative models of acute care that incorporate

the principles of comprehensive assessment into the routine care of hospitalized elderly patients.[9]

In descriptive studies, the benefits of outpatient geriatric assessment include reduced medical care costs, prolonged survival, increased use of home health care services, improved long-term care placement, and improved diagnostic accuracy. In a landmark publication, Williams and colleagues[10] demonstrated the value of a multidisciplinary evaluation in preventing inappropriate placement of elderly patients in nursing homes. After assessment of 332 patients referred for consideration for placement, 22% were enabled to remain at home and only 35% were found to need nursing homes. An independent follow-up assessment showed that 84% of the 332 patients were appropriately placed for their needs.[10] The impact of this study is evident in the subsequent proliferation of geriatric assessment units in the United States.[11]

Controlled trials of ambulatory geriatric assessment have provided conflicting results. In one study, conducted at an academic medical center, 117 carefully selected frail elderly patients were randomized either to outpatient care in a geriatric assessment center or to usual assessment and care by a group of internists known to be interested in caring for the elderly.[12] Over a 1-year period of follow-up, the patients receiving geriatric assessment in the geriatric center had fewer hospital admissions and fewer hospital days compared with the control group; annual hospital costs were also lower for the treatment group and overall institutional costs were slightly lower. The geriatric assessment center had no effect on institutionalization, functional status, or health status.[12] In another study, 240 elderly veterans were randomized to either a specialized geriatric clinic or usual care in a general medicine clinic. Over an 18-month period, the geriatric assessment group experienced less decline in self-rated functional health but had a trend toward higher mortality.[13] Attrition of patients during the study, however, limited interpretation of the results. In a study of consultative geriatric assessment for ambulatory patients in a health maintenance organization, 600 elderly patients were randomly assigned to one of three groups: (1) consultation by a geriatric assessment team, (2) consultation by a "second opinion internist," and (3) only traditional health maintenance organization services (control patients).[14] The geriatric assessment team identified previously recognized problems in 35% of patients and advised changes in medication regimens for more than 40%. However, at 1-year follow-up, there was no significant difference among the groups in other measures of health status. The authors concluded that geriatric assessment with limited follow-up did not benefit most older ambulatory patients in this setting; furthermore, for ambulatory consultative assessment to be effective, patients should be selected for their likelihood of benefiting from the intervention.[14]

Despite the uncertain effectiveness of ambulatory assessment programs, two studies have demonstrated the effectiveness of home-based assessment and management. In one, 600 nontargeted elderly patients older than the age of 75 were randomized to receive either quarterly home assessment visits by trained nurses or usual care.[15] The nurses assessed the patients' home health needs and made arrangements for appropriate medical or social services. Although the study did not measure the impact of the intervention on patient functional status, the group receiving the home assessment visit used more in-home social services than the control group and experienced a lower mortality. There was also a nonsignificant trend toward fewer hospitalizations and nursing home placements.[15] In the other study, patients in two general practices older than the age of 70 were randomized to receive at least one extra visit per year from a home visitor (equivalent to a public health nurse) or no extra visit.[16] The intervention group used more in-home nursing visits and home health care and had a significantly lower mortality rate over 2 years of follow-up. Only those patients living in urban areas benefited from the intervention. There was no improvement in functional status or the number of physician visits.[16] These two studies suggest that in-home assessment, when coupled with triage for social support and medical care, may have a beneficial effect on health outcomes.[17] Although there is no convincing evidence from controlled trials that comprehensive ger-

iatric assessment will lead to improved functional status, reduced rates of nursing home placement, or prolonged survival, descriptive studies indicate that diagnostic precision, therapeutic decision making, and appropriate diagnostic evaluation and treatment are achievable.

COMPONENTS OF A COMPREHENSIVE GERIATRIC ASSESSMENT

Case Finding (Screening)

The components of a comprehensive geriatric assessment include case finding approaches and in-depth evaluations of geriatric syndromes. These are complemented by a targeted medical history, physical examination, and laboratory evaluation. The comprehensive assessment is targeted at patients aged 75 years and older or those with a history of recent decline in physical or mental functioning.

The case finding approach, which includes the use of screening instruments, can be incorporated into the primary practice of a podiatrist. Standardized, valid, and reliable assessment instruments are available to measure mental (cognitive) function and activities of daily living.[18] The assessment instruments described here are easily taught to office staff and can be administered to patients and their families in approximately 30 minutes. The case finding assessment may be truncated with a "review of functions" that explores the patient's ability to perform basic and instrumental ADL (Table 22–1).[19] The importance of changes in patient independence in ADL is underscored by both clinical and epidemiologic studies. In longitudinal studies of community-dwelling elderly, functional dependency measured in terms of ADL is an independent predictor of morbidity and death over 3 years of observation.[20] In hospitalized medically ill patients, factors most predictive of 6-month mortality include decreased functional status, diagnosis on admission, and decreased mental status; however, functional status is a stronger independent predictor of hospital length of stay, mortality, and nursing home placement than is a principal admitting diagnosis.[4] Similar results have been found in

TABLE 22–1. **Geriatric Review of Functions**

Target Area	Assessment Procedure	Abnormal Result	Suggested Intervention
Vision	Test each eye with Jaeger card while patient wears corrective lenses (if applicable).	Inability to read greater than 20/40	Refer to ophthalmologist.
Hearing	Whisper a short, easily answered question such as "What is your name?" in each ear while the examiner's face is out of direct view.	Inability to answer question	Examine auditory canals for cerumen and clean canals if necessary. Repeat test; if result is still abnormal in either ear, refer for audiometry and possible prosthesis.
Nutrition	Weigh the patient. Measure height.	Weight is below acceptable range for height	Do appropriate medical evaluation.
Mental status	Administer Mini-Mental State Examination.	Score < 24	If score is < 24, search for causes of cognitive impairment. Ascertain onset, duration, and fluctuation of overt symptoms. Review medications. Assess consciousness and affect. Obtain consultation.
Depression	Administer Geriatric Depression Scale (short form).	Score > 5	If > 5, check for antihypertensive, psychotropic, or other pertinent medications. Consider psychiatric consultation.
Activities of daily living and instrumental activities of daily living	Administer ADL and IADL scales.	No to any question	Corroborate responses with patient's appearance; question family members if accuracy is uncertain. Determine reasons for the inability (motivation compared with physical limitation). Institute appropriate medical or social consultation.
Home environment	Ask: "Do you have trouble with stairs inside or outside your home?"; ask about potential hazards inside the home with bathtubs, rugs, or lighting.	Yes to any question	Home safety evaluation and consultation
Social support	Ask: "Who would be able to help you in case of illness or emergency?"		List identified persons in the medical record. Identify available resources for the elderly in the community.

From Lachs MS, Feinstein AR, Cooney LM, et al: A simple procedure for general screening for functional disability in elderly patients. Ann Intern Med 112:700, 1990.

elderly patients who are admitted to medical intensive care units; functional dependency at admission, in one study, is an independent predictor of mortality during 1-year follow-up.[21]

Psychosocial factors have emerged as important prognostic variables in the surgical literature. In a prospective study of predictors of functional recovery 1 year following hospital discharge for hip fracture, recovery was poorer among elderly patients who had chronic or acute cognitive impairments and depressive symptomatology while hospitalized; patient contact with the social network following hospital discharge was associated with greater recovery.[5] In another study of the determinants of recovery 12 months after hip fracture, poor cognitive status and postsurgical self-rated health were predictive of mortality; among survivors, good prefracture physical functioning and cognitive status were associated with recovery and physical function.[22] In addition, high postoperative depression scores were associated with poorer recovery in both functional and psychosocial status. Delirium (acute confusional state) in hospitalized medically ill patients was associated with prolonged length of stay, greater likelihood of institutionalization, and death; furthermore, delirium was often related to preventable or treatable conditions.[23]

BASIC AND INSTRUMENTAL ACTIVITIES OF DAILY LIVING

The most widely used measures of basic ADL are the Katz Index of ADL and the Lawton Physical Self-Maintenance Scale (Table 22–2).[24, 25] The Katz Index includes ratings of patient independence in bathing, dressing, transferring (from bed to chair), toileting, continence, and feeding. With progressive physical impairment, the ADL are lost in hierarchical order (from bathing to feeding). Assessment of independence in ADL may be made by objective (performance based) measurement or by subjective reports of the patient and/or proxy (family member). Although self-reports are most often used, particularly for community-based studies and long-term follow-up, measurement bias can be problematic.[26] Most studies suggest that patients, compared with proxies (family members or nurses), tend to overestimate their functional independence. Thus it is advisable to confirm self-reports through collateral interviews with family members or other caregivers.

The percent of community residents aged 65 and older who receive help with some ADL is age related. Community residents aged 65 to 74 are unlikely to be dependent in any of the six Katz Index ADL—only 5% have daily incontinence while less than 5% are dependent in bathing, dressing, or transferring. In contrast, among those 85 years of age and older, daily incontinence is reported in nearly 15%, dependence in bathing in 21%, and dependence in toileting and transferring in nearly 10%.[27] Among nursing home residents, however, dependence in at least one ADL is present in nearly all patients; even those in the age group 65 to 74 are likely to be dependent in multiple ADL.[27] Impairments of ambulation and mobility are also important measures of functional status. Mobility problems are implied when patients are dependent in transferring or toileting, tasks that require independent ambulation.

The measurement of patient ADL has practical implications. Patients who are dependent in basic ADL are unlikely to remain healthy while living alone. Either increased caregiving support (e.g., home health aide) or institutionalization will be needed. In addition, an impairment in performance of ADL is often a clue to the presence of one of the geriatric syndromes (e.g., dementia) described below.

The instrumental ADL (IADL) are more complex tasks than the basic ADL (see Table

---

TABLE 22–2. **Activities of Daily Living**

Activity	Independent	Needs Assistance	Unable to Perform
Basic Activities of Daily Living			
Bathing	_____	_____	_____
Dressing	_____	_____	_____
Grooming	_____	_____	_____
Transfer	_____	_____	_____
Toileting	_____	_____	_____
Continence	_____	_____	_____
Feeding	_____	_____	_____
Instrumental Basic Activities of Daily Living			
Telephone use	_____	_____	_____
Shopping	_____	_____	_____
Food preparation	_____	_____	_____
Housekeeping	_____	_____	_____
Laundry	_____	_____	_____
Transportation	_____	_____	_____
Medications	_____	_____	_____
Finances	_____	_____	_____

From Lawton MP, Brody EM: Assessment of older people: Self-maintaining and instrumental activities of daily living. Gerontologist 9:180–181, 1969. Copyright © 1969, The Gerontological Society of America.

21–2).[25] Completion of IADL requires a high degree of cognitive and/or physical functioning (e.g., handling finances and housekeeping). In many chronic degenerative diseases (e.g., osteoarthritis or dementia), impairments of patient IADL precede impairments of basic ADL. Patients who need assistance with transportation, shopping, preparing meals, housework, and personal finances are likely to have impaired physical or mental health and appear to have a poorer prognosis than functionally independent patients. In one study, the results of a five-item instrument based on IADL rapidly identified elderly community residents with impaired functional capacity.[28] Patient dependence in performing housework, traveling, shopping, meal preparation, and handling finances was predictive of deteriorating physical or mental health.[28] Inability to comply with self-administration of medication has important implications. Noncompliance with medication is common among demented and depressed patients and may result in iatrogenic illness.

COGNITION SCREENING

Cognitive dysfunction due to dementia or delirium is common among the frail elderly and is associated with postoperative complications of prolonged hospitalization, institutionalization, and mortality.[23] Approximately 25% of elderly patients become delirious during the course of hospitalization. The delirium is often a consequence of the acute illness or a result of medical, surgical, or anesthetic interventions. For example, in the perioperative period, delirium may follow the administration of psychotropic drugs or anesthetic agents (particularly those with anticholinergic properties) and prolonged hypotension or hypoxemia.[23]

Approximately 5% of the community-dwelling American population aged 65 years or older is demented. The prevalence of dementia increases to at least 20% to 30% in persons aged 80 years and older. The diagnosis of dementia is supported by evidence of cognitive impairment during a screen with an instrument, such as the Mini-Mental State Examination (MMSE) (Table 22–3)[29] or the Short Portable Mental Status Questionnaire (SPMSQ) (Table 22–4).[30] Although none of the cognitive screening instruments is ideal, the MMSE has enjoyed the widest acceptance owing to its ease of administration, testing of all major components of cognition, and sensitivity to change over time.[31] A score below 24 of 30 is consistent with cognitive dysfunction. The cutoff point for dysfunction is lowered to 21 or 22 for very old or uneducated patients. Briefer instruments such as the SPMSQ are easier to administer, although less sensitive (i.e., more false-negative results) than the MMSE. A score of more than two errors of 10 points on the SPMSQ is abnormal.

Screening for cognitive impairment in a podiatric practice is important. Cognitive dysfunction is associated with higher risks of bad outcomes from surgery (e.g., prolonged hospitalization, nursing home placement, and mortality). Successful rehabilitation from acute or chronic illness is prohibited by the patient's inability to learn and retain new information, such as appropriate care of wounds and foot dressings. Furthermore, patients who are unable to manage self-care owing to cognitive impairment will require supervision from family members, which adds to their level of burden and may place the patient at risk for institutionalization, particularly if social supports are inadequate. Although demented patients often appear alert and cooperative, they may not be competent to give informed consent for foot surgery and may be unable to follow subsequent therapeutic instructions. Therefore, a screening assessment of cognitive function is recommended before podiatric services are provided to very old patients.

DEPRESSION SCREENING

Depressive symptoms are common in the elderly population. Approximately 10% of community-dwelling elderly persons express depressive symptoms, and 3% to 5% have clinically diagnosable depression. The prevalence of depression is higher in elderly patients in hospitals and nursing homes. Depression is associated with poor responses to medical and surgical interventions and an increased risk of suicide, particularly among white males. The diagnosis of depression may be obscured by atypical symptoms and signs in elderly patients, justifying a screening test for this treatable condition. Numerous screening

TABLE 22–3. **Mini-Mental State Examination**

Maximum Score	Score	Item
		Orientation
5	( )	What is the (year) (season) (date) (day) (month)?
5	( )	Where are we? (state) (county) (town) (hospital) (floor)
		Registration
3	( )	Name three objects: 1 second to say each. Then ask the patient all three after you have said them. Give 1 point for each correct answer. Then repeat them until he or she learns all three (for later checking).
		Attention and Calculation
5	( )	Serial 7s. Give 1 point for each correct. Stop after five answers. Alternatively, spell ''world'' backward.
		Recall
3	( )	Ask for the three objects repeated above. Give 1 point for each correct answer.
9	( )	Show patient a pencil and a watch, and ask for their names. (2 points) Repeat the following; ''No ifs, ands, or buts.'' (1 point) Follow a three-stage command: ''Take a paper in your right hand, fold it in half, and put it on the floor.'' (3 points) Read and obey the following: ''Close your eyes.'' (1 point) Write a sentence. (1 point) Copy a simple design. (1 point)

_____   Total score

Reprinted with permission from Folstein MF, et al: ''Mini-Mental State'': A practical method for grading the cognitive state of patients for the clinician. J Psychiatr Res 123:196–198, 1975, Pergamon Press plc.

instruments have been validated for use in the general population. In the elderly, the Geriatric Depression Scale, a 30-item questionnaire, is recommended as a screening measure for detection of depression because of its high sensitivity and specificity, its ease of administration, and its simple format, which allows it to be used in patients with limited education and mild cognitive impairment (Table 22–5).[32] A score of more than 11 is consistent with a diagnosis of depression. The Geriatric Depression Scale has been truncated to a 15-item questionnaire, which retains good sensitivity and specificity (the 15 questions are numbers 1 through 4, 7 through 10, 12, 14, 15, 17, and 21 through 23).[33] With the short form, scores of more than 5 are consistent with depression.

SOCIAL SUPPORTS

A variety of social supports and family network instruments have been devised, but few have been widely applied in clinical practice. Social isolation or inadequate social support networks are important predictors of nursing home placement in both ambulatory and hos-

---

TABLE 22–4. **Short Portable Mental Status Questionnaire**

Instructions: Ask questions 1–10 in this list and record all answers. Ask question 4A only if patient does not have a telephone. Record total number of errors based on 10 questions.

+	–		
		1.	What is the date today? _____ Month Day Year
		2.	What day of the week is it? _____
		3.	What is the name of this place? _____
		4.	What is your telephone number? _____
		4A.	What is your street address? _____
		5.	How old are you? _____
		6.	When were you born? _____
		7.	Who is the President of the U.S. now? _____
		8.	Who was President just before him? _____
		9.	What was your mother's maiden name? _____
		10.	Subtract 3 from 20 and keep subtracting 3 from each new number, all the way down.

_____   Total Number of Errors

To Be Completed by Interviewer
Patient's Name: _____   Date: _____
Sex: 1. Male ☐   Race: 1. White ☐
2. Female ☐   2. Black ☐
3. Other ☐
Years of Education: _____   1. Grade School ☐
2. High School ☐
3. Beyond High School ☐
Interviewer's Name: _____

From Pfeiffer E: A Short Portable Mental Status Questionnaire for the assessment of organic brain deficit in elderly patients. J Am Geriatr Soc 23:440, 1975. Copyright © 1975, American Geriatrics Society.

---

pitalized elderly patients.[5] Because of the importance of the social support network, a structured interview of the patient and family is useful to identify primary and secondary family caregivers and other community supports who can assist the patient with personal care needs during times of illness. Cognitively or physically impaired patients are often a source of caregiver strain. High strain among caregivers can have untoward effects on their physical and mental health. High caregiver strain is also associated with the potential of elder abuse (neglect) and unnecessary placement of patients in nursing homes. Hence, an assessment of the caregiver's general health and attitudes about caregiving may identify high levels of strain. Several caregiver strain instruments have been validated. The Zarit Burden Scale has been the standard instrument for assessment of caregiver burden associated with care of a demented patient.[34] The Caregiver Strain Index, however, was validated with caregivers of elderly patients who were recently discharged from the hospital after treatment of

TABLE 22–5. **Geriatric Depression Scale**

Choose the best answer for how you felt over the past week.

1. Are you basically satisfied with your life?	yes/no
2. Have you dropped many of your activities and interests?	yes/no
3. Do you feel that your life is empty?	yes/no
4. Do you often get bored?	yes/no
5. Are you hopeful about the future?	yes/no
6. Are you bothered by thoughts you can't get out of your head?	yes/no
7. Are you in good spirits most of the time?	yes/no
8. Are you afraid that something bad is going to happen to you?	yes/no
9. Do you feel happy most of the time?	yes/no
10. Do you often feel helpless?	yes/no
11. Do you often get restless and fidgety?	yes/no
12. Do you prefer to stay at home, rather than going out and doing new things?	yes/no
13. Do you frequently worry about the future?	yes/no
14. Do you feel you have more problems with memory than most?	yes/no
15. Do you think it is wonderful to be alive now?	yes/no
16. Do you often feel downhearted and blue?	yes/no
17. Do you feel pretty worthless the way you are now?	yes/no
18. Do you worry a lot about the past?	yes/no
19. Do you find life very exciting?	yes/no
20. Is it hard for you to get started on new projects?	yes/no
21. Do you feel full of energy?	yes/no
22. Do you feel that your situation is hopeless?	yes/no
23. Do you think that most people are better off than you are?	yes/no
24. Do you frequently get upset over little things?	yes/no
25. Do you frequently feel like crying?	yes/no
26. Do you have trouble concentrating?	yes/no
27. Do you enjoy getting up in the morning?	yes/no
28. Do you prefer to avoid social gatherings?	yes/no
29. Is it easy for you to make decisions?	yes/no
30. Is your mind as clear as it used to be?	yes/no

The following answers count one point; scores > 11 indicate probable depression.

Answers:

1. NO	11. YES	21. NO
2. YES	12. YES	22. YES
3. YES	13. YES	23. YES
4. YES	14. YES	24. YES
5. NO	15. NO	25. YES
6. YES	16. YES	26. YES
7. NO	17. YES	27. NO
8. YES	18. YES	28. YES
9. NO	19. NO	29. NO
10. YES	20. YES	30. NO

Reprinted with permission from Yesavage JA, et al: Development and validation of a Geriatric Depression Scale: A preliminary report. J Psychiatr Res 17:41, 1983.

medical and surgical illnesses (Table 22–6).[35] This instrument can be administered rapidly to family caregivers. A score of greater than or equal to 7 suggests a high level of strain and the need for social service intervention. As with other instruments, these case finding tools are not diagnostic tests. Screening abnormalities should be confirmed by more detailed evaluation.

Geriatric Review of Functions

The "Review of Functions" (see Table 21–1)[19] is an alternative to the use of numerous instruments for case finding. This abbreviated assessment screens for the presence of significant disabilities. The formal instruments can be used to further quantify patient deficits. Deficits are commonly seen in patients with one of the various geriatric syndromes. Thus, when a screening evaluation suggests evidence of a geriatric syndrome, a more extensive evaluation is warranted.

Geriatric Syndromes

Common geriatric problems are age associated and often multifactorial (Table 22–7).

TABLE 22–6. **Caregiver Strain Index**

I am going to read a list of things which other people have found to be difficult in helping out after somebody comes home from the hospital. *Would you tell me whether any of these apply to you?* (GIVE EXAMPLES)

	Yes = 1	No = 0
Sleep is disturbed (e.g., because _____ is in and out of bed or wanders around at night)	_____	_____
It is inconvenient (e.g., because helping takes so much time or it's a long drive over to help)	_____	_____
It is a physical strain (e.g., because of lifting in and out of a chair; effort of concentration is required)	_____	_____
It is confining (e.g., helping restricts free time or cannot go visiting)	_____	_____
There have been family adjustments (e.g., because helping has disrupted routine; there has been no privacy)	_____	_____
There have been changes in personal plans (e.g., had to turn down a job; could not go on vacation)	_____	_____
There have been other demands on my time (e.g., from other family members)	_____	_____
There have been emotional adjustments (e.g., because of severe arguments)	_____	_____
Some behavior is upsetting (e.g., because of incontinence; _____ has trouble remembering things; or _____ accuses people of taking things)	_____	_____
It is upsetting to find _____ has changed so much from his/her former self (e.g., he/she is a different person than he/she used to be)	_____	_____
There have been work adjustments (e.g., because of having to take time off)	_____	_____
It is a financial strain	_____	_____
Feeling completely overwhelmed (e.g., because of worry about _____; concerns about how you will manage)	_____	_____
Total Score (count yes responses)	_____	

Scores > 6 indicate a greater level of stress.

From Robinson BC: Validation of a caregiver strain index. J Gerontol 38:345, 1983. Copyright © 1983, The Gerontological Society of America.

TABLE 22–7. **Geriatric Syndromes: Key Points**

Syndrome	Key Points
Dementia	Prevalence of 5% in patients ≥ 65 years; Alzheimer's disease and vascular dementia account for ≥ 80% of causes; screening needed to detect reversible causes.
Delirium	Occurs in about 25% of hospitalized elderly patients; a disorder of attention and alertness; most commonly caused by infections (pneumonia, urosepsis), stroke, drug intoxications.
Urinary incontinence	Prevalence of 20%–30% in patients ≥ 75 years old; underreported by patients; most cases are treatable.
Sensory impairments	
Hearing impairment	Prevalence of hearing impairment is about 30% in patients aged > 65 years; office screening detects treatable hearing loss; hearing aids are usually helpful.
Visual impairment	Prevalence of about 13% in patients aged > 65 years; common causes (glaucoma, and cataracts) are treatable.
Depression	Prevalence of depressive symptoms is about 10% in patients aged ≥ 65 years; atypical presentations (somatic symptoms, dementia) sometimes occur; treatment of major depression is usually helpful.
Iatrogenic illness (polypharmacy)	Risk of adverse drug effects (e.g., delirium, anorexia) increases with the number of medications prescribed; careful review of patient's medications is needed to prevent adverse effects
Failure to thrive	Functional decline, weight loss, and social withdrawal are seen in patients with dementia, delirium, depression, drug reactions, and chronic disease; protein–calorie malnutrition may increase mortality risk.

The insidious and progressive nature of these syndromes, and their broad differential diagnoses, creates diagnostic challenges. The geriatric syndromes are a variety of common, but easily missed, causes of disability in elderly persons: dementia, sensory impairments (vision, hearing, and balance), immobility, iatrogenic illness (polypharmacy), depression, falls, and "failure to thrive." The assessment and management of patients with a geriatric syndrome often require the collaboration of several health care professionals.

DEMENTIA

Dementia is most often suspected when the family or other caregiver reports a decline in the patient's intellectual functioning, most often memory loss. Often a decline in performance of IADL is an early manifestation of dementia. The patient's poor performance on screening cognitive instruments, such as the MMSE (see Table 21–3), supports the history of dementia. Alzheimer's disease is the most common cause of dementia in the elderly population.[36, 37] Multi-infarct or vascular dementia is the second most common etiology. Multi-infarct dementia can be distinguished from Alzheimer's disease by its presentation of an acute onset of confusion, stepwise deterioration in cognitive function, focal neurologic symptoms and signs, and a history of stroke.[38] Imaging studies of the brain (e.g., computed tomographic scan and magnetic resonance imaging) are usually abnormal in patients with multi-infarct dementia (evidence of strokes) and show nonspecific atrophy in patients with Alzheimer's disease. A small percentage of cases of dementia have treatable or reversible causes. Among these, primary hyperparathyroidism, normal-pressure hydrocephalus, medication effects, and depressive pseudodementia are the most important. Although the medical history and physical examination may suggest one of these reversible diagnoses, a laboratory diagnostic evaluation is required for definitive diagnosis.

Dementia is far more common than delirium as a cause of cognitive dysfunction in ambulatory patients. However, delirium is suggested by a history of recently disturbed cognition and is characterized by a disorder of attention, rapid fluctuation of symptoms and signs (especially at night), disruption of the normal sleep–wake cycle, and abnormal psychomotor activity. The most common etiologies of delirium in ambulatory patients are systemic illnesses such as infections, stroke, hypoxemia, and drug intoxication.[23, 39]

INCONTINENCE

Urinary incontinence, the involuntary loss of urine in sufficient amount or frequency to constitute a social and/or health problem, increases in prevalence with advancing age.[40] Twenty to 30% of community-dwelling elderly persons aged 75 and older report at least occasional episodes of urinary incontinence. Incontinence may be associated with metabolic and systemic diseases (e.g., diabetes mellitus and delirium) or with dysfunction of the lower urinary tract.[41] Although incontinence has multiple etiologies, most patients have one of the common clinical types—stress, urge, overflow, or functional. Urinary incontinence is almost always treatable and often curable. Patients, however, underreport symptoms of incontinence to physicians, and most physicians and health care professionals fail to ask older patients about incontinence. Because of the potential adverse effects of urinary incontinence—skin breakdown, recurrent urinary tract infections, social isolation, depression, economic costs, and predisposition to institutionalization—a detailed evaluation of incontinence is usually warranted.

SENSORY IMPAIRMENTS

About 30% of community-dwelling elderly have a hearing impairment. The prevalence of hearing impairment approaches 50% in persons older than the age of 85 years. Hearing impairment interferes with physical, psychosocial, and overall functioning. It is often treatable and occasionally curable. The most common cause of hearing loss is presbycusis, a progressive loss of high-frequency sound (sensorineural hearing loss). Speech discrimination may also be impaired. Hearing loss occurs with conductive disorders and disturbances of the central auditory nervous system (mixed hearing loss). Mild hearing loss is noted with cerumen impactions of the external ear canal, a condition easily diagnosed and treated.

Other causes of hearing loss are chronic otitis media, otosclerosis, and trauma (perforated tympanic membrane). Screening for hearing impairment is easily accomplished during an office examination and can be quantitated with pure tone audiometry. The hand-held audioscope allows testing by office personnel and has a good sensitivity and specificity.[42] Abnormalities that are detected by history or screening procedures require further evaluation by trained specialists. Hearing aids are often effective in improving sensory hearing loss, but elderly patients are often unwilling to use them. Communication with hearing-impaired elderly persons can be improved even without the use of hearing aids.[43] In particular, background noise should be eliminated and the examiner should directly face the patient. Speech should be in normal tone of voice or slightly louder (but not shouting), clear, and a little slower than normal.[43] In the office, a headset with microphone provides good amplification of sound.

Approximately 13% of elderly patients have visual impairment. The prevalence is nearly 30% in the age group 85 years and older. Most elderly patients require eyeglasses for reading, and many have low vision or legal blindness (a vision of less than 20/200 after best correction). The most common causes of severe visual impairment in the elderly are cataracts, glaucoma, and macular degeneration. Cataracts cause progressive, but painless, loss of vision (unilateral or bilateral). Night vision is often greatly impaired. Cataracts can be removed and replaced with a lens implant in an ambulatory setting.[44] Indeed, the high success rate of cataract surgery today exemplifies the value of screening for visual impairment. Macular degeneration is less often treatable. Photocoagulation with laser therapy, however, may prevent severe visual loss in patients with choroidal neovascularization.[44]

Approximately 3% of elderly patients have glaucoma, which causes vision loss due to damage to the optic nerve from an increased intraocular pressure. Glaucoma produces visual field defects, which may be insidiously progressive until vision is markedly impaired. Glaucoma is easily detected by physical examination of the eye and measurement of intraocular pressure. A variety of effective medications will decrease the intraocular pressure and lessen the risk of visual loss. Laser therapy is occasionally needed.

A loss of balance and symptoms of light-headedness or disequilibrium often accompany sensory impairments, particularly peripheral neuropathies, inner ear disease, and visual and hearing impairments. The multifactorial etiology of imbalance underscores the need for an in-depth evaluation of patients with this symptom.[45]

DEPRESSION

Elderly patients may develop depression for the first time in late life, with atypical symptoms.[46] Illness dominated by somatic symptoms, anorexia with weight loss, and functional dependency (e.g., urinary and stool incontinence) may be the predominant manifestations of major depression in very old patients. Although depressed elderly patients may not appear dysphoric or tearful, they may express depressive symptoms such as hopelessness and anhedonia and suicidal ideation. Depression may represent a primary affective disorder (e.g., major depressive episode and bipolar disorder) or an adjustment disorder, bereavement, medication side effect, or other major disease (e.g., dementia, Cushing's disease).[46] Adjustment disorders are frequently seen following acute medical illnesses such as delirium, systemic infections, malignancy, and heart failure. Adjustment disorders or bereavement often responds to outpatient treatments, including psychotherapy and group therapy. Major depressive illnesses will more often require pharmacologic treatment or electroconvulsive therapy. Depression is sometimes associated with medications. Antihypertensive drugs (reserpine, methyldopa, and propranolol) have been most commonly associated with depression. Psychoactive agents including barbiturates, benzodiazepines, and hypnotic agents can also cause or exacerbate symptoms of depression. Large doses of corticosteroids, antiparkinsonian drugs, and opioid analgesics are also associated with depression.

Major depressive episode is characterized by a dysphoric mood, anhedonia, diminished interest or pleasure in activities, significant weight loss or weight gain, insomnia or hypersomnia, psychomotor agitation or retardation, fatigue, feelings of worthlessness, inability to think or concentrate, and recurrent thoughts of suicide.[47] The symptoms of major depression are very likely to improve with antidepressant therapies, either antidepressant medication or electroconvulsive therapy.

FALLS AND IMMOBILITY

Each year, falls occur in approximately one third of community-dwelling persons aged 75 years and older. Accidents and falls are the sixth leading cause of death in persons older than 65 years of age. Falls due to various causes are often associated with nonfatal soft tissue injuries and fractures.[48] More than 200,000 elderly persons suffer hip fractures each year, many secondary to falls. The risk of falls in the elderly is related to the number and severity of chronic medical conditions.[49]

The maintenance of normal balance and gait requires integration of sensory (perception), central nervous system, and musculoskeletal functions. Disturbances of the central or peripheral nervous system, commonly seen with degenerative neurologic diseases, or disturbances of the musculoskeletal system, commonly seen with osteoarthritis and soft tissue injuries, increase the older person's risk of falls related to impairments of gait and balance.[50] Because the majority of falls are multifactorial in etiology, a systematic approach to the patient with recurrent falls is likely to lead to multiple diagnoses and specific interventions. For example, in arthritis of the knees, physical therapy to increase leg-muscle strength, assistive devices (e.g., knee brace, quad cane, and walker) to improve gait, and analgesics to relieve pain may improve patient mobility and lessen the risk of subsequent falls. Adverse effects of medications should be considered. Psychotropic medications have been associated with hip fractures in older persons; benzodiazepines with long half-lives (e.g., diazepam) can cause an ataxic gait, thereby predisposing patients to falls. Gait and balance abnormalities commonly follow hospitalization for acute illnesses. Restriction of physical activity and muscular deconditioning are common during hospitalization. The hospitalized elderly patient may benefit from physical therapy to strengthen lower-extremity muscles and increase flexibility of the joints.

Falls are also associated with postural hypotension, which may result from chronic diseases, medications, immobility, and dehydration.[51] Postural hypotension is often amenable to simple interventions such as a high-salt diet, change in medications, and exercise. Falls are sometimes seen in patients with postprandial reduction of blood pressure, a phenomenon that occurs even in healthy elderly persons and lasts for 30 or more minutes after a meal that contains carbohydrates.[52] The prevention of falls is potentially achievable through a comprehensive assessment that includes a balance and gait evaluation, interventions to improve patient mobility and gait and balance, and interventions to reduce environmental hazards (e.g., unstable furniture, frayed rugs, and poor lighting) in the home. Often a team approach to the assessment of the patient with recurrent falls is needed; physical and occupational therapists are invaluable in the assessment and management of these patients.

IATROGENIC ILLNESS

Iatrogenic illness complicates 36% of patient admissions to a general medical service, with a disproportionately higher incidence among the elderly.[53] Physiologic changes of aging, multiple medical illnesses, impaired homeostatic mechanisms, and the presence of polypharmacy predispose elderly patients to iatrogenic illnesses. Iatrogenic illnesses can result from hospitalization itself, diagnostic and surgical procedures, and even failure of physicians to communicate with patients or colleagues. Iatrogenic complications can occur in the office, the hospital, or the long-term care setting and can range from pressure sores (due to forced immobilization) to hematomas (from venipuncture and arterial catheterization), nosocomial infections, dehydration and hypotension (following preparation for gastrointestinal studies), and acute renal failure (resulting from intravenous administration of contrast agents). Adverse events occur more commonly in elderly hospitalized patients, in whom drug complications are the most common single type of adverse event.[54] Drugs most commonly related to adverse events in hospitalized patients include antibiotics, antitumor drugs, anticoagulants, and cardiovascular and antiseizure medications.[54]

Although the elderly account for only 12% of the American population, they consume nearly 25% of the national total for drugs and drug sundries.[55] An estimated 80% to 90% use two or more medications daily, and 40% of persons older than age 60 use over-the-counter preparations daily. In fact, over-the-counter drugs account for 40% of drugs taken by the elderly, a rate seven times greater than in younger adults. However, an estimated 40% of elderly patients rely on at least one medication for maintaining their ADL. Thus, medications are a two-edged sword for the elderly: on one hand they improve the quality of life, and on the other hand they increase the risk for iatrogenic complications. Although changes in drug disposition and tissue effects occur with aging, studies suggest that the greatest predictor of an adverse drug reaction is the total number of medications consumed by the patient.[56] Polypharmacy, the prescribing of multiple medications, is related to characteristics of patients, their families, and health care providers.[53] Resolution of polypharmacy and the prevention of iatrogenic illness is achievable through the careful review of all medications (prescription and over-the-counter) consumed by the elderly patient, an assessment of medication compliance, and simplification of the drug regimen to reduce the risks of adverse drug effects and patient noncompliance. Most importantly, instructions for medications should be given verbally and in writing to the patient and family caregiver. Computer software programs provide information on potential drug–drug interactions and can help reduce the incidence of iatrogenic illness.

FAILURE TO THRIVE

Failure to thrive (FTT) in the elderly is a term used to describe a gradual decline in physical and/or cognitive function of an elderly patient, usually accompanied by weight loss and social withdrawal, that occurs without immediate explanation.[57, 58] Clinically, patients with FTT often appear physically well but have a history of weight loss and impaired functioning. FTT is not a specific diagnosis but rather a syndrome that has been described as a paradigm of the frail elderly.[59] Patients with a diagnosis of FTT are most likely to be encountered initially in the ambulatory care setting, where a systematic approach to evaluation and treatment is likely to uncover the cause and result in effective interventions. The nonspecific manifestations of disease, the multiple co-existing illnesses, and the functional dependency of the frail elderly predispose them to FTT. Social isolation, inadequate social supports, and low socioeconomic status also contribute to the risk of FTT. Many of these patients seek medical attention because of unexplained weight loss. They often have psychiatric disease, occult malignancies (particularly of the gastrointestinal tract), or no apparent cause even after 1 year of follow-up.[60]

In population-based studies of Americans, body weight tends to decrease slightly after age 60. The loss of weight is largely attributable to decreases in skeletal muscle and total body water. The nutritional status of most older persons is normal, although subgroups of older persons at risk of undernutrition include those with low income and white men living alone.[61] Low body weight is a risk factor for mortality among older persons. Weight loss is an antecedent of protein–calorie malnutrition, which is an independent predictor of mortality in nursing home patients. The diagnosis of protein–calorie malnutrition is based on both objective measurements of nutritional status (low levels of serum albumin, plasma hemoglobin, and serum cholesterol) and clinical examination (muscle atrophy and generalized muscle weakness).[58] The most common etiologies of FTT and involuntary weight loss appear to be dementia, depression, delirium (particularly related to systemic illness in hospitalized patients), drug reactions, and chronic diseases such as heart failure, thyrotoxicosis, and malignancies. A systematic and comprehensive evaluation of the patient with FTT will usually reveal the underlying etiology. The management of FTT is directed at its etiology and contributing factors, including treatment of reversible dementia and major depression or changes in medications. In addition, nutrition counseling, food supplements, financial assistance, referrals to community health agencies, and increased family support to improve caregiving are important.

THE FOCUSED MEDICAL HISTORY, PHYSICAL EXAMINATION, AND LABORATORY EVALUATION

A comprehensive geriatric assessment includes a review of functions, a detailed history of co-morbid illnesses, a careful review of prescription and nonprescription medications, and a medical history and physical examination that focuses on the patient's functional limitations. This assessment is enhanced by an understanding of normal aging. The review of systems focuses on changes in musculoskeletal, cardiovascular, and gastrointestinal functions. Particularly important are histories of dyspnea on exertion, orthopnea, chest pain, chronic cough, chronic change in bowel habits, constipation, and diarrhea. Medications are reviewed at each office visit. The history also includes a review of adult immunizations. Elderly patients are advised to have a tetanus toxoid booster every 10 years, a pneumococcal vaccine once, and the influenza vaccine each autumn. Rates of noncompliance with recommendations are unfortunately quite high despite the proven effectiveness of immunizations in old age.[62]

Physiology of Aging

Many of the physical, psychological, and laboratory abnormalities observed with usual aging result from environmental or lifestyle factors, chronic illness, and social dysfunction. Only recently have investigators controlled for environmental and social factors when studying healthy or "successful" aging.[63] With successful aging, patients are physically and cognitively intact and comparable in these characteristics with younger patients. Often, however, the distinction between normal aging and disease is not clear. Physiologic changes of aging in cardiovascular and renal function, however, are well defined. For example, arterial stiffness increases with age and systolic blood pressure increases to compensate for the loss of aortic compliance. A compensatory hypertrophy of the left ventricle often ensues, as does isolated systolic hypertension (systolic blood pressure $\geq$ 160 mm Hg with diastolic blood pressure $<$ 90 mm Hg). The maximum heart rate achievable with exercise or stress (often estimated as 220 minus age) decreases with normal aging.[64]

A slowly progressive decline in creatinine clearance (which estimates glomerular filtration rate) occurs after 30 years of age. An average 80-year-old man has approximately 70%

of the creatinine clearance of a 30-year-old man. The serum creatinine value may be deceptively normal, however, since muscle mass and hence serum creatinine levels decline with usual aging. The rate of decline of renal function is highly variable. Some men with no prior history of hypertension or genitourinary diseases demonstrate no decline in creatinine clearance with aging.[65] Some studies suggest that the aged kidney is less efficient in excreting and conserving salt and in concentrating and diluting free water. Certain medications can exacerbate age-related changes in renal function (e.g., hyponatremia caused by thiazide diuretics and oral hypoglycemic agents).

COMMON ABNORMALITIES OF AGING

About 80% of elderly patients have at least one chronic disease that can limit their independence in ADL; 30% have three or more illnesses. The incidence of chronic illnesses that usually require medical treatment, such as cardiovascular disorders, is increasing. Many of the chronic diseases are potentially preventable through modification of lifestyle during adulthood. Hypertension, for example, is associated with obesity, excess alcohol consumption, and a high dietary salt intake. Isolated systolic hypertension is associated with arteriosclerosis, which may be exacerbated by cigarette smoking, hypercholesterolemia, and poorly controlled diabetes mellitus. Other common changes of aging that may be related to environmental or lifestyle factors include loss of vision due to cataracts (ultraviolet light), hearing impairment due to sensorineural hearing loss (trauma), heart murmurs due to calcification of the aortic and mitral valves (arteriosclerosis), skin lesions due to sun exposure, and vascular insufficiency due to atherosclerosis.

Physical examination of the elderly patient often reveals evidence of age-related abnormalities. Cardiovascular illnesses are particularly common. Isolated systolic hypertension is found in at least 10% of Americans aged 65 and older. It is associated with an increased risk of stroke, heart failure, and mortality. Treatment of isolated systolic hypertension with antihypertensive medications reduces the incidence of strokes and heart failure.[66] Postural hypotension is found in 6% to 25% of elderly patients.[51] Medications, immobility, and dehydration are among the most common and treatable causes of postural hypotension. A reduction in blood pressure after an average meal, lasting for at least 30 minutes, is observed in the majority of patients aged 75 years and older.[52] Some of these patients become symptomatic, perhaps as a result of an interaction between meal, medications, and impaired baroreflexes.[67] Irregular heart rates are also common in elderly patients and are often due to benign atrial and ventricular ectopy. The incidence of chronic atrial fibrillation increases with age, approaching 5% in the elderly population. Recently, low doses of warfarin reduced the incidence of stroke in patients with nonrheumatic atrial fibrillation, indicating the importance of diagnosing this condition.[68] Low doses of aspirin may be efficacious for patients who cannot take warfarin.[69] Systolic murmurs (both aortic and mitral) are very common and usually benign in otherwise asymptomatic patients. Vascular bruits and diminished peripheral pulses, however, suggest the presence of occlusive arterial disease.

Abnormalities of the eyes, ears, nose, and throat are common. In addition to the impairments of vision and hearing previously described, the present cohort of elderly patients has a high prevalence of disorders of dentition and oral hygiene. Missing teeth, ill-fitting dentures, and periodontal disease are common health problems in this population. Impaired mastication, losses of taste and smell, and undernutrition may result from these conditions.[58] Difficulty swallowing occurs in patients with generalized weakness (e.g., from deconditioning, impaired mastication, and neurologic diseases, such as stroke and Parkinson's disease).

Chest abnormalities are commonly observed with usual aging. Kyphosis is seen in patients with vertebral compression fractures resulting from osteoporosis or from osteoarthritis of the cervical and thoracic spines. Abnormal breath sounds, including dry rales, are often present in the absence of overt pulmonary or cardiac diseases.

Degenerative changes of the hip and knee joints are commonly seen with advancing age. Limited range of motion in those joints may impair gait and predispose patients to falls and disuse atrophy of lower extremity muscles. In addition, chronic pain may result from tendinitis, bursitis, and arthritis of the large joints.

The neurologic examination may uncover the common findings of dementia, neuropathy, and gait impairments. Diminished vibratory sensation in the toes is common with aging, even in the absence of diseases. Decreases of proprioception, deep tendon reflexes, and pain sensation usually indicate a neuropathy or other significant neurologic lesion (e.g., lumbar spinal stenosis). Discogenic disease, particularly of the lumbar spine, is also common in this population.

Common Laboratory Findings

There are no significant alterations in commonly ordered laboratory studies with successful aging. Most laboratory abnormalities result from chronic illnesses rather than aging. Anemia is common, most often caused by iron deficiency and less often by chronic disease and malnutrition. Macrocytic anemias, secondary to cobalamin or folate deficiencies, are important to recognize because they are easily treated. Impaired glucose tolerance or type II diabetes mellitus is common with usual aging. Glucose tolerance is likely to be normal in physically fit and nonobese elderly persons. The sedimentation rate is often slightly elevated with advancing age. The normal serum alkaline phosphatase value may be mildly elevated, but high levels are associated with serious diseases, such as Paget's disease of the bone, chronic liver disease, or metastatic cancer. The serum albumin value with healthy aging is within normal limits. The total protein (globulin) level is often slightly elevated. Very high globulin levels are seen in patients with benign and malignant gammopathies. The urinalysis is usually normal with healthy aging; persistent proteinuria, microscopic hematuria, and pyuria suggest an underlying urologic disorder. The chest radiograph of elderly patients with usual aging reveals slight hyperinflation, mild interstitial fibrosis, and osteoporosis of the spine. Even with "successful" aging, degenerative changes of the thoracic spine are commonly observed. The electrocardiogram remains normal with successful aging, al-

TABLE 22–8. **Interdisciplinary Geriatric Assessment: Team Members and Roles**

Team Member	Role
Physicians	
Geriatrician	Perform in-depth evaluation of geriatric syndromes; medical consultation (reduced polypharmacy, optimizing medical treatments); coordination of discharge planning; ongoing medical care.
Neurologist	Perform detailed evaluation of dementia, delirium, gait impairment, muscle weakness, neuropathy.
Psychiatrist	Evaluate for depression, affective disorder, competence, ethical dilemma.
Nurse specialist	Perform detailed review of functions (basic and instrumental activities of daily living, cognition, mood, special senses, nutrition, home environment); administration of screening instruments; health maintenance review (immunizations, dental care, foot care, smoking habits, alcohol consumption, Papanicolaou smear and breast examinations); medication review.
Social worker	Obtain demographic data (education, religion, housing); obtain legal/financial information (guardianship, durable power of attorney); review advance directives (living will, durable power of attorney for health care); assess social support network (family caregivers, formal supports); evaluate family dynamics (family dysfunction, caregiver stress, potential abuse); arrange referrals to community agencies (home care, adult day care, meals-on-wheels); arrange transfer to nursing home or rehabilitation hospital.
Physical therapist	Evaluate gait and mobility; maintain or improve strength, flexibility, and endurance of muscle and range of motion of joints; recommend assistive devices for ambulation; administer treatment modalities.
Occupational therapist	Evaluate and improve ability to perform activities of daily living; fit splints for upper extremities; environmental assessment (home visit) and recommendations; teach use of assistive and safety devices.
Dietitian	Assess nutritional status; recommend nutritional interventions (e.g., special diets and food supplements); monitor enteral and parenteral alimentation.
Speech pathologist	Evaluate patients with aphasia or dysphagia.
Neuropsychologist	Perform extensive psychometric testing to help quantitate and differentiate psychiatric disorders.

though atrial and ventricular ectopy are commonly observed. Thyroid abnormalities are very common in elderly patients. Both thyrotoxicosis and hypothyroidism may have atypical or absent symptoms and signs. An elevated serum level of a high-sensitivity thyroid-stimulating hormone may indicate primary hypothyroidism, whereas an elevated level of thyroid hormone and a depressed thyroid-stimulating hormone level may indicate hyperthyroidism.

GERIATRIC ASSESSMENT: IN-DEPTH AND OFFICE EVALUATIONS

When an in-depth evaluation of a geriatric syndrome is needed, an assessment by a core interdisciplinary team (geriatrician, nurse specialist, and social worker) will facilitate appropriate diagnostic evaluation and management. In most urban centers, ambulatory geriatric assessment centers are widely available and are often affiliated with a teaching hospital.[11] Many health care professionals may become involved in the assessment and management of elderly patients (Table 22–8). In addition, patients may benefit from referral to community-based case managers. A growing number of entitlement programs enable medically indigent patients to obtain needed home care services, which may allow them to continue residing in the community rather than entering nursing homes.

A case study illustrates the usefulness of an interdisciplinary geriatric assessment: A 98-year-old Italian-American woman was referred to the ElderHealth Center at University Hospitals of Cleveland with a history of recent forgetfulness, frequent falls at home, and recent mild weight loss. Her history included constipation, transient chest pain, impaired vision, polypharmacy, cellulitis of the lower extremities, impaired mastication and edentulousness, venous insufficiency with stasis dermatitis of

TABLE 22–9. **Social Assessment**

Primary caregivers (relationship)
Formal supports
- Primary physician
- Home care
- Community agencies

Patient demographics
- Educational level
- Financial status
- Cultural/ethnic preferences

Patient coping skills

the lower extremities, a normocytic anemia, and mild azotemia. In the course of her assessment she was evaluated by a nurse, social worker, geriatrician, ophthalmologist, and dietitian. Bereavement was treated with supportive counseling. An anemia workup revealed a benign hemoglobin abnormality (thalassemia minor), which required no further treatment. Venous insufficiency was treated with leg elevation. Home evaluation revealed safety problems as a likely cause of her falls and led to the prescribing of assistive devices to aid ambulation. The chest pain was functional and related to recent bereavement; antianginal medications were discontinued. Constipation was treated successfully with a high-fiber diet, increased exercise, and hydration. Vision improved with cataract extraction and intraocular lens implant. The azotemia improved with a change in medications and did not progress during medical follow-up. Six months after the evaluation, the patient was markedly better: forgetfulness and bereavement had resolved, symptoms related to osteoarthritis were controlled with safe doses of acetaminophen, independence in basic ADL returned, and quality of life had improved.

In the practice of primary podiatry, case finding instruments can be easily administered to frail elderly patients. Self-assessment forms can be used to obtain much of the information in the geriatric review of functions. For detailed case finding, the following instruments are recommended for office use: basic ADL (see Table 22–2), IADL (see Table 22–2), cognition screening with the Folstein Mini-Mental State Examination (see Table 22–3) or Pfeiffer Short Portable Mental Status Questionnaire (see Table 22–4), and depression screening with the Geriatric Depression Scale (see Table

22–5). Through interviews, the primary caregiver and significant formal and informal caregivers are ascertained (Table 22–9). Patients with impairments of physical, cognitive, or psychosocial functioning should be considered for appropriate referral to geriatric assessment centers.

REFERENCES

1. Havlik RJ, Liu MG, Kovar MG, et al (eds): Health Statistics on Older Persons, United States, 1986. Vital and Health Statistics, Series 3, No. 25. DHHS, publication No. (PHS) 87-1049. Public Health Service, Washington, DC, US Government Printing Office, June 1987.
2. National Institutes of Health Consensus Development Conference Statement: Geriatric assessment methods for clinical decision-making. J Am Geriatr Soc 36:342–347, 1988.
3. Rubenstein LZ, Rubenstein LV: Multidimensional assessment of elderly patients. Adv Intern Med 39:81–108, 1991.
4. Narain P, Rubenstein LZ, Wieland GD, et al: Predictors of immediate and six-month outcomes in hospitalized elderly patients: The importance of functional status. J Am Geriatr Soc 36:775–783, 1988.
5. Magaziner J, Simonsick EM, Kashner TM, et al: Predictors of functional recovery one year following hospital discharge for hip fracture: A prospective study. J Gerontol 45:M101–M107, 1990.
6. Winograd CH: Targeting strategies: An overview of criteria and outcomes. J Am Geriatr Soc 39S:25S–35S, 1991.
7. Rubenstein LZ, Josephson KR, Wieland GD, et al: Effectiveness of a geriatric evaluation unit: A randomized clinical trial. N Engl J Med 311:1664–1670, 1984.
8. Applegate WB, Miller ST, Graney MJ, et al: A randomized controlled trial of a geriatric assessment unit in a community rehabilitation hospital. N Engl J Med 322:1572–1578, 1990.
9. Collard AF, Bachman SS, Beatrice DF: Acute care delivery for the geriatric patient: An innovative approach. Q Rev Bull 11:180–185, 1985.
10. Williams TF, Hill JG, Fairbank ME, et al: Appropriate placement of the chronically ill and aged: A successful approach by evaluation. JAMA 226:1332–1335, 1973.
11. Epstein AM, Hall JA, Besdine R, et al: The emergence of geriatric assessment units: The new technology in geriatrics. Ann Intern Med 106:299–303, 1987.
12. Williams ME, Williams TF, Zimmer JG, et al: How does the team approach to outpatient geriatric evaluation compare with traditional care: A report of a randomized controlled trial. J Am Geriatr Soc 35:1071–1078, 1987.
13. Yeo G, Ingram L, Skurnick J, et al: Effects of a geriatric clinic on functional health and well-being of elders. J Gerontol 42:252–258, 1987.
14. Epstein AM, Hall JA, Fretwell M, et al: Consultative geriatric assessment for ambulatory patients: A randomized trial in a health maintenance organization. JAMA 263:538–544, 1990.
15. Hendrickson C, Lund E, Strongard E: Consequences of assessment and intervention among elderly people: A three-year randomized controlled trial. Br Med J 289:1522–1524, 1984.
16. Vetter MJ, Jones DA, Victor CR: Effects of health visi-

tors working with elderly patients in general practice: A randomized controlled trial. Br Med J 288:369–372, 1984.

17. Applegate W, Deyo R, Kramer A, et al: Geriatric evaluation and management: Current status and future research directions. J Am Geriatr Soc 39S:2S–7S, 1991.

18. Applegate WB, Blass JP, Williams TF: Instruments for the functional assessment of older patients. N Engl J Med 322:1207–1214, 1990.

19. Lachs MS, Feinstein AR, Cooney LM, et al: A simple procedure for general screening for functional disability in elderly patients. Ann Intern Med 109:699–706, 1990.

20. Guralnik JM, LaCroix AZ, Branch LG, et al: Morbidity and disability in older persons in the years prior to death. Am J Public Health 81:443–447, 1991.

21. Mayer-Oakes SA, Oye RK, Leake B: Predictors of mortality in older patients following medical intensive care: The importance of functional status. J Am Geriatr Soc 39:862–868, 1991.

22. Mossey JM, Mutran E, Knott K, et al: Determinants of recovery 12 months after hip fracture: The importance of psychosocial factors. Am J Public Health 79:279–286, 1989.

23. Francis J, Martin D, Kapoor W: A prospective study of delirium in hospitalized elderly. JAMA 263:1097–1101, 1990.

24. Katz S, Ford AB, Moskowitz RW, et al: Studies of illness in the aged: The index of ADL: A standardized measure of biological and psychosocial function. JAMA 185:914–919, 1963.

25. Lawton MP, Brody EM: Assessment of older people: Self-maintaining and instrumental activities of daily living. Gerontologist 9:179–186, 1969.

26. Rubenstein L, Schairer C, Wieland GD, et al: Systematic biases in functional status assessment of elderly adults: Effects of different data sources. J Gerontol 39:686–691, 1984.

27. Kovar MG, Hendershot G, Mathis E: Older people in the United States who receive help with basic activities of daily living. Am J Public Health 79:778–779, 1989.

28. Fillenbaum GG: Screening the elderly: A brief instrumental activities of daily living measure. J Am Geriatr Soc 33:698–706, 1985.

29. Folstein MF, Folstein SE, McHugh PR: "Mini-mental state": A practical method for grading the cognitive state of patients for the clinician. J Psychiatr Res 12:189–198, 1975.

30. Pfeiffer E: A short portable mental status questionnaire for the assessment of organic brain deficit in elderly patients. J Am Geriatr Soc 23:433–441, 1975.

31. Siu AL: Screening for dementia and investigating its causes. Ann Intern Med 115:122–132, 1991.

32. Yesavage JA, Brink TL, Rose TL, et al: Development of a geriatric depression screening scale: A preliminary report. J Psychiatr Res 17:37–49, 1983.

33. Sheikh JI, Yesavage JA: The geriatric depression scale (GDS): Recent evidence and development of a shorter version. Clin Gerontol 9:165–173, 1986.

34. Zarit SH: Relatives of the impaired elderly: Correlates of feeling of burden. Gerontologist 20:649–655, 1980.

35. Robinson BC: Validation of a caregiver strain index. J Gerontol 38:344–348, 1983.

36. Evans DA, Funkenstein HH, Albert MS, et al: Prevalence of Alzheimer's disease in a community population of older persons: Higher than previously reported. JAMA 262:2551–2556, 1989.

37. Katzman R: Alzheimer's disease. N Engl J Med 314:964–973, 1986.

38. Hachinski BC, Iliff LD, Zilhka E, et al: Cerebral blood flow in dementia. Arch Neurol 32:632–637, 1975.

39. Lipowski CJ: Delirium in the elderly patient. N Engl J Med 320:578–582, 1989.

40. National Institutes of Health Consensus Development Conference Statement. Urinary Incontinence in Adults, p 7. Bethesda, MD, National Institutes of Health, 1988.

41. Palmer RM: Ambulatory management of urinary incontinence in the frail elderly. Geriatrics 45 (3):61–66, 1990.

42. Lichtenstein MJ, Bess FH, Logan SA: Validation of screening tools for identifying hearing-impaired elderly in primary care. JAMA 259:2875–2878, 1988.

43. Voeks SK, Gallagher CM, Langer EH, et al: Hearing loss in the nursing home: An institutional issue. J Am Geriatr Soc 38:141–145, 1990.

44. Bienfang DC, Kelly LD, Nicholson DH, et al: Ophthalmology. N Engl J Med 323:956–967, 1990.

45. Baldwin RL: The dizzy patient. Hosp Pract 19 (10):151–162, 1984.

46. Fitten LJ, Morley JE, Gross EL, et al: Depression: UCLA Geriatric Grand Rounds. J Am Geriatr Soc 37:459–472, 1989.

47. Blazer D: Depression in the elderly. N Engl J Med 320:164–166, 1989.

48. Hindmarsh JJ, Estes EH: Falls in older persons: Causes and interventions. Arch Intern Med 149:2217–2222, 1989.

49. Tinetti ME, Williams TF, Mayewski R: Fall risk index for elderly patients based on number of chronic disabilities. Am J Med 80:429–434, 1986.

50. Tinetti ME: Performance-oriented assessment of mobility problems in elderly patients. J Am Geriatr Soc 34:119–126, 1986.

51. Lipsitz LA: Orthostatic hypotension in the elderly. N Engl J Med 321:952–957, 1989.

52. Peitzman SJ, Berger SR: Postprandial blood pressure decreases in well elderly persons. Arch Intern Med 149:286–288, 1989.

53. Palmer RM, Ouslander JG: Iatrogenic illness. Geriatr Med Today 6 (3):80–91, 1987.

54. Brennan TA, Leap LL, Laird NM, et al: Incidence of adverse events and negligence in hospitalized patients: Results of the Harvard Medical Practice Study I. N Engl J Med 324:370–376, 1991.

55. National Ambulatory Medical Care Survey, United States, 1980. Vital Health Stat, vol 13, No. 1, 1983.

56. Gurwitz JH, Avorn J: The ambiguous relation between aging and adverse drug reactions. Ann Intern Med 114:956–966, 1991.

57. Braun JV, Wykle MH, Cowling WR: Failure to thrive in older persons: A concept derived. Gerontologist 28:809–812, 1988.

58. Palmer RM: "Failure to thrive" in the elderly: Diagnosis and management. Geriatrics 45 (9):47–55, 1990.

59. Berkman B, Foster LWS, Campion E: Failure to thrive: Paradigm for the frail elder. Gerontologist 29:654–659, 1989.

60. Marton KI, Sox HC, Krupp JR: Involuntary weight loss: Diagnostic and prognostic significance. Ann Intern Med 95:568–574, 1981.

61. Davis MA, Randall E, Forthofer RN, et al: Living arrangements and dietary patterns of older adults in the United States. J Gerontol 40:434–442, 1985.

62. Woolf SH, Kamerow DB, Lawrence RS, et al: The periodic health examination of older adults: The recommendations of the U.S. Preventive Services Task Force: I. Counseling, immunizations, and chemoprophylaxis. J Am Geriatr Soc 38:817–823, 1990.

63. Rowe JW, Kahn RL: Human aging: Usual and successful. Science 237:143–148, 1987.
64. Weisfeldt ML: The aging heart. Hosp Pract 20 (2):115–130, 1985.
65. Lindeman RD, Tobin J, Shock NW: Longitudinal studies on the rate of decline in renal function with age. J Am Geriatr Soc 33:278–285, 1985.
66. SHEP Cooperative Research Group: Prevention of stroke by antihypertensive drug treatment in older persons with isolated systolic hypertension: Final results of the Systolic Hypertension in the Elderly Program (SHEP). JAMA 265:3255–3264, 1991.
67. Viatkevicius PV, Esserwein DM, Maynard AK, et al: Frequency and importance of postprandial blood pressure reduction in elderly nursing-home patients. Ann Intern Med 115:865–870, 1991.
68. The Boston Area Anticoagulation Trial for Atrial Fibrillation Investigators: The effect of low-dose warfarin on the risk of stroke in patients with nonrheumatic atrial fibrillation. N Engl J Med 323:1505–1511, 1990.
69. The SALT Collaborative Group. Swedish Aspirin Low-dose Trial (SALT) of 75 mg aspirin as secondary prophylaxis after cerebrovascular ischemic events. Lancet 2:1345–1349, 1991.

CHAPTER 23

PODIATRIC SURGERY

Steven M. Krych

The primary care podiatrist's role in surgical intervention is recognition of need, acknowledgment of one's own competency and the abilities of others, and the direction of the patient to a skilled surgeon for surgical care. A primary care practitioner must have the knowledge, training, ability, and capability to evaluate a patient and decide which treatment regimen is best for that patient.

Surgery is often thought of by most practitioners as the final solution to pathology. The reality is that surgical intervention is part of a bigger overall concept of care, the total care of the patient. When a patient presents to a primary care podiatrist with a complaint that is amenable to a surgical procedure, the primary care podiatrist's role is to determine whether this would be the appropriate intervention for this particular patient. It is of utmost importance to consider risks, benefits, short-term prognosis, long-term prognosis, concomitant diseases, and concomitant skeletal and/or bodily manifestations of the disease process, as well as the social and economic factors that interplay in decision making. An example may be a patient who presents with a soft tissue mass. As the current literature suggests, magnetic resonance imaging is the diagnostic test of choice for soft tissue masses in most parts of the human body. However, the foot is easily evaluated with other, less costly techniques. Therefore, the primary care podiatrist needs to be aware of all the available clinical, laboratory, and imaging techniques to help determine what type of pathologic process is occurring. The primary care podiatrist must also establish strong relationships with other medical practitioners in the community, ranging from internists, general practitioners, and specialists to orthopedic surgeons and other surgically trained or biomechanically trained podiatrists in the area. A strong and mutually beneficial relationship among those practitioners recognizing their expertise, capabilities, and abilities will strengthen the practitioner–patient relationship and improve the outcomes for all patients concerned.

SKIN BIOPSY AND PLASTIC TECHNIQUES

Biopsy techniques range from the shave biopsy of skin to the wide excisional biopsy. The technique used often depends on the lesion and its location. An example is verruca plantaris on a non–weight-bearing surface of the sole of the foot. In this instance, decision making can be combined with biopsy and treatment. Often, blunt dissection and basilar curettage of the lesion is recommended. Another consideration would be full-thickness semi-elliptical excision with primary closure of the wound. Each of these techniques has shown significant positive results. It is important, however, to understand the different types of healing that occur with the various techniques that are used. In blunt dissection, curettage of just the epidermis and not the dermal subcutaneous junction will allow for less scarring. In sharp dissection, the surgeon will violate the dermal-epidermal junction and a scar will form, with its size related to the type of closure that is performed. Orientation of the skin incision along skin tension lines and following the rule that three times the width of the lesion equals the length of the incision line will help provide for finer scarring. In a case of a lesion beneath the weight-bearing area or overlying a bony prominence, it is often necessary to do partial-thickness procedures to decrease the amount of scarring or to consider some type of full-thickness rotational flap. Rotational flaps from a non–weight-bearing area often work well. The key to this technique is maintenance of the broad pedicle from which the flap receives blood flow. Plastic skin closure with acceptable scar formation is related to the surgeon's technique, placement, design, tissue handling, and closure and to patient factors such as age, skin type, and compliance. It is also related to postoperative management, control of edema, weight-bearing stresses, and shear stresses.

In summary, soft tissue techniques should not be considered lightly. Although the skin is the most forgiving of all soft tissue structures, it is important to realize that techniques and control of patient compliance have a very strong relationship to the outcome. In general, skin incisions paralleling skin tension lines will heal with a finer scar when compared with a skin incision perpendicular to tension lines. Skin tension lines were first discussed by Durlacher in 1834, then modified by Langer in 1861 and further studied by Cox in 1941.[1] Since these pioneering works, several authors have proposed techniques for identifying appropriate incisional placement. A basic technique for identifying appropriate incision orientation is by pinching the skin immediately over the area of the proposed incision. A skin fold along the skin tension line would be essentially straight, whereas a skin fold oblique to the skin tension line will have an S-shaped fold. Again, the skin is one of the most accommodating of all the tissues that podiatric surgeons will work with. It is a fallacy to expect the skin to hold any correction, and therefore the skin should be considered a rapidly responding tissue to stress.

INGROWING TOENAILS

The toenail is an appendage of the skin, and as such it has some of the same characteristics as skin. Increasing stress to the area or increased age or decreased blood flow will cause slowing of the cellular turnover and therefore hypertrophy of the nail. Hyperkeratosis can also form adjacent to the nails by pinching the skin against the toenail.

Surgical correction of nail problems can be one of the most gratifying experiences for the patient and the physician or it can be one of the most frustrating. Treatment of diseased nails is often given a lower priority and emphasis than some of the more exotic surgical procedures. Nail surgery, however, requires the same basic elements as all surgical procedures (Table 23–1).

TABLE 23–1. **Basic Elements of All Surgical Procedures**

1. Knowledge of anatomy
2. Attention to detail
3. Visualization
4. Identification of abnormal anatomy
5. Flawless technical performance

Matricectomy Techniques

Each practitioner should have the ability to correct nail disorders through a minimum of three techniques. Debulking, including wedge resection of the toenail, is the initial treatment of choice, particularly in patients who have some type of vascular compromise. When debulking or wedge resection techniques have failed, permanent partial matricectomy or total permanent removal can be considered in patients with an intact vascular system. There are two basic techniques: sharp surgical dissection (sharp technique) or blunt curettage with chemical application (phenol technique). Several steps are the same for each technique (Table 23–2).

SHARP TECHNIQUE

The surgical excision of the matrix and hypertrophied ingrowing toenail is quite easy. In fact, it is one of the first surgical techniques described in treating the human foot in the podiatric literature. There are two basic advantages to surgical excision. One is complete removal of all related nail growth tissue from both the proximal matrix and the nail bed matrix and surgical excision of hypertrophied labial tissue. There are, however, some disadvantages. The primary disadvantage is the need to protect and not violate the underlying periosteum and the distal phalanx of bone. This is a problem particularly on the nail bed because of the close adherence of the nail bed tissue to the underlying periosteum.

Step 1. Begin the incision dorsally at the level of the clear skin line just proximal to the nail plate. The nail plate should be sharply incised through the proximal skin, and the incision should extend distally to the tip of the

toe. Care should be exercised on this step because overzealous pressure will violate the periosteum beneath the nail bed.

Step 2. Identify the skin change line of the hypertrophied ungual labia and create a semielliptical incision paralleling this line. There will be a noticeable difference in the underlying tissue consistency when cutting through the hypertrophied labial tissue. The flesh will be scarred and hypertrophied and often indurated to a greater degree than the other surrounding tissue. The granulation tissue itself will be soft and easily removable.

Step 3. Remove the skin and nail matrix sharply. Starting proximally, fillet the tissue distally, resecting skin, matrix, nail bed, and scar in toto. Sharp dissection at this point is necessary because of the fibrous periosteal attachments of this distal skin.

Step 4. Inspect the proximal incision area for removal of remaining matrix. The nail is an appendage of the skin, and violation of the periosteum is not an indicated part of this procedure.

Step 5. Free the skin margins to allow mobilization and closure.

Step 6. Close the wound using techniques of choice.

Step 7. Apply a dressing and prescribe postoperative care. This component requires postoperative pain management and surgical wound postoperative follow-up. Therefore, follow-up instructions should be given to the patient when he or she is given postoperative pain medications. As in any surgical wound, the wound needs to be protected from stresses as well as from exposure to the elements. It is often reported that with skin wounds, once the hematoma has formed the wound is impervious to violation from the exterior. This is true in general, but with ingrowing toenail procedures involving sharp techniques the wound has a hardened, keratinized nail on one side of the incision line and soft mobilized skin on the other side of the incision line. These tissues will create shearing forces along the incision line, and it is important to protect this wound for up to 2 weeks to allow for primary wound healing.

PHENOL TECHNIQUE

Step 1. Identify the apex of the deformity.
Step 2. Maintain hemostasis of the digit.

TABLE 23–2. **Steps for Sharp Surgical Technique and Phenol Technique**

1. Identification of the apex of the nail deformity
2. Physical removal of the offending portion of the nail
3. Identification and removal of retained proximal matrix
4. Identification and removal of hypertrophic granulation tissue and scar

---

Step 3. Remove the offending nail at the apex of the deformity.

Step 4. Identify the matrix dermal attachment and resect remaining matrix.

Step 5. Curette the granulation tissue and hypertrophied ungual labial along the exaggerated skin lines.

Step 6. Apply 89% phenol (carbolic acid) solution to the proximal matrix, nail bed, and area of removed granulation tissue.

Step 7. Swab the wound to remove debris and excess phenol.

Step 8. Apply a dressing. This technique usually does not require postoperative pain management but does require that the patient perform daily dressing changes and wound cleansing.

Postoperative Care

Regardless of whether the sharp or phenol technique is used, a normal healing course of 10 days to 2 weeks should be expected. If after 2 weeks redness, swelling, pain, or drainage is present, there is a high likelihood of retained material and the wound should be anesthetized and explored. Postoperative care is distinctly different for these two techniques in that the patient must maintain a clean and freely draining wound for the phenol technique and a dry, protective surgical dressing for the sharp technique. The literature is divided as to which of these techniques is best for all cases.[3–5] I believe that the phenol technique is the better technique for most cases because it is less invasive and when performed properly does not violate the dermal envelope of the nail bed.

MORTON'S NEUROMA

Morton's neuroma is an impingement of the common digital nerves between the metatarsal heads and the transversely running soft tissue structures. It is commonly seen in the second and third interspace. It is often bilateral and is commonly due to impingement of the nerve by its anatomical neighboring tissue.

Nonsurgical Techniques

Nonsurgical treatment of this problem depends on the etiology or the foot type. If the neuroma is in the second interspace, often there is juxtaposition of the metatarsal heads or lessening of the space between the second and third metatarsal heads with clawing of the digits. In a case such as this, functional control of the foot using an orthotic and/or changing from a narrow shoe to a wide shoe may provide relief. In a more flexible foot the range of motion of the third, fourth, and fifth metatarsals sequentially increases, and the range of motion of the second metatarsal is limited and often fixed relative to the foot. Therefore, in a third interspace neuroma where there is more motion between the lesser metatarsal heads, some other forms of nonsurgical care may result in a positive response (e.g., the use of a metatarsal raised pad). The metatarsal raised pads will allow for maintenance of the space between the third and fourth metatarsal heads and, when weight bearing occurs, will produce an upward force at the proximal neck or shaft of the metatarsals and not allow for shearing stresses that often occur with this foot type. Orthotics often will help by controlling the rearfoot motion, thereby locking the midtarsal joint and maintaining the relationships of the metatarsals. A wider toe box may not help a patient with a third intermetatarsal space neuroma, whereas it may help one with a second intermetatarsal space neuroma. A wider shoe will allow for more motion of the foot within the shoe, exacerbating the symptoms.

Injection of a combination of corticosteroid and local anesthetic provides temporary anesthesia and decreases the local swelling of the nerve. However, this technique is used more as a diagnostic technique than a therapeutic technique. The literature is mixed as to whether this is a necessary step in the treatment of the lesion. The theory is that blocking the nerve and injecting the corticosteroid will break the pain and inflammation cycle and give the patient temporary relief from symptoms.

Surgical Techniques

Surgery for neuroma can be very gratifying in some cases and frustrating in others for both the surgeon and the patient. Better results can be expected with proper preoperative workup, differential treatment, and postoperative follow-up. Surgical performance can be improved with visualization, meticulous dissection, and appropriate closure.

When it is determined that the best option is excision of the neuroma, the following techniques can be used. The most common surgical procedures are the dorsal longitudinal approach and the plantar longitudinal approach.[6, 7]

DORSAL LONGITUDINAL APPROACH

The dorsal longitudinal approach is begun by a longitudinal skin incision just proximal to the metatarsophalangeal joint and extending distally to the skin change lines of the toe web. The fat and superficial vessels are identified and divided longitudinally to identify the metatarsophalangeal joints, as well as the longitudinally running neurovascular structures. If properly placed, this incision should be central to avoid the neurovascular structures. At the level of the metatarsal heads, at the most proximal aspect of the skin incision, there is always some transverse venous structure immediately beneath the skin and superficial fat. Once the skin and superficial fat are divided, the digital arteries and veins are identified running longitudinally from deep to superficial in the web space. The transverse fibers of the deep transverse intermetatarsal ligament are found just proximal to the surgical necks of the metatarsal heads. The nerve is identified just deep to these fibers, running longitudinally and then dividing into digital branches distal to the transverse intermetatarsal ligament. Occasionally these divisions occur proximal to the intermetatarsal ligament, and the surgeon should take care to identify the branches going to the digits since often there are multiple branches. The single common digital nerve trunk must be identified first. It is most common then to transect the nerve proximally and then, pulling the common digital trunk distally, to follow the branches into the digits. The advantages of the dorsal approach are avoidance of plantar scarring, no weight bearing or shear stresses on the skin incision, and hiding of the distal portion of the scar in the web space. The primary disadvantage of this approach is working in a narrow, deep cavity. Transection of the nerve sharply without fragmentation of the nerve tissue proximally is often difficult without the assistance of either a laminar spreader or a neuroma metatarsal spreader during surgery. Additionally, there is a possibility of postoperative maceration of the web space and sacrificing of the deep intermetatarsal ligament.

PLANTAR LONGITUDINAL APPROACH

The plantar longitudinal incision is placed just proximally to the metatarsal heads and extends 1 to 3 cm distally. It is important to palpate and/or mark the metatarsal heads so as to avoid placement of the scar over the weight-bearing surface. This will help to avoid a weight-bearing scar. The most proximal aspect of the incision is the most important part in creating a manageable scar. Immediately beneath the skin there will be fat and multiple fibrous structures running vertically within the fat. Just distal to the metatarsophalangeal joint there are longitudinally running structures. The nerve will be readily identifiable adjacent to the digital venous and arterial structures, which should be identified just distal to the superficial intermetatarsal ligament. This ligament is thinner than the deep intermetatarsal ligament but is always found creating a sheath around the nerve. Anatomically, there is a deep intermetatarsal ligament and a superficial intermetatarsal ligament, with the superficial intermetatarsal ligament being the most plantar. It is usually thin but may be hypertrophied secondary to bursal formation and irritation by the hypertrophied nerve.

The nerve is identified, the superficial intermetatarsal ligament is transected, and the most proximal aspect of the nerve is identified. Traction is then placed on the nerve from proximal to distal, and the nerve is sharply transected at its most proximal aspect so that the nerve will retract proximally into the fat of the intermetatarsal space. If there is some regrowth of the nerve, it will not be able to approximate the metatarsophalangeal joints. The nerve is then followed distally, and the branches to the digits are transected. Dorsal to the nerve are the deep transverse intermetatarsal ligament and third metatarsal artery, which should be visualized but not violated.

Wound closure is performed with extra care and in layers so that the resulting scar is as small as possible. Minimal or no weight bearing is recommended for 2 to 3 weeks following surgery to decrease the swelling and stresses applied to the scar during the healing process. Often, ambulation creates edema and shearing stresses that cause hypertrophy and prolongation of the scarring process.

The advantage of the plantar approach is that the structures are superficial, requiring limited dissection. Therefore, there is direct visibility of the nerve even in patients with severely contracted digits, no violation of the deep metatarsal ligament, and a shallow incision site. The disadvantages are related to the need for longer postoperative immobilization and protection from weight bearing secondary to hypertrophy of the scar.

DEFORMITIES OF THE SECOND, THIRD, AND FOURTH DIGITS

Lesser toe surgery is probably the most common surgical procedure performed by podiatrists in the United States. However, because it is common, physicians dealing with deformities of the second, third, and fourth digits may take a cavalier approach to treatment of this problem. The following is an attempt to help identify the levels of deformity, types of deformity, relationships to other toes, the foot type, systemic disease, and their influence on this type of surgery.

Digital deformities of the second, third, and fourth toes can be found at the distal interphalangeal joint, such as in the mallet toe; at the proximal interphalangeal joint, as in the hammer toe; at the distal interphalangeal joint and the proximal interphalangeal joint, as in the curly toe; at the metatarsophalangeal joint, as in the contracted toe; and in the distal interphalangeal joint, proximal interphalangeal joint, and metatarsophalangeal joint, as in the claw toe. The types of deformity at these levels can be a sagittal plane deformity of flexible type, usually caused by soft tissue contracture; a sagittal plane deformity of rigid type, which is usually due to bony ankylosis; a transverse plane deformity, which is reducible and often due to soft tissue; and a transverse plane nonreducible deformity, which is bony.

Often the relationships to the other toes and metatarsals dictate which type of treatment is necessary. Is the particular toe that the patient is complaining of aligned with the other toes? Is it overlapping or underlapping other toes? What are the relationships of the toes to their respective metatarsals? At what level is the deformity? What is the foot type? (It is important to consider whether it is a flexible flatfoot, a rigid flatfoot, a flexible cavus foot, or a rigid cavus foot.) Is systemic disease present? If so, is the systemic disease of the nature and type that the deformities are progressive? All of these possibilities must be considered, because significantly different treatment regimens are used to correct the various combinations of disorders.

Of the central three digits, the most commonly involved digit is the second.[8] This is usually because the second toe and the second ray are longer than the remainder of the digits and because of the rotational or shearing forces found during gait. The incidence of hammer toes increases with age, with persons older than 60 years of age the more predominant patient population.[9] The proposed etiology is that the long flexor tendons, in an effort to stabilize the foot against the ground, overpower the intrinsic muscles secondary to a longer lever arm and cause subluxation of the interphalangeal joints, progressing to the metatarsophalangeal joints. These imbalances can be congenital, pathologic, or traumatic.

Clavi are a dermatologic protective response due to the impingement of the skin between the shoe, ground, or adjacent digits and the bony prominence of the digit. Treatment ranges from wearing shoes with enlarged toe boxes, using padding, and debriding hypertrophic skin to surgical reconstruction.

Evaluation and Treatment

The decision as to appropriate treatment is based on a disease process, concomitant pathology, and disability associated with digital deformities.

Clinical evaluation of lesser toe deformities includes range-of-motion examination, muscle strength examination, neurologic examination, vascular examination, and gait examination. It is assumed that all patients for whom surgery is discussed have also had standard weight-bearing radiographs. Radiographs are reviewed to determine bony pathology and alignment of the digits.

In all cases nonsurgical methods should be used before consideration of surgery. Once these nonsurgical management techniques have been given appropriate trials and the patient and podiatrist have decided they are not satisfied with those regimens, surgical correction is indicated.[8, 10, 11]

Surgical Procedures

The basic principles of surgical correction of lesser toe deformities are listed in Table 23–3.

The most commonly performed digital procedure is the proximal phalanx head resection or Post's procedure. This is used for simple isolated hammer toes without contracture of the metatarsophalangeal joint. If contracture of the metatarsophalangeal joint, contracture of the distal interphalangeal joint, or transverse plane deformities are present, adjunctive procedures are necessary. Flexor tendon transfer is commonly used for flexible contraction of the metatarsophalangeal joint. Distal interphalangeal joint arthroplasty or fusion, flexor tendon lengthening at the proximal interphalangeal joint, metatarsophalangeal joint release, plantar metatarsophalangeal joint release, and metatarsal neck osteotomy are all adjunctive procedures that are necessary with progressively serious pathology. These adjunc-

TABLE 23–4. **Etiology of Hallux Abductovalgus**

Reverdin 1878—wearing of pointed toe shoes
Young 1909—os intermetatarsum
Silver 1923—weak or paralyzed abductor hallucis
Root and Weed 1977—hypermobility of the first ray
Mann/Coughlin 1991—shoe gear, round metatarsal head and oblique medial angulation of the first metatarsal cuneiform joint

tive procedures are used sequentially for more severe deformities. K-wires, implants, screws, and other fixation materials are used to maintain, not to create, correction. Fusion of the interphalangeal joints is indicated when rigidity or stability is needed. It must be used with caution. If a fusion is created, the flexibility of the digit is decreased; therefore, if the patient has some type of neuropathy he or she will be at increased risk for soft tissue injury and complications.

After reviewing this chapter on foot surgery the reader should realize that digital surgery is not as simple as some persons believe. Digital procedures can be very satisfying to both the surgeon and the patient; however, proper surgical preparation and performance in surgery are essential.

HALLUX ABDUCTOVALGUS

Etiology

The proposed causes of hallux abductovalgus deformity are numerous and have been modified as the knowledge of the foot has evolved (Table 23–4). A good understanding of the predisposing factors, both extrinsic and intrinsic, is imperative to effectively treat and maintain correction of this deformity. Over the years, many etiologies of hallux abductovalgus have been popularized and fallen out of popularity. One of the difficulties with hallux abductovalgus is that there is no single type of hallux abductovalgus and no single type of patient complaint. Often the patient may not have a large deformity but it may be very symptomatic and therefore confounding to many patients and physicians.

Four stages of hallux abductovalgus have been proposed. There are a multiplicity of in-

TABLE 23–3. **Basic Principles of Surgical Correction of Lesser Toe Deformities**

1. Direct surgical intervention should be done at the level of the apex or apices of the deformity.
2. If the deformity is dynamic, treatment of the dynamic process must be part of the treatment plan.
3. If the deformity is secondary to bony deformity, it must be treated.
4. If the deformity does not appear corrected at the time of surgery, it will not be corrected.
5. The correction of the lateralmost toe or isolated toe in a foot with contracture of the next largest toe indicates a high probability, over time, that the next largest uncorrected toe will become symptomatic.
6. If the patient has a progressive systemic disease, isolated correction of digital deformities without addressing and treating the systemic disease is not indicated and will have deleterious results.

fluences on the creation and the rate of progression of hallux abductovalgus, ranging from the extent of subtalar joint pronation, the activity performed, the type of terrain, the type of shoe, and neurologic diseases. It is probably true that all these factors play a role in the development of hallux abductovalgus or at least aggravate predisposing factors.

Treatment

There are a number of ways to treat hallux abductovalgus. Change in the type of shoe and wearing of bunion shields and pads, orthotics, and arch supports should always be considered and discussed before surgery. Surgery for correction of hallux abductovalgus should be recommended for patients who have not benefitted from these nonsurgical measures.

There are over 150 surgical procedures and/or modification procedures described in the literature.[13] Several of the common surgical treatment regimens are reviewed, including the following basic procedures:

1. Capsule-tendon balancing procedures[14, 15]
2. Arthroplastic procedures[16, 17]
3. Osteotomies of the distal metatarsal head[18, 19]
4. Osteotomies of the proximal metatarsal

There is no one type of hallux abductovalgus. Hallux abductovalgus surgery needs to be directed to the apex or the apices of deformity, and subtle signs often overlooked by many caregivers will help differentiate excellent results from good results.

SURGICAL PROCEDURES

Evaluation

Once it has been determined that the patient is a surgical candidate, evaluative procedures should be performed. These should include, but not be limited to, the neurovascular examination, gait examination, muscle strength examination, biomechanical examination, radiographic examination, and, if possible, a reproducible gait plate examination. From these examinations the primary care podiatrist can determine which type of surgery is indicated.

Techniques

Each practitioner should be familiar with the simple bunionectomy techniques described in the literature by Silver and McBride, joint arthroplastic procedures described by Keller and McKeever, and metatarsal osteotomy procedures described by Reverdin, Austin, and Balacescu. These procedures are all straightforward treatments for the patient with common hallux abductovalgus. If information from the examination shows that the patient's disorder is not amenable to the above-listed procedures, then referral is indicated.

Arthroplastic Procedures. Arthroplastic procedures are used when degenerative changes of the first metatarsophalangeal joint are found. If the changes are limited to the periphery of the joint, a cheilectomy or debridement of the peripheral hypertrophic bone combined with a decompression osteotomy will often suffice. However, if there are significant degenerative changes, the cheilectomy will not be an effective treatment option. A decompression procedure can be performed on the proximal phalanx or the first metatarsal. The general concept is that shortening the first ray will decrease the compression forces of the first metatarsophalangeal joint. Often the first metatarsal, or proximal phalanx, is relatively long and therefore causes accelerated degenerative changes secondary to function. This is an option if there are no significant degenerative changes of the metatarsal head or the base of the proximal phalanx. In cases where there are central degenerative changes, surgical options are resectional arthroplasty, Keller arthroplasty, implant arthroplasty, or fusion.

Resectional arthroplasty, or the Keller bunionectomy, has withstood the test of time. It is a viable option for a partially destroyed first metatarsophalangeal joint where medial or lateral instability is not a problem. Keller first described the use of the procedure alone in hallux abductovalgus surgery. Over time its indications have narrowed, and it is often used in combination with proximal metatarsal osteotomies.

Osteotomies. Akin, in 1925, introduced a new operative procedure for hallux valgus that is the classic closing base wedge phalangeal osteotomy. It consists of a closing base wedge of the proximal phalanx with resection of the medial eminence of the bunion. The Akin procedure has been modified over the years to include not only the wedge resection but also a shortening osteotomy and derotational osteotomies. The Akin osteotomy can be used as an adjunct with other procedures; however, its primary indication is to correct the high distal articular set angle in cases of hallux interphalangeus. Several studies have reported that the use of the Akin procedure alone does not correct bunion deformity.

Reverdin, in 1981, described a closing base wedge of the head of the first metatarsal to correct the outward deviation of the great toe. Today we know this outward deviation of the great toe to be the proximal articular set angle, and the Reverdin procedure is the treatment of choice for this disorder. Many modifications of this osteotomy have been created, and one of them is the Austin bunionectomy. The Austin bunionectomy is a Chevron osteotomy of the distal metatarsal head of the first metatarsal. It is an ideal procedure because it can be modified in many ways to close down the intermetatarsal angle or to plantarflex or dorsiflex the metatarsal head. It is a stable osteotomy, and multiple fixation techniques can be used to hold the correction. The point to remember, however, is that even with the best osteotomy and with maximum transposition of the head, the most intermetatarsal angle correction that can be expected will be 6° to 8°. Therefore, the highest intermetatarsal angle for which an Austin bunionectomy would be indicated would be 12° to 14°.

Base wedge osteotomies are indicated in patients with metatarsus primus varus greater than 14° and a stable first metatarsal cuneiform joint. It is often used in combination with distal procedures. Either a closing base wedge osteotomy or a crescentic osteotomy will suffice. The advantage of the closing wedge osteotomy is the medial hinge, which when maintained allows for a point of fixation and will necessitate only one other point of fixation. The advantage of the crescentic osteotomy is that it usually allows for less shortening of the first metatarsal. Both procedures are technically difficult to perform; therefore, the podiatrist who participates in these procedures should have appropriate training in these techniques.

SOFT TISSUE AND BONE TUMORS

Other areas that need to be considered in primary care are soft tissue and bone tumors. Malignant tumors of the foot are rare; however, many carry a poor prognosis. The treatment of a patient with a tumor of the foot begins with a proper history, clinical examination, laboratory evaluation, and biopsy. It does not limit further definitive treatments. Most bone tumors of the foot are primary tumors and not metastasis. Because of this, most diagnoses are made only after surgical excision of the tumor. There are currently no reliable published reports that definitely describe the presentation, workup, and differentiation of tumors of the foot. A general tumor workup should consist of a thorough history and examination, a chest radiograph, and a laboratory examination including the complete blood cell count with differential count, erythrocyte sedimentation rate, and alkaline phosphatase, alkaline acetate, serum potassium, and serum calcium values. If this workup proves to be positive, it should be followed with a gallium bone scan of the whole body and magnetic resonance imaging of the suspected area using a head coil; bilateral studies should be obtained, using sagittal and axial planes of both T1- and T2-weighted films.

Indications for biopsy are a lesion that does not respond to usual treatment modalities, sudden changes of an existing lesion, or rapid development of a new lesion.

TRAUMA

There is a high likelihood of trauma to the foot because of its location. Common foot injuries are lacerations, abrasions, puncture wounds, gunshot wounds, crush injuries, and open fractures.

As in any injury, it is extremely important to establish a baseline of function. It begins in a nonanesthetized patient by determining whether the neurovascular status is intact. For digital injuries, a simple visual examination and checking of sharp and dull differentiation, two-point discrimination, and capillary refill time are important. In more proximal injuries, these assessments plus physical examination of the injury are of utmost importance.

Lacerations

Careful documentation of lacerating trauma, depth of wound, and transected vital structures all impact on the treatment. In general, the golden rule of closure applies to lacerations. If the traumatic event is less than 8 hours old and the wound is clean with no foreign material, debris, or necrotic tissue, then the wound can be closed. If, however, the lacerations include bone, capsule, tendon, or joint space, then delayed primary closure is indicated after appropriate wound lavage and antibiotic regimen.

Puncture Wounds

Penetrating wounds must be differentiated by the type of penetrating object. The most common puncture wounds are those caused by nails, glass, and wood splinters. Other examples include gunshot wounds, knife wounds, and aerosolized material. Most gunshot wounds are considered high-velocity wounds; in these cases, the bullet can be left in place, unless it involves a joint or marginally viable structure or unless it can be easily retrieved with minimal tissue damage. This rule does not apply to close-range gunshot wounds, because the packing included in the shell causes burns and can implant a lot of foreign material. These wounds must be treated with open debridement.

The following guidelines apply to the treatment of puncture wounds:

1. Is the patient's tetanus prophylaxis up to date?
2. Did the penetrating object bring anything with it into the wound?
3. Which structures did the penetrating object violate?
4. What is the time frame of injury? Less than 8 hours? Between 24 and 48 hours?
5. Does the patient have a disease process or a social situation that will negatively affect the healing of the wound?
6. What kind of function can be regained?

In all cases concomitant injury must be ruled out. Therefore, radiographs of the foot, including three separate views, are necessary. Radiographic evidence of bony involvement will imply the need for at least a prolonged course of antibiotics following open incision and drainage. When foreign bodies are identified and because of the nature of the puncturing event (i.e., lower velocity wounds with larger amount of peri-injury tissue damage), a fairly large area of peri-injury tissues must be resected. The limiting factor regarding how much tissue must be excised relates to the puncturing event or object. An example is a relative increase in soft tissue damage incurred by a clean sharp puncture from a knife vs. the blunt trauma of entrance and exit of a nail. The nail puncture would require more debridement secondary to the peripheral tissue damage. When bone or capsule is involved, both must be opened and/or drained and left open until infection is determined not to take place.

Crush Injuries

Crush injuries are common in the foot. The most common is the subungual hematoma. Crush injuries can be differentiated clinically because of time delay and tissue necrosis. The key to determining the extent of the injury is the history. Severity of soft tissue injury increases the risk of infection and dictates treatment.

Reflex Sympathetic Dystrophy

One of the long-term complications of lower-extremity injury is reflex sympathetic dystrophy. In reflex sympathetic dystrophy a patient presents with pain that is apparently out of proportion to the injury. It involves an entire limb and includes redness, swelling, and hyperesthesia. Following the acute disability, there is usually significant stiffness, muscular atrophy, and loss of function. If it is allowed to progress, this limb may become cold, pale, and nearly useless. Clinical suspicion and radiographic evidence are used for diagnosis.

REFERENCES

1. Cox HT: The cleavage lines of skin. Br J Surg 29:234, 1941.
2. Miller SJ: Surgical principles. In McGlamry ED (ed):

Fundamentals of Foot Surgery. Baltimore, Williams & Wilkins, 1987.

3. Frost L: Root resection for the incurvated nail. J Natl Assoc Chir 40(3):19–28, 1950.

4. Kuwada GT: Long-term evaluation of partial and total surgical and phenol matricectomies. J Am Podiatr Med Assoc 81:35–36, 1991.

5. Tait GR, Tuck JS: Surgical or phenol ablation of the nail bed for ingrowing toenails: A randomized controlled trial. J R Coll Surg Edinburgh 32:358–360, 1987.

6. Gaynor R, Hake D, Spinner SM, Tomczak RL: A comparative analysis of conservative versus surgical treatment of Morton's neuroma. J Am Podiatr Med Assoc 79:27–30, 1989.

7. Greenfield J, Rea J Jr, Ilfeld FW: Morton's interdigital neuroma. Clin Orthop 185:142–144, 1984.

8. Sorto LA: Surgical correction of hammer toes. J Am Podiatr Med Assoc 64:930–940, 1974.

9. Gould N, Schneider W, Ashikaga T: Epidemiological survey of foot problems in the continental United States. Foot Ankle 1(1):8–10, 1980.

10. Turain I: Deformities of the smaller toes and surgical treatment. J Foot Surg 29(2):176–178, 1990.

11. Coughlin J: Lesser toe deformities. Orthopedics 10(2):63–75, 1987.

12. Root ML, Orien WP, Weed JH: Normal and Abnormal Function of the Foot. Los Angeles, Clinical Biomechanics Corp, 1977.

13. Ruch JA, et al: First ray hallux abductovalgus and related deformities. In McGlamry ED (ed): Comprehensive Textbook of Foot Surgery. Baltimore, Williams & Wilkins, 1987.

14. Silver D: Operative treatment of hallux valgus. J Bone Joint Surg 5:225–232, 1923.

15. McBride E: Conservative operation for bunions. J Bone Joint Surg 10(4):735–739, 1928.

16. Keller WL: The surgical treatment of bunions and hallux valgus. NY Med J 80:741, 1904.

17. McKeever D: Arthrodesis of the 1st MPJ for hallux valgus, hallux rigidity and metatarsus primus varus. J Bone Joint Surg [Am] 34:1, 1952.

18. Beck E: Modified Reverdin technique for hallux abductovalgus. J Am Podiatr Med Assoc 64:657, 1974.

19. Austin DW: A new osteotomy for hallux valgus. Clin Orthop 157:25–30, 1981.

20. Balacescu, J: Un cas de hallux valgus simetric. Rev Chir Orthop 7:128–135, 1903.

CHAPTER 24

INTERPRETATION OF LABORATORY VALUES

Christiane H. Gardner
Patricia M. Sullivan
Brad G. Samojla

The marked increase in the number and availability of laboratory tests has inevitably resulted in an increasing reliance on these studies. It is essential to bear in mind the limitations of these procedures. More importantly, the accumulation of laboratory data cannot relieve the practitioner of the responsibility of careful observation and study of the patient.

Several of the laboratory tests that are described in this chapter are common components of screening batteries in asymptomatic patients. Although there is little doubt that most of these tests provide useful information about the status of the health of a patient, these tests should be ordered rationally and selectively. Clinical situations for tests contributing to patient care include screening before surgery, testing patients suspected of having an abnormality, and monitoring the response to treatment of those with an abnormal test.

Indiscriminate use of laboratory tests causes needless discomfort and anxiety for a patient and certainly contributes to the escalating costs of health care. The purpose of this chapter is to assist the podiatrist in choosing those laboratory tests that are most appropriate for the patient's medical problem.

HEMATOLOGY

Complete Blood Cell Count

The complete blood cell count and the leukocyte differential count are two of the most common clinical laboratory tests obtained in medical practice. These tests have been advocated as routine components of the diagnostic investigation of persons who are sick and also as part of a screening program for those who are well.

A complete blood cell count is generally done with a Coulter counter, which measures the total leukocyte count, erythrocyte count, hemoglobin level, hematocrit, red blood cell indices (mean corpuscular volume, mean corpuscular hemoglobin, mean corpuscular hemoglobin concentration), and platelet count.[1]

BLOOD CELL COUNTS

White Blood Cell Count

The white blood cell count denotes the number of white blood cells in 1 cubic millimeter of whole blood. In a normal healthy person, the white blood cell count is between 5000 and 10,000 cells/mm[3]. Newborns have a high normal white blood cell count of 10,000 to 20,000 cells/mm[3], which gradually decreases to adult values by age 15. During childhood, the total count is usually around 8000 cells/mm[3] and the range is between 4000 and 13,000 cells/mm[3]. The adult values achieved at about age 15 are maintained throughout the remainder of a person's life.[2] Measurement of the total number of circulating white blood cells is important in the diagnosis and prognosis of the disease process because specific patterns of white blood cell response can be expected in different types of diseases. Since white blood cells are affected by so many diseases, the white blood cell count serves as a useful guide to the severity of the disease process, with the exception of primary diseases of the white blood cells. White blood cell and differential counts by themselves are of little value as aids to diagnosis, unless the results are related to the clinical condition of the patient.[3]

Leukocytosis is defined as a white blood cell count above 10,000 cells/mm[3]. Leukocytosis is usually due to an increase in only one type of white blood cell. When leukocytosis occurs, it is given the name of the type of cell that shows the largest increase. An example of this is lymphocytic leukocytosis or lymphocytosis.[4] Leukocytosis is more likely to occur in acute infections than in chronic disorders. In certain diseases, such as measles or sepsis, the increase of white blood cells is so great that the blood picture is suggestive of leukemia. The absence of anemia helps to distinguish severe infections from leukemia; however, a bone marrow study may be warranted to rule out leukemia.[5] Other causes for leukocytosis besides acute infections may include trauma or tissue injury as occurs in surgery; malignant disease; uremia; corticosteroid therapy; emotional stress; exercise; or inflammation.[3]

Leukopenia is a decrease of white blood cells below 4000 cells/mm[3] and is generally due to a decrease in neutrophils (neutrophilia).[2] The most common causes of leukopenia are viral infections; bone marrow damage such as aplastic anemia or damage from irradiation; splenomegaly; certain drugs (antimetabolites, barbiturates, antibiotics, and antihistamines); alcoholism; and diabetes. It has been shown that alcoholic and diabetic disease states tend to decrease the mobilization of white blood cells, which may contribute to increased susceptibility to pneumonia and other infections.[5] The primary care practitioner should be alert to white blood cell counts less than 500 cells/mm[3]. This value is considered the panic value because the body is essentially left unprotected from invading organisms. These patients must be protected from infection by use of strict reverse isolation techniques.[3]

There are several nonpathologic causes for leukocytosis and leukopenia. Spontaneous fluctuations in the white blood cell count appear to occur throughout the day, consisting of an early morning low level and an afternoon peak level.[2] Food, exercise, and psychological stress can all cause an increase in the overall white blood cell count.[5] Several medications can also result in an increase or decrease in the white blood cell count. It is imperative that information from the history and physical examination be combined with the laboratory values, rather than relying solely on laboratory results to formulate a diagnosis.

Red Blood Cell Count

The two primary functions of the red blood cells are to carry oxygen from the lungs to the tissues of the body and to transfer carbon dioxide from the body tissues back to the lungs. This process is achieved by the hemoglobin molecule, which is contained within the red blood cell. The red blood cell is shaped like a biconcave disk, which results in a greater surface area for oxygen to bind with hemoglobin. The red blood cell is also capable of changing its shape so that it may pass through small capillaries.[5] In adults, the red blood cells are formed within the bone marrow (erythropoiesis) of the ribs, femur, sternum, and pelvis.[6] Normally, the rate of production of the red blood cells determines the red blood cell count and the hemoglobin level in the blood and shows little variation among persons.[7] The red blood cells in the circulating blood have a life span of approximately 120 days.[8] At the end of their life span, these cells are removed from the circulation by phagocytes in the liver, spleen, and bone marrow. The red blood cell count is the number of red blood cells in 1 cubic millimeter of whole blood. Normal values for men range from 4 to 6 million cells/mm[3]. Women may have a slightly lower count, and newborns a higher count.[5] As with the white blood cell count, there are variations in the red blood cell count that have physiologic causes and are not pathologic. Exercise appears to increase red blood cell counts, as does altitude. The higher the altitude, the greater the increase in the number of the red blood cells.[9] Many drugs decrease red blood cells. Examples of those drugs that decrease the red blood cell count are gentamicin and methyldopa.[5]

When a person's hemoglobin level falls below normal it indicates that peripheral tissues are not receiving adequate amounts of oxygen; thus, a state of hypoxia exists. This condition stimulates the production of erythropoietin, a hormone that stimulates the production of red blood cells in the bone marrow.[7] The most common cause for a decreased red blood cell count is anemia. This decreased value may be due to decreased blood cell production, increased red blood cell destruction, blood loss, or dietary insufficiency of iron and certain vitamins essential for the production of red blood cells.[5] Other causes of decreased red blood cell counts include bone marrow depression, severe infections, malaria, and lead poisoning. Increased values are usually found with polycythemia, dehydration, and certain kidney diseases and lung diseases (i.e., emphysema, asthma, and chronic obstructive pulmonary disease).[7]

HEMATOCRIT

When anticoagulated whole blood is centrifuged, the space occupied by the packed red blood cells is termed the *hematocrit* and is expressed as the percentage of red blood cells in a given volume of whole blood. Owing to the simplicity and reproducibility of the test, it is the favored test for evaluating anemias or other pathologic changes within the body.[1, 4] The values for the hematocrit closely parallel the values for the hemoglobin and red blood cell count. Roughly, the hematocrit value should be three times the hemoglobin value ($\pm 3\%$).[8] Many researchers believe the hematocrit value is a better measure of anemia than hemoglobin, especially if serum iron values are normal.[1] Normal ranges for hematocrit are 40% to 54% for men and 37% to 47% for women.[8] Increased values are found in polycythemia, severe dehydration, and angina and after surgery or trauma. Decreased values are found in anemias, leukemia, and cirrhosis. The hematocrit is usually normal immediately following an acute hemorrhage but may be decreased for as long as 72 hours after hemorrhage.[10] Infusion of 1 unit of whole blood (450 mL total volume) will raise the hematocrit by approximately 3%.[11] Normal values for the hematocrit vary with age and sex. Newborns have a higher value (50% to 62%) and adults older than the age of 50 tend to have slightly lower than normal values. As with the red blood cell count, persons living at high altitudes will usually have higher hematocrit values.[9]

HEMOGLOBIN

Hemoglobin is an iron protein substance that is synthesized within newly formed red blood cells and remains there for the life of the cell. It is composed of a single protein called globin and a molecule called heme, which contains iron. Hemoglobin is the vehicle for the transportation of oxygen and carbon dioxide within the body. Each gram of hemoglobin can carry 1.34 mL of oxygen.[5] The oxygen-carrying capacity of the blood is directly proportional to the hemoglobin concentration and not to the number of red blood cells, since not all red blood cells carry the same amount of hemoglobin.[5] This is why the hemoglobin value is more important than the red blood cell count in the evaluation of anemia. Normal hemoglobin values are 13.5 to 17.5 g/dL for men and 12 to 16 g/dL for women.[8]

There are different forms of hemoglobin, and these forms are usually measured together as the total hemoglobin.[1] A familiar variant of hemoglobin is hemoglobin S, which is associated with sickle cell anemia. Other forms of hemoglobin are associated with heavy smoking. In this case, the normal hemoglobin value may consist of upward of 20% of carboxyhemoglobin. Carboxyhemoglobin has a 200 times greater affinity for carbon monoxide than for oxygen.[12] Obviously, in this case the smoker's "normal" value is well below normal. Only by knowing the patient's history of smoking can the practitioner correctly interpret the hemoglobin results and, if deemed necessary, order further tests such as a carboxyhemoglobin test. Increased values of hemoglobin may be seen in polycythemia, congestive heart failure, and chronic obstructive pulmonary disease. Decreased levels of hemoglobin are seen in anemia (especially iron-deficiency anemia), severe hemorrhage, and cirrhosis. Altitude again has the effect of causing increased levels of hemoglobin, while pregnancy tends to lower the levels.[5]

RED BLOOD CELL INDICES

The red blood cell indices are used to define the size and hemoglobin content of the red blood cell. They consist of the mean corpuscular volume, mean corpuscular hemoglobin, and mean corpuscular hemoglobin concentration. These indices are used as an aid in differentiating anemias. When they are used together with an examination of the red blood cells on the stained smear, a clear picture of red blood cell morphology is ascertained. By examination of these indices, the volume and hemoglobin content of the red blood cells are characterized. By virtue of these indices, anemias are classified by cell size (i.e., macrocytic, normocytic, microcytic) or by a combination of cell size and color (i.e., microcytic, hypochromic).[1,4]

Mean Corpuscular Volume. The mean corpuscular volume (MCV) indicates the average volume of the red blood cells and is the best index for classifying anemias. The MCV indicates whether the red blood cell appears normocytic, microcytic, or macrocytic. Normal values for MCV are 80 to 96 μm^3.[1] If the MCV is less than 80 μm^3, the red blood cells are microcytic. If the MCV is greater than 96 μm^3, the red blood cells are macrocytic.[1] If the MCV falls within the normal range, the red blood cells are normocytic. Decreased values can be found in iron-deficiency anemia, thalassemia, and anemia of chronic blood loss, while increased values are seen in liver diseases, alco-

holism, antimetabolite therapy, and vitamin B_{12} deficiency.[5]

Mean Corpuscular Hemoglobin Concentration. The mean corpuscular hemoglobin concentration (MCHC) is a calculated measure of the average concentration of hemoglobin in the red blood cells. It is obtained from both the hematocrit and hemoglobin values and is expressed as a percentage of cell volume.[8] *Normochromic* is the term given to the red blood cells falling within normal values (33% to 36%). Values below 33% indicate hypochromia, while values greater than 36% indicate hyperchromia. A decreased MCHC indicates that the red blood cells contain less hemoglobin than normal, and this may occur in iron deficiency, chronic blood loss, and thalassemia. An increased value for MCHC usually indicates spherocytosis.[4] Because this index is a measure of the concentration of hemoglobin within red blood cells, it is especially valuable for monitoring therapy for anemia.[1]

Mean Corpuscular Hemoglobin. The mean corpuscular hemoglobin (MCH) indicates the average weight of hemoglobin in the red blood cell. It is calculated from the red blood cell count and the hemoglobin value and is expressed in picograms. Normal values are 27 to 33 pg.[1] The value for the MCH should always correlate with the MCV and MCHC. This index offers little more information than can already be obtained from the MCV and MCHC.

PLATELETS

Platelets (thrombocytes) are the smallest of the formed elements in the blood. They are fragments that bud from the cytoplasm of megakaryocytes (large multinucleated cells found in the bone marrow) at the approximate rate of 100,000 per day and have a life span of 8 to 11 days.[8] At any given moment, about 80% of the platelets are in circulation and 20% are located in the spleen.[13] The bone marrow does not contain a reserve of platelets, and if the circulating platelets are rapidly destroyed or lost, thrombocytopenia exists for several days until enough new platelets are formed. Platelets are vital to hemostasis and function in several ways: maintaining the integrity (leak-free state) of blood vessels, forming plugs to stop blood loss from injured vessels, and promoting thrombin production.[14] The normal range for the platelet count is 150,000 to 450,000 cells/mm³.[1] This measurement is helpful in evaluating bleeding disorders that occur in liver disease, thrombocytopenia, and uremia and with anticoagulant therapy. An increased platelet count is termed *thrombocytosis* and is found in polycythemia, idiopathic thrombocythemia, cancer, and chronic myelogenous leukemia and following a splenectomy. A decreased number of platelets *(thrombocytopenia)* occurs in acute leukemia, in idiopathic thrombocytopenic purpura, during cancer therapy, and in certain allergic conditions.[1, 4] Generally, platelet counts of greater than 50,000 cells/mm³ are not associated with spontaneous bleeding.[5] Aspirin irreversibly renders platelets ineffective by acetylating cyclo-oxygenase.[13] The platelet count only assesses the amount of platelets, not their function. If a patient's platelet count is normal, do not assume the platelets are functioning normally. The best test for determining the function of the platelets is the bleeding time.[15]

Differential Blood Cell Count

The differential white blood cell count is performed to determine the relative number of each type of white blood cell present in the blood. More information can be obtained from a detailed examination of the stained peripheral blood smear than from any other single laboratory test. Most larger laboratories today use electrical impedance hematology analyzers, which not only report cell counts and calculate red blood cell indices, but also provide a histogram differential white blood cell count (absolute and relative percentages of lymphocytes, neutrophils, and mononuclear cells), as well as note the presence of any atypical white blood cells. The analyzers also describe the presence of any abnormal red blood cells, indicating size and shape abnormalities.[1] On request, most laboratories will perform the differential blood cell count manually.

WHITE BLOOD CELL DIFFERENTIAL COUNT

The white blood cells are differentiated according to the five types of white blood cells:

segmented and band neutrophils, eosinophils, basophils, lymphocytes, and monocytes. In adults, more than half of the circulating white blood cells are granulocytes, or cells whose cytoplasm contains visible granules enclosing various chemicals or enzymes. Granulocytes are categorized according to the staining properties of the granules and include neutrophils, eosinophils, and basophils.

Neutrophils. The segmented neutrophils are the most numerous and the most important type of white blood cell. They provide the primary defense against microbial invasion through the process of phagocytosis. In their immature stage of development, the segmented neutrophils are referred to as "bands." Band neutrophils do not contain the lobulated nucleus, which is the identifying feature of the neutrophils. Rather, band cells have nuclear material that is thicker and often U shaped.[4, 8] The mature neutrophil is released into the peripheral blood as the segmented neutrophil. When the demand for neutrophils in the body increases, more stored neutrophils are released. When all the stored neutrophils are released, then band cells begin entering the circulation. This is reflected by an increased percentage of bands in the differential cell count and is described as a "shift to the left." Normally, segmented neutrophils make up 50% to 60% of the total white blood cell count while band cells account for 0% to 3%.[4] Conditions that may cause an increase in the percentage of neutrophils include bacterial infections, inflammatory diseases such as rheumatoid arthritis, tissue necrosis, and metabolic disorders such as uremia. Several drugs have also been shown to cause a neutrophilia, such as epinephrine, heparin, and digitalis.[5] A decrease in neutrophils, or neutropenia, occurs in any condition that depresses bone marrow activity, such as acute viral infections and leukemia. It should be remembered that a neutropenia of less than 500 cells/mm³ dramatically decreases a patient's ability to fight infections, and proper precautions should be taken.

Eosinophils. These cells are granulocytes that have a two-lobed nucleus and moderately large, refractile granules that stain deep red with the acidic stain eosin.[4] Eosinophils are not bactericidal; rather, they become active in the later stages of inflammation and ingest antigen–antibody complexes.[16] The hallmark of these cells is their activity in allergic reactions and parasitic infections. Normally, eosinophils constitute an average of 3% of the total white blood cell count.[4] An increase in eosinophils is seen in response to allergies, parasitic diseases, myelogenous leukemia, and polycythemia. A reduction in eosinophils occurs with any stress or following corticosteroid administration.

Basophils. Basophils are also granulocytes and contain large, coarse granules that stain deep blue with basic dyes. These granules are rich in histamine and are believed to be involved in certain acute allergic reactions. Although basophils normally constitute less than 1% of normal circulating white blood cells, an increase may be seen in patients with chronic myelogenous leukemia and polycythemia vera.[4, 16]

Lymphocytes. Lymphocytes are recognized on peripheral blood smears as mononuclear cells with a small amount of blue cytoplasm. The basic function of lymphocytes is to react with antigens, thereby initiating the immune response. It has been found, through analysis of antigens and receptors on the surface of these cells, that there are two main types of lymphocytes: T and B cells. These two types of cells are morphologically similar and can only be distinguished by their surface markers.[17] The T lymphocyte is so named because it resides within the thymus for a short period of time, where it differentiates for cell-mediated immunity.[8] The T lymphocyte functions in cell-mediated immunity by organ transplant rejection, producing certain autoimmune diseases and detecting or destroying new growth. The bursa-dependent (B) lymphocyte is believed to be derived from the bone marrow and is not dependent on the thymus.[8, 17] The B lymphocyte is responsible for humoral immunity and functions chiefly to produce immunoglobulins. Normally, lymphocytes constitute 20% to 40% of the total white blood cell count. Approximately 80% of blood lymphocytes are T cells and 12% to 15% are B cells.[17] The remaining small percentage of lymphocytes lack the characteristic surface receptors of the T and B cells and are called null cells.[8] An increase in lymphocytes is seen in certain infections, such as infectious mononucleosis,

infectious hepatitis, and syphilis, as well as blood diseases such as lymphocytic leukemia. A decrease in circulating lymphocytes commonly occurs with acute, stressful illnesses such as myocardial infarction, pneumonia, and sepsis as well as a variety of malignancies.[3, 17]

Monocytes. Monocytes characteristically are large with abundant blue-gray cytoplasm and an elongated, indented, or folded nucleus.[4] Derived from the same precursor cell as the granulocytes, monocytes mature in the bone marrow, circulate in the peripheral blood briefly, and then enter the tissues to become macrophages. These phagocytic cells remove injured and dead cells, microorganisms, and insoluble particles from the blood. Monocytes are also able to produce the antiviral agent called interferon.[3] Monocytes normally make up 2% to 6% of the total white blood cell count.[8] Increases are seen in certain infections such as tuberculosis and subacute bacterial endocarditis as well as some collagen vascular diseases and malignancies. Monocytopenia is observed in many acute infections, with aplastic anemia, and as an effect of immunosuppressive drugs.[2]

RED BLOOD CELL MORPHOLOGY

Much diagnostic information can be gained by examining red blood cells on a peripheral blood smear. It is useful in diagnosing blood disorders such as anemia, thalassemia, and leukemia. Normal red blood cells have a small area of central pallor and show only slight variation in size (normally 6 to 8 μm in diameter).[16]

Size. Variation in the size of the red blood cells is known as anisocytosis. Microcytes are cells that are decreased in size and are found in thalassemia and a variety of anemias. Macrocytes are cells that are increased in size and may be found in liver disease, pernicious anemia, and folic acid deficiency.[8]

Color. Normally, the red blood cells have a tendency to absorb acid stains. The depth of staining is a rough guide to the amount of hemoglobin within the red blood cell. Normochromic cells are those red blood cells containing normal amounts of hemoglobin. Hypochromia is used to describe those red blood cells with a large area of central pallor. This area of central pallor is due to a decrease in the amount of hemoglobin present and is seen most characteristically in patients with iron-deficiency anemia. Hyperchromic red blood cells contain an increased amount of hemoglobin and show no area of central pallor. These deeply staining cells may indicate megaloblastic anemia.[1, 4, 8]

Shape. Variation in the shape of red blood cells is known as poikilocytosis. Normally, the red blood cell assumes the shape of a biconcave disk; however, several distinctive shapes of red blood cells are related to specific disease states. Sickle cells (drepanocytes) are crescent-shaped red blood cells that come to a point at one end. These cells are associated with hemoglobin S and are found in sickle cell anemia.[4, 8] Burr cells are described as red blood cells with uniformly spaced pointed projections on the outer surface. These cells occur in acute blood loss, cancer of the stomach, and uremia. Spherocytes are not biconcave and do not possess the central area of pallor. They are associated with hemolytic anemia and hereditary spherocytosis. Target cells are thinner than normal with a small amount of hemoglobin in the center. The most common cause of target cells is liver disease; however, they are also prevalent in sickle cell anemia as well as thalassemia. Finally, schistocytes are red blood cell fragments that occur in hemolytic anemia, uremia, and disseminated intravascular coagulation and are also associated with artificial heart valves.[1, 4, 5, 8]

Inclusions. Red blood cells may also be noted to contain inclusions, which may indicate a specific disease state. Basophilic stippling refers to fine blue granules enclosed within the red blood cell. The granules are attributed to a precipitation of RNA and are found in lead poisoning, alcoholism, and megaloblastic anemia.[8] Nucleated red blood cells are the precursors of the non-nucleated mature red cells in the blood and when seen on a blood smear are often mistaken for lymphocytes. In the healthy adult, these cells are confined to the bone marrow and appear in circulating blood only in diseases, such as thalassemia major, where there is an extreme demand on the bone marrow to produce red blood cells.[1, 7] With the influx of immigrants from Third World countries, malaria is no longer an unusual finding. In malaria, the parasite resides within the red blood cell and takes on a fine, granular stippling appearance that is referred to as Schüffner's dots.[5]

PLATELETS

Platelets are examined on the blood smear for morphology and approximate number present. A normal blood smear (normal red blood cell count and normal platelet count) should show 8 to 20 platelets per field in an area of the smear where the red blood cells are almost touching one another.[13] This estimate of the platelet count should correspond with the actual count obtained. Normal platelets are non-nucleated and 2 to 3 μm in diameter.[8] They appear light blue and contain small purple-red granules when stained with Giemsa's solution. In disease states affecting platelets, large atypical platelets may be seen, often with decreased or absent granules.[13]

Coagulation Studies

Before any surgical procedure, the physician must be familiar with the status of the patient's ability to coagulate blood. A thorough history can do much to arouse suspicions as to the patient's ability to form an adequate clot to stop bleeding. If a patient complains of bruises, bleeding gums, or difficulty in postsurgical healing, it is wise to take this seriously.[13] For a patient about to undergo an operation, the prothrombin time, partial thromboplastin time, and platelet count constitute an adequate screening. A bleeding time may be indicated if the history is suggestive of inadequate platelet function.

PLATELET COUNT

The platelet count and peripheral blood smear examination have been discussed previously. A normal platelet count is 150,000 to 450,000 cells/mm^3.[1] If a patient's platelet count is within normal range yet a history suggestive of a possible bleeding disorder is obtained, a screening battery including a bleeding time should be ordered.

BLEEDING TIME

This simple test is used in screening for disorders of platelet function and for von Willebrand's disease. The time taken for bleeding from a standardized skin wound to cease is referred to as the bleeding time. It is a measure of platelet function as well as a measure of how quickly small arteries and veins will constrict and close off to stop bleeding and furthermore is independent of the coagulation mechanism.[18] Most laboratories now use the Ivy bleeding time, in which a sphygmomanometer cuff is placed around the upper arm and inflated to maintain a constant pressure of 40 mm Hg. A disposable spring-loaded device containing one or two blades, which are released when the trigger is pressed, is placed on the flexor surface of the forearm. A timer is started and at 30-second intervals, the drops of blood are blotted with filter paper. When blood no longer stains the paper, the timer is stopped. Normal values for this test are 2.5 to 7.5 minutes.[18]

Again, it must be remembered that aspirin, nonsteroidal anti-inflammatory drugs, and a large number of other drugs can prolong the bleeding time as long as 20 to 30 minutes. A patient scheduled for a bleeding time should be advised to discontinue aspirin for 7 days before the test.[2, 5] Bleeding time is prolonged when the level of platelets is decreased or when the platelets are not functioning adequately. Several disease states can cause an increase in the bleeding time, such as thrombocytopenia, leukemia, aplastic anemia, and severe liver disease.[19]

PROTHROMBIN TIME

Prothrombin is one of the 12 known factors necessary to stop bleeding. It is a protein produced in the liver from vitamin K. In the prothrombin time (PT) test, the time taken for recalcified citrated plasma to clot in the presence of tissue thromboplastin is measured. Normal PT is 10 to 14 seconds.[19] This test is sensitive to defects in the extrinsic clotting system and is a useful screening procedure for deficiencies in factors II, V, VII, and X.[13] This test is commonly ordered in conjunction with the management of coumarin anticoagulant therapy. Coumarin acts in the liver to delay coagulation by interfering with the action of vitamin K–dependent factors (II, VII, IX, and X). Coumarin takes 16 to 48 hours to cause a measurable change in the PT.[5] It is imperative

to establish a baseline by measuring the PT before beginning coumarin therapy. Conditions that may cause an increase in the PT include vitamin K deficiency or poor absorption, liver disease, and biliary obstruction.[15, 19]

ACTIVATED PARTIAL THROMBOPLASTIN TIME

The activated partial thromboplastin time (APTT) is the single most useful test available for routine screening of coagulation disorders. The APTT measures those coagulation factors present in the intrinsic system, including factors VIII, IX, XI, and XII.[15, 19] This test is most frequently used to monitor heparin therapy. The best known action of heparin is the inactivation of thrombin, which prevents it from acting on fibrinogen, which, in turn, prevents the formation of the fibrin clot.[13] The normal value for the APTT is 35 to 45 seconds, with results of 45 to 50 seconds considered borderline and results over 50 seconds considered abnormal.[19]

Although all coagulation tests are affected by heparin, including the prothrombin time, the APTT has been found to be the most sensitive test to monitor the pharmacologic effect of heparin. Unlike coumarin, heparin provides an immediate anticoagulant effect, yet because heparin does not remain in the blood very long, the APTT should be measured before each injection. Ideally, the APTT is maintained at two to two and one-half times the normal limit; again, it is important to establish a baseline APTT before instituting heparin therapy.[5, 19] Conditions that may cause a prolonged APTT include hemophilia, liver disease, and vitamin K deficiency.[19]

Erythrocyte Sedimentation Rate

The erythrocyte sedimentation rate (ESR) is a measure in millimeters of how far the red blood cells will cling together, fall, and settle toward the bottom of a specially marked test tube in an hour's time. Anticoagulated blood is placed in a vertically oriented, graduated, small-bore tube and allowed to sit undisturbed for 1 hour. At the end of 1 hour, the value of the ESR is read directly from the graduated markings on the tube. It is important that the

ESR tube be exactly perpendicular since a tilt of as little as 3° can cause errors up to 30%.[8, 16] This test is based on the fact that inflammatory and necrotic processes cause an alteration in plasma proteins, resulting in an aggregation of red blood cells, thus making them heavier and more likely to fall when placed in a vertical tube.[8] Normal values are 0 to 15 mm/h for men, 0 to 20 mm/h for women, and 0 to 10 mm/h for children.[8] Pathologic changes in the blood can cause an unreliable ESR result; for example, anemia generally causes an elevated ESR, while polycythemia decreases the value.

Nonspecific increases in plasma proteins (globulin and fibrinogen) occur when the body responds to injury, inflammation, or pregnancy. Consequently, an elevated ESR accompanies most acute inflammatory disease (either local or systemic) and flareups of chronic inflammatory states. The ESR can be used to monitor the course of and therapy for chronic inflammatory conditions such as rheumatoid arthritis.[20]

Sickle Cell Anemia

Sickle cell anemia is a cause of significant morbidity and mortality among black persons. This type of anemia is caused by an abnormal form of hemoglobin known as hemoglobin S. If both genes for hemoglobin S are inherited, the patient has sickle cell anemia, while sickle cell trait exists if only one gene is inherited. In sickle cell anemia, the hemoglobin becomes more viscous and tends to precipitate with decreased oxygen tension, causing the red blood cells to sickle. Not only are these abnormally shaped cells unable to pass as easily through capillaries, they also are more fragile, reducing their survival time. Although patients with sickle cell trait usually present with no clinical symptoms, they may develop sickle cells if they become severely hypoxic.[21]

A screening test is usually performed on any person with a familial history of sickle cell anemia. The purpose of the test is to detect the presence of hemoglobin S by removing oxygen from the red blood cells. Red blood cells with normal hemoglobin will retain their shape, while those containing hemoglobin S will sickle. This test does not differentiate between the disease and the trait forms of sickle cell anemia; for this, electrophoresis of the hemoglobin is required.[16, 22]

CHEMISTRY

The blood transports many substances that participate in and reflect ongoing metabolic processes, but only a few are routinely measured. Some substances are analyzed to provide information about specific organ systems, and others reflect the combined effects of several metabolic processes. A discussion of some of the more common tests ordered by primary care physicians follows. It is by no means an exhaustive essay on blood chemistries but rather focuses on those tests that are routinely ordered.

Electrolytes

A common group of substances studied are the electrolytes. Almost all metabolic processes are dependent on or affected by electrolytes. Maintenance of osmotic pressure, maintenance of proper body pH, and regulation of the heart and other muscles are just a few of the body functions for which electrolytes are responsible. Abnormal levels of these anions or cations may be either the cause or the result of a variety of disease states. The most commonly tested electrolytes are potassium (K^+), sodium (Na^+), chloride (Cl^-), and bicarbonate (HCO_3^-).[23]

POTASSIUM

Potassium is the most abundant intracellular electrolyte. It functions in nerve conduction and muscle contraction, including the cardiac muscle, and assists in maintaining acid–base balance when combined with HCO_3^-. The normal serum level is 3.5 to 5 mEq/L, and this level must be strictly maintained.[24] The kidneys are responsible for excretion of K^+ through the distal tubules. Levels below 2.5 mEq/L or over 7.0 mEq/L may lead to changes in muscle irritability, respiration, and myocardial function, accompanied by characteristic electrocardiographic changes. Either an increase or decrease in K^+ will enhance the action of digitalis.[25]

Potassium enters the serum when cellular membranes are damaged, resulting in a leakage of K^+ out of the cell. Increased K^+ levels (hyperkalemia) occur when the kidneys are unable to excrete the K^+ and it accumulates in the serum.[24] Hyperkalemia can be caused by inadequate excretion owing to renal failure, oliguria and anuria, Addison's disease, crush injuries, and burns, which cause renal shutdown. Extrarenal causes include hypoaldosteronism, dehydration, internal hemorrhage, uncontrollable diabetes, and surgical tourniquets, which cause cellular damage. Numerous medications that can elevate the K^+ level include penicillin, K^+-sparing diuretics, heparin, epinephrine, and histamine.[25] A hemolyzed blood specimen may falsely elevate K^+ levels.[24] Clinical signs and symptoms include tachycardia initially, but if the hyperkalemia persists, bradycardia may occur. Other indicators of hyperkalemia include abdominal cramps and tingling, twitching, and numbness of the extremities.[25]

Hypokalemia (decreased K^+ levels) is most commonly due to diuretics, especially thiazides, loop diuretics, and carbonic anhydrase inhibitors. These medications will cause excess K^+ to be excreted in the urine. Other causes of hypokalemia include vomiting, diarrhea, malnutrition, excessive ingestion of glucose, metabolic alkalosis, overhydration, and stress. Medications that can cause hypokalemia include corticosteroids, antibiotics such as gentamicin and amphotericin, and insulin, laxatives, and salicylates.[16, 24] Signs and symptoms of hypokalemia are vertigo, hypotension, nausea, vomiting, diarrhea, abdominal distention, muscle weakness and cramps, confusion, and mental depression.[25]

SODIUM

Sodium is the most abundant extracellular electrolyte. It functions in neuromuscular conduction and enzyme activity, aids in maintaining acid–base balance by combining with Cl^- or HCO_3^-, and helps maintain water balance and osmotic pressure. The serum level of Na^+ is 135 to 145 mEq/L. This concentration is maintained by the kidneys and endocrine system.[24]

Hypernatremia (increased Na^+ concentration) is due to dehydration, severe vomiting and diarrhea in which water loss is greater than sodium loss, congestive heart failure, diabetes insipidus, and hepatic failure. Certain medications, such as cortisone preparations, cough medicines, laxatives, and methyldopa, can cause hypernatremia. Restlessness, thirst, flushed skin, tachycardia, and edema are all indicators of hypernatremia.[23, 25]

Hyponatremia (decreased Na^+ levels) is usually the result of overhydration, which causes dilution of the Na^+ concentration, or an increase in Na^+ loss. Causes of hyponatremia include burns, diarrhea, vomiting, Addison's disease, nephritis, and malabsorption. Signs of hyponatremia are apprehension, anxiety, muscular twitching and weakness, headache, hypotension, and tachycardia.[25]

CHLORIDE

Chloride is an extracellular anion. It functions to maintain water balance and fluid osmolarity in conjunction with Na^+. It also helps to maintain acid–base balance and combines with hydrogen in the stomach to produce acidity. It will combine with cations such as Na^+ to be excreted through the kidneys.[23, 24]

Normal values of Cl^- are 95 to 105 mEq/L.[24] High serum Cl^- levels are observed in dehydration and in conditions causing decreased renal blood flow, such as congestive heart failure. Clinical signs include weakness, lethargy, and deep, rapid, vigorous breathing. Low serum Cl^- levels may be due to vomiting, heat exhaustion, diabetic acidosis, acute infection, and diuretic usage. Hyperexcitability of the nervous system and muscles, tetany, slow and shallow breathing, and hypotension secondary to fluid and Cl^- loss are all indicators of low Cl^- levels.[26]

BICARBONATE

Bicarbonate is the most important buffer compound in the blood and serves to transport CO_2 from the tissues to the lungs. HCO_3^- is easily regulated by the kidney, which excretes it when there is an excess and reabsorbs it when needed. In most instances, HCO_3^- concentrations are determined by testing for the total amount of CO_2.[23] Blood HCO_3^- levels normally range from 24 to 26 mEq/L.[24] Concentrations of HCO_3^- are usually increased when there is severe vomiting, with excessive ingestion of antacid preparations, with use of diuretic or corticosteroid medications, and when breathing prevents the release of proper amounts of CO_2. Levels may be decreased with rapid breathing, with liver or kidney disease, and with diarrhea.[23, 25]

Blood Glucose

SERUM GLUCOSE

Glucose is a common blood test ordered by podiatrists. It is the main source of energy for cells and is formed from the digestion of carbohydrates and the conversion of glycogen in the liver. Hormones are responsible for regulating the level of glucose. Glucagon will increase the breakdown of glycogen, which will increase blood glucose levels. Insulin is responsible for increasing cellular membrane permeability to glucose, allowing the cells to utilize glucose for metabolism. Adrenocorticotropic hormone, adrenocorticosteroids, epinephrine, and thyroxine all stimulate glucose metabolism.[16, 27] Normal fasting values for glucose range from 70 to 110 mg/dL.[8]

Hypoglycemia, a glucose level of less than 50 mg/dL, is the result of inadequate dietary intake or excessive levels of insulin. This condition may be seen in Addison's disease, pancreatic islet cell cancer, which causes excessive insulin excretion, alcoholism, and lung cancer and may follow strenuous exercise. Clinical indications of hypoglycemia include nervousness, weakness, confusion, diaphoresis, and tachycardia.[28]

Hyperglycemia occurs when fasting glucose levels are greater than 110 mg/dL. This condition is most commonly due to diabetes, which could be a result of inadequate insulin levels or cellular resistance to insulin. A diagnosis of impaired glucose tolerance is made when fasting glucose levels are between 110 and 140 mg/dL, while a level greater than 140 mg/dL is indicative of diabetes.[28] Other causes include adrenal gland hyperfunction, stress, crush injuries, burns, acute pancreatitis, and pancreatic cancer. Clinical signs of hyperglycemia are polydipsia, polyphagia, polyuria, and weight loss. If the level exceeds 500 mg/dL, Kussmaul's breathing will result from the acidosis.[28]

GLYCOSYLATED HEMOGLOBIN

The diabetic patient is perhaps one of the most challenging patients the podiatrist must face in daily practice. Most diabetic patients today self-monitor their blood glucose levels, and the physician routinely orders blood glucose levels during patient visits; yet, until the correlation of glycosylated hemoglobin levels with long-term glucose levels, these results gave little indication of a patient's glucose level over several weeks.

Red blood cells contain several different types of hemoglobin, one of which is hemoglobin A_1 (HbA_1), which undergoes change or glycosylation to HbA_{1a}, HbA_{1b}, and HbA_{1c} within the red blood cell. The amount of glycosylated hemoglobin stored by a red blood cell depends on the amount of glucose available to it during the cell's 120-day life span.[5] The greater the amount of glucose in the blood, the greater is the percentage of glycosylated hemoglobin. This test indicates blood glucose activity during the 6 to 8 weeks before the test. The result is of particular value in monitoring a patient with diabetes to ascertain if the patient's blood glucose level is properly controlled, and therefore it is also a measure of success or failure of treatment. A patient whose diabetes has recently come under good control will still have a high percentage of HbA_1. This level will decline gradually as newly formed red blood cells with normal HbA_1 replace older red blood cells with high concentrations of HbA_1.[5, 29]

This test is usually performed every 2 months for insulin-dependent diabetics and every 6 months for non–insulin-dependent diabetics. A diabetic patient without complications should have a result of less than 10%.[29] Currently there are two tests available for measuring glycosylated hemoglobin; one measures HbA_1 while the other measures specifically HbA_{1c}. The value for the HbA_1 determination will generally run 2% to 4% higher than the HbA_{1c}. It should be kept in mind that hemoglobin variants, uremia, and anemias can cause a false test result.[29] Although most laboratories can easily perform this test, new technology will move the availability of this test into the physician's office.

Individual Blood Chemistry Tests

PROTEIN

Proteins consist of amino acids linked together by peptide bonds. There are three general categories of proteins: tissue or organ proteins, plasma proteins, and hemoglobin. Relatively little protein circulates in the blood except for hemoglobin. Plasma proteins are used for nutrition and also maintain the osmotic pressure of the blood. Serum protein measurement usually includes the total protein level and specific analysis of either albumin or globulin. Serum normally contains 6 to 8 g/dL of total protein.[16, 30]

The two major proteins are albumin and globulin. Albumin makes up 52% to 68% of the total protein level, or 3.8 to 5.0 g/dL.[31] It is formed in the liver and functions to maintain osmotic pressure, as well as serving as the transport medium in the blood for ions, pigments, hormones, bilirubin, enzymes, and certain drugs. Except in dehydration, elevated levels of albumin do not occur. Decreased albumin levels are associated with severe liver disease, malabsorption, diarrhea, chronic renal failure, malnutrition, cirrhosis, massive burns, and widespread malignancy. If there is a decrease in the serum albumin concentration, fluid will leave the vessels and diffuse into the surrounding tissue, causing edema.[30, 31]

Globulins are really many specific proteins that are often classified into subgroups. Electrophoresis can separate globulins based on the order of descending mobility as α_1, α_2, β, and γ globulins (immunoglobulins are not included and are studied as part of the immune system). Results are reported as the percent of total protein each group makes up. The subdivisions of globulins can be used to identify the cause for increased or decreased globulin levels. For example, an increase in γ-globulins may be seen in collagen diseases, rheumatoid arthritis, Hodgkin's disease, multiple myeloma, or liver disease.[30]

CALCIUM

Calcium (Ca^{2+}) is another important cation in the body. Normal serum Ca^{2+} levels are 4.5 to 5.5 mEq/L. About half of the total calcium circulates as free ions, which participate in blood coagulation, control of skeletal and cardiac muscle contractility, and maintenance of membrane function. The remaining Ca^{2+} is protein bound and has no physiologic role.[25]

There are two hormones that regulate the serum level of Ca^{2+}: parathyroid hormone and calcitonin. Parathyroid hormone will cause the serum level of Ca^{2+} to increase by releasing Ca^{2+} from bone and increasing the amount of Ca^{2+} absorbed by the intestines and kidneys. Calcitonin acts to lower the serum Ca^{2+} levels by increasing the amount of Ca^{2+} excreted by the kidneys. There are several other factors that contribute to the Ca^{2+} level. Vitamin D is required for Ca^{2+} absorption by the small intestine. Estrogens will cause Ca^{2+} to be deposited into bones, while androgens cause bone decalcification, thereby raising Ca^{2+} levels.[16]

The most common causes of hypercalcemia (increase in blood Ca^{2+}) are hyperparathyroidism and cancers that have metastasized to bone. Lesser causes are Addison's disease, Paget's disease, bone fractures, and hyperthyroidism. Clinical signs include lethargy, headaches, weakness, anorexia, and nausea. Hypocalcemia (decreased Ca^{2+} levels) is associated with diarrhea, malabsorption of Ca^{2+}, burns, and an inadequate intake of vitamin D and calcium. Hypoparathyroidism, chronic renal failure, alcoholism, heparin, and certain drugs such as gentamicin and antacids can cause a decrease in the levels of serum Ca^{2+}. Tetany, spasms of the larynx, and paresthesia are all clinical signs of hypocalcemia.[25, 32]

CHOLESTEROL

Cholesterol is a lipid synthesized in the liver and is found in red blood cells, cell membranes, steroid hormones, and bile acids. Approximately 70% of the total cholesterol is bound to fatty acids, while the remaining 30% is free floating.[16, 33] High cholesterol levels are associated with atherosclerosis and increased risk of coronary artery disease. A desirable cholesterol level is less than 200 mg/dL. A moderate risk of coronary artery disease is associated with levels between 200 and 240 mg/dL, while values over 240 mg/dL are considered high risk.[34] Increased levels of cholesterol are related to obstructive jaundice, hypothyroidism, nephrosis, uncontrolled diabetes, and high stress. Decreased levels are due to decreased absorption of cholesterol from the gastrointestinal tract, liver disease, and hyperthyroidism. Several factors that can contribute to a falsely high reading are a high-cholesterol diet before blood sampling, severe hypoxia, and hemolysis.[34]

URIC ACID

Uric acid is a breakdown product of purine metabolism. The normal values are 4.0 to 8.5 mg/dL for males and 2.7 to 7.3 mg/dL for females.[16] Uric acid is formed from protein breakdown, and two thirds is excreted in the urine while the remaining one third is excreted in the feces. Elevated levels may be due to excessive cellular degeneration, as seen in cancer, starvation, alcoholism, and chemotherapy. Decreased excretion of uric acid owing to renal failure will also result in increased levels. Increased serum uric acid concentrations often present as gout. It must be remembered that a normal serum uric acid level does not exclude the diagnosis of gout, just as an elevated level does not definitively indicate gout.[35] The only test that can absolutely diagnose an acute gouty attack is a joint aspiration that demonstrates sodium urate crystals. Decreased uric acid levels are associated with Wilson's disease, anemia, burns, folic acid deficiency, and certain medications, including coumarin.[35, 36]

Enzymes Useful in Clinical Diagnosis

Enzymes are catalysts that enhance reactions without directly participating in them. Individual enzymes exist to enhance nearly all of the reactions that maintain body functions. Certain metabolic reactions occur in so many tissues that the enzymes involved exist in many cell types. Other enzymes occur only in one specialized cell type, such as the liver. A major goal of enzyme analysis is to localize disease processes to specific cell types or organ systems. Enzymes that are unique to a specific cell type are especially useful. Isoenzymes are different forms of a single enzyme that may have special chemical or immunologic characteristics. The following is a discussion of those enzymes and isoenzymes whose values are commonly checked by primary care physicians.

CREATINE PHOSPHOKINASE

Creatine phosphokinase (CPK) has a normal value in males of 50 to 180 IU/L and in females of 50 to 160 IU/L.[37] CPK catalyzes the reversible exchange of phosphate between creatine and adenosine triphosphate. There are three subdivisions of CPK: MM isoenzyme, MB isoenzyme, and BB isoenzyme. CPK is commonly found in the heart (MB) and skeletal muscles (MM) and to a lesser degree in the brain (BB). Increased levels of CPK are found with anything that damages skeletal or cardiac muscle, such as myocardial infarction, skeletal muscle disease, vigorous exercise, and deep intramuscular injections. Once it has been determined that the CPK level is elevated, the isoenzymes can be used to identify the cause of the elevation.[16]

The MM isoenzyme is elevated in muscular dystrophy, delirium tremens, and crush injuries, following surgery involving muscle, and after prolonged vigorous exercise.[16, 38] The MB isoenzyme is elevated in acute myocardial infarction and severe angina, following cardiac surgery, and after cardiac defibrillation. The MB isoenzyme can be diagnostic of acute myocardial infarction in a patient with chest pain. The CPK-MB will start to increase 4 to 6 hours after an acute myocardial infarction and peaks within 18 to 24 hours. The peak value is six times normal. The level will return to normal 3 to 40 days after the infarction. If the CPK-MB has not increased in 48 hours after the onset of chest pain, it is unlikely that the patient is suffering from myocardial infarction.[25, 39] The BB isoenzyme is most notably increased secondary to a head injury.

LACTIC ACID DEHYDROGENASE

Lactic acid dehydrogenase (LDH) is used for anaerobic metabolism and converts pyruvate to lactate. It is an intracellular enzyme common in the kidneys, heart, skeletal muscle, brain, liver, lungs, and red blood cells. Normal values in males are 63 to 155 units, while in females they are 62 to 130 units. Increased levels indicate cellular damage, which allows the enzyme to leave the cells.[38] LDH has five isoenzymes, which helps to determine where the elevated value is originating. LDH_1 constitutes 25% to 40% of the total LDH. It is found primarily in the heart, red blood cells, kidney, and brain. LDH_2 constitutes 35% to 46% of the total LDH and is also found primarily in the heart, red blood cells, kidney, and brain. Isoenzyme LDH_3 is 17% to 23% of the total LDH. It is located in the brain and kidney. LDH_4 is 2% to 4% of the total LDH and is found in the liver, skeletal muscle, and kidney. The fifth isoenzyme is LDH_5, which constitutes 0.5% to 1.5% of the total serum LDH.[16] This isoenzyme is most abundant in the liver, skeletal muscle, and ileum. Increased LDH_4 and LDH_5 values indicate liver disease; in acute hepatitis, these isoenzymes are elevated before jaundice is present.[16]

The LDH level can also be used in the diagnosis of an acute myocardial infarction. The level will start to rise 12 to 24 hours after the infarction and will peak in 2 to 5 days. It will remain elevated for 6 to 12 days. The LDH levels will remain elevated longer than the CPK level after a myocardial infarction. Normally, the LDH_2 isoenzyme concentration is greater than the LDH_1 isoenzyme. An elevated LDH combined with an LDH_1 greater than LDH_2 concentration is very valuable in the diagnosis of an MI.[39]

Increases in LDH may be due to acute myocardial infarction, cerebrovascular accident, cancer, acute pulmonary infarction, acute hepatitis, and skeletal muscle disease. Drugs such as codeine, morphine, or meperidine can cause an elevated LDH value. Levels may be falsely elevated owing to strenuous exercise or hemolysis of the red blood cells.[39, 40]

ACID PHOSPHATASE

cmAcid phosphatase is found predominately in the prostate gland. The male hormone testosterone causes the prostate to secrete acid phosphatase into the bloodstream. It is measured primarily to evaluate the presence and extent of prostatic cancer. Normal values are 1 to 1.9 IU/L. Acid phosphatase is elevated with metastatic carcinoma of the prostate, Paget's disease, and multiple myeloma.[16]

ALKALINE PHOSPHATASE

Alkaline phosphatase is found in the liver, bone, and, to a lesser extent, intestine, kidney,

and placenta. Normal values are 11.7 to 45.0 IU/L.[38] The isoenzymes can be used to determine if the elevated level is due to bone (ALP_2) or liver (ALP_1). If the alkaline phosphatase value is elevated owing to liver disease, the ALP_1 will be elevated. It is the inability of the liver to excrete alkaline phosphatase due to biliary obstruction that causes the level to increase. In bone disease, the increase in the alkaline phosphatase value is proportional to the rate of bone turnover.[16] In addition to cancer, other causes of increased levels are hepatitis, Paget's disease, healing fractures, rickets, leukemia, and the latter stages of pregnancy. Drugs that can cause an elevation in alkaline phosphatase include thorazine, erythromycin, oxacillin, indomethacin, colchicine, and oral contraceptives.[41]

Liver Function Tests

The liver performs many critical functions for the body. It metabolizes medications, stores glucose, and produces bile acid and is involved in blood coagulation as well as the filtration of blood. Many of these hepatic activities are reflected in many measurable constituents of the blood. Of course, no diagnostic test can take the place of a thorough history and physical examination.[42]

SERUM BILIRUBIN

Bilirubin is the breakdown product of hemoglobin in the red blood cells and is measured to confirm the presence and severity of jaundice. It is divided into two subgroups: direct or conjugated bilirubin, which is water soluble and excreted in the urine, and indirect or unconjugated bilirubin, which is bound to albumin and excreted through the bile. Normal values for total bilirubin are 0.2 to 1.0 mg/dL.[43] If the total bilirubin value is increased, the next step is to measure the direct bilirubin, with indirect bilirubin being the difference between the total and direct bilirubin. Normal values are 0.0 to 0.2 mg/dL for direct bilirubin and 0.2 to 0.8 mg/dL for indirect bilirubin.[43] Indirect bilirubin is elevated owing to an increase in red blood cell destruction associated with internal hemorrhage, sickle cell anemia, pernicious anemia, or septicemia.[16] The level can also be elevated owing to liver damage, which prevents conjugation of the bilirubin. An increase in direct bilirubin is the result of obstruction of the liver preventing the bilirubin from being excreted in the bile. The direct bilirubin will accumulate in the liver and spill out into the serum.[41] Regardless of whether the direct or indirect bilirubin value is elevated, the patient will appear jaundiced owing to the deposition of bilirubin in the tissue.[10]

PROTHROMBIN TIME

Prothrombin time can be used not only to determine the effectiveness of the patient's clotting mechanism but also to indicate hepatic function. It is especially important in patients with liver disease who are bleeding or about to have surgery.[44] Prothrombin is formed by the liver and is converted to thrombin through the coagulation mechanism to form a fibrin clot. The requirements for prothrombin production are an adequate intake and absorption of vitamin K as well as a healthy liver to synthesize the prothrombin. If the liver is not functioning properly, it will be unable to synthesize prothrombin, causing an increase in the PT. As discussed previously, there are several factors that may cause an elevated PT, and these include liver disease, vitamin K deficiency, anticoagulant therapy, and several drugs.

AMINOTRANSAMINASES

Determinations of many serum enzymes have been used to ascertain the extent of liver damage. The two most useful of these enzymes are aminotransaminases known as serum aspartate aminotransferase (AST) and alanine aminotransferase (ALT). AST, previously known as serum glutamic oxaloacetic transaminase (SGOT), is found in tissues of high metabolic activity such as heart and liver and to a lesser extent in skeletal muscle, kidney, and pancreas.[16] The normal value for AST is 5 to 40 μm/mL.[45] The levels will increase when cell injury occurs and the enzyme is released. Increased levels are also associated with acute myocardial infarction or liver disease. During an infarction the AST level may increase by as much as 10 times normal. It peaks in 24 hours after the myocardial infarction and returns to normal by the fourth day. In liver disease, the AST will reach levels 20 to 30 times normal and remain elevated for a longer period of time.[44] Acute hepatitis, acute cirrhosis, infections, and hepatic necrosis can all cause elevated AST levels.[45]

Alanine aminotransferase (ALT), previously known as serum glutamic pyruvic transaminase (SGPT), is present primarily in the liver and to a lesser extent in kidney and skeletal muscle.[16] The ALT levels will tend to be similar to AST levels, except that ALT levels increase before AST levels in acute hepatitis, yet do not always increase during a myocardial infarction. With extensive liver necrosis such as acute viral hepatitis, serum enzyme levels may reach levels of 1000 to 3000 μm/mL.[44]

LABORATORY DIAGNOSIS OF HEPATITIS

No section on liver function would be complete without a discussion of the causes, types, and diagnostic testing of hepatitis. Any health care professional is at risk of contracting hepatitis, which can be a life-threatening disease. It is recommended that every health care professional be vaccinated against hepatitis B. Hepatitis is a viral infection predominately affecting the liver. Classically, two types of viruses have been implicated as etiologic agents: hepatitis A virus and hepatitis B virus. Non-A, non-B virus has also been described. The discussion that follows will concentrate on the more common viruses, types A and B.[16]

Hepatitis A. Hepatitis A is due to an RNA virus and is not as lethal as hepatitis B. It is usually transmitted by the fecal-oral route and has an incubation period of 2 to 6 weeks.[46] Hepatitis A commonly affects children and young adults. The manifestations of the disease in children are usually mild, or the patient can be asymptomatic. In adults, however, hepatitis A often causes an overt febrile illness.[47] There is no chronic hepatitis A, nor is there a chronic carrier state as is seen with hepatitis B. The patient initially produces an IgM antibody 4 to 6 weeks after the infection. The IgM antibody will decline a few months after the infection. As the IgM antibody is declining, an IgG antibody is formed. This antibody will remain present in the blood for years and possibly a lifetime, providing immunity against future hepatitis A infections.[46]

Hepatitis B. Hepatitis B is a DNA virus that can cause a more serious infection than hepatitis A. The severity of the infection can range from an asymptomatic carrier state to a chronic state or even an acute fulminant disease state. It is spread through parenteral routes, including blood transfusions, blood products, and needle sticks. The incubation period ranges from 4 to 26 weeks, and the acute disease can last from weeks to months.[47]

The progression of hepatitis B can be monitored using a series of antigen–antibody levels. Hepatitis B surface antigen (HBsAg) will appear 4 to 12 weeks after inoculation and is the first indication of the presence of acute disease. It is present 1 to 7 weeks before the onset of symptoms and will decline in 3 to 6 months.[46] The next antigen to be detected is the hepatitis B antigen (HBeAg). This is detected only in HBsAg-positive serum and indicates the peak of viral replication and a high degree of infectivity. If this antigen persists, it indicates a chronic carrier state (approximately 10% of patients with hepatitis will become chronic carriers). The hepatitis B core antibody (HBcAb) is the first antibody to appear and indicates resolution of the infection. This antibody is detected 8 to 16 weeks after inoculation. The hepatitis B surface antibody (HBsAb) is the last to appear.[46, 47] Its appearance indicates previous exposure to hepatitis B and resultant immunity to future hepatitis B infections.

Renal Function Tests

Many diseases affecting the kidneys or the lower urinary tract can often be detected from clues derived from laboratory tests. Urinalysis obviously provides information about the status of the kidneys, and this information when combined with knowledge gained from determining circulating blood levels of excreted material can offer the physician a vast array of data regarding the status of renal function.

Blood Urea Nitrogen

Blood urea nitrogen (BUN) is formed in the liver as an end product of protein catabolism and is excreted through the kidney. The determination of the BUN level is a common test with which to measure the function of the kidneys. Normal values for BUN are 7 to 18 mg/dL.[16] When levels of BUN are high, the condition is called uremia. The most common cause of uremia is impaired excretion, resulting from renal failure. Uremia may also indicate dehydration or result from a high-protein diet.[16]

Creatinine

Creatinine is an end product of the breakdown of muscle creatine phosphate. It is produced at a constant rate based on the person's muscle mass. Creatinine is filtered at the glomeruli and excreted in the urine. The creatinine excretion is not dependent on the patient's hydration status.[16] Normal levels of creatinine range from 0.6 to 1.3 mg/dL for males and 0.5 to 1.0 mg/dL for females.[16] Increased creatinine levels are due to impaired renal function, chronic nephritis, systemic lupus erythematosus, and diabetic nephropathy. Elevated BUN levels in a patient with normal creatinine levels usually indicate a nonrenal cause of uremia. Nonrenal causes of increased creatinine include crushing injuries, degenerative disease causing massive muscle damage, or acromegaly.[16]

URINALYSIS

Not only do kidneys function to rid the body of nitrogenous waste products, they also serve to maintain the homeostasis of fluid, electrolytes, and acid–base status. The kidneys receive 1 liter of blood every minute, and through filtration, reabsorption, and secretion, they excrete 500 to 2000 mL of urine daily.[16] Urinalysis is probably the oldest clinical laboratory test, and its importance is often overlooked in favor of more sophisticated laboratory procedures. Just as the peripheral blood smear can offer incredible insight as to the status of the blood, urinalysis offers the opportunity to obtain an impressive array of data from a single specimen. As with all laboratory tests, a good urinalysis result begins with a good specimen. A first morning specimen is best, since this urine reflects a prolonged period without fluid intake and so will be more concentrated. A clean-catch specimen should be obtained to avoid contamination. Ideally, the specimen should be examined within 2 hours after collection. If this is not practical, the specimen should be refrigerated to avoid bacterial overgrowth.[16]

General Characteristics of Urine

Urinalysis should begin with visual observation of color and appearance. Urine should range in color from yellow to light amber and should be clear or transparent. Intensity in color closely parallels the degree of concentration. Very dilute urine is almost colorless, while very concentrated urine will be a deep yellow-orange and sometimes brown. Concentration of the urine can be quantitated by determining specific gravity or osmolality. Normal specific gravity ranges between 1.002 and 1.030, with water (specific gravity of 1.000) used as a reference point. The higher the concentration of the urine, the higher the specific gravity.[48] The odor of urine has been described as aromatic or nutty. Several foods such as asparagus and garlic can produce abnormal odors of urine. The urine of a patient with uncontrolled diabetes is often described as fruity owing to the abnormal presence of ketones. Bacteria impart the characteristic odor of ammonia. Although normal urine should appear clear, cloudiness within the specimen gives an indication as to the amount of urinary sediment. This sediment will be examined more closely on microscopic examination.[48]

Reagent Strips (Dipsticks)

Reagent strips are available with single or multiple test sections. The most important screening tests performed with reagent strips are pH, sugar, protein, hemoglobin, and ketones. The strips can be easily used in an office or clinic setting; however, a few precautions should be taken. The strips should be stored in a tightly covered container and protected from moisture and light. When used, the strips should be dipped into the specimen for a few seconds, removed, and the color changes compared against the reference guide provided with the strips.[16]

pH. The urine pH has a normal value of 4.5 to 8.0 and is a measure of the free hydrogen ion concentration in the urine.[49] The kidneys function to maintain the urinary pH by reabsorption of sodium and excretion of hydrogen and ammonium. An acidic urine pH less than 7 is found in acidosis, uncontrolled diabetes, starvation, and dehydration. An alkaline urine pH greater than 7 is found in patients with urinary tract infections, renal tubular necrosis, renal failure, systemic alkalosis, and salicylate intoxication.[16]

Renal calculi will form based on the pH of the urine. By altering the pH it is possible to prevent the formation of these stones. Calcium phosphate, calcium carbonate, and magnesium phosphate stones occur in alkaline urine. A patient with a history of these stones may benefit from an acidic urine. Uric acid, cystine, and calcium oxalate stones occur in acidic urine. Precipitation of these stones may be prevented by alkalyzing the urine.[49]

Sugars. Normally, there should be no sugar present in the urine.[16] The presence of glucose in the urine, a condition known as glucosuria, is an abnormal finding. Glucose is normally reabsorbed by the proximal tubules and not excreted. If an excess amount of glucose is present in the blood (defined as greater than 160 to 180 mg/dL), the kidneys will be unable to reabsorb all the glucose and some will "spill" into the urine. Diabetes mellitus, brain injury, myocardial infarction, and a lowered renal threshold to glucose are all causes of glucosuria. Stress, excitement, or testing after a heavy meal may all result in false-positive results.[49]

Protein. Normally, protein should be absent from the urine. Proteinuria, the presence of protein in the urine, indicates renal dysfunction, specifically, glomeruli dysfunction.[16] This occurs when antibody–antigen complement is deposited in the capillaries of the glomeruli. Proteinuria may be associated with nephritis, nephrosis, polycystic kidney, renal cancer, kidney stones, or ascites. Extrarenal causes of proteinuria include fever, trauma, severe anemia, leukemia, hyperthyroidism, and intestinal obstruction.[49]

Hemoglobin. The presence of free hemoglobin in the urine is known as hemoglobinuria and is usually associated with a rapid hemolysis of red blood cells outside the urinary tract. A false-positive result will occur with the presence of myoglobin, a muscle protein, in the urine.[16] A positive hemoglobin on the reagent strip without any red blood cells present on microscopic examination is suggestive of myoglobinuria. Hemoglobinuria is seen with burns, crush injuries, transfusion reactions to incompatible blood, fever, poisons, and drugs (e.g., bacitracin, amphotericin, coumarin, or aspirin).[49]

Ketones. Ketones are produced by the metabolism of fatty acids in the liver, and only a negligible amount appears in the urine. If there is an alteration in carbohydrate metabolism, such as carbohydrate deprivation (starvation) or decreased utilization of carbohydrates (diabetes), fat will become the predominate fuel, thereby increasing the amount of ketones produced.[16, 49] Causes for ketonuria (excess ketone in the urine) include diabetes mellitus, starvation, digestive disturbances, dietary imbalance, and prolonged vomiting. Ketonuria found in diabetic patients indicates poor control.[49]

Examination of Urinary Sediment

Microscopic examination is needed to observe cells and other formed elements within the urine. The most common technique is to centrifuge part of the specimen and examine a drop of the wet sediment. This drop of sediment is examined for the presence of red blood cells, white blood cells, epithelial cells, casts, crystals, and bacteria.

Red Blood Cells. Normally, only zero to two red blood cells are seen per high-power field. Except for during menses, the presence of an increased number of red blood cells in the urine is abnormal. Red blood cells trapped in tubular protein (casts) suggests that the source of bleeding is renal and usually is due to damaged glomeruli.[16] If there are red blood cells in the urine that are not associated with casts, then it is much more difficult to determine whether the source of bleeding is the kidney, bladder, or urethra, and further testing is required. Increased numbers of red blood cells are seen in renal disease, kidney stones, acute infections, tumors, and trauma.[49]

White Blood Cells. Normal persons have an occasional (zero to three) white blood cell per high-power field.[16] An increased number of white blood cells in the urine (predominantly neutrophils) occurs in renal disease and diseases of the urinary tract. White blood cells found within protein casts always indicate inflammation or infection involving the renal tubules, peritubular tissue, or glomeruli.[16, 50] Urine with an increased number of white blood cells should be sent for a culture and sensitivity examination.

Epithelial Cells. Epithelial cells from the urethra or bladder are a common finding in the examination of urinary sediment. These cells are classified as either transitional epithelial cells, which are found in the trigone area of the bladder and along the urinary tract, or as squamous epithelial cells, which line the urethra.[50] The presence of these cells in the urine in large quantities, such as clumps or sheets, is abnormal, and further examination is necessary.[16] The increased presence of epithelial cells in urine may be helpful in evaluating aminoglycoside therapy. The most commonly used indicator for nephrotoxicity and aminoglycoside usage is the serum creatinine level. Unfortunately, by the time the level of serum creatinine rises, significant damage to the kidney has already occurred. Some clinicians have used urinalysis results in conjunction with serum creatinine and creatinine clearance levels to monitor the therapy. By examining a baseline urine sample before initiating aminoglycoside therapy and reexamining the urine at intervals during the therapy, the presence and quantity of epithelial cells can be noted. A large increase in the number of cells noted during therapy may indicate early renal damage. Although this is by no means absolutely reliable, it is yet another indicator of potential renal damage and warrants consideration.[51]

Casts. Casts are formed in the renal tubules by precipitation and gelling of the Tamm-Horsfall mucoprotein, which is secreted by renal epithelial cells. The Tamm-Horsfall mucoprotein forms the matrix of all urinary casts.[16] Although normal urine may contain a small number of clear protein casts, an increased number of casts usually indicates widespread renal disease. Casts are identified based on their matrix, inclusions, pigments, and cells trapped within the cast material.[16, 52]

Hyaline casts are clear, colorless casts that are difficult to see unless illumination is reduced.[22] They are increased in renal disease and transiently with exercise, fever, congestive heart failure, and diuretic therapy.[22] Waxy casts are homogeneously smooth casts and are also known as renal failure casts. Their presence is associated with tubular inflammation and degeneration, acute or chronic allograft rejection, and end-stage renal failure. Granular casts are cellular casts that have degenerated and may represent combinations of inflammation or hemorrhage. This is seen with pyelonephritis and chronic lead poisoning. Fatty casts contain lipid and are associated with proteinuria.[52]

Crystals. Crystals present in the urine are usually of no medical consequence unless there is a history of stones or of therapy with drugs known to crystallize in the kidneys.[16] The acidity or alkalinity influences which crystals are present. Some of the more common clinically significant crystals are uric acid, oxalate, cystine, and tyrosine. Uric acid crystals take on many forms (plates, prisms, hexagons) and are usually colored and easily dissolvable with heating. Their presence may indicate uric acid calculi or gout. Oxalate crystals are colorless, octahedral crystals and appear as small squares with a cross in the middle. Their presence may indicate severe chronic renal disease. Cystine crystals are found in acidic urine and appear as highly refractile plates. Although they are rare, their presence indicates an error in metabolism known as cystinuria (excretion of excessive amounts of the amino acid in the urine).[22] Crystals in the shape of needles are tyrosine crystals that are found in association with acute liver failure.

MICROBIOLOGY

The primary function of the microbiology laboratory is to assist physicians in the diagnosis and treatment of patients with infectious disease. In general, the process of microorganism culture, identification, and the determination of sensitivity to drugs is a simple one. A properly obtained specimen is sent to the laboratory in special transport medium. Once the specimen arrives at the microbiology laboratory, it is immediately processed. The initial analysis includes direct visual examination, a microscopic examination (i.e., Gram's stain) if indicated, and culturing of the specimen in an appropriate medium.[53] The inoculated medium is then placed in an incubator, and after a specified period of time (generally 24 to 48 hours) any microorganisms that have grown are identified.

By virtue of our specialty, podiatrists are faced most commonly with bacterial infections secondary to cutaneous ulcerations, postoperative wounds, and, to a lesser extent, fungal infections of the skin and skin structures. What follows is a discussion on the guidelines for obtaining a proper specimen, the role of the Gram's stain in forming a presumptive diagnosis, and how culture and sensitivity can guide treatment.

Obtaining a Specimen

The proper collection of a specimen for culture is the most important step in the recovery of microorganisms responsible for an infection. A culture will provide useless or even misleading information if it is improperly collected or transported to the laboratory. The culture specimen is obtained from exudates or from swabbing tissue. The specimen must be obtained from the actual infection site. One must be leery about a superficial culture because it has been shown numerous times that superficial cultures are loaded with a variety of microorganisms that are not contributing to the infection. In some situations, it can be quite a difficult decision as to what to culture. In these uncommon circumstances superficial cultures are obtained but should always be compared with deeper cultures if possible. When necessary, aspiration needles may be used to avoid contamination. Lastly, in the very unlikely situation that a wound looks infected, but all cultures fail to report significant growth, one must not automatically rule out infection. In these situations other diagnostic aids, such as leukocyte indium-111 and technetium-99m bone scans, are necessary.

It is essential to obtain a sufficient quantity of the specimen. Too frequently, dry swabs are submitted to the laboratory with the hope that something will grow. Not only is this an exercise in futility, but it can also be expensive for the patient. Sterile containers should be used for the collection of all specimens. Swabs are commonly attached to tubes containing transport medium. The swab is inserted into this medium after the specimen has been collected to prevent drying. Unfortunately, once a swab has entered the transport medium, it cannot be used for a Gram's stain. A second swab should be used, or a portion of the specimen should be placed on a microscope slide before inserting the swab into the medium. Finally, the specimen must be adequately labeled with the patient's name, source of the specimen, physician's name, date, and time. Although this may seem elementary, it is not unusual for laboratories to receive improperly identified specimens, which must then be discarded.[51, 53] Ideally, specimens should be received by the laboratory within 1 hour after obtaining representative material. In general, the order of obtaining specimens is as follows: (1) anaerobic cultures, which are taken first to avoid prolonged exposure to the air; (2) aerobic cultures; and (3) the material for the Gram's stain.[51]

If possible, specimens should be obtained before the administration of antibiotics. Although pathogens are still recovered after the administration of antibiotics has begun, their growth may be substantially altered. If antibiotics have been given, the laboratory should be notified as to the type and dosage.

The Gram's Stain

The Gram's stain can provide an incredible amount of information very quickly. Although the culture takes 24 to 48 hours or longer to recover an organism, the Gram's stain procedure requires about 10 minutes and provides important clues, such as size, shape, staining characteristics, and the presence of polymorphonuclear cells (Fig. 24–1). Often, this information alone is enough to begin empiric antibiotic therapy.

It is important to recall what structures will pick up or stain with Gram's stain. Some microorganism cell walls will retain the stain (gram positive) while others will lose it (gram negative). The presence of polymorphonuclear leukocytes should also be sought when examining a Gram-stained specimen. The cytoplasm of the leukocyte will appear light pink, while the nucleus will stain purple. Lastly, while not ideal, this staining procedure can also be used to visualize fungi and yeast, which will stain faintly purple.

Gram's staining also assists with the quality control of the culture by revealing which organisms failed to grow or by suggesting contamination. If growth occurs that is different from what was seen on the smear, it may be indicative of a contaminant. Although the Gram's stain can provide a great deal of information about the physical characteristics of bacteria, it cannot demonstrate their viability. The best test for viability is the culture.[16, 51]

Culture and Sensitivity

Despite the time it takes for culture results to be reported, this is the most definitive procedure available for identifying and isolating pathogenic organisms. For the optimal recovery of bacteria, it is essential to culture the specimen as soon as possible after delivery to the laboratory. Once the specimen arrives at the laboratory, the technician chooses the medium, selected on the basis of the anatomic source of the specimen and knowledge of the normal flora as well as potential pathogens commonly encountered in those sources. Although it is unlikely that the practitioner will be directly responsible for selecting the appropriate isolation medium, he or she can assist the laboratory by labeling the specimen with the anatomical source and by providing information as to antibiotic therapy and whether an unusual infectious disease is suspected.[53]

There are many requirements that must be met for successful diagnosis by cultures. Organisms causing the infection must be capable of growing in vitro. The specimen material must be representative of the disease. The specimen must be collected in such a way as to maintain the viability of the pathogens. Finally, culture reports must be interpreted with an understanding of the bacteria that are normally present in and on the body. Fluids from joints, blood, and urine are normally sterile. The skin normally contains a large variety of normal flora, including *Staphylococcus epidermidis* and *Micrococcus*.[53] It must be emphasized that not every pathogen can be detected by culture.[16]

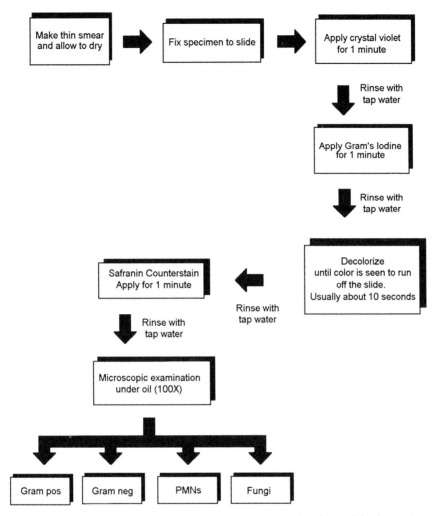

FIGURE 24–1. Procedure for Gram's stain. After a thin smear of specimen is placed on a slide, the specimen may be fixed by air drying for 5 to 10 minutes. The most important step in the staining process is the decolorization. Care must be taken not to over-decolorize, otherwise all bacteria may appear pink. Gram's stain may stain other cells, such as polymorphonuclear leukocytes and fungus, and these should be noted if observed.

When all of these requirements are met, the physician can be confident of a successful culture. For a more thorough explanation of microbiological procedures, the reader is referred to any text on diagnostic microbiology.

Once the pathogen has been identified, its sensitivity to several antibiotics must be determined so that the appropriate antibiotic therapy may be instituted. Several factors have led to the growing dependence on antimicrobial sensitivity testing. Organisms acquired in hospitals or nursing homes tend to be more resistant to a wide variety of antibiotics. Patients who have received prior antibiotic therapy tend to develop more resistant pathogens. Finally, the inappropriate use of the new broad-spectrum antibiotics in place of a more conservative drug for simple infections has led to increased resistance of several pathogens.[51] Although antimicrobial sensitivity testing is not indicated for every infection, certain situations should lead the physician to consider ordering this test. If the isolated pathogen has an unpredictable antimicrobial susceptibility spectrum (e.g., *Staphylococcus*) or if the patient is immunodepressed and has an impaired defense against pathogens, then antimicrobial sensitivity testing should be employed.

The two primary methods of antimicrobial sensitivity testing are the Kirby-Bauer or disk diffusion method and the antimicrobial dilution test. The disk diffusion method used to be the most effective way to test susceptibility to antimicrobial drugs. The pathogen must first be isolated and then inoculated onto an agar plate that will support its growth. Several different antibiotic-impregnated disks are placed on the inoculated surface so that the drug diffuses into the agar. After about 18 hours, the plate is examined for growth patterns, which reveal whether the high concentration of drug around the disk prevents bacterial growth. The circle of agar clear of bacterial growth is called the zone of inhibition, and the diameter is measured in millimeters. This measurement must then be compared with the standard set by the National Committee on Clinical Laboratory Standards to determine if that zone represents sensitivity or resistance to the pathogen.[53] Although this method remains a useful and important technique for assessing antimicrobial sensitivity, it is not without its drawbacks, including the time delay involved in isolating a pure culture for inoculation and the inability to use this method with anaerobic pathogens.[51, 53]

A second method of determining antimicrobial sensitivity is the antimicrobial dilution test, in which the antibiotic to be tested is incorporated into broth or agar in varied concentrations. The broth or agar is then inoculated with the isolated pathogen and incubated for about 18 hours. The medium is then examined. Cloudiness indicates that bacterial growth has not been inhibited by the concentration of antibiotic within the broth or agar. The lowest concentration of antibiotic in milligrams per milliliter that prevents the in vitro growth of bacteria (i.e., no cloudiness) is known as the minimal inhibitory concentration (MIC). If it becomes necessary for the physician to know the minimum bactericidal concentration (MBC), or the amount of antibiotic needed to totally kill the pathogen, all of the broth used in the above test that did not show growth is plated onto an antibiotic-free agar and incubated for 18 hours. The lowest concentration of antibiotic to show no growth is the MBC. In practice, the MBC is indicated for patients on anticancer drugs or who are otherwise immunosuppressed.[16, 22, 51, 53]

Although the laboratory can determine the antibiotic susceptibility and MIC and MBC of the pathogen, it cannot measure the effectiveness of the antibiotic once it is inside the body. Those conditions that can affect a drug's therapeutic effectiveness include poor absorption from the site of administration, protein binding, excessively rapid elimination of the drug, inactivation by other drugs, or metabolic alteration of the drug by the liver or kidney.[16]

Mycology

Two of the most common presentations in a podiatrist's office are tinea pedis infection and onychomycosis. Although in most instances history and clinical presentation point to the diagnosis, it may become necessary to isolate the responsible pathogen. It is not unusual for an examination of a potassium hydroxide (KOH) mount to indicate the presence of a rapidly growing mold or species of *Candida* when the clinical presentation suggested a dermatophyte infection.[54] Since KOH preparations are so quick and easy to perform and can be so revealing, the use of this method along with the culture for confirmation of clinical impressions is encouraged. The two basic techniques for identification of dermatophytes are microscopic examination and culture.

MICROSCOPIC EXAMINATION

The use of a KOH mount for rapid diagnosis of dermatophyte infections is a common and easy procedure. Before obtaining a specimen, the area is cleansed with 70% alcohol to remove contaminating surface bacteria.[5] A small portion of skin scales or nail scrapings taken from a representative sample of involved tissue is placed into one or two drops of 10% KOH on a glass slide. The mixture should then be either gently warmed over a flame and a coverslip applied or allowed to incubate at room temperature for 10 to 15 minutes.[56, 57] The slide is then examined under a microscope utilizing low power. The hyphae can be seen more easily if the light is reduced by lowering the condenser of the microscope. The dermatophyte hyphae are multicelled with thin, smooth walls and are often found in fragments. The most common dermatophytes implicated in tinea pedis and onychomycosis are *Trichophyton rubrum*, *T. mentagrophytes*, and *Epidermophyton floccosum*.[54]

CULTURE

As with bacteria, the microscopic examination of fungi gives a clue as to classification based on physical characteristics; however, culture is the only definitive means of identifying the responsible organism. Mycobiotic and Mycosel agars are the media of choice for the recovery of dermatophytes. These agars use Sabouraud dextrose agar as a base with chloramphenicol and cycloheximide added to prevent bacterial overgrowth.[54] Microscopic examination of any growth must be done to confirm the species. A commonly used medium in physicians' offices is the dermatophyte test medium. This medium contains a phenol-red indicator that will turn red in the presence of alkaline metabolites produced with fungal growth.[54] This color change does not occur with most strains of *Candida*.[55] This medium is not specific to dermatophyte growth, and colonies should be examined microscopically to confirm the species. After inoculation into any of the above agars, the culture is incubated at room temperature for 2 to 4 weeks. All cultures should be held for 30 days before being reported as negative.[54]

Most dermatophytes will form colonies after 1 to 2 weeks of incubation. Visual examination of the colonies will reveal fluffy or granular colonies that are usually white, gray, or a shade of yellow or brown. *T. rubrum* and *T. mentagrophytes* often produce deep red pigments that diffuse into the agar. As has been discussed, microscopic examination of any growth should be performed to confirm the species.[53]

LABORATORY DIAGNOSIS OF ARTHRITIS

Carefully selected laboratory studies can be very helpful in the diagnosis of the specific type of arthritis. Unfortunately, the laboratory results can be confusing and often misleading. An elevated erythrocyte sedimentation rate indicates inflammation and little else. Serum uric acid levels can be elevated by low doses of aspirin or other medications, giving a potentially false impression of gout. Latex fixation tests for rheumatoid factor may also be positive in other disease states, such as cirrhosis or tuberculosis.[56] The following section will discuss those laboratory studies used most often in the diagnosis of the arthritides.

Synovial Fluid Analysis

Perhaps the most useful test in rheumatology is the examination of synovial fluid, since it provides valuable information as to the process occurring within the joint. In fact, examination of the synovial fluid is mandatory for the diagnosis of septic arthritis and crystal-induced arthritides.[20] There is simply no other definitive method of diagnosing septic arthritis than to demonstrate organisms within the synovial fluid. Synovial fluid is produced by dialysis of plasma across the synovial membrane and secretion of a hyaluronate–protein complex. The concentration of total protein found within the synovial fluid is approximately one half that of plasma, while concentrations of glucose and uric acid are comparable to plasma.[57, 58]

Once the synovial fluid specimen has been obtained, the gross appearance of the fluid should be noted. Normal synovial fluid appears clear with a straw or light yellow color. Red or pink fluid indicates the presence of red blood cells caused by either a hemarthrosis or poor aspiration technique. Inflammatory fluid generally assumes an opaque and sometimes purulent appearance. Edema, due to its low protein content, produces a nearly colorless fluid.[20, 57]

White blood cell counts and differential counts should be performed on all synovial fluid specimens. Often, an increase in the white blood cell count is a good indicator of the degree of inflammation or the presence of a bacterial infection. Total white blood cell counts are performed by examining the undiluted fluid and counting the white blood cells using a counting chamber. The upper limit of normal is 200 cells/mm³. Septic arthritis is often associated with a white blood cell count over 20,000 cells/mm³ and sometimes greater than 100,000 cells/mm³; however, low counts are common in early bacterial arthritis caused by gonococcal infections.[20, 56, 57] White blood cell counts over 20,000 cells/mm³ may also be seen in association with acute gout and rheumatoid arthritis. A differential count of the white blood cells will provide a few additional clues as to the type of arthritis present. Normal synovial fluid contains approximately 65% monocytes, 15% lymphocytes, and 20% neutrophils. Noninflammatory fluid or synovial fluid from a joint with degenerative joint disease will generally contain less than 50% neutrophils.[58] Fluids from joints with rheumatoid arthritis, acute gout or pseudogout, or infective processes exhibit a high percentage of neutrophils, often as high as 95%.[20]

The glucose level in synovial fluid is a commonly ordered test. Normally, glucose in synovial fluid is approximately 80% of the serum glucose concentration. In severe inflammation, the glucose levels drop secondary to an increase in glucose consumption by the cells and tissues of the joint. Unfortunately, a low synovial fluid glucose result only gives an indication of the level of inflammation within a joint and not the cause of the inflammation. Other tests should be ordered in conjunction with a synovial fluid glucose test to determine the cause of the inflammation.[57]

All fluids should be sent for Gram's stain and culture if septic arthritis is suspected. Obtaining a positive synovial fluid culture is enhanced by plating the fluid on the appropriate medium while still warm. The fluid should not be refrigerated, especially if a culture may be required; and whenever possible, the specimen should be delivered to the laboratory within 1 hour after aspiration since white blood cells will begin to degenerate after this time.[20]

Because the serum uric acid level can be misleading, examination of synovial fluid for the presence of crystals is essential for the diagnosis of gout. The crystals of gout and pseudogout are differentiated by their size, shape, and appearance under polarized light. Only a drop of synovial fluid is necessary for examination, and often the crystals can be recovered even during asymptomatic periods. Monosodium urate crystals (the crystals of gout) are generally needle or rod shaped and are 2 to 15 μm in length. They appear bright yellow and parallel to the axis of slow vibration marked on the polarizing microscope compensator (negatively birefringent).[56, 59] These crystals are identified in approximately 90% of patients with acute gout and 75% of patients between gouty attacks. Certain crystalline corticosteroid preparations will appear identical to monosodium urate crystals.[58] These include betamethasone acetate and triamcinolone hexacetonide. Calcium pyrophosphate dihydrate crystals appear as rods or rhomboids and are positively birefringent (i.e., appear blue under polarized light).[20, 56]

Rheumatoid Factor

Rheumatoid factors are antiglobulins that are directed against a patient's own IgG. These antiglobulins have been termed *rheumatoid factors* because of their presence in the serum of over 80% of patients with rheumatoid arthritis. The exact role that these factors play in rheumatoid arthritis is uncertain. It is known that they can enhance the inflammatory response by causing an increase in complement fixation or by changing the properties of the immune complexes. Rheumatoid factor is found not only in the blood of patients with rheumatoid arthritis but also in the blood of patients with a variety of other diseases, such as chronic liver disease and subacute bacterial endocarditis. However, the incidence and titers of rheumatoid factors are higher in patients with rheumatoid arthritis than in patients with other diseases. The titer is normally higher in the elderly and when multiple vaccinations and transfusions have been given.[5, 20, 60, 61]

The test for the presence of rheumatoid factors should be ordered when rheumatoid arthritis is suspected; however, the results should be considered only part of the picture. Clinical signs and symptoms as well as radiographic findings and other laboratory values such as erythrocyte sedimentation rate and synovial fluid analysis should be combined to diagnose a patient with rheumatoid arthritis. Elevated titers of rheumatoid factor may not be seen for the first several months of rheumatoid arthritis and may not appear at all in cases of juvenile rheumatoid arthritis.[20, 60]

HLA-B27

Although all nucleated cells have HLA antigens on their surface membranes, they are most easily detected on lymphocytes. So far, at least 27 antigens have been identified. Although HLA typing was originally used to match histocompatible donors and recipients for organ transplantation, statistical associations were found to exist between individual HLA antigens and certain diseases. The best association exists between the HLA-B27 antigen and arthritic disorders. This antigen has been found in 90% of patients diagnosed with ankylosing spondylitis. Reiter's syndrome, juvenile rheumatoid arthritis, and arthritic complications of psoriasis also show a correlation with the HLA-B27 antigen.[5, 16] This antigen has only been found to occur in populations native to the northern hemisphere.[16]

ACQUIRED IMMUNODEFICIENCY SYNDROME

Acquired immunodeficiency syndrome (AIDS) is a disease state resulting from infection with the human immunodeficiency virus (HIV) and characterized by opportunistic infections, cancers that are associated with the HIV infection, and a variety of other syndromes. The clinical manifestations may vary from an acute, self-limited infectious mononucleosis–like syndrome to the development of AIDS or AIDS-related complex (ARC). The latent period between the initial infection to the onset of AIDS or ARC can vary from a few months to 15 years or longer.[62]

The number of patients identified as being infected with HIV has increased dramatically in the past few years as testing for the virus has become more widespread. Each practitioner will probably come in contact with HIV-infected patients at some point during his or her career. Health care professionals should wear gloves when examining all patients regardless of a negative history of HIV infection. Accidental needle sticks are very common, and all health care personnel should know how to avoid these accidents. Should a needle stick or similar accident occur, regardless of the patient's past medical history, the health care provider should have blood drawn immediately to test for HIV antibodies. The test must be run again 6 weeks later. If both tests are negative, he or she is said to be HIV negative.[62]

Human Immunodeficiency Virus Tests

Currently, the testing options available for the detection of HIV include culture to isolate the virus, antigen detection, or antibody screening. Although isolation of the virus or detection of the antigen provides the most specific diagnosis of HIV infection, these tests are expensive, not widely available, and often insensitive. In contrast, tests that demonstrate antibodies to HIV are sensitive and specific during most stages of the infection and are inexpensive and widely available. The two tests that are widely used are the enzyme-linked immunosorbent assay (ELISA) and the Western blot test. The ELISA detects antibodies to HIV and has proven to be highly sensitive and specific. This is the test that is used to screen all donated blood and plasma in the United States and is 99% accurate.[63] The test cannot predict if or when a patient will develop AIDS. When the ELISA is positive in asymptomatic or low-risk patients, the test should be repeated on the same sample to rule out a false-positive result. If it is positive the second time, the result should be confirmed by the more specific Western blot test.[63]

The Western blot test identifies antibodies to specific viral proteins by immunoelectrophoresis. Patients with a positive ELISA and a positive Western blot test should be considered infected and contagious. A negative result does not guarantee that the patient is not infected with HIV. If a patient has recently been exposed to the virus, the body may not have had time to develop the antibodies to HIV, and a repeat test should be performed after a period of time. The most common cause for a false-negative test result appears to be related to the very early stage of infection before the formation of antibodies. Causes for false-positive results include multiple transfusions, chronic hemodialysis, alcoholic hepatitis, and autoimmune diseases.[62, 63]

PREOPERATIVE LABORATORY EVALUATION

Certain screening tests should be included in the preoperative evaluation. Often the hospital or surgical facility will require a minimum set of laboratory studies to be performed on all patients before surgery. The purpose of these screening tests is to detect common disease states that may not have been evident on a routine history and physical examination.

We consider the following tests to be the minimum required for an apparently healthy person about to undergo surgery; however, further laboratory studies may be indicated based on the results of the history and physical examination.

As discussed previously, the complete blood cell count with differential count can provide a great deal of information. Preoperatively, this test will give a baseline indication of the white blood cells, which can be very helpful if a postoperative infection develops. The hemoglobin and hematocrit values may indicate the presence of anemia. A fasting blood glucose value of greater than 150 mg/dL may point to undiagnosed diabetes. A urine pregnancy test should be performed on all women of childbearing age. A urinalysis may indicate the presence of a subclinical urinary tract infection or an early sign of renal impairment. A screening test for sickle cell anemia should be ordered for any black patient whose family history of the disorder is questionable.

REFERENCES

 1. Nelson D, Morris M: Basic examination of blood. In Henry JB (ed): Clinical Diagnosis and Management by Laboratory Methods, p 553. Philadelphia, WB Saunders, 1991.
 2. Leavell BS, Thorup AO Jr: Fundamentals of Clinical Hematology, ed 4. Philadelphia, WB Saunders, 1976.
 3. Nelson D, Davey F: Hematopoiesis. In Henry JB (ed): Clinical Diagnosis and Management by Laboratory Methods, p 604. Philadelphia, WB Saunders, 1991.
 4. Williams W: Examination of blood. In Williams W, Beutler E, Erslev A, Lichtman M (eds): Hematology, ed 3, p 9. New York, McGraw-Hill Book Company, 1983.
 5. Fischbach FT: A Manual of Laboratory Diagnostic Tests, ed 3. Philadelphia, JB Lippincott, 1988.
 6. Williams PL, Warwick R, Dyson M, Banister LH: Gray's Anatomy, ed 37. New York, Churchill Livingstone, 1989.
 7. Erslev A: Production of erythrocytes. In Williams W, Beutler E, Erslev A, Lichtman M (eds): Hematology, ed 3, p 365. New York, McGraw-Hill Book Company, 1983.
 8. Brown BA: Hematology: Principles and Procedures, ed 3. Philadelphia, Lea & Febiger, 1980.
 9. Nelson D, Davey F: Erythrocytic disorders. In Henry JB (ed): Clinical Diagnosis and Management by Laboratory Methods, p 627. Philadelphia, WB Saunders, 1991.
10. Robbins SL, Cotran RS, Kumar V: Pathologic Basis of Disease, ed 3. Philadelphia, WB Saunders, 1984.
11. Bryant NJ: An Introduction to Immunohematology. Philadelphia, WB Saunders, 1976.
12. Friedman PA: Diseases due to environmental hazards and physical and chemical agents. In Petersdorf RG, Adams RD, Braunwald E, et al (eds): Harrison's Prin-

ciples of Internal Medicine, ed 10, p 1259. New York, McGraw-Hill Book Company, 1983.
13. Nossel HL: Bleeding. In Petersdorf RG, Adams RD, Braunwald E, et al (eds): Harrison's Principles of Internal Medicine, ed 10, p 292. New York, McGraw-Hill Book Company, 1983.
14. Miller J: Blood platelets. In Henry JB (ed): Clinical Diagnosis and Management by Laboratory Methods, p 717. Philadelphia, WB Saunders, 1991.
15. Williams W: Principles of coagulation tests. In Williams W, Beutler E, Erslev A, Lichtman M (eds): Hematology, ed 3, p 1257. New York, McGraw-Hill Book Company, 1983.
16. Widmann FK: Clinical Interpretation of Laboratory Tests, ed 9, Philadelphia, FA Davis, 1983.
17. Dale DC: Abnormalities of leukocytes. In Petersdorf RG, Adams RD, Braunwald E, et al (eds): Harrison's Principles of Internal Medicine, ed 10, p 304. New York, McGraw-Hill Book Company, 1983.
18. Hougie C: Bleeding time. In Williams W, Beutler E, Erslev A, Lichtman M (eds): Hematology, ed 3, p 1671. New York, McGraw-Hill Book Company, 1983.
19. Miller J: Blood coagulation and fibrinolysis. In Henry JB (ed): Clinical Diagnosis and Management by Laboratory Methods, p 734. Philadelphia, WB Saunders, 1991.
20. Gilliland BC, Mannik M: Disorders of the joints and connective tissues. In Petersdorf RG, Adams RD, Braunwald E, et al (eds): Harrison's Principles of Internal Medicine, ed 10, p 1974. New York, McGraw-Hill Book Company, 1983.
21. Bunn HF: Disorders of hemoglobin structure, function, and synthesis. In Petersdorf RG, Adams RD, Braunwald E, et al (eds): Harrison's Principles of Internal Medicine, ed 10, p 1875. New York, McGraw-Hill Book Company, 1983.
22. Raphael SS, Hyde TA, Mellor LD, et al: Lynch's Medical Laboratory Technology, ed 4. Philadelphia, WB Saunders, 1983.
23. Preuss H, Podlasek S, Henry J: Evaluation of renal function and water, electrolyte and acid–base balance. In Henry JB (ed): Clinical Diagnosis and Management by Laboratory Methods, p 119. Philadelphia, WB Saunders, 1991.
24. Tietz NW: Electrolytes. In Tietz NW (ed): Fundamentals of Clinical Chemistry, ed 2, p 873. Philadelphia, WB Saunders, 1976.
25. Rutsky EA: Water, electrolyte, mineral, and acid–base metabolism. In Berkow R (ed): The Merck Manual of Diagnosis and Therapy, ed 16, p 986. Rahway, NJ, Merck, 1992.
26. Coodley EL: Laboratory medicine. In Berkow R (ed): The Merck Manual of Diagnosis and Therapy, ed 16, p 2573. Rahway, NJ, Merck, 1992.
27. Caraway WT: Carbohydrates. In Tietz NW (ed): Fundamentals of Clinical Chemistry, ed 2, p 234. Philadelphia, WB Saunders, 1976.
28. Winegrad AI: Disorders of carbohydrate metabolism. In Berkow R (ed): The Merck Manual of Diagnosis and Therapy, ed 16, p 1106. Rahway, NJ, Merck, 1992.
29. Kennedy L: Glycation of hemoglobin and serum proteins. In Alberti KGMM, DeFronzo RA, Keen H, Zimmet P (eds): International Textbook of Diabetes Mellitus, p 985. Philadelphia, John Wiley & Sons, 1992.
30. McPherson R: Specific proteins. In Henry JB (ed): Clinical Diagnosis and Management by Laboratory Methods, p 215. Philadelphia, WB Saunders, 1991.
31. Grant GH, Kachmar JF: The proteins of body fluids. In Tietz NW (ed): Fundamentals of Clinical Chemistry, ed 2. Philadelphia, WB Saunders, 1976.

32. Potts JT: Disorders of parathyroid glands. In Petersdorf RG, Adams RD, Braunwald E, et al (eds): Harrison's Principles of Internal Medicine, ed 10, p 1929. New York, McGraw-Hill Book Company, 1983.

33. Ellefson RD: Lipids and lipoproteins. In Tietz NW (ed): Fundamentals of Clinical Chemistry, ed 2, p 474. Philadelphia, WB Saunders, 1976.

34. Bachorik P, Levy R, Rifkind B: Lipids and dyslipoproteinemia. In Henry JB (ed): Clinical Diagnosis and Management by Laboratory Methods, p 188. Philadelphia, WB Saunders, 1991.

35. Kelley WN: Gout and other disorders of purine metabolism. In Petersdorf RG, Adams RD, Braunwald E, et al (eds): Harrison's Principles of Internal Medicine, ed 10, p 517. New York, McGraw-Hill Book Company, 1983.

36. McCarty DJ: Crystal induced conditions. In Berkow R (ed): The Merck Manual of Diagnosis and Therapy, ed 16, p 1346. Rahway, NJ, Merck, 1992.

37. Pincus M, Zimmerman H, Henry J: Clinical enzymology. In Henry JB (ed): Clinical Diagnosis and Management by Laboratory Methods, p 250. Philadelphia, WB Saunders, 1991.

38. Kachmar JF, Moss DW: Enzymes. In Tietz NW (ed): Fundamentals of Clinical Chemistry, ed 2, p 565. Philadelphia, WB Saunders, 1976.

39. Killip TK: Diseases of the heart and pericardium. In Berkow R (ed): The Merck Manual of Diagnosis and Therapy, ed 16, p 446. Rahway, NJ, Merck, 1992.

40. Braunwald E, Alpert JA: Acute myocardial infarction. In Petersdorf RG, Adams RD, Braunwald E, et al (eds): Harrison's Principles of Internal Medicine, ed 10, p 1432. New York, McGraw-Hill Book Company, 1983.

41. Shaffer EA: Laboratory and radiologic evaluation of the liver and biliary system. In Berkow R (ed): The Merck Manual of Diagnosis and Therapy, ed 16, p 865. Rahway, NJ, Merck, 1992.

42. Isselbacher KJ: Approach to the patient with liver disease. In Petersdorf RG, Adams RD, Braunwald E, et al (eds): Harrison's Principles of Internal Medicine, ed 10, p 1771. New York, McGraw-Hill Book Company, 1983.

43. Routh JI: Liver function. In Tietz NW (ed): Fundamentals of Clinical Chemistry, ed 2, p 1026. Philadelphia, WB Saunders, 1976.

44. Isselbacher KJ, LaMont JT: Diagnostic procedures in liver disease. In Petersdorf RG, Adams RD, Braunwald E, et al (eds): Harrison's Principles of Internal Medicine, ed 10, p 1779. New York, McGraw-Hill Book Company, 1983.

45. Schaffner J, Schaffner F: Assessment of the status of the liver. In Henry JB (ed): Clinical Diagnosis and Management by Laboratory Methods, p 229. Philadelphia, WB Saunders, 1991.

46. Dienstag JL, Wands JR, Koff RS: Acute hepatitis. In Petersdorf RG, Adams RD, Braunwald E, et al (eds): Harrison's Principles of Internal Medicine, ed 10, p 1789. New York, McGraw-Hill Book Company, 1983.

47. Simon JB: Hepatitis. In Berkow R (ed): The Merck Manual of Diagnosis and Therapy, ed 16, p 897. Rahway, NJ, Merck, 1992.

48. Faulkner WR, King JW: Renal function. In Tietz NW (ed): Fundamentals of Clinical Chemistry, ed 2, p 975. Philadelphia, WB Saunders, 1976.

49. Schumann E, Schweitzer S: Examination of urine. In Henry JB (ed): Clinical Diagnosis and Management by Laboratory Methods, p 387. Philadelphia, WB Saunders, 1991.

50. Coe FL, Brenner BM: Approach to the patient with diseases of the kidneys and urinary tract. In Petersdorf RG, Adams RD, Braunwald E, et al (eds): Harrison's Principles of Internal Medicine, ed 10, p 1595. New York, McGraw-Hill Book Company, 1983.

51. Joseph WS: Handbook of Lower Extremity Infections. New York, Churchill Livingstone, 1990.

52. Cutler RE: Clinical evaluation of genitourinary disorders. In Berkow R (ed): The Merck Manual of Diagnosis and Therapy, ed 16, p 1646. Rahway, NJ, Merck, 1992.

53. Koneman EW, Allen SD, Dowell VR, Sommers HM: Color Atlas and Textbook of Diagnostic Microbiology. Philadelphia, JB Lippincott, 1979.

54. Koneman E, Roberts G: Mycotic disease. In Henry JB (ed): Clinical Diagnosis and Management by Laboratory Methods, p 1099. Philadelphia, WB Saunders, 1991.

55. Samitz MH: Microbiological diseases. In Samitz MH (ed): Cutaneous Disorders of the Lower Extremities, ed 2, p 27. Philadelphia, JB Lippincott, 1981.

56. Schumacher HR: Approach to the patient with joint disease. In Berkow R (ed): The Merck Manual of Diagnosis and Therapy, ed 16, p 1297. Rahway, NJ, Merck, 1992.

57. Hasselbacher P: Arthrocentesis and synovial fluid analysis. In Schumacher HR, Klippel JH, Robinson DR (eds): Primer on the Rheumatic Diseases, ed 9, p 55. Atlanta, Arthritis Foundation, 1988.

58. Krieg A, Kjeldsberg C: Cerebrospinal fluids and other body fluids. In Henry JB (ed): Clinical Diagnosis and Management by Laboratory Methods, p 445. Philadelphia, WB Saunders, 1991.

59. Tate G, Schumacher HR: Clinical features of gout. In Schumacher HR, Klippel JH, Robinson DR (eds): Primer on the Rheumatic Diseases, ed 9, p 198. Atlanta, Arthritis Foundation, 1988.

60. Nakamura R, Tucker E, Carlson I: Immunoassays in the clinical laboratory. In Henry JB (ed): Clinical Diagnosis and Management by Laboratory Methods, p 848. Philadelphia, WB Saunders, 1991.

61. Zvaifler N: Rheumatoid arthritis. In Schumacher HR, Klippel JH, Robinson DR (eds): Primer on the Rheumatic Diseases, ed 9, p 83. Atlanta, Arthritis Foundation, 1988.

62. Stiehm ER: Human immunodeficiency virus infection. In Berkow R (ed): The Merck Manual of Diagnosis and Therapy, ed 16, p 77. Rahway, NJ, Merck, 1992.

63. Faison BS: The AIDS Handbook. Durham, NC, Designbase, 1991.

INDEX

Note: Page numbers in *italics* refer to illustrations; page numbers followed by t indicate tables.

ISBN 0-7216-4363-9